Health & Medical Horizons

1986

MACMILLAN EDUCATIONAL COMPANY
A Division of Macmillan, Inc.
NEW YORK
COLLIER MACMILLAN PUBLISHERS
LONDON

Health & Medical Horizons 1986 is not intended as a substitute for the medical advice of physicians. Readers should regularly consult a physician in matters relating to their health and particularly regarding symptoms that may require diagnosis or medical attention.

Macmillan Educational Company
A Division of Macmillan, Inc.
866 Third Avenue, New York, N.Y. 10022
Collier Macmillan Canada, Inc.

ISBN 0-02-943960-4

Library of Congress Catalog Card Number 82-645223

Manufactured in the United States of America

Staying Healthy

Knowing as much as you can about health can help you and your family be well and stay well. This book answers your questions and provides you with valuable, practical information—in articles prepared by experts and written in clear, easily understood language.

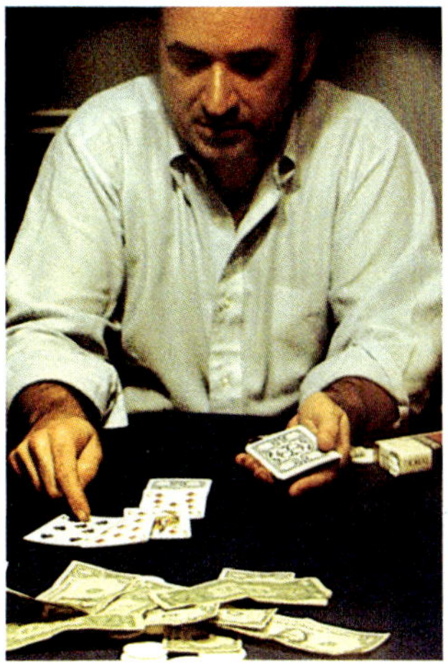

Page 30

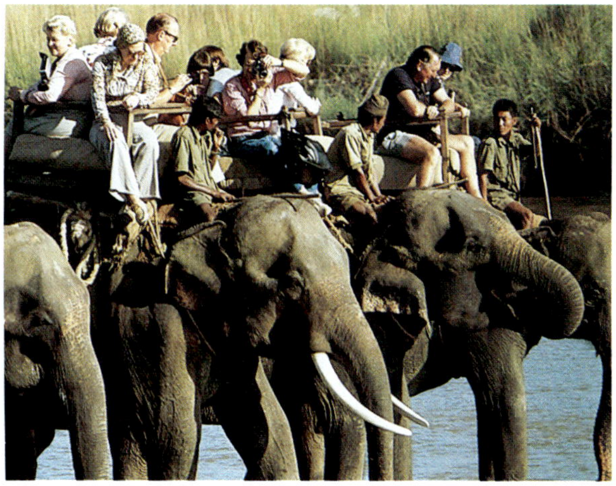

Page 92

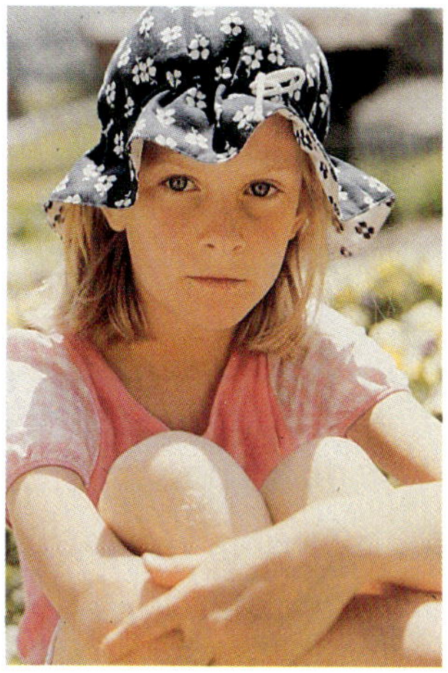

Page 104

FEATURE ARTICLES

THE FACTS ABOUT SWEETENERS — 4
Sugar, corn syrup, honey, saccharin, NutraSweet—the list goes on. How safe are these sweeteners? Are some more healthful than others?

BATHS AND SPAS — 18
There is a long history of "taking the waters" for treatment and relaxation. What are the real health benefits of hot springs and mineral waters?

GAMBLING CAN BE AN ADDICTION — 30
The obsessive need to gamble can lead to debt, divorce, and suicide, but the right treatment can help avert disaster.

AIDS: TWO EPIDEMICS — 42
A deadly and fast-spreading disease has spawned a second epidemic of fear that may be out of proportion to the risk. What we now know—and still need to learn—about AIDS.

EXERCISING AT HOME: WHAT YOU NEED TO KNOW — 54
Tips on the best exercises and the most suitable equipment for your private workout.

COLON CANCER: PREVENTION AND TREATMENT — 64
Who is most at risk for this common type of cancer; what can be done to prevent it or detect it in an early, treatable stage.

WHAT IS GENETIC COUNSELING? — 70
A whole range of tests and techniques are now available to help a couple determine the likelihood of their having a child with a genetic disorder.

FISH IN THE DIET — 80
Fish is highly nutritious, low in calories and fat, and even has a special ingredient that may lower the risk of heart disease.

STAYING HEALTHY WHEN TRAVELING — 92
What to do about motion sickness, jet lag, and other minor annoyances of traveling. The significant health risks of visiting developing countries.

THE SKIN: A VITAL ORGAN — 104
The unique qualities of the body's largest organ. The effects of the sun. Different types of skin cancer.

HYPOCHONDRIA — 116
An all-encompassing preoccupation with disease can disrupt a person's life.

HEART ATTACKS: REDUCING DEATHS — 124
Dramatic breakthroughs in understanding why heart attacks happen—and techniques to actually stop an attack in progress—have helped reduce deaths and disability.

HOW LONG CAN WE LIVE? — 136
Life expectancy is steadily improving. Is there a limit to the human life span? Will we ever be able to halt the aging process?

THE NEW VACCINES — 148
Vaccines have already saved countless lives. Now, new methods are being explored to make vaccines against herpes, AIDS, and even cancer.

UNDERSTANDING MEMORY — 156
The physical, biochemical, and behavioral forces that help explain why we remember and why we forget.

REHABILITATION CENTERS — 166
Their ambitious goal: to help patients with chronic or disabling conditions lead normal physical and social lives.

Contents Continues

SPOTLIGHT ON HEALTH

A series of concise reports on practical health topics.

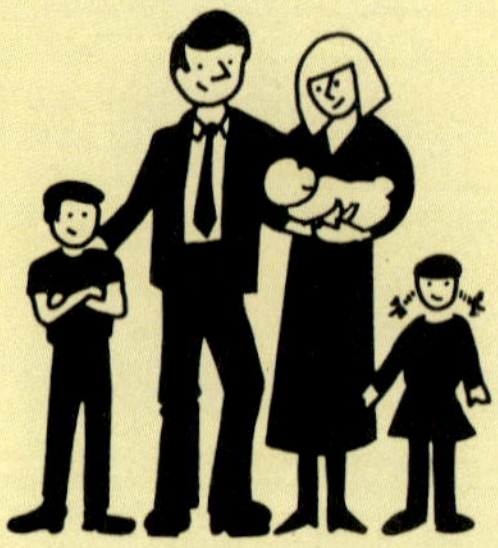

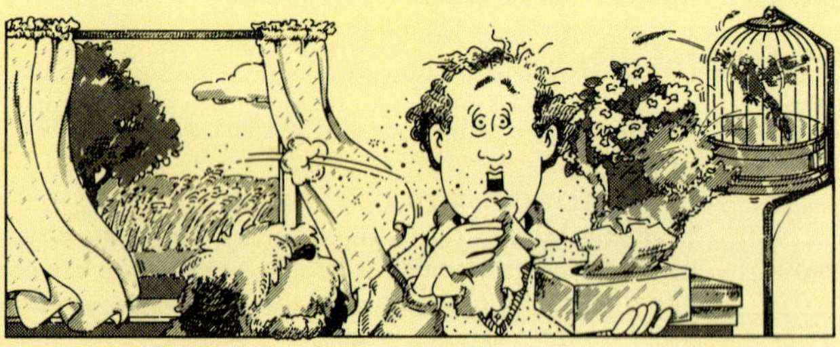

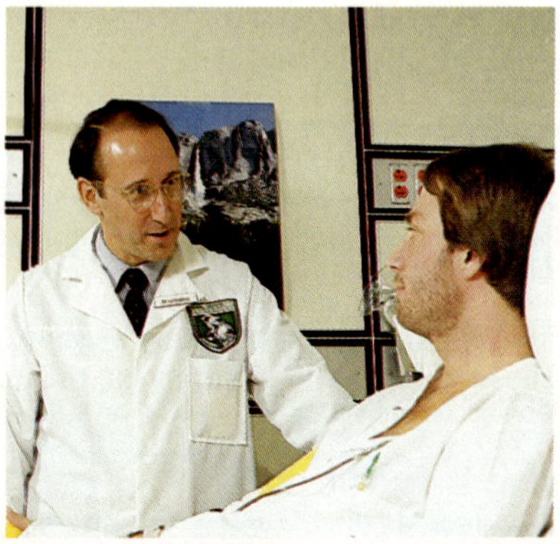

Health and Medical News

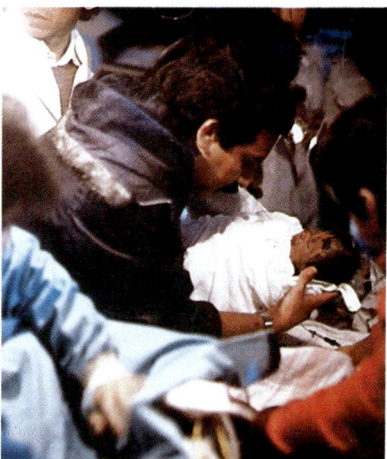

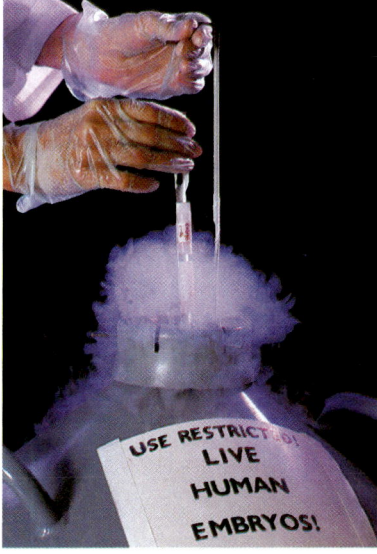

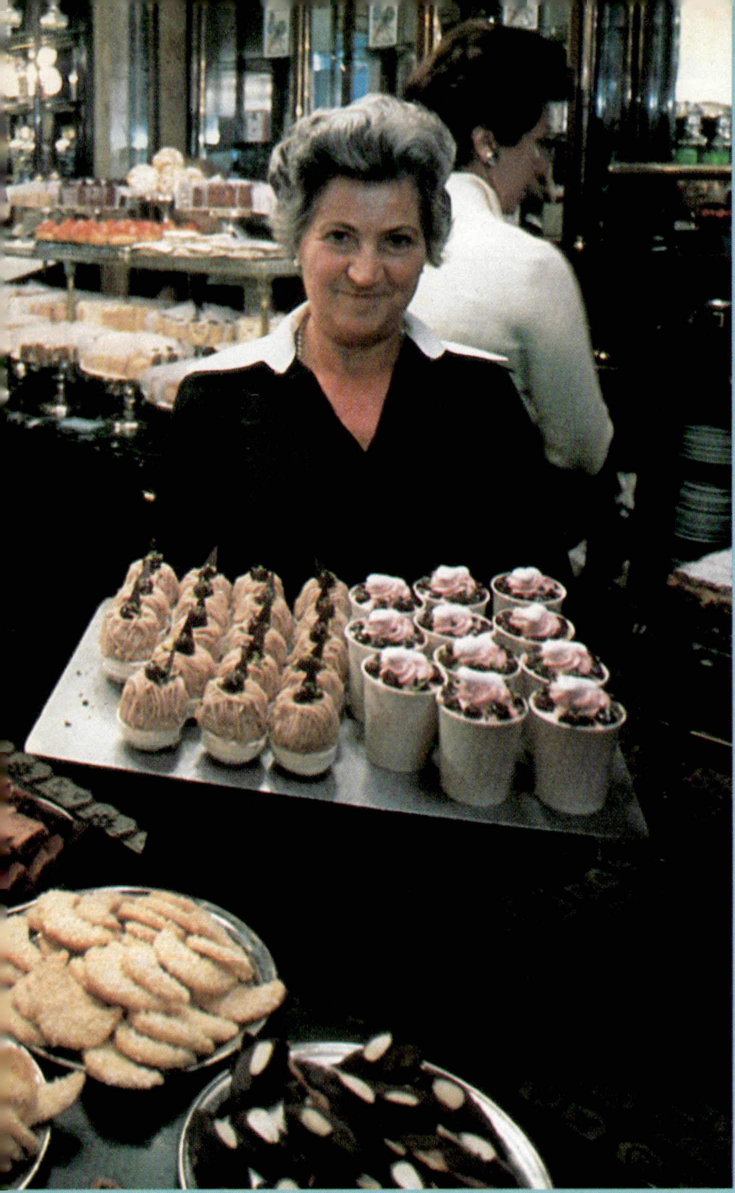

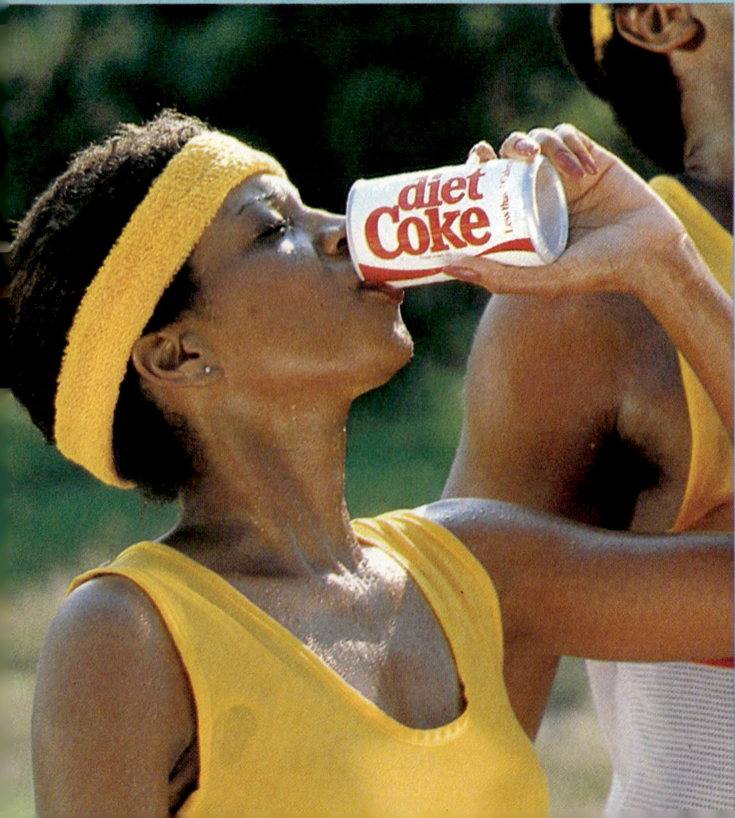
diet
Coke

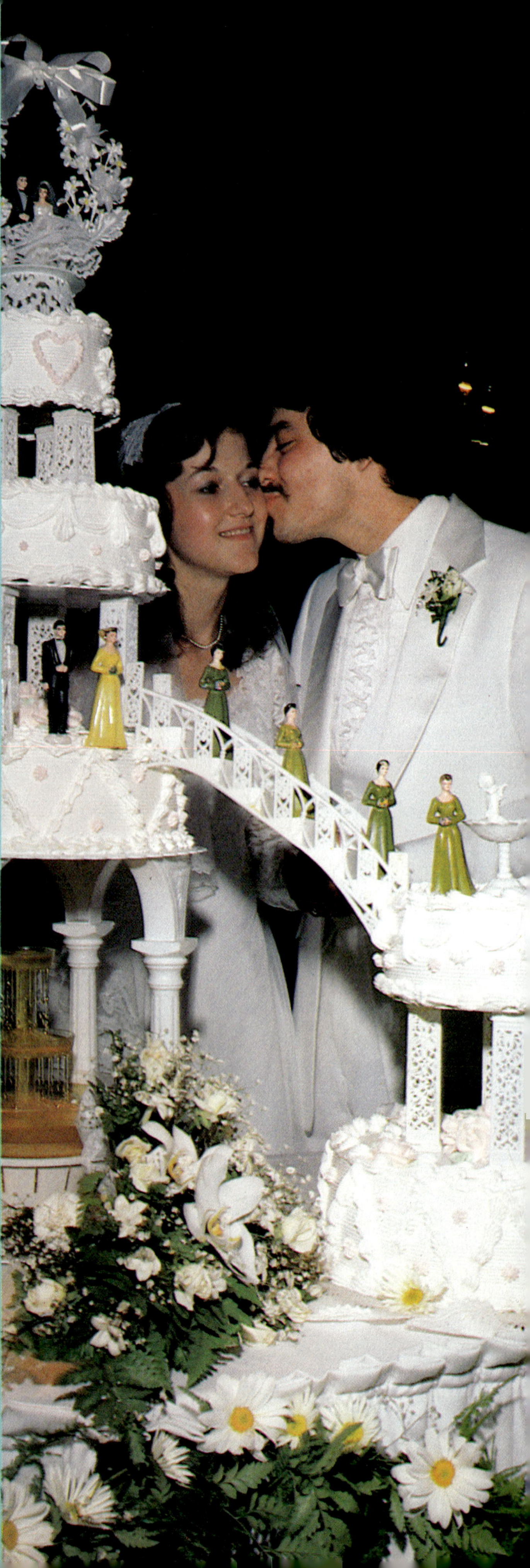

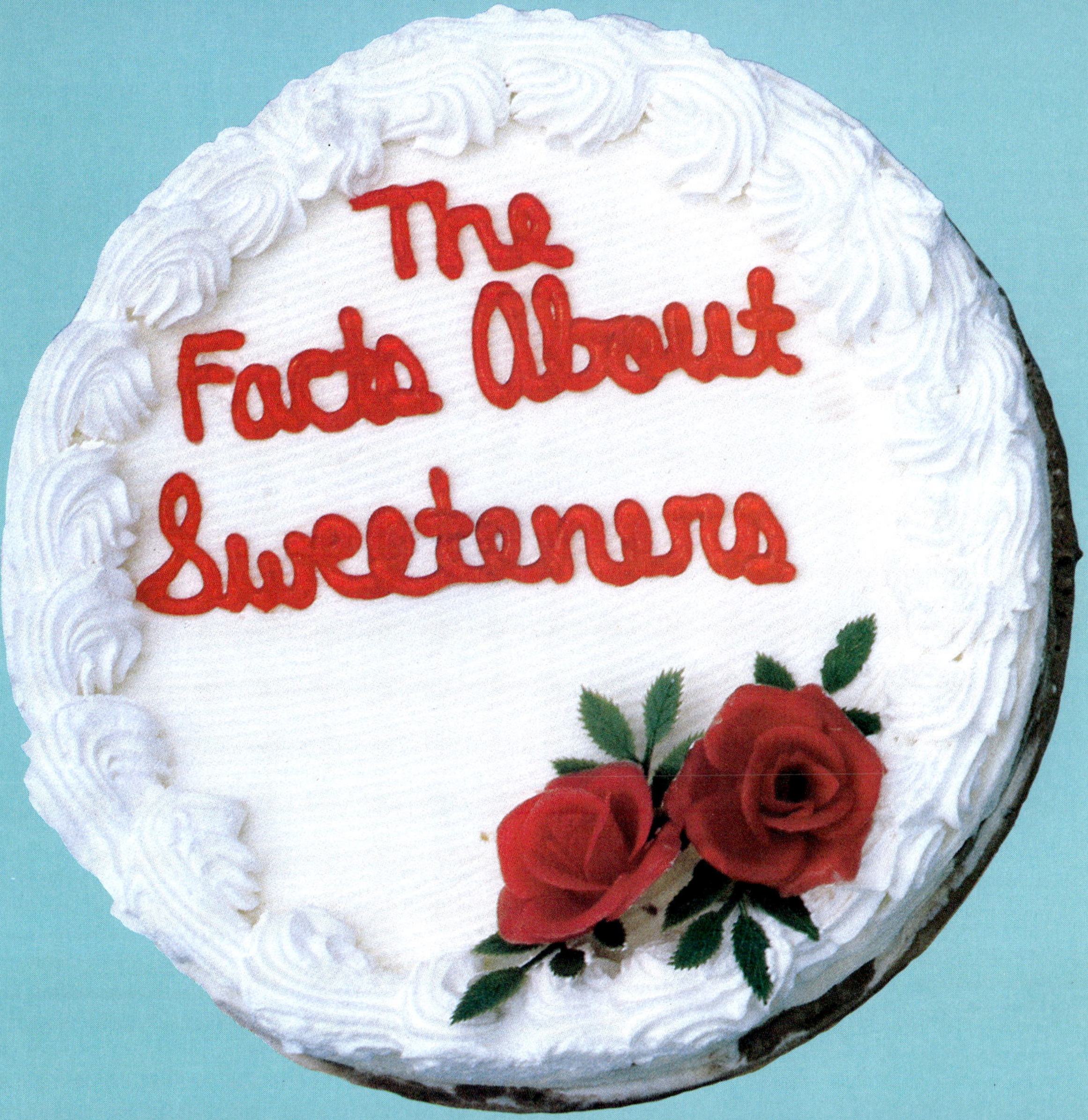

Susan Walton

Newborn babies, if offered samples of the four basic flavors—salty, bitter, sour, and sweet—invariably favor one: sweet. Photographs of taste experiments show cheerful babies drinking sugar water and crabby babies stuck with the other flavors.

Tastes change and diets become more varied, but most people keep their sweet tooth throughout life. They indulge it with cookies, candy, and cakes—delectable ways to get at the sweetness of sugar, honey, molasses, or synthetic sweeteners like saccharin.

More sweeteners of more kinds are being used than ever before. Although the amount of refined white sugar people consume has been dropping slowly in the United States, the use by food companies of a less expensive sweetener called high-fructose corn syrup is on the increase—in soft drinks and even in foods that once went unsweetened, like salad dressings and sauces. Artificial sweeteners are also enjoying boom times. According to the Calorie Control Council, a coalition of industry groups, at least 68 million Americans over the age of 18 now include saccharin or aspartame in their diets. This is a rise of more than 60 percent since 1978.

Doubts are sometimes voiced, however, about the safety of sweeteners. Some people believe that sugar is inherently bad for you. Other people won't touch refined sugar but happily eat honey, molasses, or other "natural" sweeteners that they think are more healthful. Some people shun all natural sweeteners but avidly use artificial ones to help cut calories. Then there are the people who avoid artificial sweeteners for fear of cancer or other diseases.

Are they right to worry? A look at the scientific evidence suggests that except for individuals who have serious problems handling sugar (as in diabetes) or a sensitivity to a particular sweetener (such as difficulty in digesting it) most of the worries are not well-founded. Sugar has, however, been firmly linked with tooth decay. Also, eating a lot of sugar could have a negative effect on general health if it caused a person to pass up foods with needed nutrients. Sugar provides energy but nothing else, which is why it's often called a source of empty calories. The question of individual sensitivity aside, there is as yet no firm evidence conclusively linking artificial sweeteners to disease in humans.

SWEET WORDS

Aspartame, an artificial sweetener, made from two naturally occurring substances, that is about 200 times sweeter than table sugar.

Brown sugar, refined white table sugar that has had some molasses added back in.

Confectioner's sugar, finely powdered white sugar (sucrose); also called powdered sugar.

Cyclamate, an artificial sweetener taken off the U.S. market in 1970.

Fructose, or levulose, the sweetest naturally occurring sugar; found in fruits and honey.

Glucose, or dextrose, the sugar most important to the body's metabolism.

High-fructose corn syrup, a liquid sweetener made from cornstarch by an enzyme process.

Lactose, the sugar found in milk.

Maltose, a sugar about half as sweet as table sugar; important in brewing, it is also used in beverages and baby foods.

Maple syrup, a sweet golden-brown syrup obtained from the sap of certain maple trees.

Molasses, the syrup that is separated from sugarcane (or sugar beet) juice in the production of white sugar.

Saccharin, the oldest artificial sweetener, about 500 times sweeter than table sugar.

Sorghum, a sweet syrup made from the sorghum plant, a member of the grass family.

Sorbitol, a sugar alcohol about half as sweet as table sugar; commonly used as a sweetener in dietetic foods.

Sucrose, ordinary white table sugar, consisting of one molecule of glucose and one of fructose.

The Taste for Sweetness

The statistics on sweetener consumption aren't that surprising when you consider that people's fondness for sweets is basically inborn, not learned. This is true of many animals as well—for example, horses, bears, and guinea pigs. There are other animals that do not show a liking for sweets; these sourpusses include the cat family, chickens, gulls, armadillos, and hedgehogs. Chickens are not only indifferent to most types of sugar but find one, xylose, "terribly offensive," according to Morley Kare and Gary Beauchamp of the Monell Chemical Senses Center in Philadelphia.

The precise reason why people are born liking sweets may never be known. Kare and Beauchamp theorize that plant eaters with a taste for sweets had an evolutionary advantage because sweetness in plant foods tends to signal that they contain substantial food energy, which is low in many edible plants. Other researchers have noted that a high sugar content is characteristic of fruits when they are ripest and most nourishing. Our taste for sweets is probably inherited from our prehuman as well as human ancestors.

Actually, taste is not the only reason sugar is added to foods. It can be an important preservative—notably in jellies and jams—and it enhances the action of yeast in bread and helps make cured meats juicier.

Susan Walton is a free-lance writer who specializes in health topics.

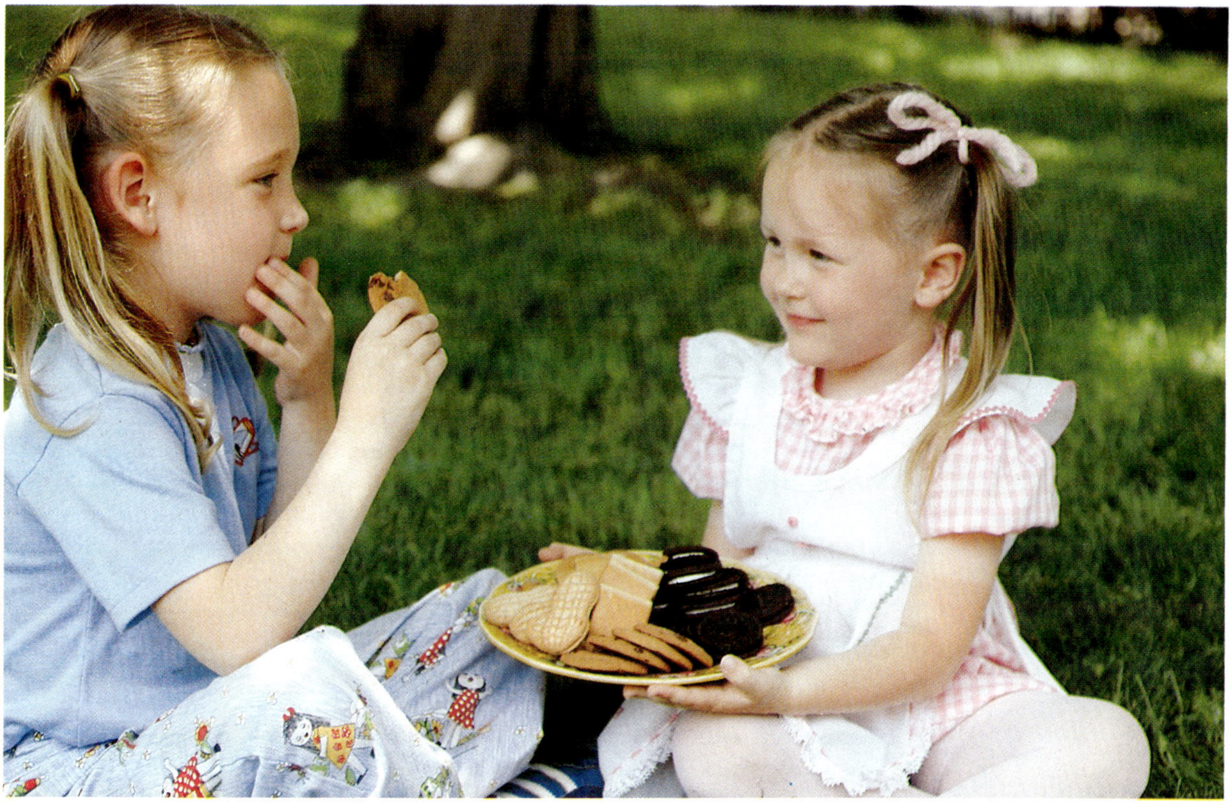

Children are born liking sweets, and most people retain their sweet tooth into adulthood.

The Sweetness of Nature

Several types of sugar are found in nature. (See the box on the opposite page for brief descriptions of various natural and artificial sweeteners.) All of the natural sugars are simple carbohydrates—as opposed to starches, which contain bigger molecules (made up of the same building blocks as sugars) and are called complex carbohydrates. There are two basic groups of sugars: simple sugars, or monosaccharides, and double sugars, or disaccharides. Double sugar molecules consist of two simple sugars linked together.

In the digestive system, double sugars and starches are broken down into simple sugars—glucose, fructose, and galactose. The simple sugars then enter the bloodstream and travel to the liver, where fructose and galactose are converted to glucose. Glucose is then carried to all tissues of the body. Glucose is critical to cell function and the maintenance of life. When it reacts with oxygen, it produces energy, carbon dioxide, and water. Glucose is one of the body's, and especially the brain's, most important sources of energy.

Ordinarily, when people talk about sugar, they mean sucrose, the most common sweetening agent. White table sugar is almost pure sucrose; so, for that matter, is brown sugar. Sucrose is a disaccharide, made up of two simple sugars, glucose and fructose. Sugarcane and sugar beets are the most concentrated sources of sucrose, but it is found in other vegetables and fruits as well. A teaspoon of sucrose contains about 16 calories.

Corn sweeteners, produced from cornstarch or potato starch, are often

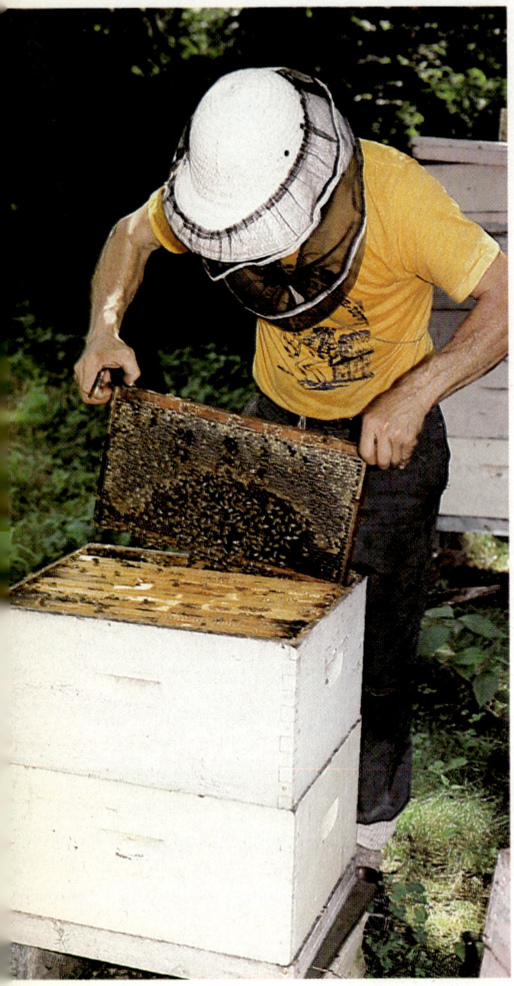

Honey is the world's oldest sweetener; in antiquity it was seen as a precious substance. Here a beekeeper gathers honey from the honeycombs that the bees have constructed in an artificial hive.

used in food processing. In the past, they were made up chiefly of glucose, which limited their usefulness because glucose is less sweet than sucrose. Technological developments have enabled producers to use an enzyme to chemically change much of the glucose found in corn syrup into fructose, the sweetest naturally occurring sugar. The resulting substance, called high-fructose corn syrup, contains 42 percent or more fructose. Consumption of this sweetener—almost all of it as an ingredient in beverages and processed foods—has grown dramatically in recent years, from 2.1 pounds per person in the United States in 1973 to 42.7 pounds in 1985. Pure fructose in solid form is still quite expensive to produce, and it accounts for a very small portion of the sugar people eat.

Closely related to the sugars is the class of sweeteners called polyols or sugar alcohols. These are also found in nature and are less sweet than sucrose and fructose. They include sorbitol, which is about half as sweet as sucrose and is a common sweetener in "sugar-free" products. Another sugar alcohol, xylitol, found in fruits, berries, and mushrooms, is also used as a sweetener, chiefly in dietetic foods. Mannitol, widely used in the pharmaceutical industry, occurs naturally in foods such as endive and celery.

Imitating Sugar

Then there are the synthetic, or artificial, sweeteners—compounds that taste sweet but have fewer calories or are more concentrated sources of sweetness than the naturally occurring sweeteners. Artificial sweeteners were once used almost solely by people with diabetes who had to limit their intake of sugar because their bodies could not metabolize it properly. Now, dieters, too, often rely on synthetic sweeteners to satisfy their sweet tooth.

Saccharin, which is about 500 times sweeter than sucrose, is perhaps the best-known artificial sweetener. Discovered in 1879, saccharin, along with cyclamate, became extremely popular in the 1960's, when diet soda began to join regular soda on grocery shelves. Saccharin has a bitter aftertaste that makes it unpalatable to some people. It has also been the subject of a heated—and still unresolved—safety controversy. A label warning of a possible cancer risk is now required in the United States on products containing saccharin.

Cyclamate (or cyclamates, since there is more than one form) is about 30 times sweeter than sucrose. Discovered by accident in 1937, it was used as a sugar substitute, often in combination with saccharin, until it was pulled from the U.S. market in 1970 following research that implicated the combination as a possible cause of bladder cancer.

Aspartame is the latest commercially available find in the quest for a sugar substitute. Discovered in 1965, aspartame is about 200 times sweeter than sucrose and, unlike saccharin, leaves no bitter aftertaste. Sold as NutraSweet and Equal, it is made by combining two naturally occurring amino acids (the building blocks of proteins). Aspartame is the only artificial sweetener approved for use in food products in both the United States and Canada. Both saccharin and cyclamate are available to Canadian consumers in powdered form, but they may not be used in commercially prepared foods.

Sweet History

The wide array of sweeteners available today is a relatively recent development. Our earliest ancestors probably satisfied their sweet tooth with fruit and honey. French cave paintings 30,000 years old show people using smoke to drive bees out of their hives. Indeed, the presence of cavities in teeth from our prehuman forebears who lived over a million years ago suggests to paleontologists that "hominids" of that time were fond of honey.

Egyptian pictographs portray beekeeping as early as 2600 B.C., and pots of honey were routinely placed in tombs with the deceased. (Honey was also used in embalming.) The Vikings fermented honey and drank it as mead. Honey was used as a medication in a number of traditional systems of medicine, including the Ayurvedic system in India.

Throughout most of historical time, honey has been a precious substance, eaten regularly only by the rich and seldom tasted by the poor. Its use in religious ceremonies reflected its prestige. Honey was virtually the only sweetener in biblical and classical times in Europe and the Middle East, and its importance was reflected in the biblical Promised Land, flowing with milk and honey.

The traditional New England process of making maple sugar from the sap of maple trees was depicted by Grandma Moses in Sugaring Off *(1943).*

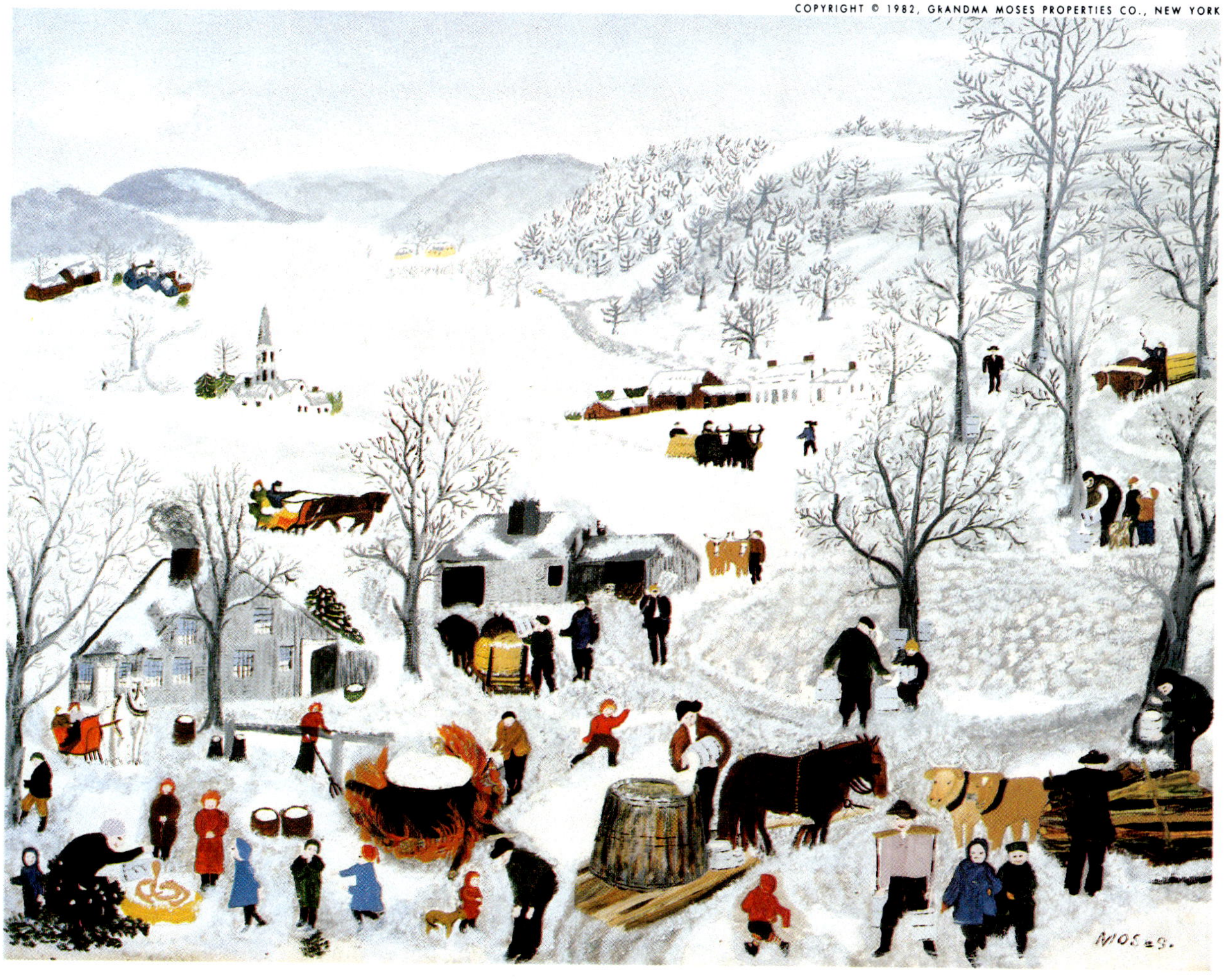

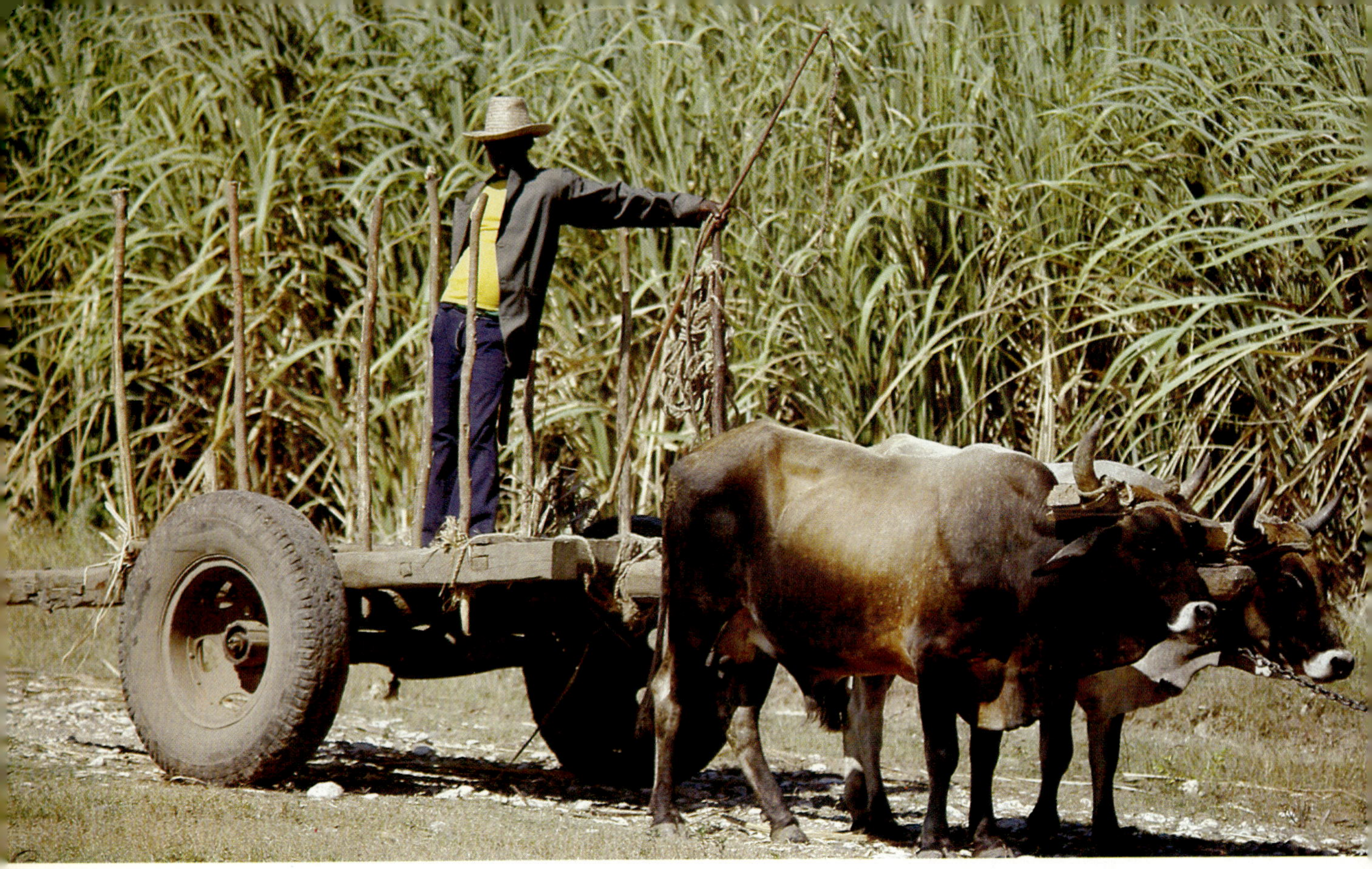

Sugar began as a scarce commodity. The growing of sugarcane probably originated in the South Pacific, possibly in New Guinea. Sugarcane was apparently cultivated in India before 3000 B.C. A member of Alexander the Great's invading army encountered it there and left the first written reference to sugarcane in a European language.

Around A.D. 600 sugarcane cultivation began to move toward the Mediterranean, where the Arabs adopted it. The tales of the *Arabian Nights*, many of which date back to the eighth and ninth centuries, often refer to sugar. War carried sugarcane further; Arab conquests brought it into Syria, Cyprus, Crete, Egypt, Morocco, Sicily, and Spain. Venice apparently became a reexporting center for sugar before the end of the tenth century. Crusaders returning from Palestine brought a taste for sugar back home to many parts of Europe, beginning about 1100. Sugar became known as an expensive but highly desirable product, and in the following centuries increasing amounts of it were imported into Western Europe.

Christopher Columbus, whose father-in-law owned a sugar plantation, carried cane to Hispaniola on his second journey to the New World in 1493. Within a few years sugarcane cultivation was widespread in the West Indies. The need for labor in the cane fields became a major impetus behind the slave trade, and rum made from the molasses that was produced in processing the cane was used to pay for the slaves. Successful planting of sugarcane in what is now the United States is generally reckoned to have begun in Louisiana in 1751.

It was not until the beginning of the next century that commercial production of sugar from the sugar beet began. The first beet sugar factories were established in Germany about 1802, and development of the new source of sugar received a big push when the British blockade of the

Making Sugar

Sugarcane was the earliest source of sugar, later joined by sugar beets. At left, a field of sugarcane in Jacmel, Haiti, is worked with the help of oxen. At right, a worker in Costa Rica manufactures dulce, a sweet drink produced by making a slight variation in the standard processing of brown sugar.

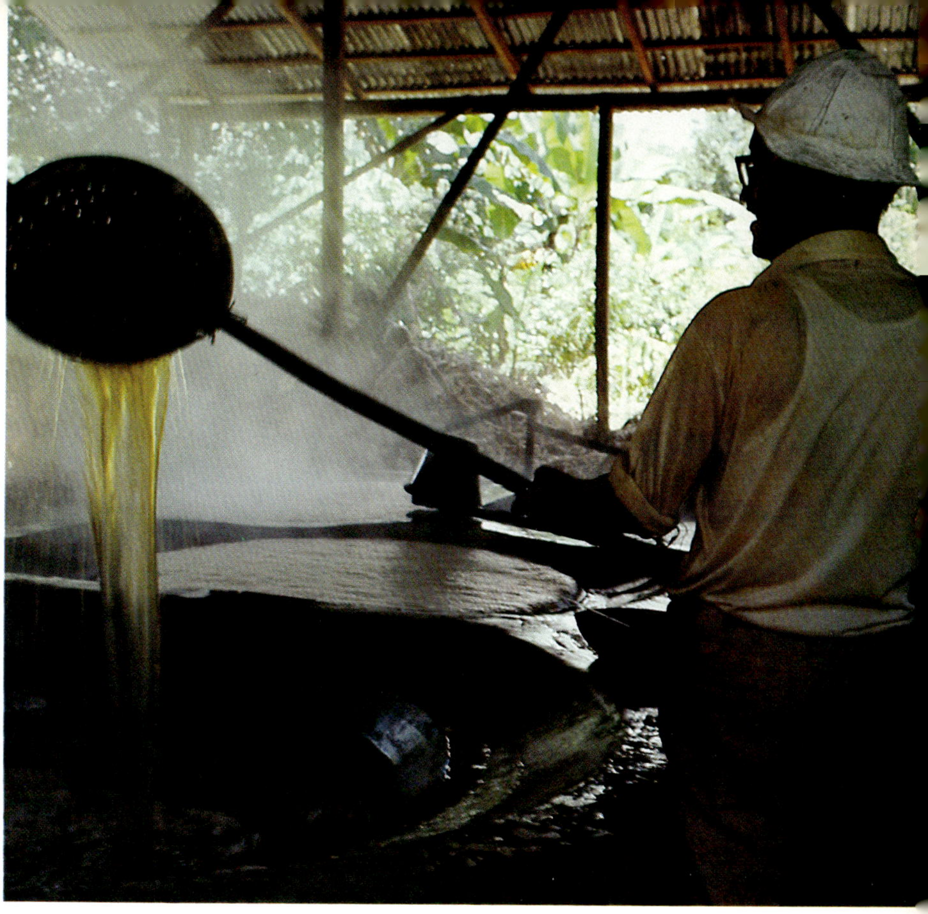

Continent during the Napoleonic wars prevented cane sugar from reaching France. Production of sucrose from beets has grown until it now accounts for more than a third of the world's supply.

Sugar and Health

Worries about sugar's effects on health are not new. In 1633 a London physician wrote, "Sugar in it self be opening and cleansing, yet being much used produceth dangerous effect in the body: as namely, the immoderate use thereof, as also of sweet confections and Sugar Plummes, heateth the blood, ingendreth obstructions, cachexias, consumptions, rotteth the teeth, making them look blacke; and withal, causeth many times a loathsome, stinking breathe."

Nutrition. In language less colorful than that of 17th-century England, some modern writers have also questioned the health effects of both naturally occurring and synthetic sweeteners. Dietary guidelines that urge people to reduce their sugar intake have further undermined sugar's reputation. But the rationale behind such advice implies that sugar itself, in moderation, isn't harmful. The basic problem is that since sugar does not contain essential nutrients, people who satisfy their appetite with sweets instead of more nutritious foods may end up with an inadequate diet. (Sugar, as a carbohydrate, does provide energy, but many other sources of carbohydrates, unlike sweets, do contain substantial nutrients.) Nutritionists hope that people who reduce their sugar intake will turn to foods that make a more positive contribution to health.

Molasses, a by-product of sugar refining (usually from cane), is the only sweetener to offer significant nutritional benefits. The lowest grade—blackstrap molasses (what is left of the cane syrup after all the sugar that can be economically removed has been taken out)—is the most nutritious kind, providing calcium, potassium, phosphorus, and iron. The higher-grade types more usually used in baking are richer in sugar and lower in nutrients, but their calories are still less empty than table sugar.

Honey, contrary to the claims of enthusiasts, is not much better than sugar. It does contain a few nutrients, but the amounts are so small as to be nutritionally insignificant. Brown sugar, touted by some as a more "natural" product, is actually little more nutritious than white sugar, and less natural. This is because commercial brown sugar is usually no more than white sugar with some of the molasses added back in—an additional step in the refining process.

But even if sugar doesn't do you a whole lot of good, it doesn't follow that it does a lot of harm. Although scientists have probed for links between sugar and a range of ailments, the evidence to date connects sugar firmly with only one disease—dental caries, or tooth decay.

Tooth decay. The connection between sugar and cavities was noted a long time ago, but it took a while for scientific evidence to accumulate. Aristotle noted that soft, sweet figs adhered to the teeth, putrefied, and damaged the teeth. Elizabeth I was famous for her sweet tooth and later for her blackened and decaying teeth.

Dental caries (tooth decay) is so far the only disease that has been firmly linked to sugar consumption.

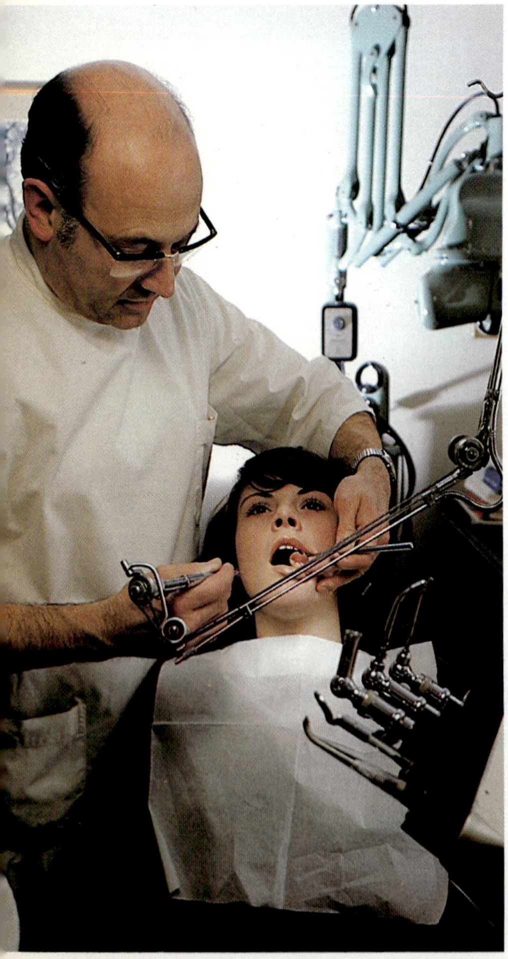

Surveys by the World Health Organization and other agencies show that high sugar consumption goes hand in hand with high rates of dental caries. This does not prove anything in itself, because increased sugar consumption tends to accompany other changes in diet, but there is additional evidence for the role of sugar in tooth decay.

The process by which sugars and other carbohydrates affect the teeth is well understood. A key role is played by plaque, a thin film consisting largely of bacteria and bacteria by-products that constantly forms on the teeth. When a person eats a food that contains sugars or starches, the bacteria in plaque produce acids that can destroy tooth enamel. The plaque, which is sticky, holds the acids to the teeth for a period of about 20 minutes. During that time, the acids eat away at the tooth enamel. When enough enamel is gone, a cavity is formed. There is a simple way to avoid the whole process: after eating, brush your teeth well. Since other carbohydrates have the same effect as sugars on plaque, not all tooth decay is caused by sucrose—but scientists generally believe that sugars promote tooth decay much more than do starches.

Sugar's effect on teeth depends on how much is consumed, and under what circumstances. If you eat sugary foods often, even in small amounts, you are exposing your teeth to acid damage more often. If the foods are sticky—Aristotle was right about the figs—the exposure will last longer. Sugar that stays in the mouth a long while, as in hard candy and cough drops, also gives acid more time to attack the teeth. Whether you eat carbohydrates by themselves is also important; those eaten as part of a well-balanced meal are less damaging to the teeth, and some kinds of cheeses and other foods appear to have an anticaries effect that could conceivably cancel out the harmful qualities of sugar.

Diabetes. Sugar is also linked with diabetes in the minds of many, and, indeed, people with diabetes generally restrict their intake of sugar. However, research has not shown that eating sugar directly causes diabetes. According to Drs. Donald J. Rose and John J. B. Anderson of

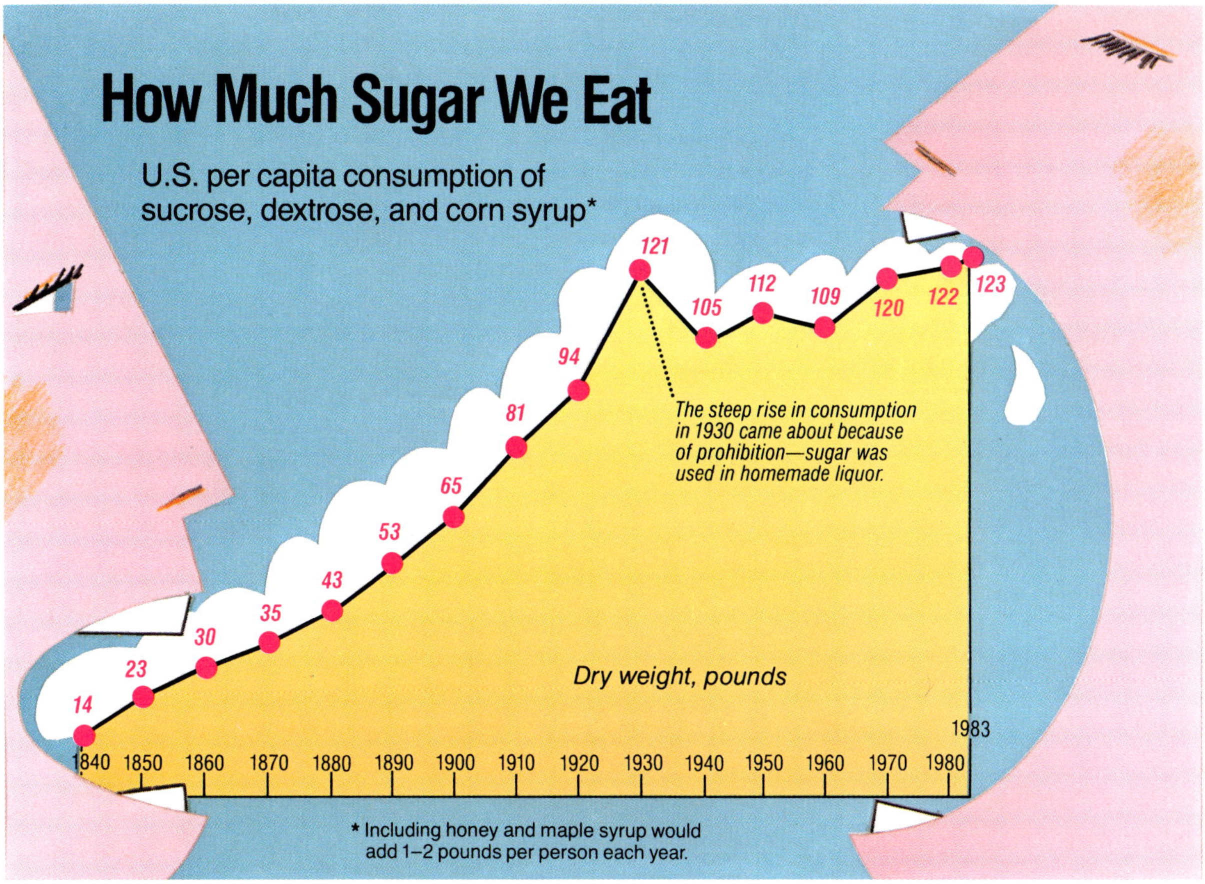

Source: U.S. Department of Agriculture

the University of North Carolina, "There is no epidemiological evidence that increased sugar intake leads to the development of diabetes mellitus, despite the belief prevalent over the past 100 years that the overconsumption of sugars has led to the increased prevalence of diabetes."

Hypoglycemia, or low blood sugar—which can be a warning sign of diabetes—does not seem to be brought on by sugar consumption either, although some have suggested a link. In one type of this fairly rare condition, the body overreacts to sugar in the blood by producing too much insulin, which in turn drives the blood-sugar level down below normal levels. People who suffer from the problem must avoid ingesting too much sugar at one time, but that does not mean the disorder was caused by sugar.

Heart disease. Some researchers have connected high sugar consumption with coronary heart disease. In 1957 the British physician John Yudkin published a paper noting that countries with high rates of sugar consumption also have high rates of heart disease. But Rose and Anderson point out that heart disease has multiple causes, and it isn't possible to distinguish the effects of eating sugar from other factors when doing comparisons between countries. Most researchers believe that there is as yet no solid evidence of a direct link between sugar and coronary heart disease—except in some individuals with a genetic disorder in which high sugar intake results in undesirable increases in fatty substances in the blood and a consequently increased risk of developing heart disease. It can be noted that coronary heart disease has actually declined in the United States in recent years, while consumption of sugars has gone up.

Doesn't sugar make you fat? Many people view sugar as what one researcher called a uniquely fattening food. Strictly speaking, it isn't. A calorie is a calorie, so sugar isn't more fattening than a lot of entirely unsweetened, high-calorie foods. Nor are the obese particularly high sugar consumers. An analysis by Dr. Edwin L. Bierman of the University of Washington School of Medicine found that fat people actually tended to eat less sugar than their slim counterparts. Bierman also noted that those who hope to lose weight simply by reducing sugar could cut back on any source of calories and achieve much the same effect.

But even if sugar is not uniquely fattening, this does not absolve sweets of all blame. They tend to have a high concentration of calories, and some people find them simply too tasty to resist. Eating just a couple of small chocolate bars can mean taking in hundreds of calories with little nutritional benefit.

Sugar and Behavior

One of the most intriguing charges leveled against sugar is that it makes people prone to disruptive behavior. This idea received widespread publicity several years ago, when lawyers defending a man accused of

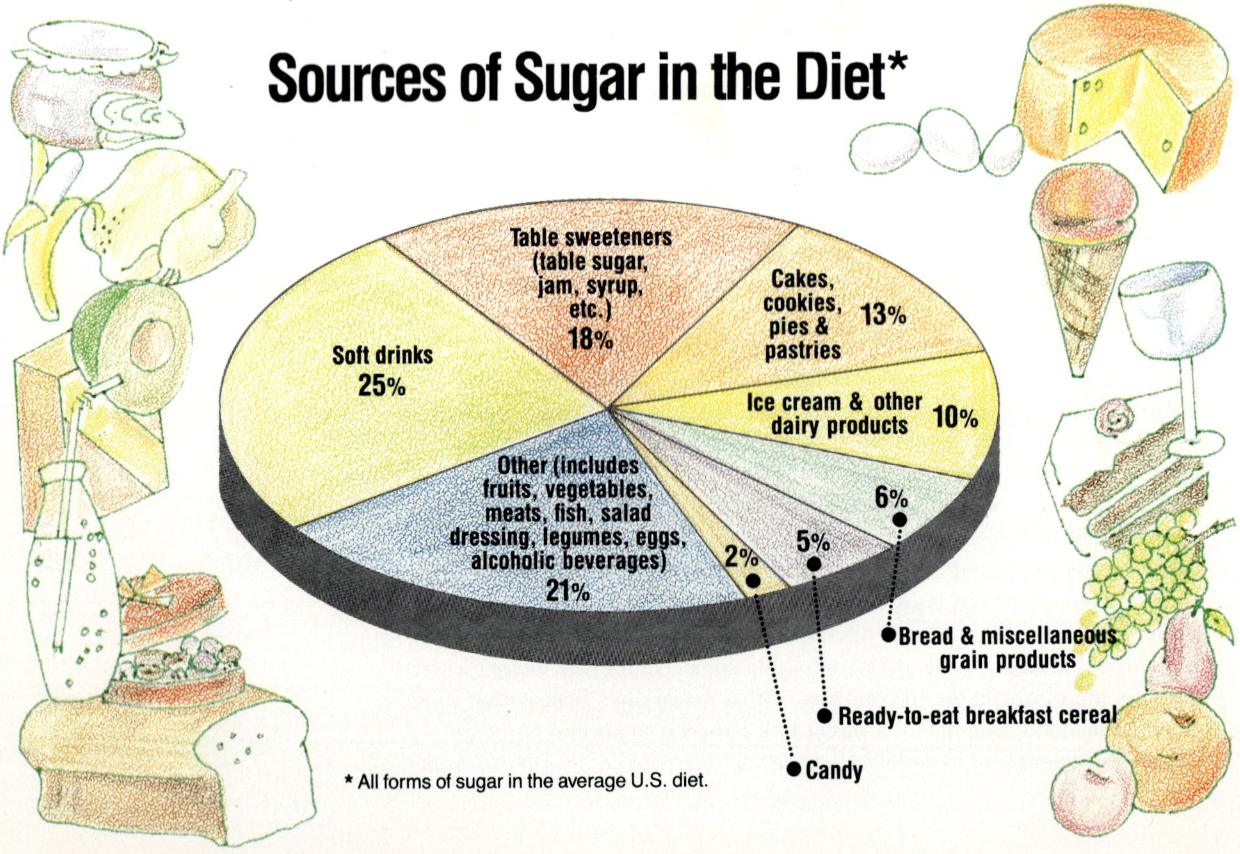

Source: Center for Science in the Public Interest, Washington, D.C.

shooting two San Francisco politicians relied on the so-called Twinkie defense. They argued that their client's behavior was unbalanced at least partly because he consumed a lot of sweet, highly refined foods. Medical research, however, suggests that if sugar has any effect on behavior, it is generally likely to be minor.

There has been much interest in the theory that eating excess sugar contributes to hyperactivity in children. But a study by Dr. Mortimer D. Gross of the University of Illinois Medical Center did not support this claim. Gross described one hyperactive boy whose symptoms did become noticeably worse after he ate sucrose, while glucose, lactose (milk sugar), and saccharin produced no change. To follow up on this, Gross tested 50 hyperactive children whose mothers believed that sucrose worsened their symptoms. Some of the children received lemonade sweetened with sucrose, and some drank saccharin-sweetened lemonade. Gross observed no difference in behavior between the two groups. He suggested that the sensitivity the first child showed to sugar is a real but rare condition.

At a 1984 symposium on diet and behavior sponsored by the American Medical Association and other groups, scientists reported only a few instances in which sugar appeared to have a negative effect on behavior. Dr. Keith Conners of Children's Hospital in Washington, D.C., found that children's learning ability decreased after a combination of a high-carbohydrate meal and a sugar-rich food. But the effect was not present if the children ate a high-protein meal followed by sugar; if the children ate sugar after a balanced meal, their learning actually improved. Another study, by Dr. Ron Prinz of the University of South Carolina, found that children whose sucrose consumption was high—25 to 35 percent of their daily calorie intake—did worse than average on a test measuring attention span. But Prinz suggested that the problem was more likely caused by a generally inadequate diet than by eating a lot of sugar.

In a study reported in 1982, Dr. Judith Rapoport of the U.S. National Institute of Mental Health monitored the physical activity and behavior of hyperactive boys who were given sugar-containing drinks. She found that the boys became calmer and less active when they drank the sugar mixture than when they did not receive it.

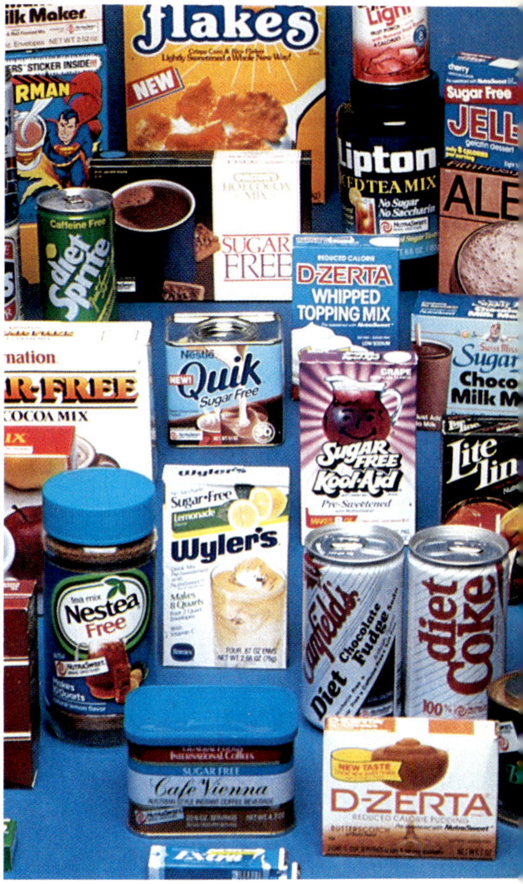

Aspartame (known as NutraSweet) is the latest artificial sweetener to be marketed; increasing numbers of companies are using the substance, which does not have the unpleasant aftertaste of saccharin, in their diet products.

Artificial Sweeteners and Health

Saccharin, cyclamate, and aspartame have all generated argument over their safety. In one case, the result was a ban.

Saccharin and cancer. Saccharin, the first artificial sweetener to be widely used, has been as controversial as it has been popular. The debate began when scientists reported that male rats fed high doses of saccharin had an increased incidence of bladder cancer. Many consumers questioned, however, whether they would ever ingest proportionate amounts of saccharin comparable to the amounts that the rats received, which were very high indeed.

But U.S. law does not allow for such distinctions; all food additives known to cause cancer in humans or animals must be removed from the market. After much debate, Congress passed a bill exempting saccharin from the ban pending further study. In mid-1985 the exemption came up for renewal and Congress extended it until May 1987.

A U.S. National Academy of Sciences report released in 1978 reviewed all the studies on saccharin that had been published up to then. It concluded that saccharin is a weak carcinogen, or cancer-causing substance, in animals and a potential carcinogen in humans. Pregnant women and young children were advised to avoid the sweetener, since the developing fetus and young children are most apt to be harmed by it. Taking into account more recent data, an American Medical Association report published in November 1985 found that the available evidence did not indicate that saccharin increases the risk of bladder cancer in humans. The report noted, however, that data concerning saccharin's effects on pregnant women and young children were sparse.

Cyclamate ban. Cyclamate too has a less-than-perfect record as a potential health risk, but the studies pointing to these dangers have been questioned by many scientists. In the late 1960's a study showed that a mixture of ten parts cyclamate and one part saccharin produced an increased incidence of bladder cancer in rats, a conclusion that led to the U.S. cyclamate ban.

The search for new sweeteners continues; here Herbert Seltzman and Yung-Ao Hsieh of the Research Triangle Institute work on the synthesis of a substance 58 times sweeter than sucrose.

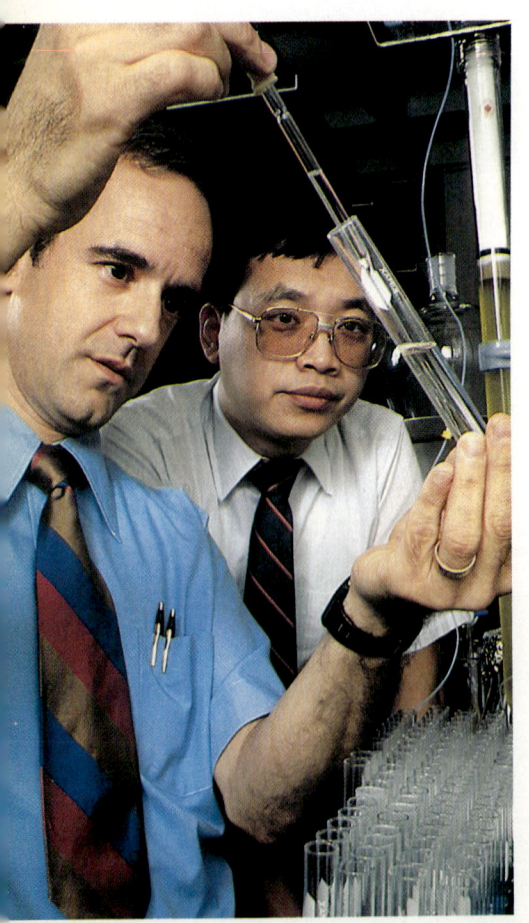

In 1985 a new review of the evidence concluded that cyclamate probably does not cause cancer by itself. However, the review, issued by a committee of the U.S. National Research Council, did find that the sweetener might enhance the cancer-causing effects of other substances and recommended further study of this possibility. The committee identified several problems in determining just what cyclamate's effects are. One is that much research has focused on mixtures of cyclamate with saccharin. Another is that most of the studies done on cyclamate alone were carried out on animals and on living cells in laboratory dishes, and scientists are uncertain as to what extent the findings apply to humans.

Studies have not settled another critical question—whether cyclamate can give rise to disorders other than cancer. Some research has suggested that it causes genetic damage and atrophy of the testicles. The U.S. Food and Drug Administration (FDA) has said that it will consider these studies before making a final decision on whether to allow cyclamate back on the market.

Is aspartame safe? Although many scientists argue that aspartame has been thoroughly studied and found safe, others contend that it may have an adverse effect on health and behavior if consumed in large enough amounts.

In evaluating aspartame, scientists have looked at the effects of the compound itself, and at its two component amino acids, aspartic acid and phenylalanine. They also have investigated the effects of the type of alcohol called methanol, which forms when aspartame is kept too long and starts to break down. Methanol can be toxic at high doses, but the FDA has set a suggested daily limit for methanol consumption that would be equivalent to the methanol that could form in 18 cans of diet soda.

Much of the concern has focused on phenylalanine. One worry is that the amino acid could cause mental retardation in fetuses and infants, similar to that found in phenylketonuria (PKU), a congenital enzyme deficiency. Persons born with PKU lack the enzyme their bodies need to utilize phenylalanine (which, as an amino acid, occurs in many food proteins). Studies show that although people with PKU must absolutely avoid aspartame, like other sources of phenylalanine, the sweetener apparently does not harm the nervous system of normal adults and children, even when consumed in fairly large amounts. Some scientists believe, however, that a great many people who do not have PKU may carry a recessive gene for it and consequently may have a higher than normal susceptibility to possible harmful effects of aspartame.

Whether phenylalanine can affect behavior is, to some investigators, an open question. Dr. Richard J. Wurtman, an endocrinologist at the Massachusetts Institute of Technology, reported on one experiment in which rats that were fed the amino acid showed increases in brain levels of phenylalanine and changes in other brain chemicals known to be involved in regulating mood and behavior. Wurtman testified before Congress that he did not think aspartame should be banned for this reason. But he did advocate a requirement that products be labeled to say exactly how much aspartame they contain.

While the quest for new artificial sweeteners goes on, many people will probably stick with plain old sugar.

Some individuals have reported other symptoms that seemed to occur after they consumed aspartame—including headaches, dizziness, nausea, diarrhea, and skin reactions. But when researchers from the U.S. Centers for Disease Control analyzed over 500 complaints in 1984, they found no specific group of symptoms associated with aspartame consumption and concluded that in most cases it was a coincidence that the problems occurred after eating aspartame. Some people, of course, may be particularly sensitive to the product and should avoid it. But according to an American Medical Association report published in July 1985, the available data suggest that, for normal individuals, aspartame consumption is safe and is not linked with serious adverse health effects.

A Sweeter Future?

Meanwhile, the quest for the perfect sweetener goes on. In April 1985, Herbert Seltzman of Research Triangle Institute in North Carolina reported on yet another candidate for the title. The substance, which was synthesized in accordance with the knowledge scientists have gained about what makes things sweet, is 58 times sweeter than sucrose, has no undesirable side tastes, leaves no aftertaste, and has shown no toxic effects in tests so far. Someday you may find D,L-aminomalonyl-D-alanine isopropyl ester, labeled with a catchy name, on your breakfast table.

Another approach is to look for new sweeteners in the library: four researchers at the University of Illinois found a reference to a "sweet herb" known to the ancient Aztecs in a 16th-century book on the New World. Relying on an illustration in the book, the researchers decided it was an herb still used in Mexico for medicinal purposes, and they isolated from it a substance a thousand times sweeter than sucrose, which they named hernandulcin. After its safety is tested and a manufacturing process developed, this substance too may appear in the marketplace.

Other candidates for sugar substitutes today include acesulfame K, already approved for use in several countries, and L-sugar, whose molecular structure is a mirror image of regular sugar. It is not so rare for scientists to find something that tastes sweet, but new sweeteners that meet the tests of safety and commercial practicality come along much less often. Whatever progress is made, though, it's a safe bet that a lot of people will stick with plain old sugar. □

Baths and Spas

Barbara Scherr Trenk

From the times of the earliest civilizations to the contemporary California hot tub, men and women have found comfort in an activity that children frequently claim to loathe: taking a bath. Soaking in pleasingly warm water can make a person feel relaxed and at peace with the world.

Claims have also long been made that bathing can alleviate a host of medical problems. Today the use of various forms of hydrotherapy (literally, treatment with water) is an accepted technique in physical rehabilitation following certain injuries and ailments. Beyond this, there is a widespread popular belief that bathing in water with special properties can have healing effects. In Europe in particular, millions of people each year seek relief from such disorders as arthritis, impotence, and constipation at spas where the waters contain certain minerals. Stories of remarkable improvement or even cures are sometimes heard. But most doctors believe that whatever benefits may result from a stay at a spa—potentially a refreshing experience—there is no solid proof that they are due to the waters' mineral content.

An Ancient Practice

The early Japanese, Greeks, Egyptians, Romans, and Hebrews are all reported to have used baths for both ritual and health-promoting purposes. No less famed a healer than the Greek physician Hippocrates advocated bathing as a form of therapy.

This art-nouveau swimming pool belongs to Budapest's Gellért public thermal baths, built in 1928.

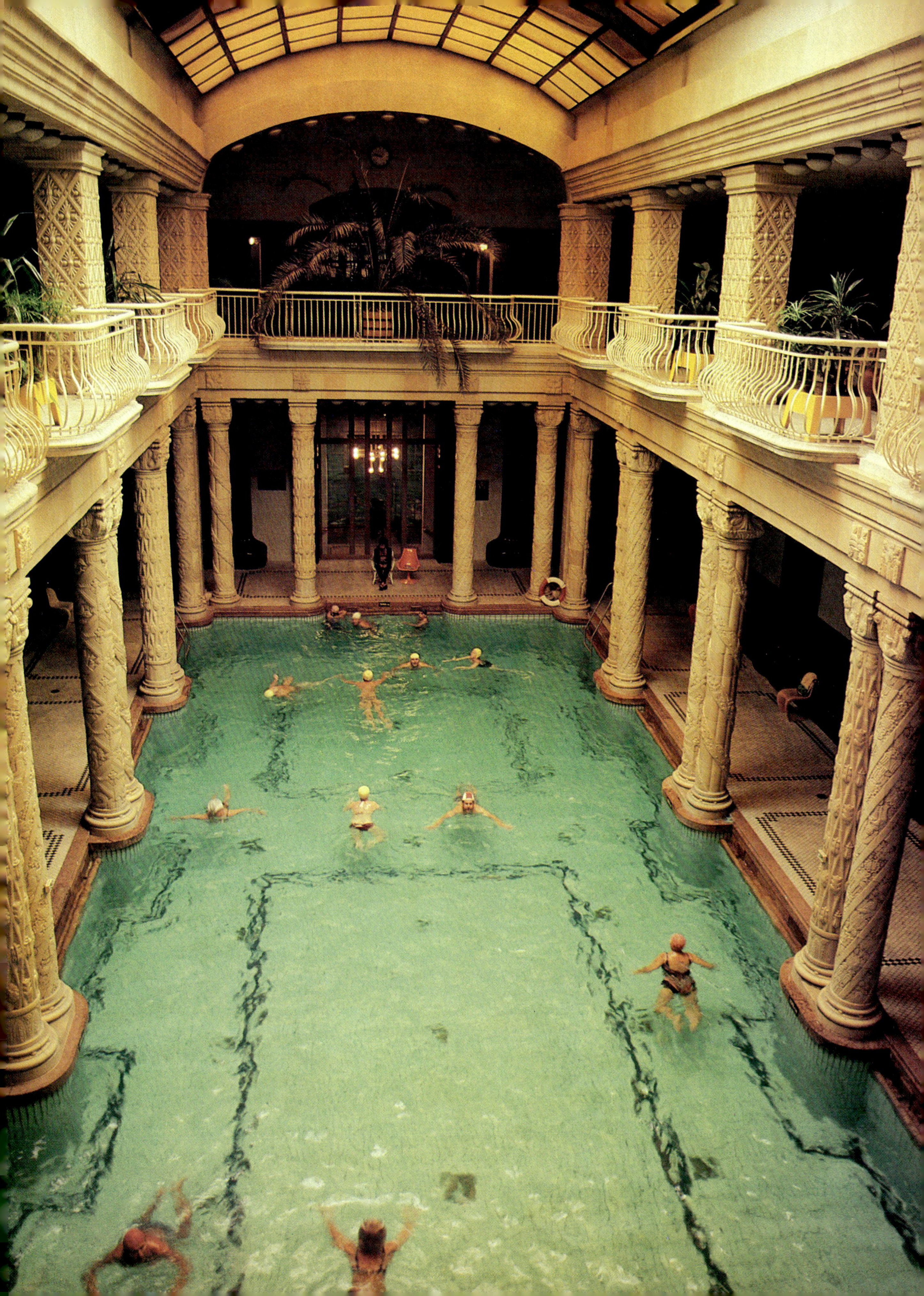

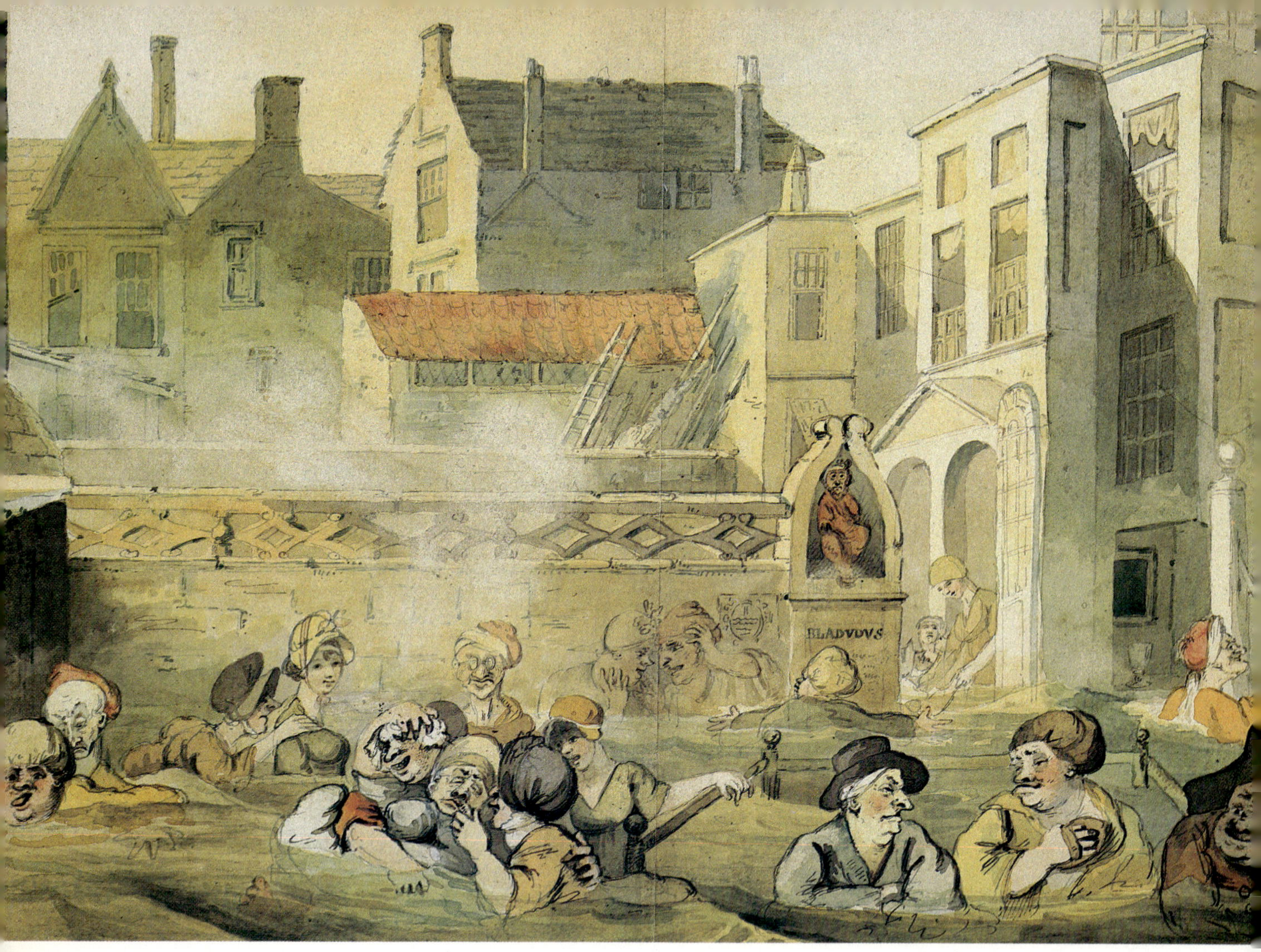

The mineral springs of Bath, in southwestern England, were originally developed by the Romans in the first century A.D.; the spa became famous as a pleasure and health resort, reaching its heyday in the 18th and 19th centuries (see caricature by John Nixon).

The Romans seem to have built baths around hot springs wherever their conquests took them. Tiberias, on the Sea of Galilee in Israel, is believed to be the oldest bathing resort on earth; in A.D. 18, Herod founded the city in honor of the Roman Emperor Tiberius near springs referred to in the biblical Book of Joshua. In the 12th century the Jewish physician and philosopher Maimonides sent his patients from Egypt to bathe at Tiberias; today travelers still come to the mineral hot springs to seek medical treatment.

As the Romans marched north and west, they found more sites for their baths. When Julius Caesar set out to conquer the Gauls, he rested at the hot springs later enjoyed by Charlemagne, now called Aix-les-Bains in the department of Savoie, France. In Britain the Romans developed a major spa around the hot mineral springs at what is now known as Bath.

Health spas, which today in the United States may be anything from a neighborhood health club to a posh fitness resort or a whirlpool bath, derive their name from the Belgian town of Spa, another site of mineral springs believed by the Romans to have therapeutic effects. In the late 18th century Spa became a fashionable resort city, with such notables as Russia's Peter the Great and the Holy Roman Emperor Joseph II paying regular visits. (The German word for spa is "Bad," meaning bath; in this case, "bad" is good when found in combination with such spa names as Neuenahr, Kreuznach, or the better known Baden-Baden.)

The belief that hot springs could promote healing was not limited to early European and Middle Eastern cultures. Native Americans in various parts of the New World used hot springs for their supposed curative effects long before European settlers reached the area. The Ute Indians traveled each spring to what is now known as Glenwood Springs, Colo., to bathe in the waters they called Yampa, meaning big medicine. Some Indian tribes feared the mineral hot springs in what is now Canada's Banff National Park, but others brought their sick there for healing. And one of the most famous U.S. mineral spring areas, Saratoga Springs, N.Y., noted for its carbonated water, was well known by the Mohawk Indians in the area; according to some sources, they first shared their healing place with Europeans in 1767 when the British superintendent of Indian affairs, Sir William Johnson, was taken there after an old wound he had suffered in the French and Indian War worsened.

Warm Water and Cold

Various cures involving the treatment of disease by the copious and frequent use of water were commonly known as hydropathy in the 19th century. A name often mentioned by those who take bath cures seriously is Father Sebastian Kneipp, a 19th-century parish priest from Worishofen, Bavaria. Kneipp claimed that water was "capable of curing every curable disease"; of course, in Kneipp's era fewer diseases were considered to be curable, and there were far fewer medical and surgical techniques to compete with the water cure. Some health spas in Europe still offer the "Kneipp cure," in which water in various forms and at various temperatures is used to treat specific diseases.

In the 1800's cold bath treatments were promoted as a substitute for the even more uncomfortable practices of leeching and bleeding.

The use of cold water as a purported cure was a popular healing practice in both Europe and North America during the 1800's. Bathing was only part of this school of treatment; cold water was also applied by wrapping patients in wet sheets or giving them sponge baths. Cold water baths were even given to treat yellow fever during an epidemic in Louisiana in the early 1800's. Trained doctors as well as charlatans practiced these techniques, and water cures were promoted as a substitute for treatment by bleeding and leeching. As late as 1892 some physicians treated typhoid fever by immersing the patient for about 15 minutes in water at a temperature of 65° Fahrenheit.

Cold water treatments became sufficiently popular in the United States for 10,000 copies of the 1847 *Water Cure Manual* to be sold. Among the types of baths described in the book were the wet-towel bath, which required only a quart of water; sponge bath; shower bath; affusion bath (in which the subject stood in a tub while cold water was poured on the neck and shoulders); and a douche bath (wherein a narrow stream of water was aimed at the seated patient from 10 or more feet away).

Among the explanations given for whatever success cold water treatments enjoyed was one that appeared in the *American Journal of the*

Barbara Scherr Trenk is a free-lance writer specializing in health subjects; her articles have appeared in American Medical News, Amtrak Express, *and* Long Island Life.

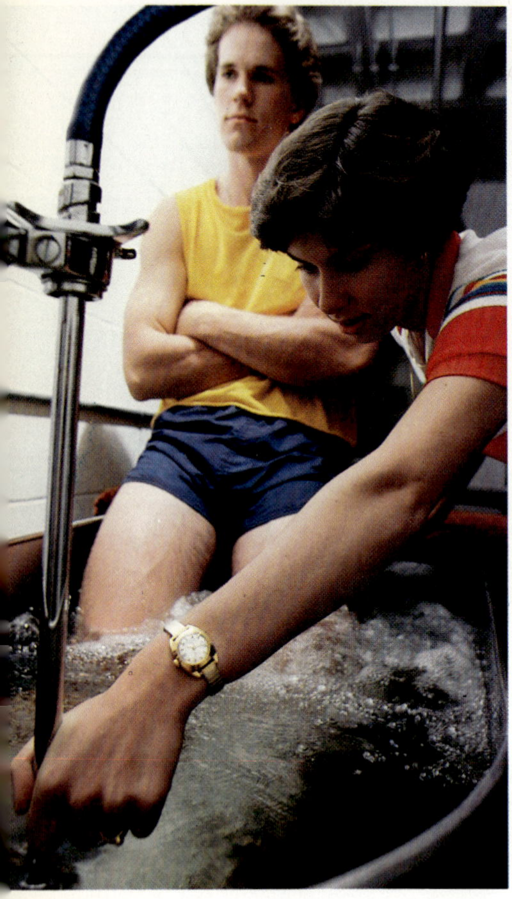

A patient sits in a heated whirlpool bath at a facility for athletic injuries in Massachusetts.

Medical Sciences in 1847: "Cold water applied to the surface promoted the union of morbific matter with oxygen and their expulsion from the body." Medical opinion now suggests it seems far more likely that the cold water simply helped to reduce high fever.

Mineral and Other Special Waters

Most contemporary American medical thought attributes any therapeutic benefits derived from bathing mainly to the water's potential relaxing effects and to its buoyancy, or "lifting" action. But some bath therapy advocates contend that there are definite curative properties in water with specific mineral content. Cures for virtually everything from gastrointestinal discomfort to infertility have been claimed for the waters of various hot springs. More than a few spas have had their reputation enhanced when a well-known person with a health problem showed improvement during or after "taking the waters"—even though the disease remission was probably just a coincidence.

For example, Princess Sophia, the wife of the Austrian Archduke Francis Charles, paid a visit to Bad Ischl in the salt region of Austria when she hadn't conceived a child after several years of marriage. She eventually became pregnant, an accomplishment she attributed to the effects of the spa waters; two years after her visit, in 1830, she gave birth to Francis Joseph, who later became emperor of Austria.

It has been suggested that at some hot springs a process of "electromagnetic ionization" of the water occurs deep in the earth. At such places—one where claims for this theory have been made is Murrieta Hot Springs in Southern California—bathing in the water is said by its advocates to parallel experimental scientific work suggesting that mild electric shocks can accelerate healing of sore areas. There is, however, no generally accepted medical evidence for such claims.

Many spas boast that their waters are mildly radioactive, attributing the waters' professed healing powers to the gas radon. Among the spas that offer this "benefit" are Aix-les-Bains in France, Cucos in Portugal, and Badgastein in the Austrian Alps. However, exposure to radon may carry an increased risk of lung cancer and leukemia. In Poland concern has been expressed in recent years for the health of the staff working in the treatment rooms of spas with radioactive waters, and attempts are being made to limit their exposure.

Adherents of thalassotherapy (from the Greek word *thalassa,* meaning sea) advocate the use of seawater for healing. In New York State, for example, Gurney's Inn at Montauk on Long Island offers baths in water pumped directly from the Atlantic Ocean. On the opposite side of the Atlantic there are 20 thalassotherapy centers along the French coastline, two of them founded by Louison Bobet, a Tour de France world champion bicyclist in the 1950's. Bobet had been seriously injured in an automobile accident and was unable to walk. About a year after the injury he visited a thalassotherapy center at Roscoff in northern Brittany. After five weeks in the program there he began to walk again, an improvement he attributed to "reeducating my muscles with physical therapy and gymnastics, always carried out in seawater." Proponents of thalassotherapy say that bathing in ocean water is beneficial because blood plasma and the sea are similar in chemical composition. In actual fact, however, seawater has a vastly higher salt content than does plasma, and there is no solid scientific evidence of thalassotherapy's effectiveness.

Yet another school of bath treatment advocates are those who make their own additions to the water of a home tub. One English naturopath claims that lime blossom, chamomile, and rosemary will benefit those with "nervous complaint." (Practitioners of naturopathy avoid the use of drugs and emphasize the use of natural agents.) But most medical authorities consider the use of such additives to be without benefit; for sensitive skins some may even be harmful.

Rehabilitation Therapy

Baths are accepted as a tool of physical therapy today, rather than an actual form of treatment, according to Steven Rose, director of the physical therapy department at Washington University in St. Louis. Rose notes that the buoyancy of the water makes motion easier for people with reduced movement ability. Temperature may have an effect as well. Some rehabilitation medicine specialists find baths a useful preliminary before exercise for arthritic patients, whose stiff joints move more easily after immersion in warm water.

Jack Rockwell, a physical therapist and athletic trainer, uses bathing as part of the treatment regimen at the sports medicine clinic he heads in Santa Rosa, Calif. For acute injuries (for example, sprained ankles and hyperextended elbows), he recommends soaking alternately for four

Bathing in sea water is part of the thalassotherapy offered by Gurney's Inn in Montauk, N.Y.; here a therapist, using an underwater hose, massages the patient.

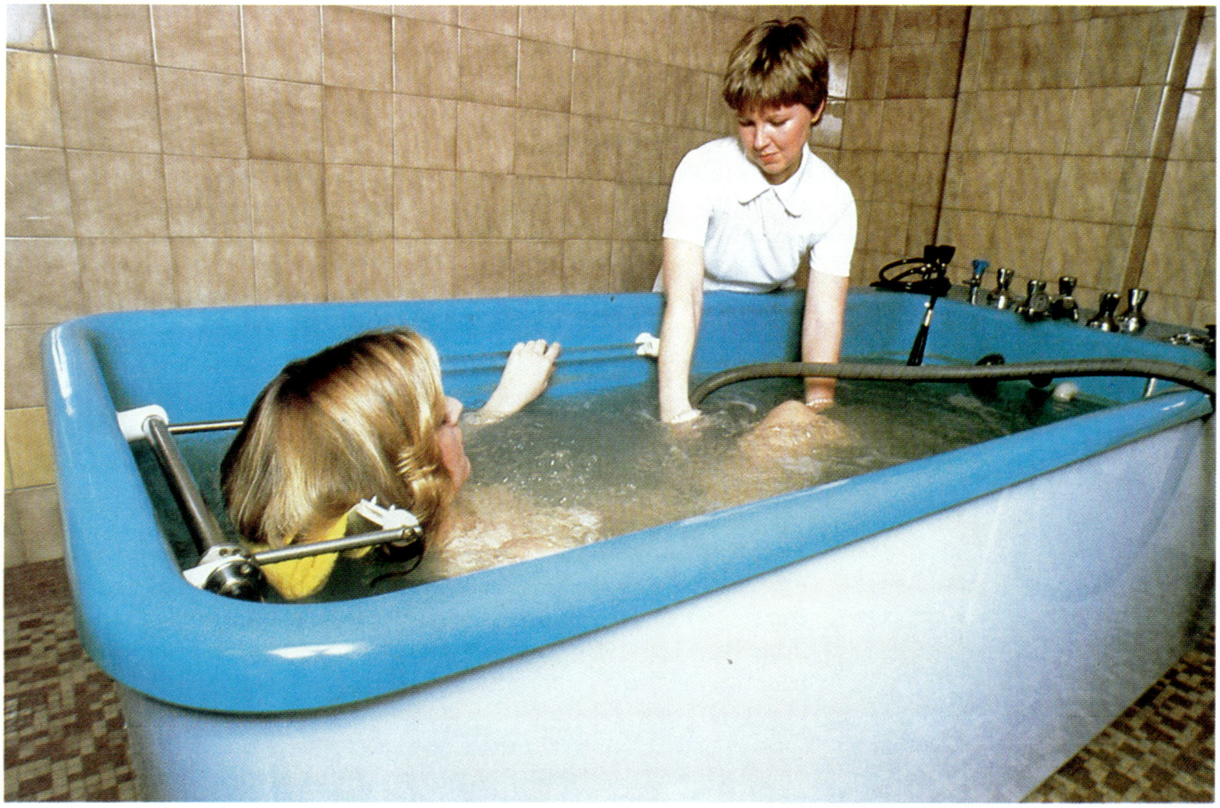

Hydrotherapy is valued by physicians for the relaxing effect of water rather than for any real curative powers it might have.

minutes in a hot water bath and one minute in cold water to promote blood flow to the area of the injury. Patients are urged to begin moving the injured part as it warms up and becomes flexible. Most of Rockwell's patients, many of whom are recovering from surgery, soak in a large Jacuzzi (whirlpool bath), in water heated to 104°F, to improve circulation and reduce muscle spasms. Basically, the only uses of hydrotherapy accepted by most physicians involve water's buoyancy and relaxing effects.

Perhaps the best-known American patient to benefit from the rehabilitative use of baths was Franklin D. Roosevelt, who became a regular visitor at Warm Springs, Ga., because the warm water eased the muscle spasms that resulted from polio. Roosevelt found swimming in the warm water to be so effective that he bought the springs, the hotel, and 1,200 acres of land around them. In 1927 he established the Warm Springs Foundation, now a state facility named the Roosevelt Warm Springs Institute for Rehabilitation.

At one time baths were commonly used to treat burn patients during the process of debriding, or removing the damaged skin; this treatment has become less common since the mid-1970's. Such leading burn care institutions as the Shriners Burn Institute in Boston now use either showers to wash away the affected skin or a process of surgical excision performed under general anesthesia.

Spa Therapy in Europe

Many hot spring spa resorts in Europe are under medical supervision and are covered by national health insurance. In recent years, however, the West German government has begun to restrict expense-paid spa visits to those people who are able to show they are in need of treatment, a measure that is causing financial problems for the spas.

In Czechoslovakia all the spas are part of the national health service, having been nationalized when the Communist Party came to power in 1948. The government takeover of the spas followed the Soviet tradition established by Lenin's 1919 decree that all "localities with curative properties are the property of the people." Today all Soviet and Czechoslovak workers are entitled to free short vacations every year at the spas and to longer stays for treatment of disease or recovery from surgery.

Balneotherapy—a word used mainly in European countries for the treatment of disorders by baths—tends to be taken more seriously by the medical profession in Europe than it is in the United States. Americans who visit spas for bath treatments are far more likely to have learned about them by reading their newspaper's travel section than to have been referred by a physician.

Medical journals in Europe—particularly in such Central and Eastern European countries as East Germany, Czechoslovakia, Poland, and Hungary—report regularly on experience with balneotherapy. Articles on this subject are seldom seen in the American medical literature, no doubt reflecting skepticism among physicians about the usefulness of bathing treatments.

Occasionally, however, articles relating to balneotherapy do appear in American journals. A paper by two Israeli dermatologists published in

1985 in the *Journal of the American Academy of Dermatology* reported on a treatment program at the Dead Sea that included bathing. It was found that 94 out of a group of 110 patients with the skin disease psoriasis showed "complete clearing or excellent improvement" after undergoing the program. The physicians believed the improvement was a result mainly of the naturally filtered ultraviolet rays in the sunlight in this area. (A continuous haze or mist over the sea filters out most of the ultraviolet rays that cause sunburn but lets through longer-wavelength rays of the kind often used in psoriasis treatments.) Bathing in the Dead Sea was considered an additional factor contributing to the patients' improvement; its waters are extraordinarily rich in natural minerals and salts.

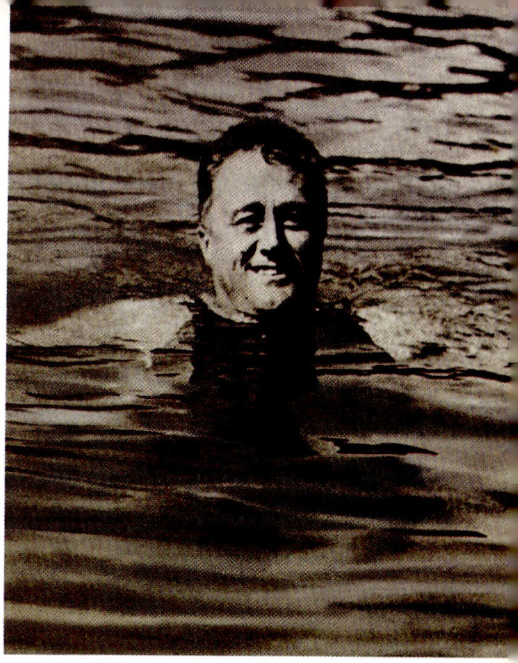

Socializing at Spas

Many mineral spring resorts in the United States have enjoyed a long history of popularity for both their social activities and their supposed therapeutic benefits. But the introduction of modern drugs for numerous diseases, as well as vaccinations that dramatically reduced the incidence of polio, led to a great decline in visits to spas for cures and treatment. Shortly after World War II a million baths a year were taken in the bathhouses at Hot Springs, Ark.; today the number is down to 100,000, and a proposal has been made to turn the empty buildings into art galleries, theaters, restaurants, and fitness centers.

While the popularity of hot spring resorts has declined since the days when Franklin Delano Roosevelt (above) swam regularly to relieve muscle spasms caused by polio, there are still many loyal spa-goers, who enjoy not only the therapeutic but also the social side of spa life.

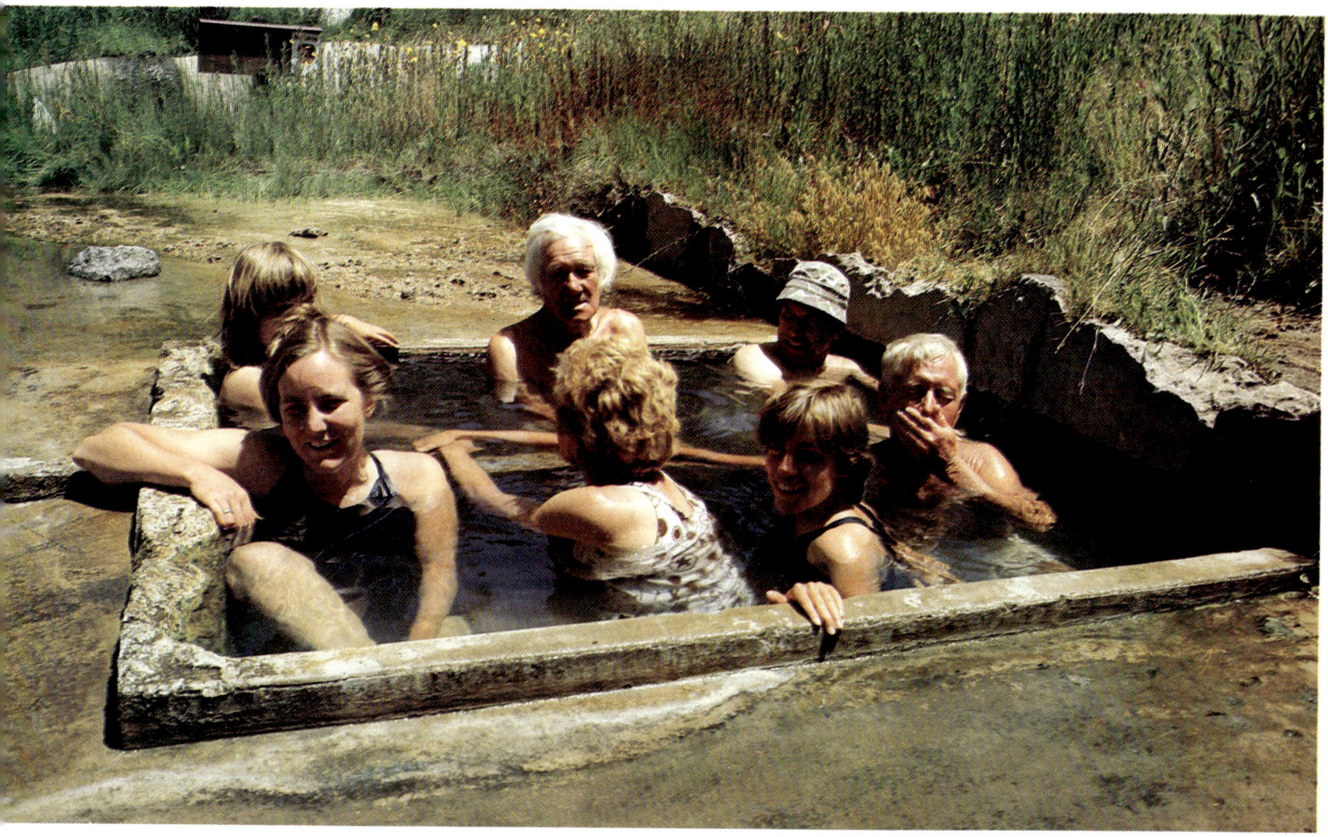

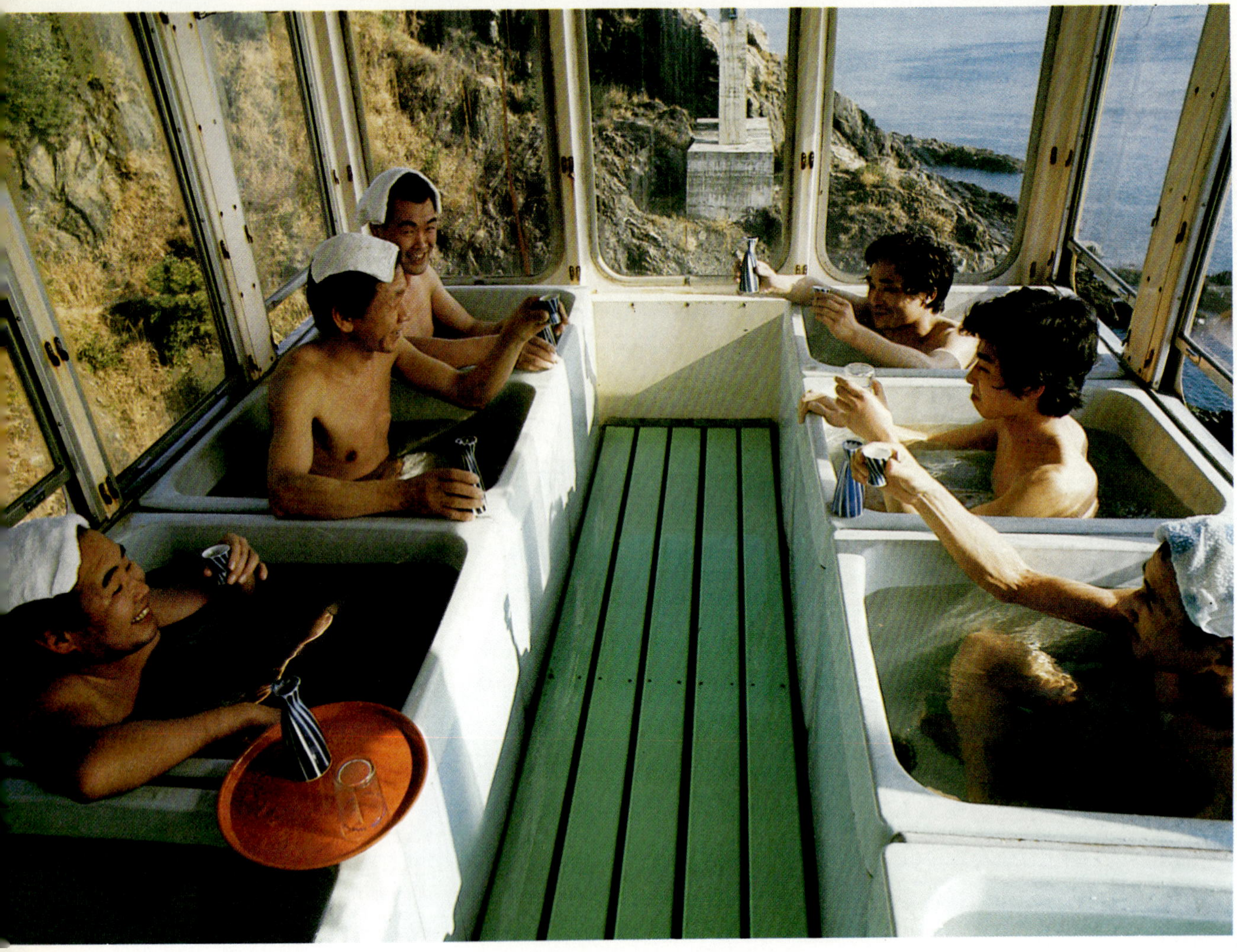

Some hot springs in the United States and Canada have become part of government-operated park systems. Berkeley Springs, W.Va., is a state park; Hot Wells, La., is operated by that state's Department of Health and Human Resources; and what is now Hot Springs National Park, Ark., was first put under federal protection as a "pleasuring ground" in 1832, thus becoming a forerunner of the modern U.S. national park.

The recreational attractions of many U.S. spas make them popular vacation spots. Saratoga Springs, N.Y., is now better known for its racing season and summer ballet and concert festivals than as a place for health treatments. The Greenbrier at White Sulphur Springs, W.Va., is a luxury resort where golf, tennis, and a cooking school are among the options that have been added to what the management characterizes as the "supposedly 'curative' waters" of the springs.

This description of the waters is quite modest when compared to the more extravagant benefits advertised by some spas. For instance, Buckhorn Natural Hot Mineral Wells in Arizona claims that its mineral-laden water helps those suffering from "arthritis, neuritis, neuralgia, gout, anemia, sciatic[a], overweight, underweight, high blood pressure, nicotine poisoning, [and] blood and skin diseases," among other conditions.

Bathing in Japan

The Japanese approach to therapeutic bathing features some interesting variations. At left, guests at the Kisyu Arita Spa toast each other as they soak in steaming tubs during a 15-minute cable car ride (customers usually stay for two rides). At right, beach lounging is given a whole new twist at the Ibusuki Spa on the island of Kyushu; guests are covered with "geothermically" heated sand as they lie on the beach.

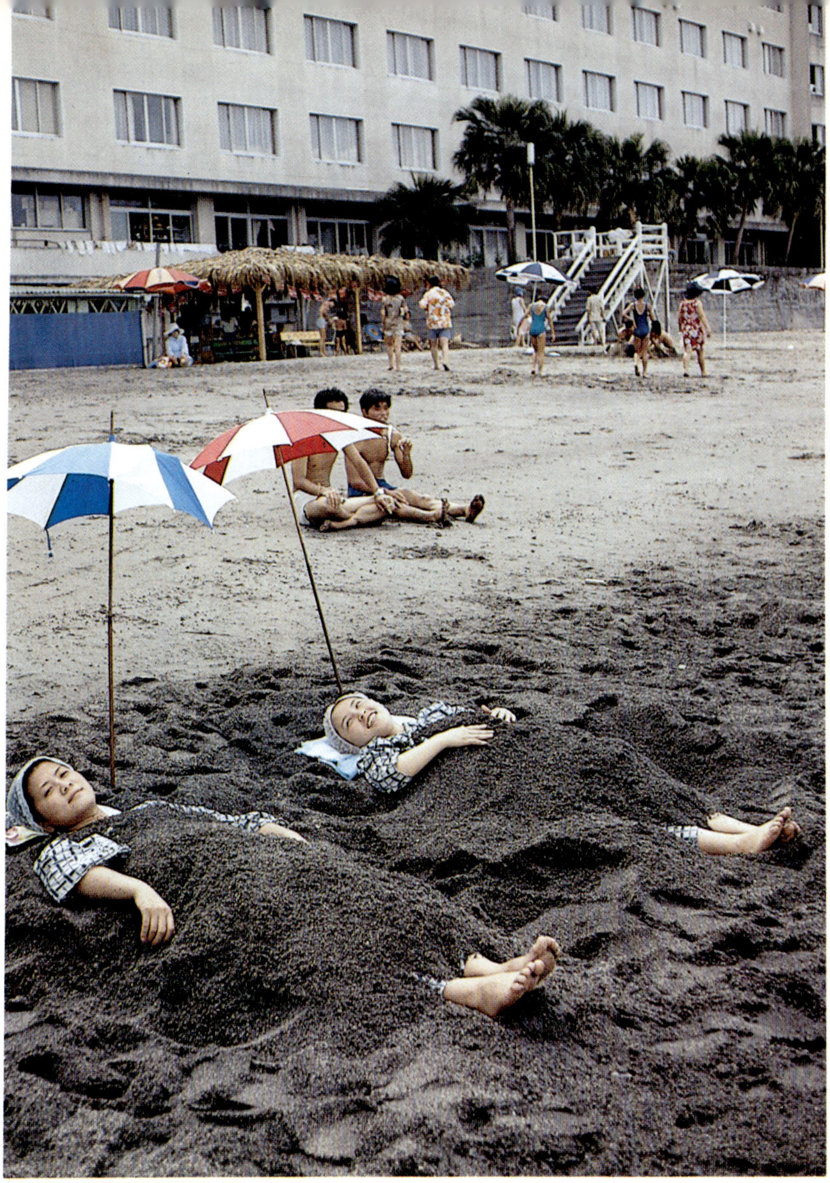

Alaskan natives (Eskimos) are said to have learned to use the Serpentine Hot Springs for healing from the miners who came to the Seward Peninsula area early in the 20th century. Now groups of Eskimos travel by chartered plane to the springs with an Eskimo healer twice a year, for several days of soaking (in a bathhouse) and socializing. Like spa bathers in many other parts of the world, the Eskimos come to the springs seeking relief from arthritis, back and hip pain, skin rashes, and strained muscles.

Gurney's Inn on Long Island claims to offer the closest thing to a U.S. version of the European therapeutic baths, although it does not pretend to be a "medicinal spa." It features 125-gallon tubs containing seawater that has been filtered to remove impurities and heated to body temperature.

Many Americans travel great distances to visit overseas spas, often using the services of package tour operators who specialize in arranging visits to such "health-giving" vacation spots. Sometimes the spas promise to combine the benefits of therapeutic baths and the comfort and luxury of a Sheraton hotel. Europe is not the only destination for this myriad of health seekers. In recent years the thousand or more thermal pools found throughout Japan have also attracted the attention of visiting Americans. In a variation on the mud baths available at some European and North

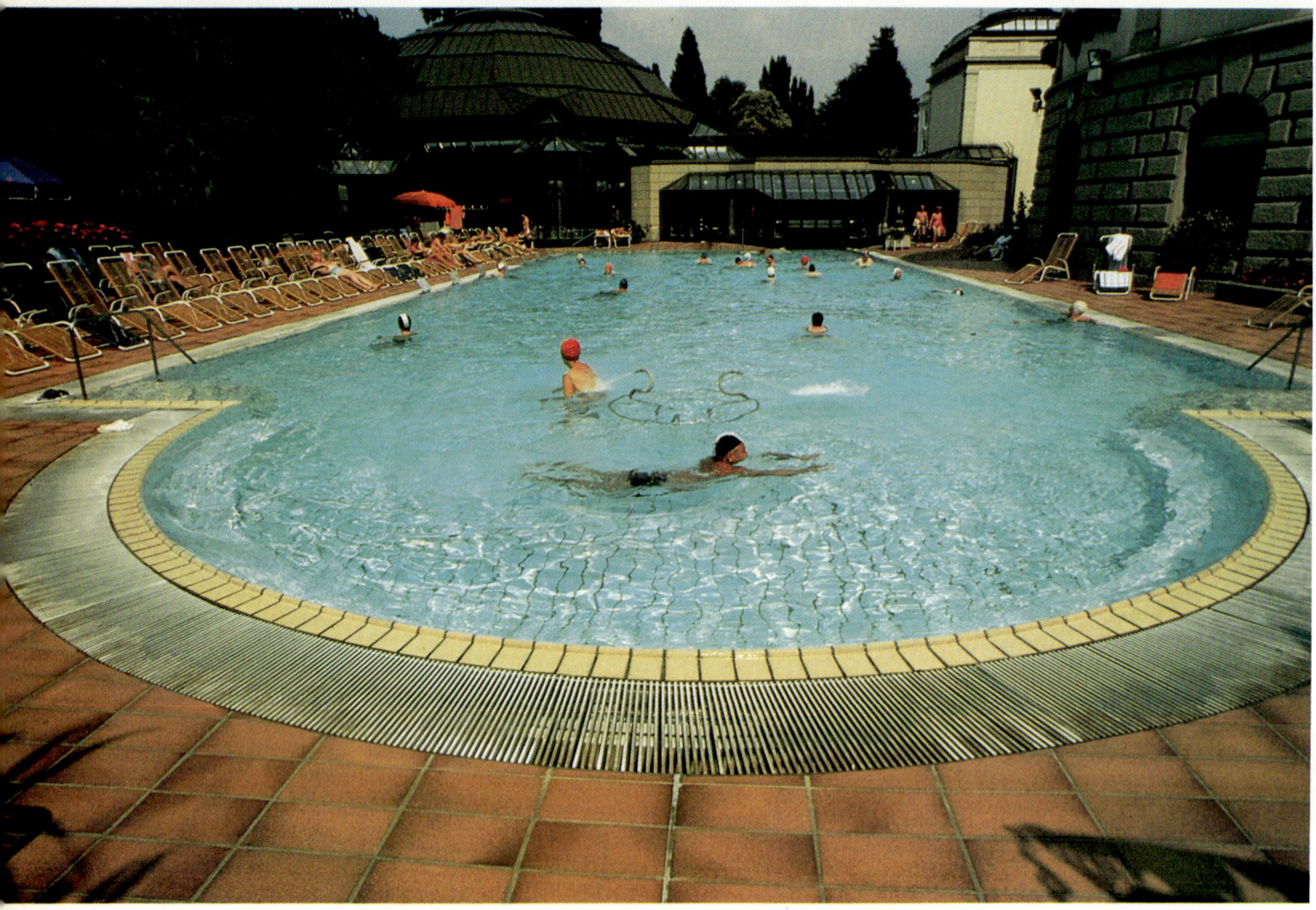

Bath treatments are taken more seriously in Europe than in the United States; some countries include visits to hot spring resorts in their national health insurance coverage. Here guests at a spa in Germany's Black Forest enjoy a night swim.

American spas, visitors to the Ibusuki Spa on Kyushu, Japan's southernmost island, sometimes try sand bathing. The guest lies on the beach and is covered with "geothermically" heated sand.

Hot Tubs and Home Baths

In recent years hot tubs (sometimes called home spas when the tub is made of a material other than wood) have become a popular way to enjoy the relaxing benefits of a hot bath. About a million U.S. homeowners have now installed these wood or acrylic tubs either inside or outside their homes. Many hotels and motels also offer such tubs for the use of guests, and in some areas an individual or a group of people can rent the use of a tub for a half hour or an hour. Even home-size whirlpool baths are available to provide the extra luxury of moving water for those who are willing to pay the price.

There are warning signs near most tubs used by the public, such as those at hotels or health clubs and those available for rental. These signs generally state that a bather should stay in the tub for no more than 15 minutes, and that pregnant women and people with heart disease, diabetes, and high or low blood pressure should not enter the tub without first consulting a physician. This is not idle advice. The temperature of the water in such tubs is usually about 104°F, far warmer than body temperature. As the water warms the skin, the blood circulates faster and the heart must work harder to accommodate this accelerated blood flow. For the same reason, exercise should not be performed in the tubs, since this would further heat the body, nor should a spa user combine hot water relaxation with the use of drugs or alcohol. Many people find a soak in a hot tub to be such a relaxing experience that they can do little but take a nap after leaving the tub. Napping is often recommended by health spas after a warm mineral bath.

For many people, even a simple warm bath at home provides a welcome escape from daily stress.

Hot tub owners who do wish to use their tubs for exercise should lower the temperature to a safe 78° to 80°F, suggests the National Spa and Pool Institute, a trade organization. At that temperature the tub becomes comparable to a heated swimming pool, an environment that many people find ideal for exercise, particularly those who are elderly or obese, suffer from arthritis, or are just not used to exercising. The buoyant effect of the water enables movements that some individuals would otherwise find difficult, and people who find walking on land painful may benefit from simply walking in a swimming pool. Of course, anyone who has a health problem should clear even a moderate program of exercise with a physician. A physical therapist can help to plan an appropriate set of water exercises, or classes may be available through a YMCA or medically oriented exercise club.

For some people, taking a bath—even at home in an ordinary tub—provides an escape from daily stress, almost like a brief vacation. Inflatable bath pillows are a boon to those who like to put their heads back to relax in the tub, and herbs and bath oils can help to turn ordinary bathing into a soothing retreat whether or not the bather has faith in the therapeutic value of specific bath preparations. Some people claim that adding oatmeal to baths helps to ease the discomfort of skin diseases; others say that apple cider vinegar in the bath water combats fatigue. Pine-scented oil is said to soften and stimulate the skin—and for the indoor bather may enhance the illusion of enjoying the benefits of a natural spring in the woods. Most people, however, find plain warm water as effective as water with any additives.

A long, luxurious soak in a warm tub may be just the answer to sore muscles, aching joints, or a stressful day. In fact, a bather may begin to understand why the Romans went to so much trouble to build comfortable bathing facilities at the same time that they were trying to conquer the world, and why there is still such widespread faith in the healing benefits of bathing in hot springs. □

SUGGESTIONS FOR FURTHER READING

BUCHMAN, DIAN DINCIN. *The Complete Book of Water Therapy.* New York, Dutton, 1979.

WECHSBERG, JOSEPH, with additional material by Ruth Brandon. *The Lost World of the Great Spas.* New York, Harper & Row, 1979.

Gambling Can Be An Addiction

Robert Custer, M.D.

"Perhaps passing through so many sensations [while gambling], my soul was not more satisfied, but only irritated by them, and craved still more sensations—and stronger and stronger ones till utterly exhausted."

Fyodor Dostoevsky, *The Gambler*, 1866

The above excerpt from a Dostoevsky novel is a vivid description of the forces that drive the compulsive gambler. It is believed that Dostoevsky wrote *The Gambler* partly because of his urgent need for money to cover his losses in the gambling casinos of Europe. Whatever the motivation, the novelist was able to give an intimate and terrifying description of an individual who, because of his compulsion, has lost control of his own destiny.

Compulsive gambling is a chronic, progressive behavioral disorder in which an individual becomes

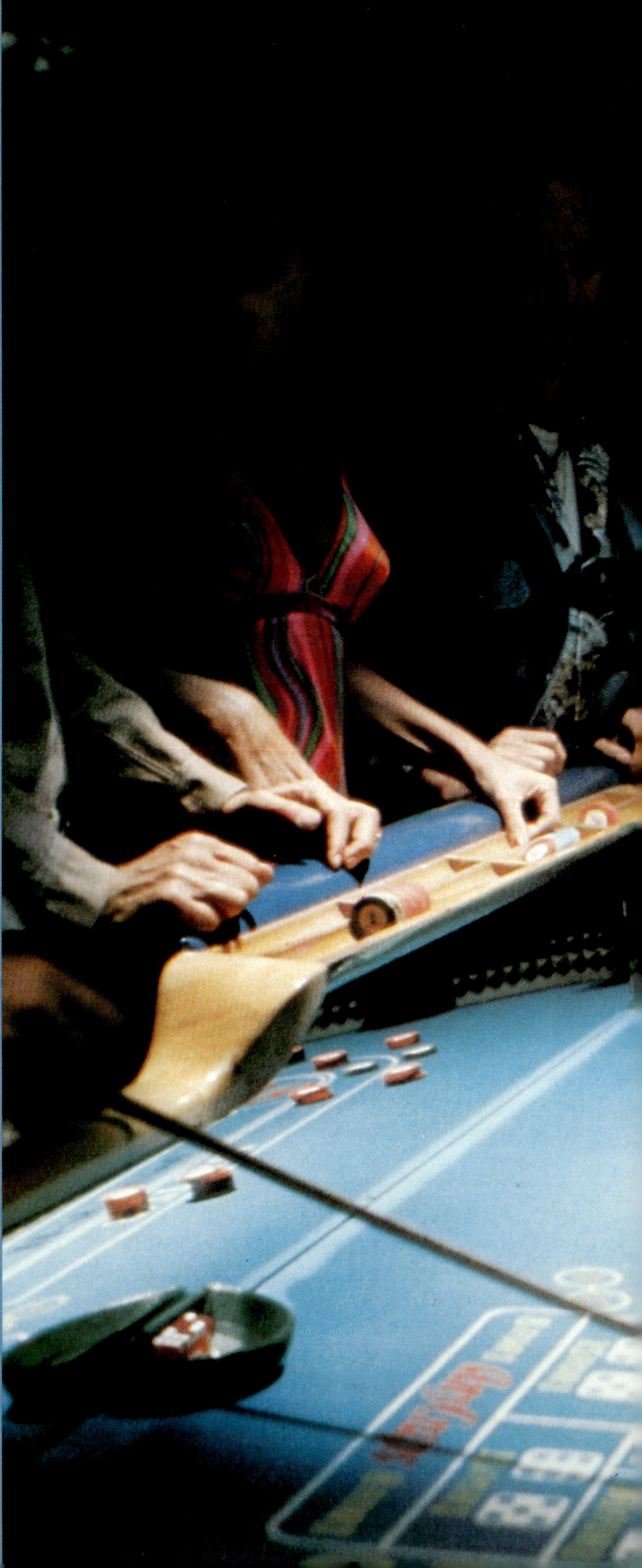

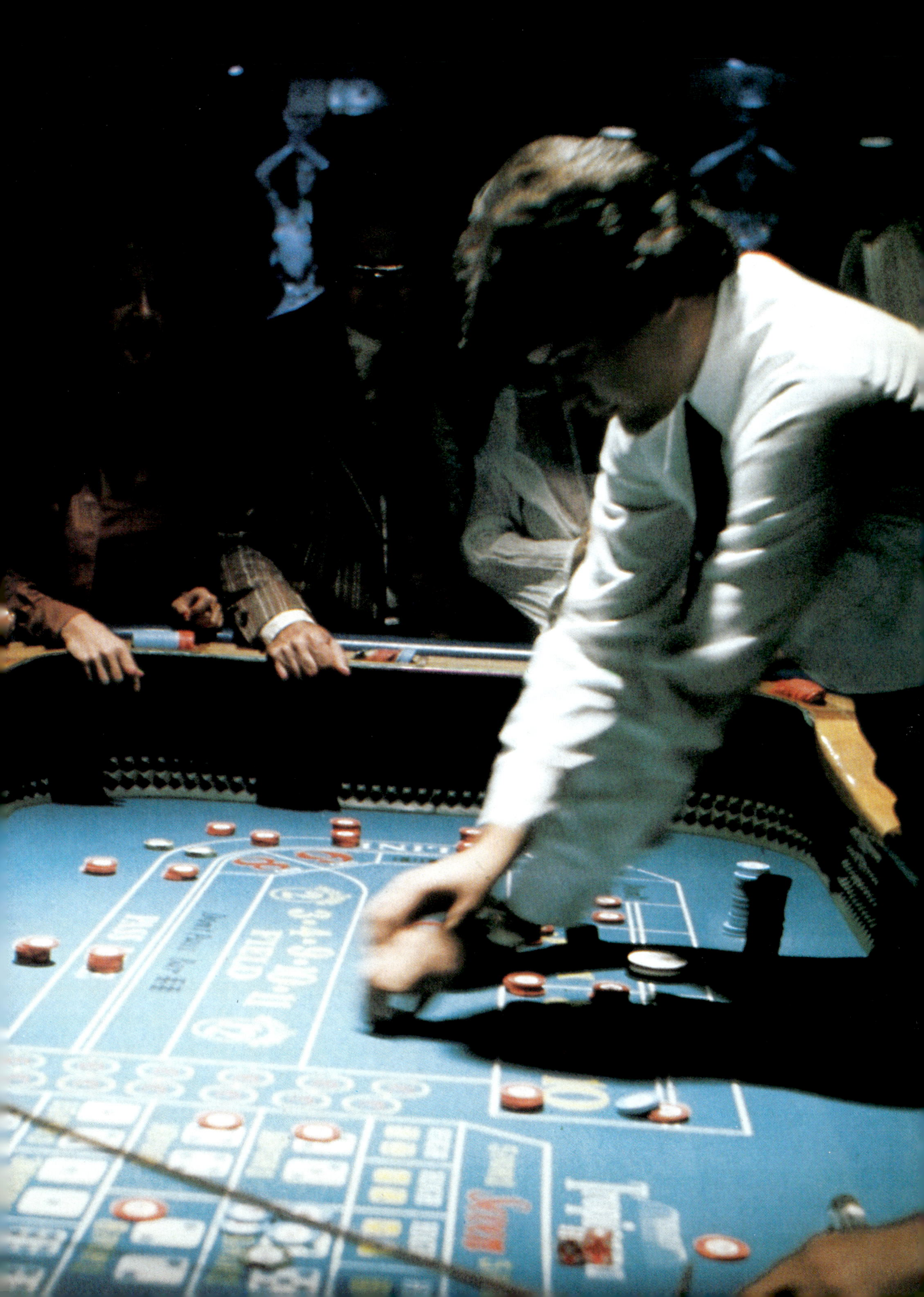
FIELD

dependent on gambling to the exclusion of practically everything else in life. Eventually the compulsive gambler loses all ability to control the gambling impulse and is literally unable to function without gambling. Typically, the final stage of the disorder finds the gambler physically and psychologically exhausted, feeling hopeless and helpless, alienated from everyone. Compulsive gamblers may be welcome nowhere, on the verge of divorce, heavily in debt, and about to be fired or to lose their business. Depression, suicidal thoughts, and suicide attempts are common. However, the compelling urge to gamble is still there.

Most noncompulsive gamblers do not realize that the compulsive gambler is unable to curb this urge, despite the consequences. The change from innocent betting to the obsessive, irresistible need to gamble occurs gradually, as gambling begins to take precedence over the needs of family and business, personal health and well-being, and even personal safety. Characteristically, the compulsive gambler had a "big win" or an early string of wins that led to an irrational and euphoric illusion of invincibility and of limitless, never-ending good fortune. The inevitable losses that follow engender a desperate need to keep on gambling to recoup the losses (known as chasing) and restore the illusions. Frantic efforts will be made to beg, borrow, or steal money to keep on gambling. With mounting losses, the frequency of gambling and the amounts involved increase. The inevitable downward spiral of gambling losses leads to social, economic, emotional, and physical collapse.

Types of Gamblers

There are approximately 130 million gamblers in the United States and Canada. They can be broken down into six distinct, if somewhat overlapping, groups: the professional gambler, the criminal gambler, three types of social gamblers, and the compulsive gambler.

The professional gambler, who makes a living by gambling, is the rarest type. The professional makes a very serious study of a particular form of gambling, manages money carefully, and bets only when the odds are favorable. Patient, knowledgeable, and unemotional, the professional approaches gambling not as fun but as work.

The criminal gambler's career is getting money by illegal means: running a numbers game or bookmaking on sporting events. This activity is just one phase of an illegal life-style. When criminal gamblers engage in legitimate gambling, they often steal money in order to pursue the activity.

Social gamblers constitute the vast majority of gamblers. There are three types of social gamblers, again with some overlap: the casual gambler, the serious gambler, and the escape gambler.

The casual social gambler might occasionally play cards with friends and wager on special sporting events like the Super Bowl. Casual gamblers occasionally purchase a few lottery tickets, bet on the office football pool, or go to the races. If you were to take gambling out of their lives, they could easily fill the void with other pursuits.

Robert Custer, a psychiatrist with the U.S. Veterans Administration, is president of the National Foundation for the Study and Treatment of Pathological Gambling.

HOW HABIT-FORMING IS GAMBLING?

Not all gambling games are alike; the more of the following characteristics a game has, the more likely it is to be addictive:

- an element of skill, real or perceived
- a short interval between wager and payoff
- an opportunity to increase the amount of money that is bet
- a high frequency of wins
- social appropriateness and acceptability
- easy availability
- a high level of excitement

WHAT GAMES FIT THE BILL?

Highly Addictive

Baccarat
Blackjack (21)
Betting on sporting events
Craps
Horse racing (including Offtrack betting)
Poker
Roulette
Stock options and commodities futures

Moderately Addictive

Dog racing
Gin rummy
Instant lottery
Poker machines

Mildly Addictive

Bingo
Bridge
Jai alai
Keno
Lotto
Slot machines
Weekly lottery

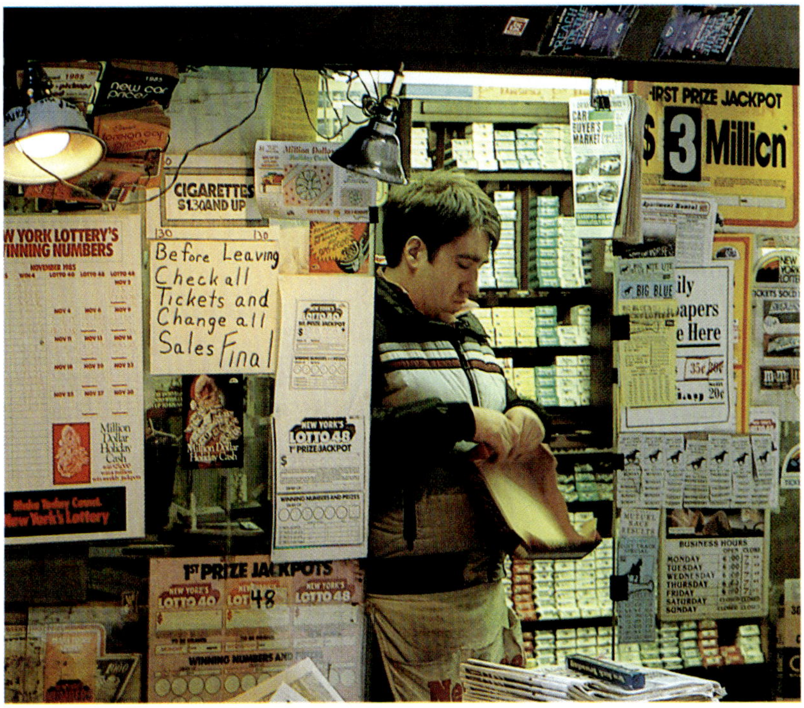

The number of compulsive gamblers is directly related to the availability of gambling—such as legal lotteries.

In contrast, the serious social gambler plays regularly, enjoys gambling, and puts much time and energy into improving gambling skills. However, such gamblers remain attentive to family, vocational, and social needs, which remain inportant to them. Gambling is a part of their lives, but it is only an avocation. Such people are chronic gamblers, but the behavior does not progress—that is, it does not take up more and more time or cost more and more money over the years.

Escape social gamblers gamble to avoid tension, frustration, anger, or worry. They gamble erratically, impulsively, and emotionally, with no consistent pattern. Such gambling may occur once every few months or not at all for years. The amount lost is usually easily tolerated and is expected.

Social gamblers can become compulsive gamblers, but only a small fraction of them are likely to do so.

How Many Are Compulsive?

The only currently available source of authoritative U.S. statistics on compulsive gambling is *Gambling in America,* the final report of the Commission on the Review of the National Policy Toward Gambling, a congressionally mandated committee established by the Organized Crime Control Act of 1970. *Gambling in America,* published in 1976, reported that there were an estimated 1.1 million compulsive gamblers in the United States, or less than 1 percent of the adult population. The report estimated that there were an additional 3.1 million potential compulsive gamblers. Medical evidence suggests that the percentage of the

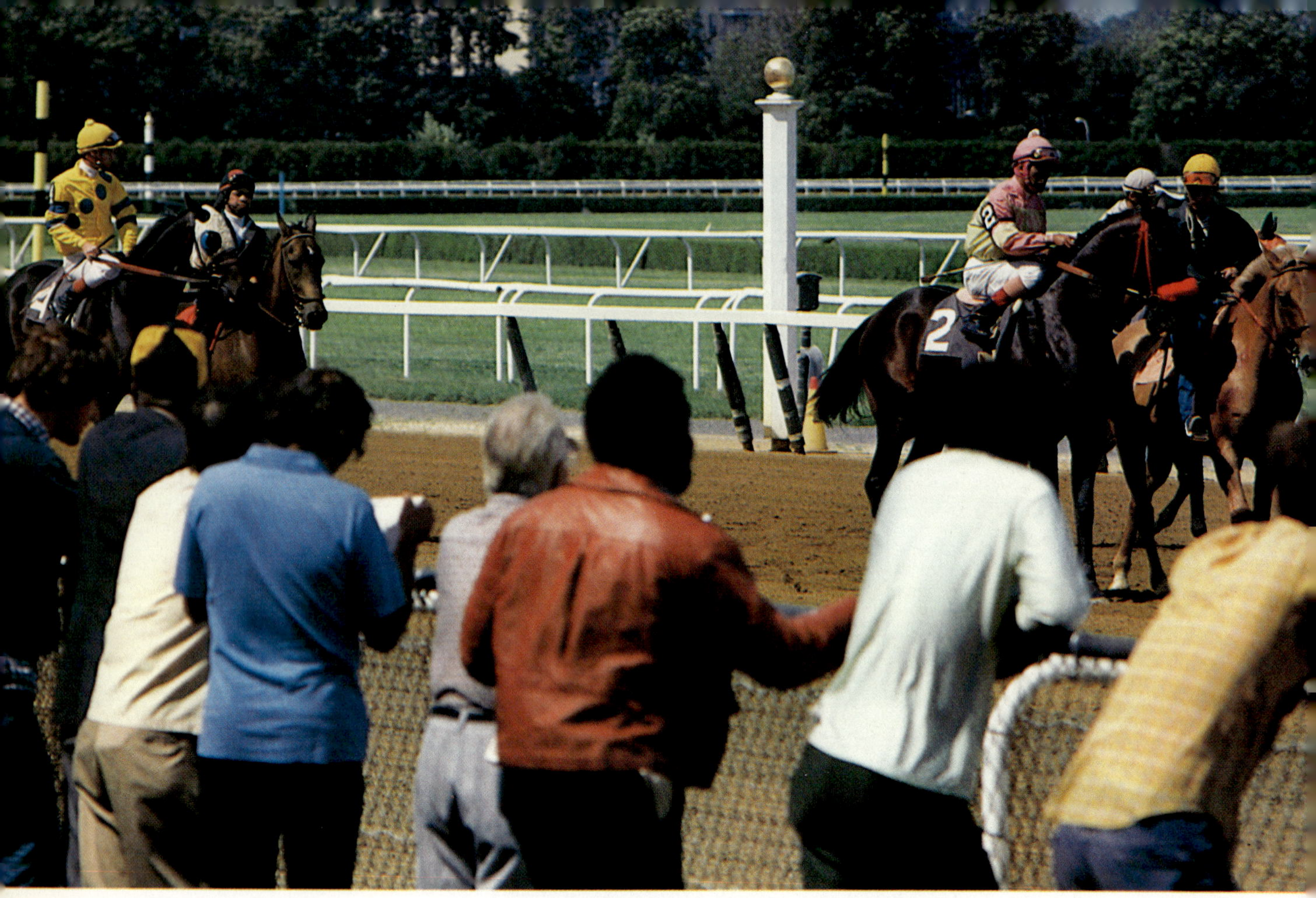

population afflicted with compulsive gambling is comparable in other countries, especially when the availability of legalized gambling is equivalent to that in the United States. About four out of five compulsive gamblers currently seeking treatment are men, but the proportion of women appears to be rising.

The American Psychiatric Association first listed pathological (compulsive) gambling as an illness in the third edition of its *Diagnostic and Statistical Manual of Mental Disorders,* published in 1980. The disorder is recognized internationally by virtue of its inclusion in the ninth revision of the World Health Organization's *International Classification of Diseases,* adopted in 1975.

As numerous as compulsive gamblers are, their number promises to grow much larger—an inevitable fallout of the expansion of legalized gambling. *Gambling in America* pointed out that there was a direct correlation between the availability of gambling and the incidence of compulsive gambling. As gambling is legalized in more places and therefore gains social respectability, more people can be expected to engage in gambling, and a certain proportion of those growing numbers will fall into the trap of compulsive gambling. Twenty years ago only a handful of places in North America permitted gambling of any kind. Today, with the authorization of lotteries, pari-mutuel betting, and the like, legal gambling of various sorts flourishes in most U.S. states and Canadian provinces.

Unfortunately, public attitudes and understanding of compulsive gambling are inadequate for what is sure to be a growing problem. Few

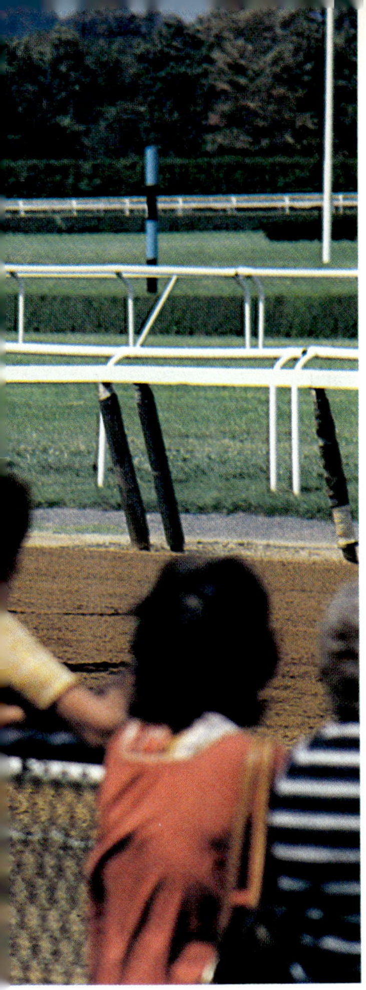

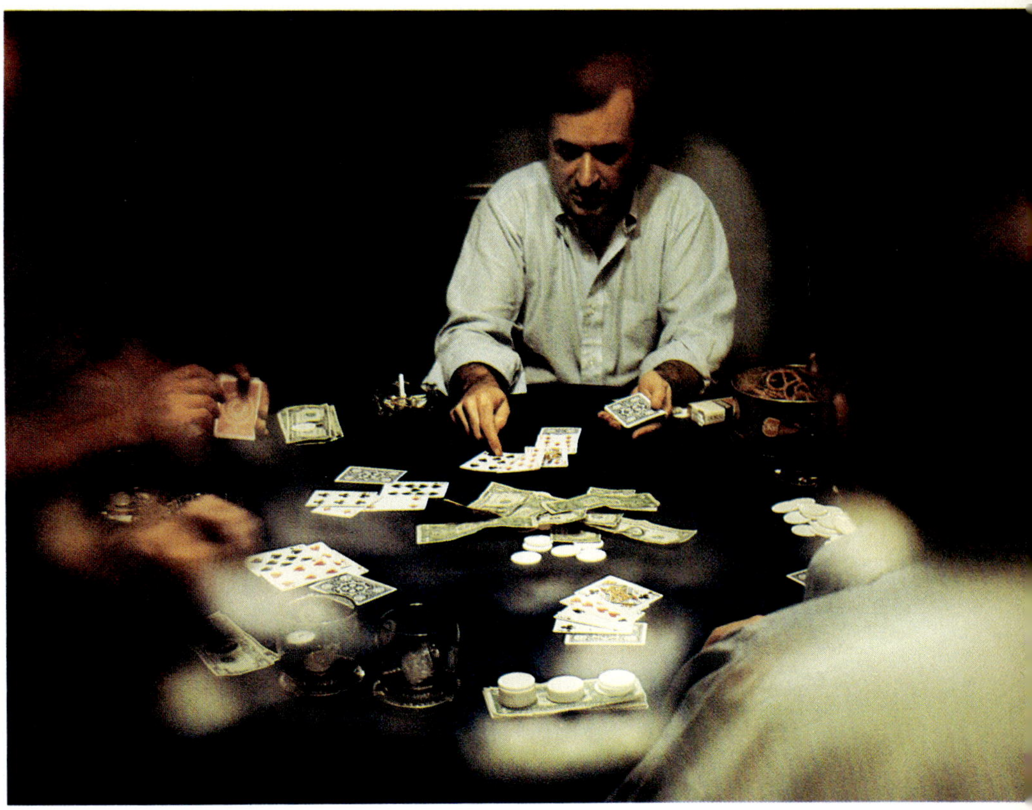

Leading to Addiction

Certain types of gambling are much more addictive than others. Among the games most likely to become a habit—and a problem—are horse racing and poker (above). Investing in stock options and commodities futures is another highly addictive form of gambling; right, the Chicago Board of Trade.

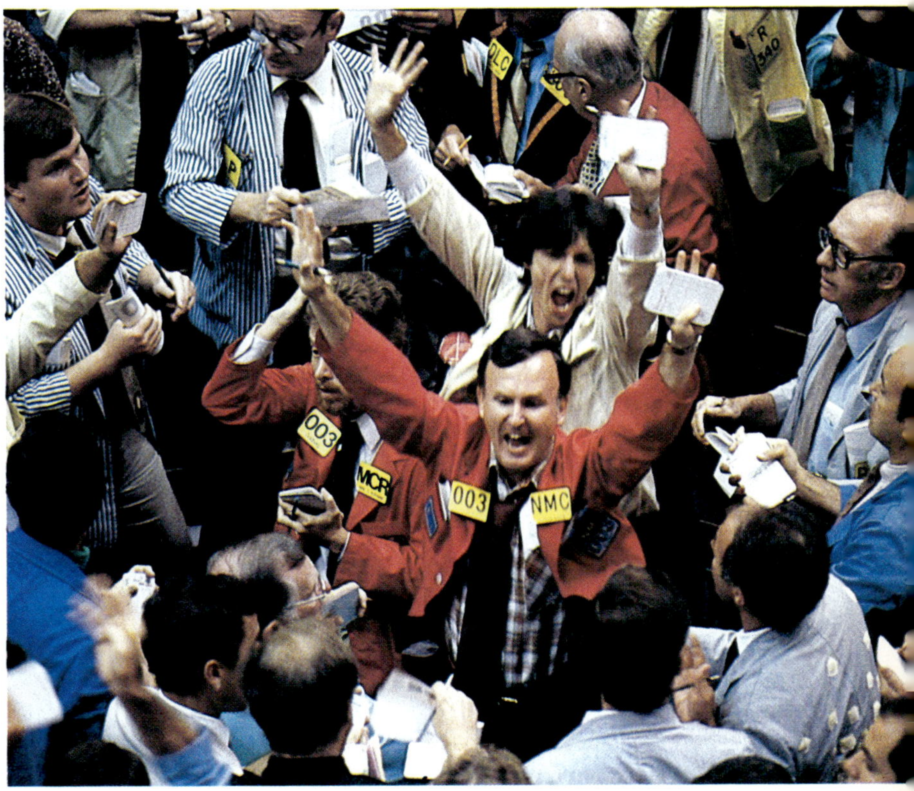

people understand that pathological gamblers are not criminals without decency or honor. In most cases, compulsive gamblers were once participants in community activities and loving spouses and parents. It is their illness that drives them to destitution, to neglect of family, perhaps to crime, and even to suicide.

Two Case Histories

Obsessive gamblers have definite personality characteristics.

A typical case history is that of a 48-year-old attorney who was arrested for embezzling money from his firm. He had every intention of paying it back—after making a killing on the horses. The lawyer had been betting on the races for many years and had come close to arrest for embezzlement in the past, but his father had provided him with funds to make restitution. After a serious losing streak, he began borrowing money from illegal sources and was driven to defraud his firm again because of frightening threats from loan sharks. His father refused to help him again, and the lawyer was forced to resign from his firm and submit to arrest. The loss of his professional status was a tremendous blow. He had always been a hardworking lawyer, although his performance had been slipping recently because of the time spent gambling. Having borrowed money

Quarterback Art Schlichter was treated for compulsive gambling.

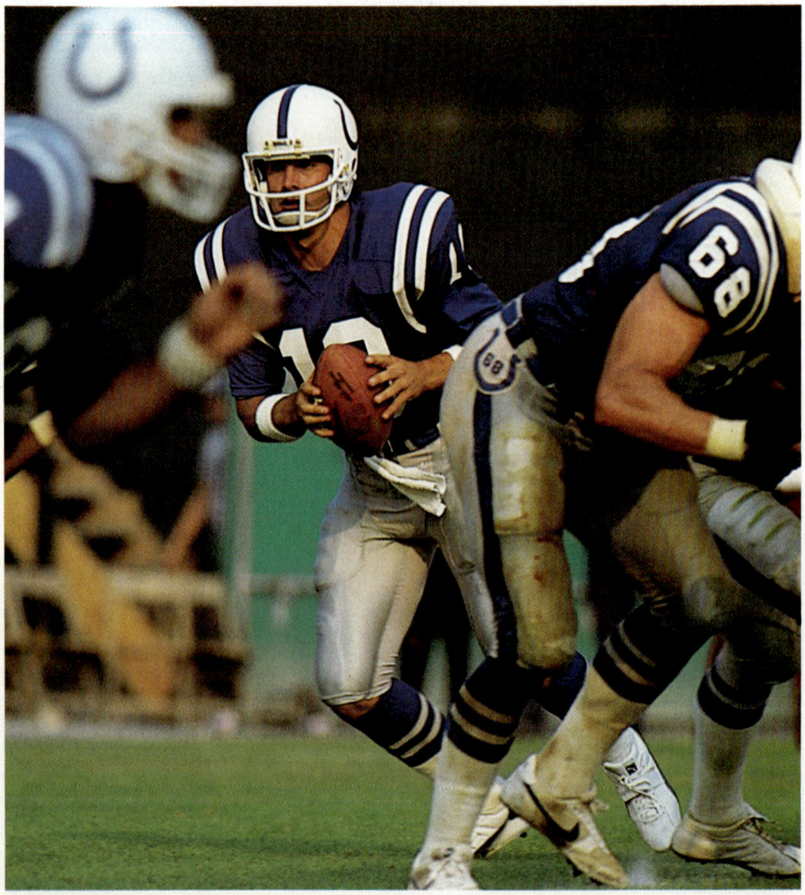

from his wife and friends, he at last had to admit his problem to them. His wife left him and moved in with her parents.

One recent compulsive gambling case many people have heard of is that of former Indianapolis Colts quarterback Art Schlichter, who was suspended from the National Football League for a year after losing $1 million or more on gambling. He had been a habitué of the racetrack during his college days and had borrowed money from his father to pay his gambling debts. After Schlichter signed a $990,000 contract with the Colts, his losses became enormous. He ran through his starting bonus and his first year's salary and then sank nearly $400,000 into debt. Finally, he went to the FBI to complain about harassment from the people who had loaned him money illegally. (They threatened to break his passing arm.) He also admitted his problem to NFL Commissioner Pete Rozelle, who suspended him. After treatment, Schlichter was reinstated by the league and for a time returned to the Colts.

Development of the Problem

There is a certain personality profile that characterizes compulsive gamblers before they ever place a bet. They tend to be of superior intelligence and are strongly competitive and industrious, with a high energy level. They often have outstanding athletic ability and good scholastic records. They also thrive on challenges and are attracted to situations that are highly stimulating. They do not tolerate boredom well, and tasks they find dull are often avoided or left incomplete.

There are three stages in the evolution of the compulsive gambler. The specific pattern and the length of time involved vary greatly for different people, but the elements are essentially similar.

The early phase. The first phase in compulsive gambling is characterized by winning. A winning streak or a single, very large win seems to be necessary for compulsion to develop. For example, a 57-year-old widow goes to the dog races for the first time and wins $740 on her first bet, or a 17-year-old high school student goes to the racetrack and wins a $500 daily double on his first $2 wager. Fortunately—or unfortunately—the luck continues. Where the average person would simply be delighted with such beginner's luck, future compulsive gamblers begin to believe that they are exceptionally lucky and are endowed with special capabilities or intuition. A tremendous win strongly reinforces this perception. The big win establishes the conviction that if such a killing can happen once, it can happen again, and the next time it could be even larger.

As winnings continue, the gambler comes to feel invincible, gifted, blessed with extraordinary judgment and wisdom. This attitude is understandable but illogical, ignoring the reality that the winning streak is a matter of pure chance. Each win tends to reinforce this irrational perception. Ego and self-esteem become bound up with success at gambling. Euphoric and ill-prepared for the losses to come, the gambler gets a psychological kick from winning that comes to exceed the rewards of family and work.

The losing phase. The laws of chance are inexorable, and the winning streak inevitably ends. For the now confident and optimistic compulsive

Recognizing the Compulsive Gambler

The American Psychiatric Association's *Diagnostic and Statistical Manual of Mental Disorders*, third edition, defines pathological gambling as follows:

First, the compulsive gambler is unable to resist the urge to gamble; this inability is chronic and worsens over time.

Second, the compulsive gambler's actions cause damage or disruption to the gambler's personal or professional life in at least three of the following ways: (1) the gambler has been arrested for forgery, fraud, embezzlement, or tax evasion committed to obtain funds for gambling; (2) debts or other financial responsibilities have not been met; (3) family or marital relationships have been disrupted by gambling; (4) money has been borrowed from loan sharks; (5) the gambler cannot account for money that has been lost; if winnings are claimed, the gambler cannot produce evidence of them; (6) absenteeism brought on by gambling has led to loss of the gambler's job or business; (7) the gambler has required assistance from others in a desperate financial situation.

Psychopaths and sociopaths often engage in similar behavior. True compulsive gamblers are unlike them in that they usually have a good work record until it is disrupted by gambling and rarely commit crimes when they have enough money to gamble.

gambler, however, losing no longer represents an expected phenomenon in the world of chance; it is a painful threat to ego, pride, and confidence. There is an urgent need to recoup the losses. Unless this is done, there is a tremendous threat to the image the gambler is trying to project and a personal wound that must be healed. Losing is intolerable. The gambler begins to chase, that is, to bet more in order to recover the losses. Wise gamblers consider this escalation to be a cardinal sin in gambling, but the compulsive gambler, certain that the next bet will be successful, ignores such precautions.

The desperation phase. The desperation phase is brief, intense, irrational, and often tragic. Caution and calm judgment are thrown to the winds. The passion for gambling becomes all-consuming, and family, friends, and work are disregarded. The gambler may begin to borrow from loan sharks or embezzle money. In some cases astonishing sums are involved—one Toronto assistant bank manager went through more than Can$10 million of his employer's money, most of it dropped at Las Vegas gaming tables, before being caught and eventually sentenced to prison. As debts mount and desperation increases, suicide becomes a real possibility. Treatment is imperative—but how?

When the passion for gambling becomes all-consuming, family, friends, and work are disregarded.

Getting Treatment

The ultimate aim of treatment, regardless of its exact nature, is simple: getting the gambler to stop gambling completely. For many people, this can be achieved only with the aid of a trained therapist; for other individuals, a self-help group like Gamblers Anonymous (GA) may provide all the support needed. The two types of treatment are not mutually exclusive. Gamblers getting professional help can also benefit tremendously from GA.

It is difficult for compulsive gamblers to accept their need for help and take action to obtain it. Only about half of those who make an appointment to begin treatment with a therapist or to attend a GA session will appear at the scheduled time. However, almost 90 percent will start treatment or show up at GA within a year of their first planned session. This phenomenon is probably a result of the gambler's ambivalence about and even denial of the need for treatment.

Once treatment with a mental health professional begins, it is directed at overcoming the problems, financial and personal, that gambling has created as well as at controlling the urge to gamble. Since by this point compulsive gamblers have consciously begun to realize that gambling has reduced them to a state of unbelievable indebtedness, it is often unnecessary to tell them that they must discontinue gambling; they already know. The trouble is that they literally do not know how to stop. The connection between the impulse to gamble and the act of gambling is so strong and well-established that the gambler is unable to break it. Treatment to interrupt the process by which impulse becomes action must be intense, prompt, and specific.

Daily therapy sessions are often necessary at first, followed by less frequent sessions for about two years. It is important that an understanding and empathetic posture be established by the therapist. If the therapist is critical, punitive, or judgmental, the patient will not open

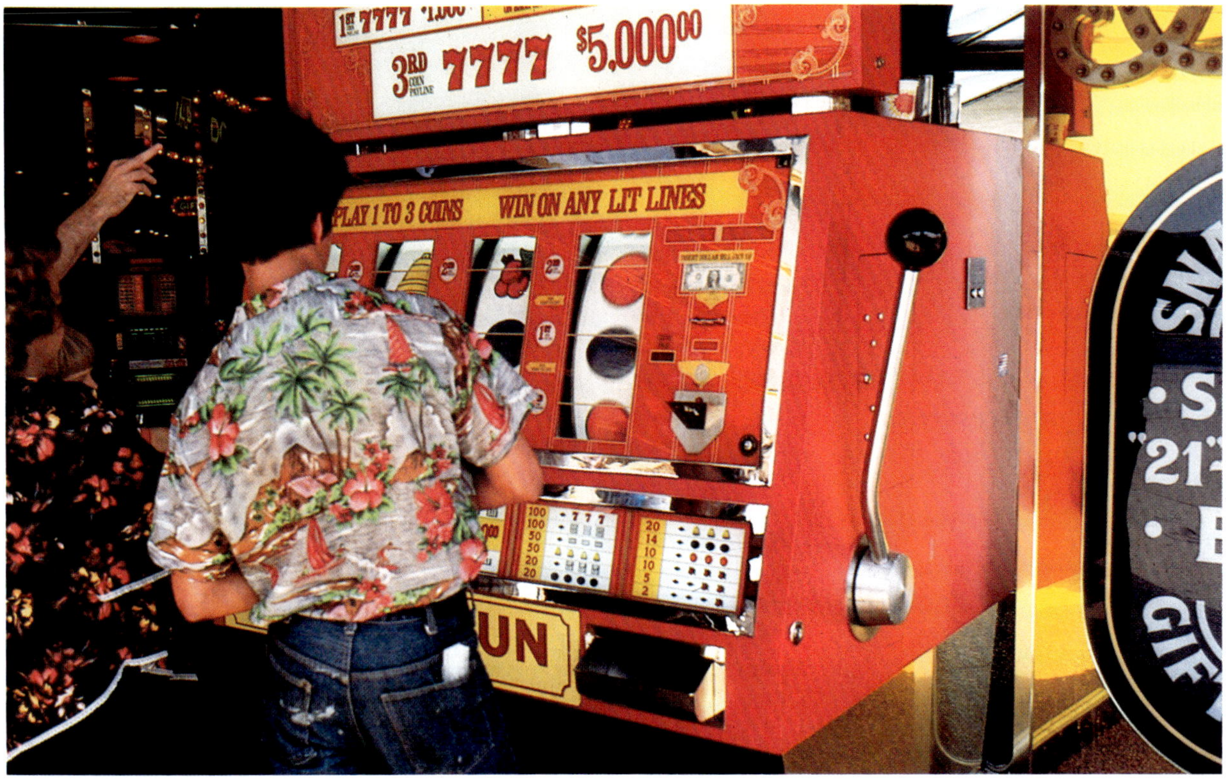

In a gambling resort like Las Vegas, playing slot machines is cheap, popular, and available 24 hours a day.

up and may leave treatment quickly. The therapist must also be tenacious and willing to try new and creative approaches for this difficult and complex disorder.

The gambler must be forced to stop behaving irresponsibly and avoiding the family, vocational, financial, and legal problems that have developed. But patience and planning are not strengths of the compulsive gambler, and the huge burden of problems plus the loss of gambling as an escape may bring on an overwhelming feeling of hopelessness. Adding to the burden is a period of withdrawal analogous to that experienced by drug addicts and alcoholics.

In order to break out of this trap, the patient must have some rapidly attainable goals. Patient and therapist need to establish and agree on a concrete treatment plan for the short and medium term. Specific, high-priority goals tend to reduce hopelessness and stress. Attainable short-term goals, like vowing not to bet on anything for one day, are more easily adhered to than such sweeping resolutions as never gambling again. Major objectives at the start of the treatment program include getting the gambler back to work and setting up a repayment plan for gambling debts.

During the initial stage of treatment, the risk of suicide must be evaluated by the therapist. This is usually done by direct questioning about past suicidal behavior, present feelings, and suicidal thoughts. Inpatient treatment may be necessary for suicidal patients, particularly if the patient has no family to provide support or family relations have been broken off. The compulsive gambler who is isolated and cannot see any way out of serious predicaments is at high risk.

Some compulsive gamblers who are not suicidal may be on the verge of committing a crime in order to resolve their financial problems. This possibility, too, needs to be explored by the therapist.

During periods of tension that are inevitable during the recovery process, the patient is more vulnerable to the temptation to gamble. The therapist must be alert to signs of tension in order to intervene and try to lower the pressure. A slip—a brief return to gambling—should not be considered a calamity. A prompt return to the treatment plan is necessary and can be effective.

Gamblers may resort to crime to cover their losses.

Reassurance by the therapist is at first invariably viewed with skepticism by the compulsive gambler. But when patients attend sessions of Gamblers Anonymous—which they may continue to do for the rest of their lives—they are provided with actual examples of people who had the same problems but proceeded to successful recovery through abstinence. For some gamblers, in fact, a referral to GA is sufficient treatment—they can recover with the help of their fellow compulsive gamblers and do not need a mental health professional. (Those gamblers with underlying psychiatric or physical disorders should seek the help of a mental health professional and physician.)

With proper, intensive treatment, including regular participation in GA (even after treatment with a therapist ends), a remarkably high proportion of compulsive gamblers recover—from 50 to 80 percent.

The Gambler's Family

The gambler's family members play a crucial role in assisting the compulsive gambler to recover. It should be remembered as well that the family, not just the gambler, suffers, and their own problems must be treated.

When family members discover the gambler's lies and deceit, there is usually intense alienation. Children and spouse lose faith and trust, no longer believing anything the gambler tells them. What is more, the family is often destitute and dependent on relatives for financial support.

The combination of financial ruin and the breakdown of marital trust can have a devastating impact on the gambler's spouse. Remaining feelings of loyalty and duty conflict with anger and resentment. Depression is common, and many marriages break up under the pressure.

The effects of this kind of stress on the children are also severe. Good students lose ground in schoolwork. Children develop behavior problems like truancy, and some take to alcohol or drugs or begin gambling themselves. Small children may regress to night terrors, bed-wetting, and sleepwalking.

It is important for families of compulsive gamblers to understand that they are witnessing symptoms of a sickness, not evidence of a basically vicious and insensitive personality. The family members should make clear—despite all the gambler's denials—that they know about the gambling problem. Any requests for money should be flatly refused, and if creditors call, family members should not assume responsibility for the gambler's debts. A referral to GA or psychiatric help, not money, is the kind of assistance needed. The gambler's spouse should make every effort to get whatever assets possible out of the gambler's control.

Compulsive gamblers are notorious for rationalizing and projecting blame onto their spouses and other family members. The family must resist guilt feelings. Assistance is available for spouses and parents from a self-help organization called Gam-Anon. Other victims in the same situation will help family members work out their problems. Older children can get help from Gam-A-Teen, the mutual help organization for children of compulsive gamblers.

Gamblers Anonymous

Gamblers Anonymous is the single most effective means of treatment for the compulsive gambler. It is a voluntary fellowship of compulsive gamblers gathered for the sole purpose of helping themselves and each other to stop gambling. There is one condition for membership in GA: being a compulsive gambler who wants to stop gambling. There is one absolute principle: referral to GA may come from anyone, but help is given only at the request of a compulsive gambler. When help is requested, it is given unstintingly.

Gamblers Anonymous has proved to be the single most effective means of treatment for compulsive gamblers.

GA is effective because its members are familiar with the types of denial and rationalization compulsive gamblers engage in and will refuse to accept them. GA members have personal experience of the serious implications of gambling and know how to demand honesty and responsibility. They are experienced at identifying and correcting the kinds of character problems that lead to compulsive gambling; at the same time they provide affection, personal concern, and support to those in a plight all of them have shared. Having faced the problem themselves, they can also help the compulsive gambler develop substitutes for the void left by the cessation of gambling. □

SOURCES OF FURTHER INFORMATION

Gam-Anon, P.O. Box 967, Radio City Station, New York, N.Y. 10101. Provides information on Canadian and U.S. chapters and on Gam-A-Teen.

Gamblers Anonymous National Service Office, P.O. Box 17173, Los Angeles, Calif. 90017. Covers Canada and United States.

National Council on Compulsive Gambling, 444 West 56th Street, Room 3207S, New York, N.Y. 10019.

National Foundation for the Study and Treatment of Pathological Gambling, 217 East Preston Street, Baltimore, Md. 21202.

SUGGESTIONS FOR FURTHER READING

COMMISSION ON THE REVIEW OF THE NATIONAL POLICY TOWARD GAMBLING. *Gambling in America.* Washington, D.C., U.S. Government Printing Office, 1976.

CUSTER, ROBERT, AND HARRY MILT. *When Luck Runs Out.* New York, Facts on File, 1985.

DOSTOEVSKY, FYODOR. *The Gambler.* New York, Norton, 1981.

LESIEUR, HENRY R. *The Chase: The Compulsive Gambler.* Cambridge, Mass., Schenkman, 1984.

AIDS
TWO EPIDEMICS

Steven D. Helgerson, M.D., M.P.H.
James F. Jekel, M.D., M.P.H.

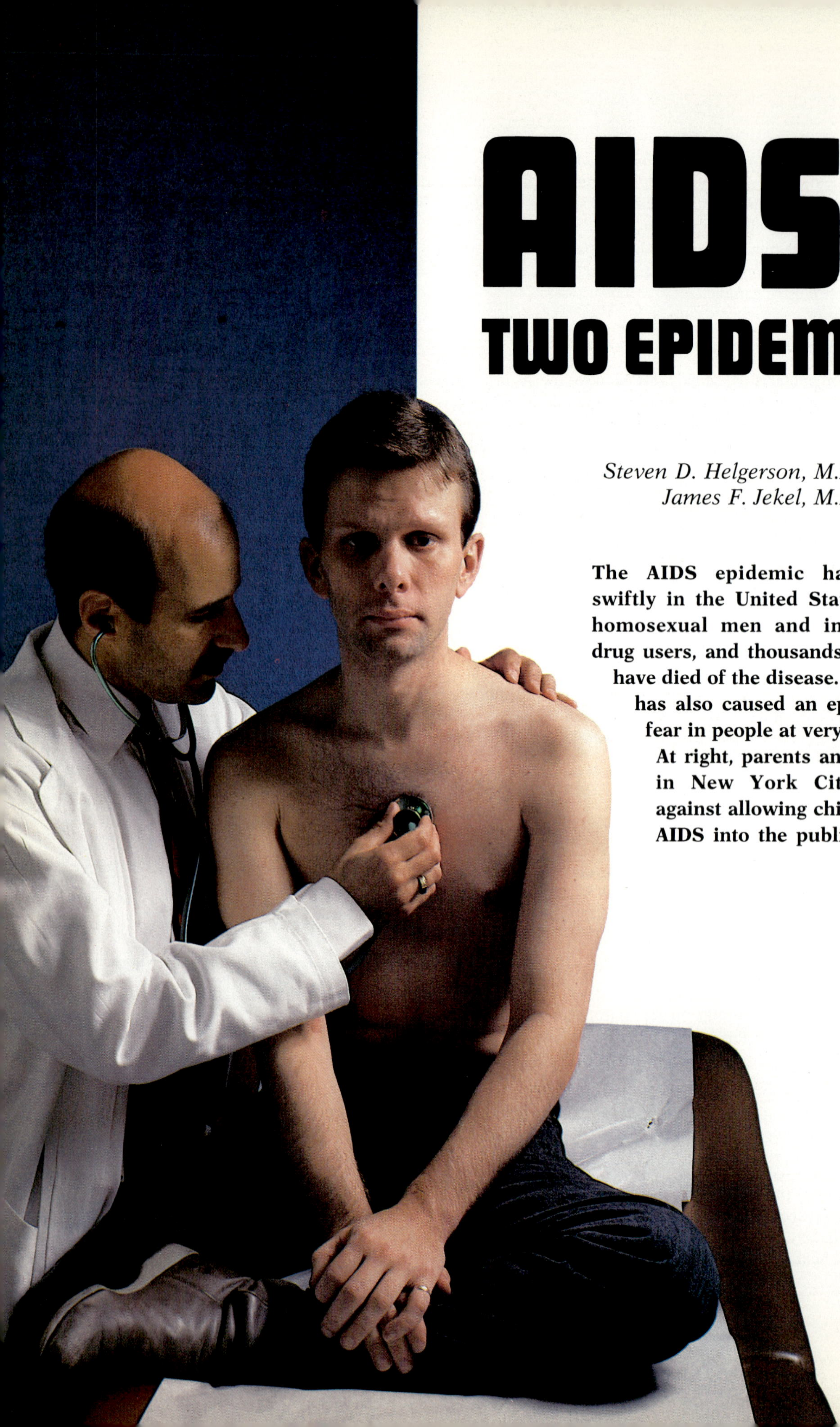

The AIDS epidemic has spread swiftly in the United States among homosexual men and intravenous drug users, and thousands of people have died of the disease. But AIDS has also caused an epidemic of fear in people at very little risk. At right, parents and children in New York City protest against allowing children with AIDS into the public schools.

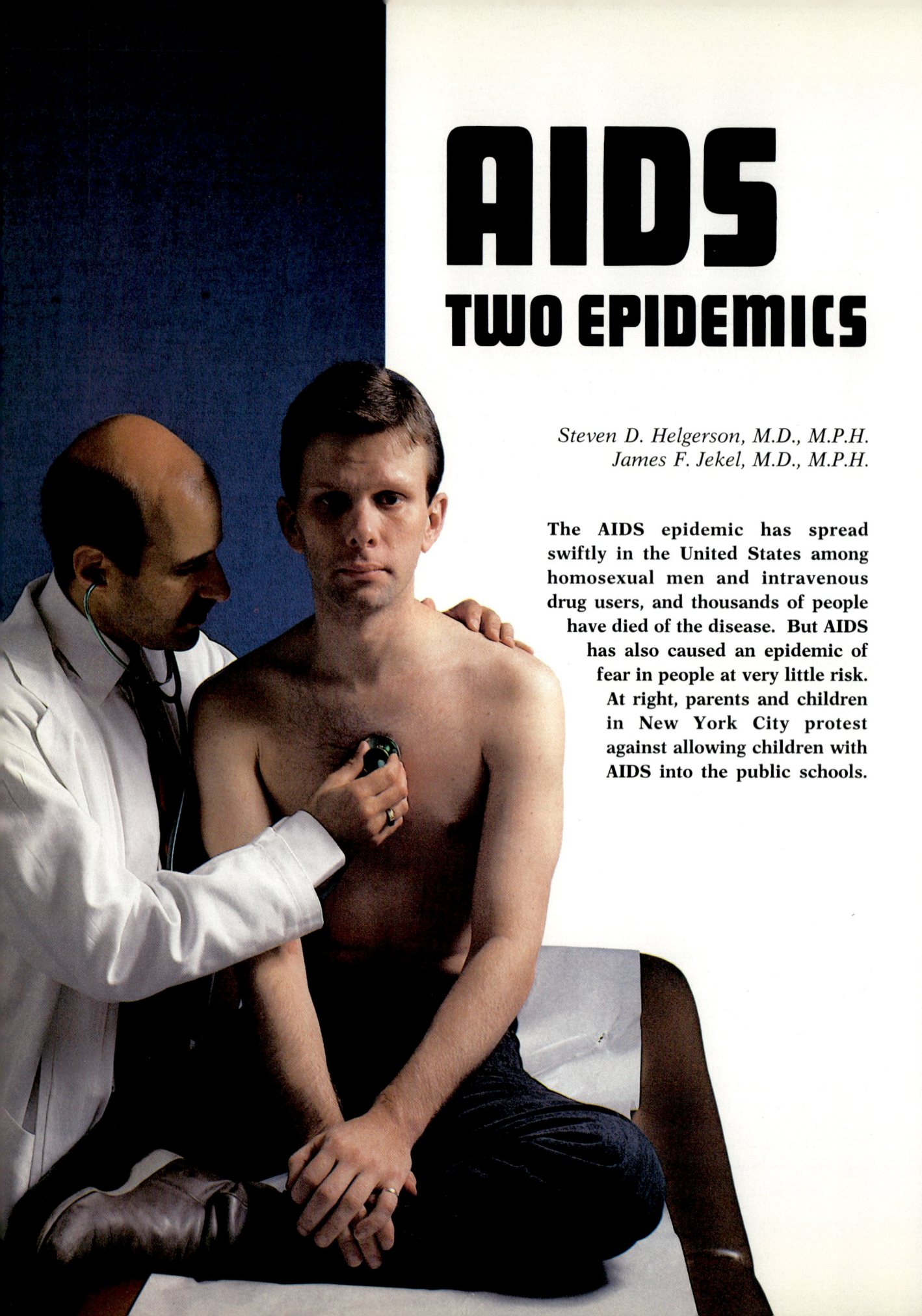

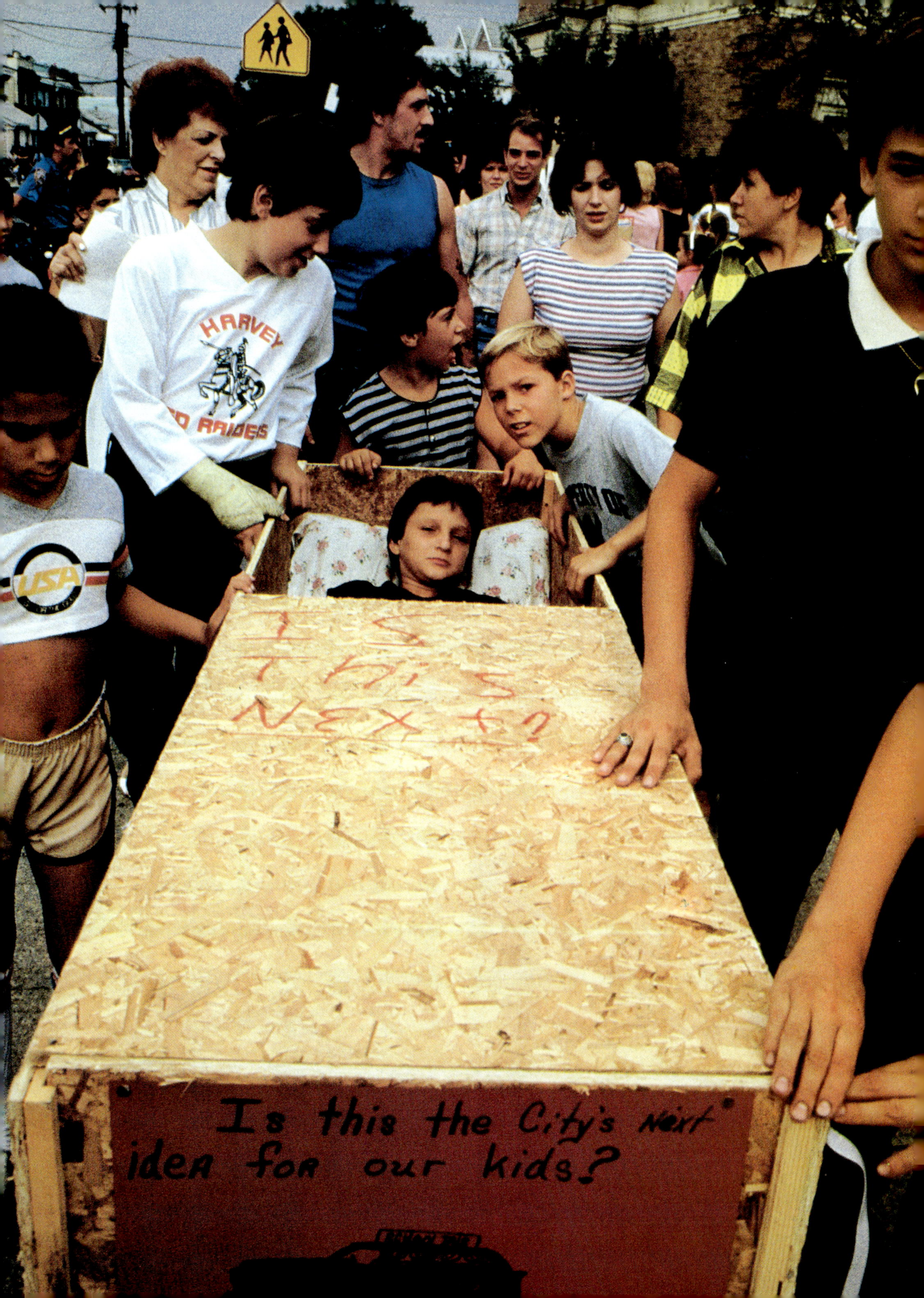
Is this next?
Is this the City's next idea for our kids?
HARVEY
USA

In the short time since AIDS was first recognized in 1981, the disease, which devastates the body's immune system, has gained an extraordinary notoriety. According to one recent poll, at least nine of every ten adults in the United States have heard of it. Media coverage of the AIDS epidemic intensified in 1985, fueled by the July revelation that movie star Rock Hudson had AIDS and by Hudson's death in October. Along with the epidemic of disease there seemed to be developing an epidemic of public fear, fed by widespread misconceptions about the chances of contracting AIDS. One magazine cover story announced that AIDS was the nation's worst public health problem, a declaration that overlooked the enormous toll of illness, injury, and death from smoking-related diseases and motor vehicle accidents.

AIDS has indeed spread quickly. By March 1986 over 18,000 cases had been reported in the United States since the epidemic was first recognized, with more than 9,500 deaths. The number of cases was expected to reach 30,000 by the end of the year. Canadian cases exceeded 500 by March 1986, with about 250 deaths. As of late 1985, more than 3,000 cases were recorded from some 50 other countries, including Western European nations, the Soviet Union, and nations in Latin America. Not included were the nations of Central Africa, which had not yet begun official reporting of their cases although the disease is known to be widespread there. (In December, Kenya became the first nation in black Africa to officially report AIDS cases to the World Health Organization.) In general, some countries' problems in data collection or unwillingness to make AIDS cases public render an accurate worldwide estimate of AIDS patients all but impossible.

The growing number of AIDS cases notwithstanding, for most people, according to the best research, the risk of contracting AIDS can be very small if some simple precautions are observed. In this and other respects, scientists have rapidly accumulated insights into the disease, as the epidemic has stimulated a virtual explosion of research. Major developments in 1985 included the blood test now being used to screen the U.S. blood supply for possible contamination with the virus causing AIDS and the finding that this virus attacks the nervous system as well as the immune system.

The virus that causes AIDS, shown here under a microscope, reproduces itself quickly in the body and attacks both the immune system and the central nervous system.

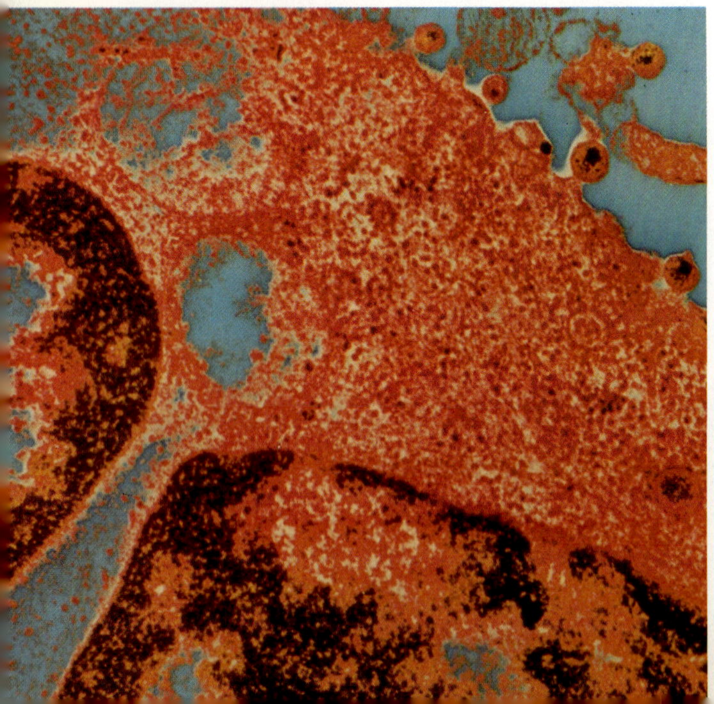

Identifying AIDS

Doctors came to know AIDS as a syndrome, that is, a set of symptoms allowing them to identify and report cases, well before the cause of AIDS was identified. The U.S. Centers for Disease Control (CDC) defined AIDS as the occurrence of certain rare infections or cancers which indicate that the body's immune system is malfunctioning in the absence of a known reason for the immune system to be weakened—for example, from the use of steroid medications or because of an inherited defect. From this set of factors the disease got its name: acquired immune deficiency syndrome.

The rare infections and cancers that afflict AIDS patients are called opportunistic because they take advantage of the fact that the body has lost its natural defense system. They seldom occur in people with healthy immune systems; in persons with AIDS, however, they not only occur but are life threatening. They include a pneumonia caused by the organism *Pneumocystis carinii;* a skin cancer known as Kaposi's sarcoma; primary lymphoma of the brain, another cancer; cryptococcal meningitis, an infection of the membranes lining the brain and spinal cord, caused by the *Cryptococcus* fungus; and toxoplasmosis, a brain inflammation caused by a parasite that commonly affects cats.

In some AIDS patients these diseases are preceded by symptoms that signal the impending collapse of the immune system. The individual may experience otherwise unexplained symptoms such as appetite and weight loss, night sweats, diarrhea, coughing, fever, extreme fatigue, and shortness of breath, and there is often a persistent swelling of the lymph nodes ("swollen glands"). This group of symptoms falls under the umbrella term "AIDS-related conditions." People with such symptoms may or may not eventually develop one of the deadly infections or cancers that means they have AIDS itself, but they remain capable of spreading the disease. Estimates for progression from AIDS-related conditions to AIDS during periods of up to five years have ranged as high as 25 to 34 percent. As far as is now known, an actual case of AIDS is always fatal.

In 1985 researchers reported clear evidence that the virus responsible for AIDS directly attacks the nervous system as well as the immune system. An estimated 30 percent of AIDS patients have symptoms of brain or spinal cord damage, and many patients show signs of dementia—including slowed thought processes, memory loss, and an attitude of general indifference. Individuals with AIDS or AIDS-related conditions may also experience slowed speech or movement, loss of muscle coordination, paralysis, and acute or chronic forms of meningitis caused by direct infection of the central nervous system with the virus. In late 1985 research was reported suggesting that the virus that causes AIDS may sometimes infect the central nervous system without first affecting the immune system.

The Virus Responsible for AIDS

The virus that causes AIDS is known under various names. First identified in 1983 by a team of researchers at France's Pasteur Institute, it was called by them LAV, for lymphadenopathy-associated virus, because they isolated the virus from a lymph node and swollen lymph nodes, or lymphadenopathy, are an early AIDS symptom. The following year researchers at the U.S. National Cancer Institute, working independently of the French team, reported isolating essentially the same virus and named it HTLV-III, for human T-cell lymphotropic virus type III. Another group of U.S. scientists pioneering in the isolation of the virus called it AIDS-associated retrovirus or ARV. A good shorthand name is "AIDS-related virus."

The AIDS-related virus belongs to a group called retroviruses (because their reproductive mechanism involves a reverse step in comparison to other viruses). Within the immune system the virus attacks the white blood cells known as T4 lymphocytes. These are "helper" cells that assist various immune system processes. The T4 cells play multiple, critical roles in the body's defenses against disease; their destruction devastates those defenses.

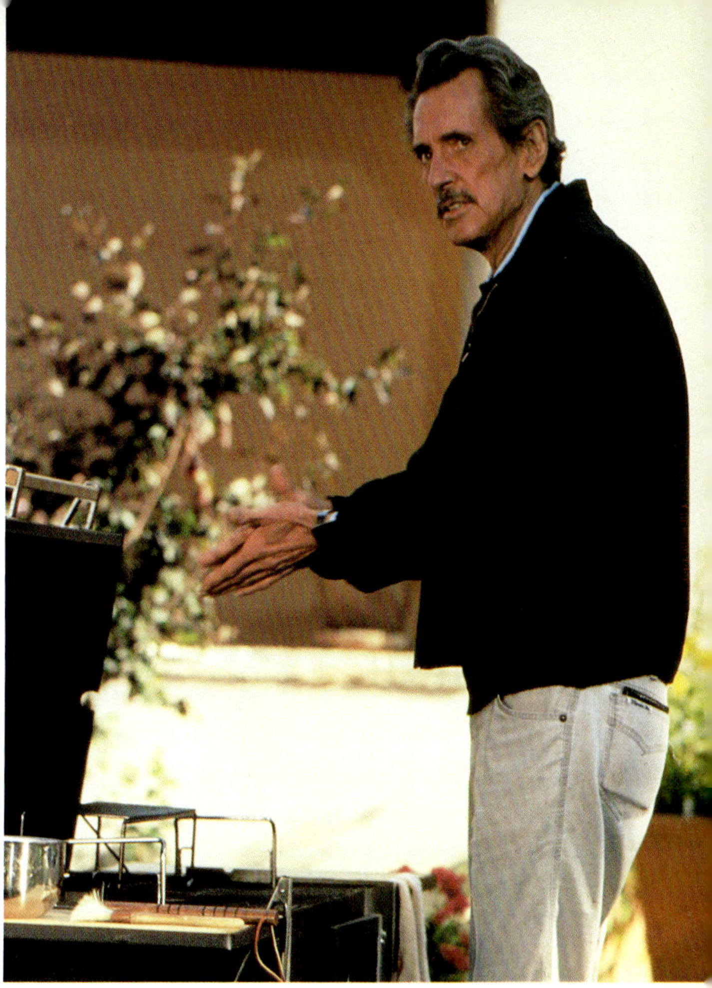

The death of actor Rock Hudson, the first celebrity known to have died from AIDS, raised public awareness of the disease and concern for its victims.

The discovery of the virus made possible, at least theoretically, the development of screening tests for its presence and perhaps even a vaccine. An easier task was developing a blood test indicating whether a person had been infected by the virus.

The Blood Test

One way in which AIDS has been transmitted is through transfusions of blood contaminated with the virus. With a blood test able to identify persons who had been infected by the virus, blood banks could greatly improve the safety of their blood supply by

---

Steven D. Helgerson is clinical assistant professor of epidemiology and public health at the Yale University School of Medicine and medical epidemiologist with the Centers for Disease Control. James F. Jekel is professor of epidemiology and public health at Yale.

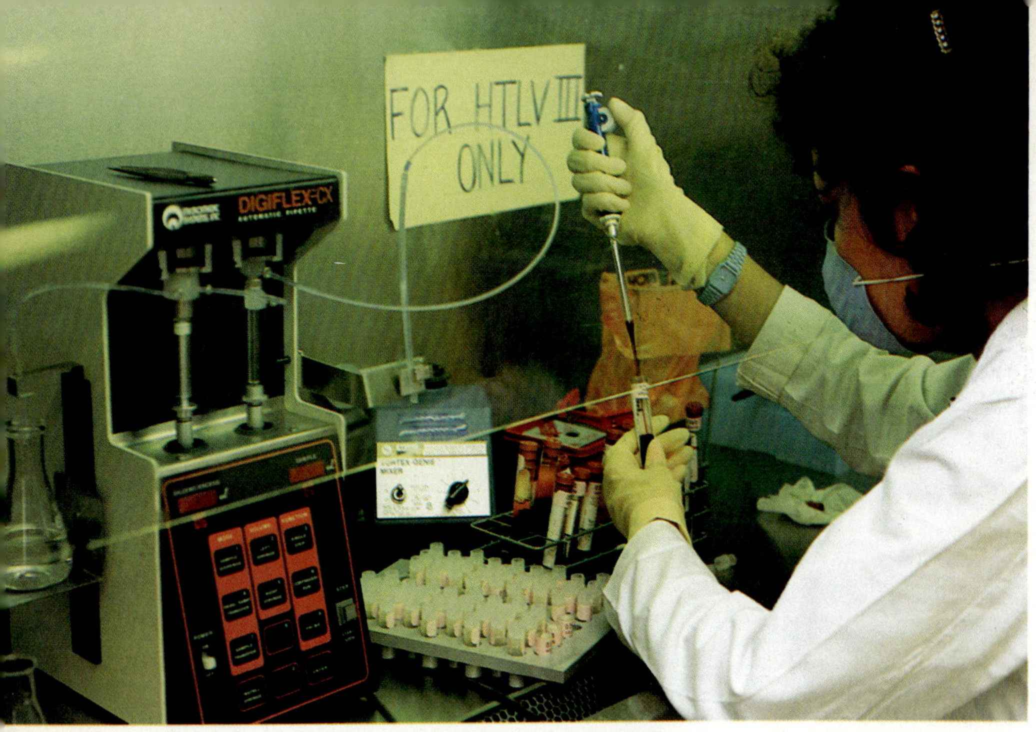

A laboratory worker in a blood bank tests a donor's blood for evidence of exposure to the virus that causes AIDS. The test significantly reduces the danger that AIDS will be transmitted through blood transfusions or blood products.

screening out donations from such individuals. In March 1985 the U.S. Food and Drug Administration (FDA) approved such a test. Its technical name is ELISA, for enzyme-linked immunosorbent assay. The antibodies produced by the body's immune system to help combat an invading disease organism are specific to that organism. The ELISA test for AIDS detects the presence in blood of antibodies to the AIDS-related virus. A positive result means that, at least at one time, the person was infected by the virus. It does not tell whether the individual is still carrying the virus or will ever develop AIDS.

The test has proved very useful to blood banks for screening out blood potentially contaminated with the virus. Blood products, such as the clotting agent called factor VIII that is given to hemophiliacs, can also be screened by this test. Use of the test was expected to virtually eliminate the risk of getting AIDS from a blood transfusion or blood product. Blood transfusion-related AIDS cases would not immediately cease to appear, however, because some people who had previously received contaminated blood might take years to show symptoms.

The test is not perfect. It will give a negative result if exposure was so recent that antibodies have not yet formed or if the amount of antibody produced is below the detectable level. As a safety precaution, people in groups considered at high risk of developing AIDS have therefore been asked not to donate blood. Moreover, there is controversial evidence suggesting that ELISA, as well as the more expensive follow-up analysis called the Western blot test that is sometimes performed to confirm ELISA's results, may miss an estimated 5 percent of blood samples that do in fact contain antibodies to the AIDS-related virus.

In itself, ELISA is of little use in diagnosing AIDS. Aside from the fact that it does not tell whether the virus is present, it sometimes suggests that antibodies are present in blood when in fact they are not; one research group estimated that over half of positive results from screening of the general population would be such so-called false positives. For blood banks, which need to be maximally cautious, it is useful that the test is very sensitive even if it sometimes yields a falsely positive result. Given this ambiguity about the meaning of a positive result, should an individual who donates blood that tests positive be notified of the result? Most authorities suggest that a donor be told of a positive finding only if ELISA testing is repeatedly positive and the results are confirmed by the more specific Western blot analysis, performed by an experienced laboratory. (The Western blot is harder to interpret.)

Who Is at Risk?

Nearly 95 percent of AIDS cases reported in the United States by January 1986 belonged to the same high-risk groups that had been identified after the CDC began investigating the disease in 1981. These groups are homosexual and bisexual men (72 percent), intravenous drug users of both sexes (17 percent), hemophilia patients (1 percent), recipients of blood transfusions (2 percent), heterosexual partners of people in high-risk groups (1 percent), and babies born to an infected or at-risk parent (1 percent).

Some 70 percent of children with AIDS were born to mothers who were intravenous drug users. One study estimated the risk of transmission from pregnant women with the virus to their unborn children to be as high as 65 percent.

Haitian-Americans, formerly designated by the CDC as a separate high-risk group, were no longer listed separately after April 1985. This change resulted from information that suggested that heterosexual contact and exposure to contaminated needles (not associated with intravenous drug abuse) played a role in transmission of the disease. However, because Haitian-Americans are more likely than the general U.S. population to have been affected by the virus, the CDC continues to recommend that Haitian entrants into the United States not donate blood. (Canada, still separately monitors reported cases occurring in "persons from an endemic area"—Haiti and Central Africa; this category made up 9.5 percent of Canadian cases as of March 1986.)

Blood test results have shown that many more people in high-risk groups have been infected with, and have antibodies to, the AIDS-related virus than have actually developed the syndrome—an estimated 1 million to 2 million people in the United States alone. How many of these will eventually develop AIDS is not known, but estimates range from 5 to 10 percent within five years. Nor is it known how many of these carriers of the disease can spread the virus to others; at present, all are presumed to be capable of doing so. Moreover, research indicates that infection of the immune system and brain by the AIDS-related virus persists for years and may be lifelong whether or not the infected person develops symptoms. Thus, people with the virus may be carriers for life.

In Canada and Western Europe, AIDS has occurred predominantly in the same high-risk groups as in the United States. As of March 1986 homosexual or bisexual men accounted for 7.8 percent of Canadian cases. In Central Africa, however, most adult cases have been in sexually active heterosexual men and women, in nearly equal numbers.

Although in some African cases the virus may have been transmitted through exposure to contaminated blood or unsterile needles, it is possible that many cases have resulted from heterosexual contact. One study of 33 female prostitutes in Rwanda found that 88 percent were infected with the virus; these women were probably an important source of infection for heterosexual men. In turn, men with AIDS—often customers of prostitutes—may have a high frequency of sexual contacts with different sexual partners, spreading the virus even further. Moreover, the high proportion of women with the disease means widespread transmission of the virus to children (who accounted for 20 percent of the recognized AIDS cases in Rwanda, compared with 1 percent of U.S. cases). In Uganda a disease the same as or very similar to AIDS and known locally as slim disease (because of the extreme weight loss that occurs) was identified predominantly in promiscuous heterosexuals infected with the AIDS-related virus. A possible hint as to how AIDS might be spread among heterosexuals came in early 1986 when U.S. researchers reported that the virus had been found in vaginal and cervical secretions in some women.

Modes of Transmission

It has become increasingly clear that the virus is transmitted through intimate homosexual and

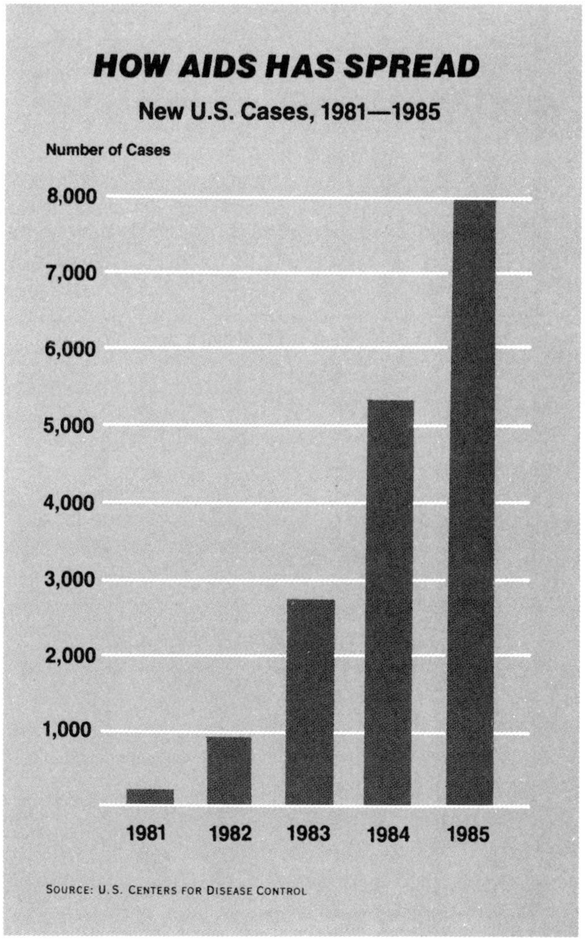

Who Has AIDS?

Distribution of U.S. Cases Through 1985

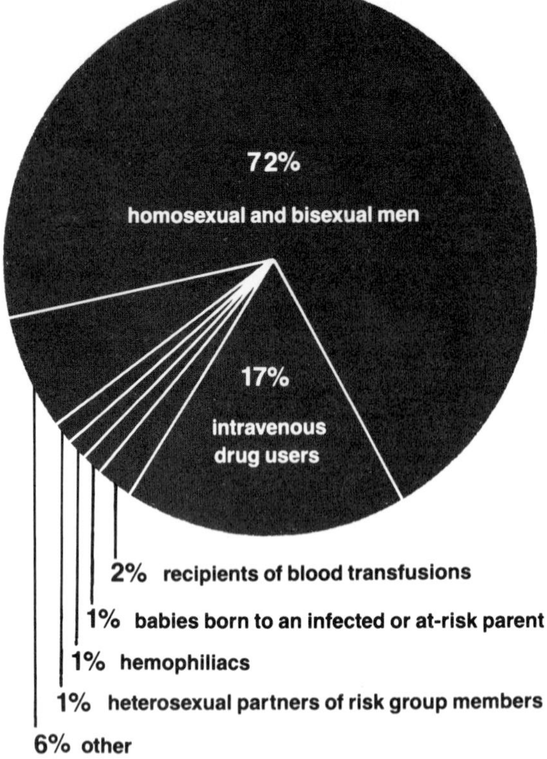

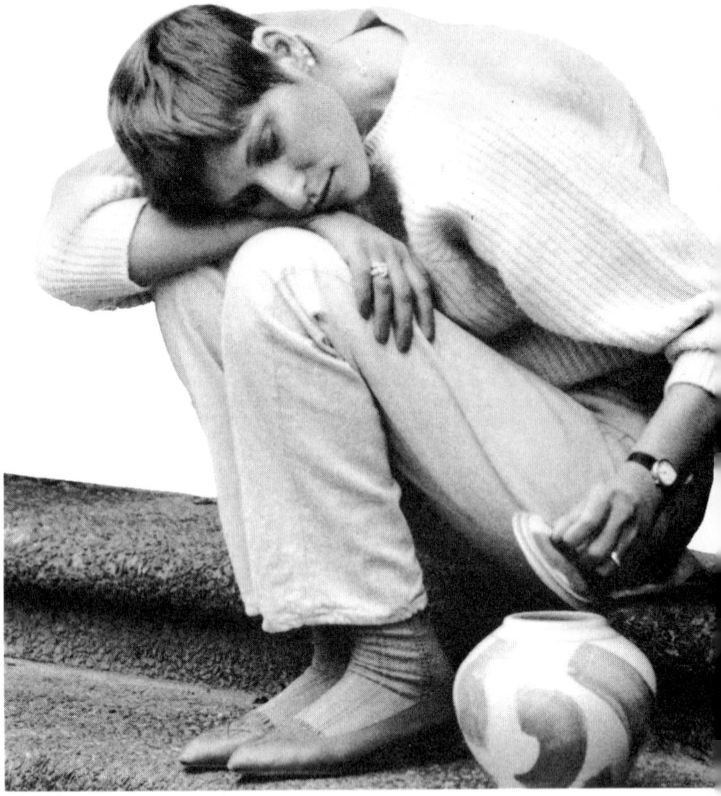

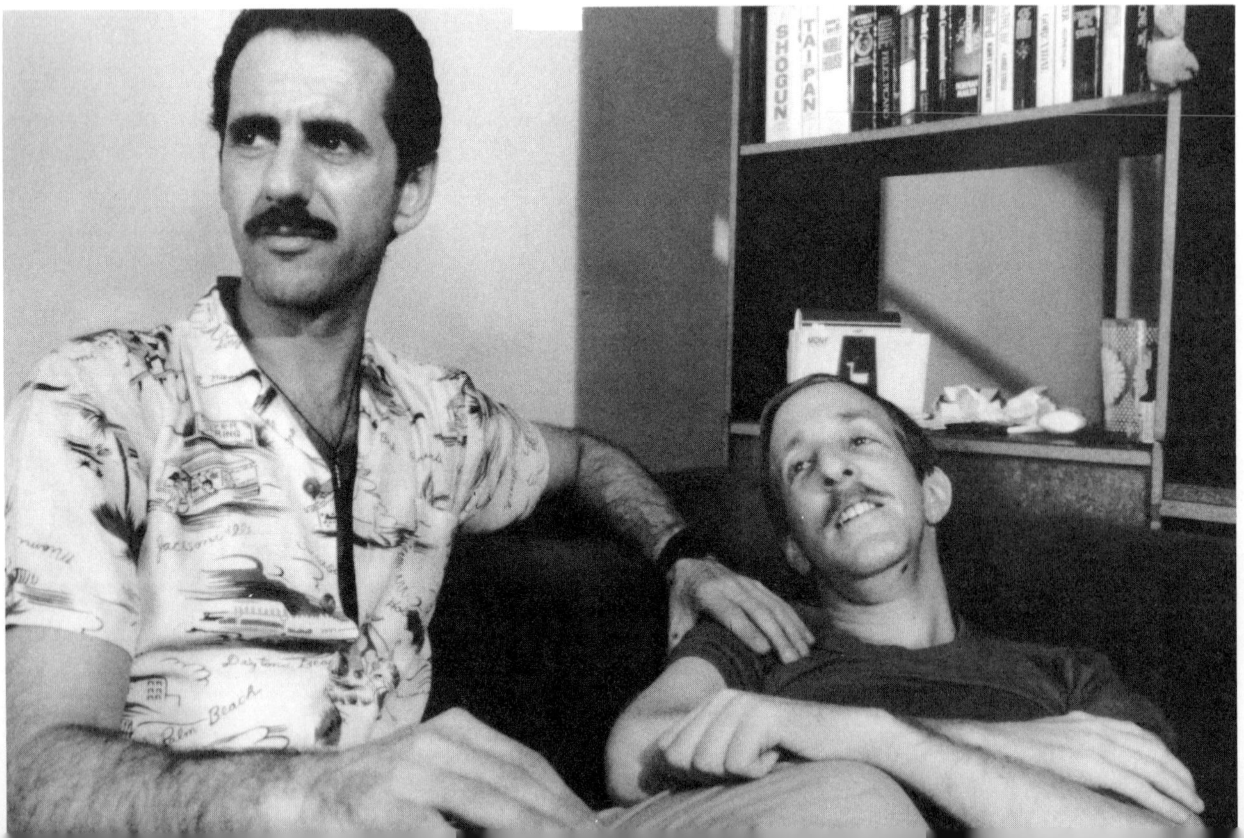

heterosexual contact, through use of a hypodermic needle contaminated with infected blood (a common means of transmission among intravenous drug users), by exposure to infected blood and blood products, or from mother to child during the perinatal period (that is, before birth and, possibly, through breast feeding after birth). There is no evidence suggesting transmission by air, water, food, mosquitoes or other blood-sucking insects, or casual contact like shaking hands, being near an infected person who coughs or sneezes, or swimming in the same pool as an infected person. Although people who advocate the isolation of AIDS patients point to the fact that the virus was reported in 1985 to occur in tears and has been detected in saliva as well, there is no evidence that the virus has been transmitted through either contaminated tears or saliva.

People living in the same household as AIDS patients are considered to have very little, if any, risk of either being infected with the AIDS-related virus or developing the disease in the absence of intimate contact. The chances of the virus being transmitted to any of the thousands of healthcare workers who have cared for AIDS patients are very low. An analysis of cases reported by early 1986 shows that only a handful of such workers in the United States not having known AIDS risk factors had been found to have antibodies to the AIDS-related virus, probably because of exposure to contaminated blood in the workplace.

Seeking a Cure

There is currently no specific treatment for AIDS, but there is a large and growing worldwide research effort to find medications that are both safe and effective. In the United States a number of drugs had been approved for testing by early 1986.

One approach to treatment is to attack the virus directly. While a wide choice of antibiotic drugs is available to combat bacterially caused diseases, there are very few drugs that act against viruses. Those being tested in AIDS patients include suramin, ribavirin (Virazole), and HPA-23. (Rock Hudson went to France in July 1985 reportedly to receive HPA-23; it was approved for experimental use in the United States in September.) Researchers who administered these drugs for two to six weeks found that the drugs seem to temporarily stop the AIDS-related virus from reproducing itself but sometimes produce serious side effects. More information may come from testing for longer periods, at differing dosages, and possibly in combination with other types of drugs.

A second treatment strategy is to help the damaged immune system work better despite persisting infection with the virus. Interleukin-2 and several types of interferon are examples of substances called immune stimulators or immunomodulators that are being investigated. Another is the drug inosiplex, which is not commercially available in the United States but is marketed elsewhere under the brand

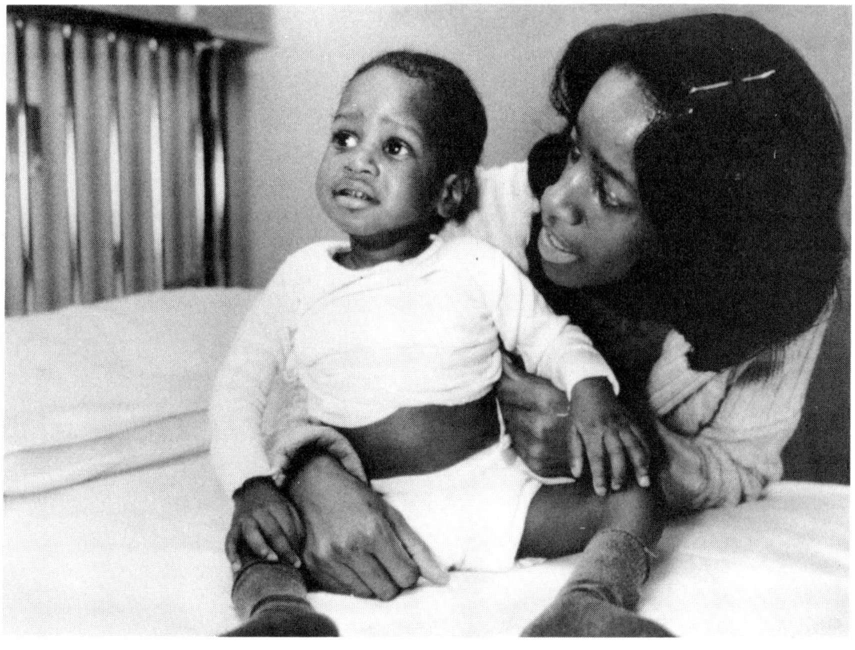

The number of AIDS cases has gone up, but the percentage of people in each risk group, shown in the chart at left, has stayed basically the same. Homosexual and bisexual men (left) have by far the highest risk. Women may contract AIDS by sexual intercourse with a bisexual man—the case of the woman above left, who has chosen her funeral urn. The baby at right was born with AIDS transmitted by his mother.

name Isoprinosine. In May 1985 the FDA made it possible for AIDS patients to obtain the drug from their doctors under test conditions, not because there was proof that it works but because rumors that it may help persons with AIDS-related conditions had sent patients to Mexico, where it could be obtained legally; a black market for the drug was said to exist in some U.S. cities. Inosiplex apparently does not have harmful side effects. Drugs are also being tested that combine the two approaches to treatment. An example of these antiviral agents that stimulate the immune system is acyclovir.

A seemingly opposite plan of attack provoked surprise and controversy when it was announced by French researchers in October 1985. They said they had obtained beneficial effects with the drug cyclosporine, which depresses the immune system and is used to prevent rejection of organ transplants. The announcement was made after only a week of testing in a handful of patients. Three of the patients had died by the end of November, but further study of this approach was planned. The French scientists hypothesized that cyclosporine might inactivate cells infected by the AIDS-related virus while permitting the immune system to recover.

Unfortunately, while careful testing of various drugs continues, some desperate AIDS patients have resorted without a physician's guidance to experimental treatments that may not help, or worse, may add to their symptoms. Physicians in the meantime are doing their best to treat the infections and cancers that signal the presence of AIDS. None of these treatments cure the underlying AIDS infection, but they do "buy time" and often provide relief of symptoms to gravely ill patients.

A major goal of scientists is the development of a vaccine to protect the healthy population from AIDS. But these efforts are still at an early stage, and the U.S. Public Health Service has cautioned that it may not be possible to eliminate the risk of AIDS before the year 2000. One problem is the variability of the AIDS-related virus, which makes it difficult to find a common vaccine that works on all forms. The commercial introduction in 1985 of the first vaccine against a retrovirus in mammals—in this case, against the virus that causes leukemia in cats—offered encouragement to researchers, although the work is not considered directly applicable to the far more complex retrovirus that causes AIDS.

In early 1986 researchers reported they had isolated and produced in a relatively pure form a "reverse transcriptase" enzyme that plays a key role in the virus's ability to infect human cells. This achievement might prove helpful in developing drugs against AIDS and perhaps even a vaccine.

The progress of AIDS research is advanced not only by cooperation among scientists but also by competition, which can be intense. A dispute between French and U.S. researchers grew into a lawsuit in December 1985. The Pasteur Institute filed suit against the U.S. government, which holds the U.S. patent on the ELISA blood test, seeking (among other things) recognition of the significance of the French virus discovery to the development of methods of detecting infection with the virus. The French also wanted a share in the royalties received by the U.S. government from the test. In early 1986 the FDA approved a similar blood test made by a U.S. company under license to the Pasteur Institute.

Educating the Public

While scientists search for drugs that can cure AIDS and a vaccine to prevent it, education remains the most important public health approach to protection against infection with the AIDS-related virus. Public health experts have urged people not to donate blood if they are in a high-risk group, to avoid infected sexual partners to the extent possible (in part by simply not having many sexual partners), to use only syringes that have been adequately sterilized, and to be aware that some types of sexual behavior, such as anal intercourse, are more conducive to the transmission of AIDS. To help combat the spread of the virus, U.S. government health officials in March 1986 advised that healthcare facilities routinely offer blood tests to individuals in high-risk groups, along with counseling on ways to avoid spreading the disease.

In November 1985 the U.S. Public Health Service announced guidelines for protecting a wide range of workers from infection. Healthcare workers were advised to wear gloves and sometimes masks when working with blood or other body fluids of AIDS patients. It was recommended that instruments used to pierce the skin (hypodermic needles and tattoo, acupuncture, and ear-piercing devices, among others) be used once and either thoroughly disinfected or discarded. The guidelines also enumerated some steps that were *not* necessary to protect the work force in general. They noted that workers with AIDS should not be restricted from using telephones, water fountains, or other public facilities, pointed out that the virus cannot be transmitted through food handled by infected workers, and recommended against routine blood test screening of workers.

Although the chance of the virus being transmitted to students or staff in schools, day care centers, or foster homes is extremely remote, in order to be prudent the CDC in August 1985 issued recommendations for these environments. Routine childhood diseases that often spread at school can have severe, even life-threatening effects for children with AIDS. But, the CDC said, for most AIDS children the benefits of attending school will outweigh the risks of their contracting harmful infections. The agency urged that decisions on the schooling or foster care of AIDS children be made on a case-by-case basis, and advised that confidentiality be maintained. The CDC did not recommend any special precautions for students and staff in schools but did reaffirm its long-standing encouragement of good hygiene to minimize the chances of anyone acquiring a communicable disease. Such elementary measures as washing one's hands and the disinfection of soiled surfaces significantly decrease the risk of transmission of infectious diseases—and the exceedingly remote possibility of exposure to the virus that causes AIDS.

A decreasing incidence of sexually transmitted diseases such as gonorrhea and syphilis has been observed among homosexual men in several U.S. cities. This development may at least in part reflect changes in sexual behavior caused by concern about AIDS and suggests that educational campaigns can be effective. Whether the trend means that the incidence of new AIDS infections is also falling is not yet known.

A Civil Liberties Issue

In the 20th century it has been common for information gained through technological advances to exceed our ability to use the information appropriately. The public response to the introduction of the blood test for the presence of antibodies to the AIDS-related virus is a good example. Despite the fact that the test does not reveal whether a person has AIDS or will ever develop it, nor whether the individual even has the virus or will transmit it, there have been numerous proposals to use the test to screen selected workers like food handlers and school employees or to generally determine people's eligibility for insurance coverage or acceptability for employment. Some proposals have been adopted.

Thus, in August 1985 the U.S. Defense Department announced that all military recruits would be screened for the presence of antibodies to the virus. In October the Pentagon said it would test all 2.1 million active-duty personnel. Those with positive test results would be assigned to limited duties or areas, unless they showed signs of disease or admitted to illicit drug use or homosexuality—in which case they would be discharged. At the community level, a 1985 ordinance in Dade County, Fla., required annual antibody testing

A billboard campaign in Los Angeles is part of the large-scale public education effort needed to overcome the rejection of and discrimination against AIDS patients and people in high-risk groups.

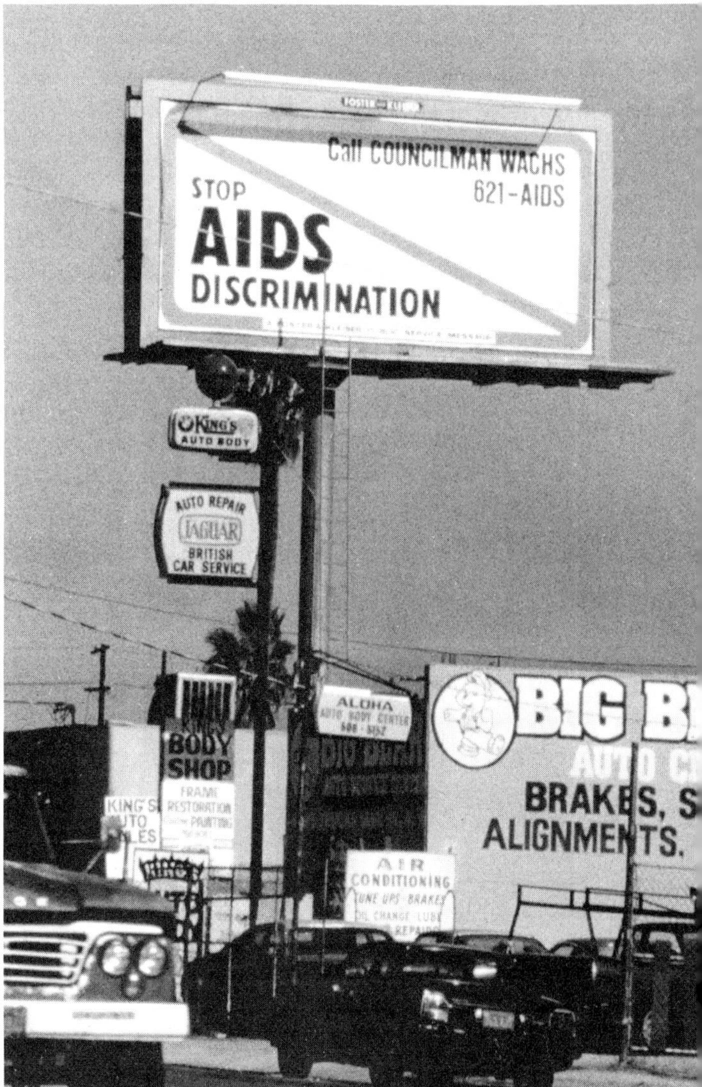

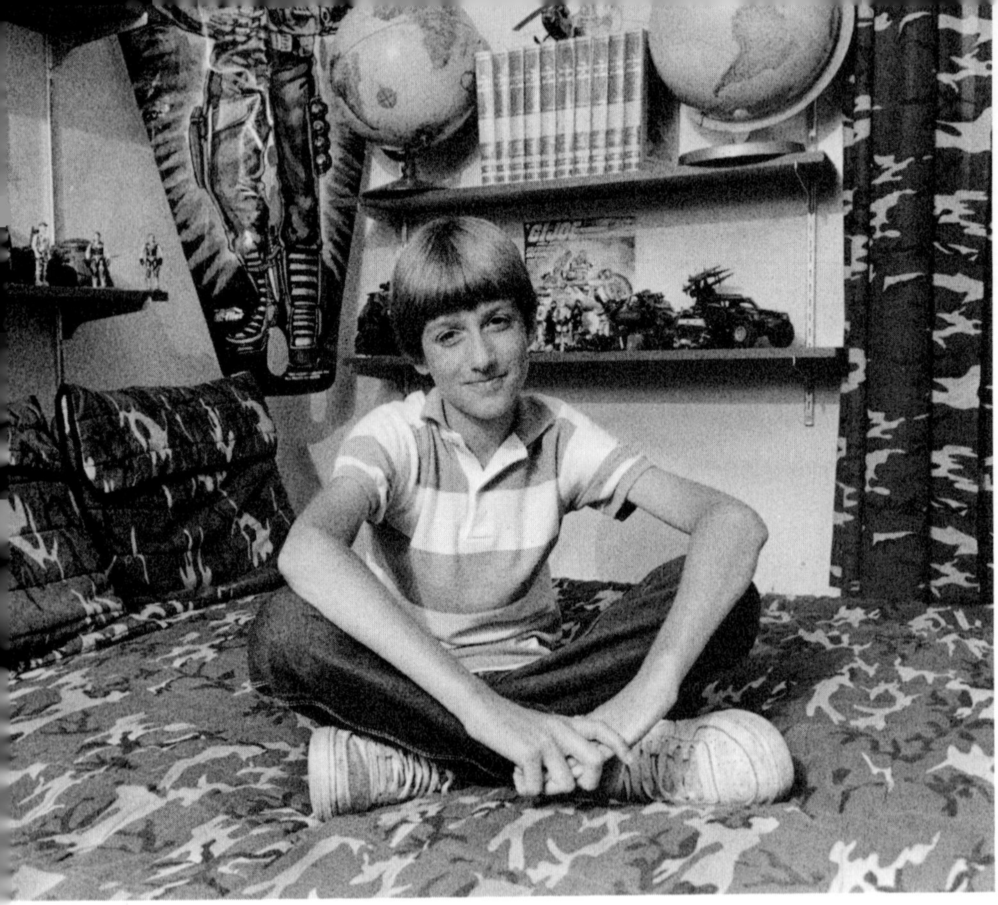

Ryan White, a hemophiliac who contracted AIDS from a contaminated blood-clotting agent, was barred from attending the local middle school in Kokomo, Ind. He listened to his classes and talked to teachers and classmates over a special telephone hookup in his bedroom.

for commercial food handlers, and the school board in Bedminster, N.J., introduced blood test screening of the school staff.

This trend has caused special concern to homosexual men, many of whom argue that blood test results could easily be used to discriminate against homosexuals in such areas as jobs and housing. Their concern is at the heart of an ethical dilemma: how should the civil liberties of individuals with AIDS or at risk of contracting it be balanced against the community's desire for reasonable protection from the disease. A 1985 decision by the Colorado Board of Health to maintain a confidential register both of AIDS cases and of persons who test positive for antibodies (based on mandatory reporting from laboratories) highlighted the fragility of this balance. Public health authorities are concerned that fear of disclosure will prevent at-risk individuals from taking the blood test; not knowing whether they have been exposed to the virus, they may be more likely to continue behavior that might spread the disease.

Some states have enacted safeguards to reduce potential abuses. In California persons who are found to carry antibodies to the virus are notified of the test results, and their names are entered on a register of deferred blood donors; there are, however, civil and criminal penalties for unauthorized disclosure of test results. California and Wisconsin passed laws in 1985 prohibiting insurance companies from using test results to evaluate applicants for coverage (although Wisconsin later modified its law to permit such use under certain conditions).

Epidemic of Fear

Although many news reports have taken pains to accurately convey researchers' findings that infection with the AIDS-related virus is unlikely for the general public, vague, groundless fears of catching AIDS have sometimes prevailed. Indeed, some people have seemed almost eager to perceive themselves at risk. A September 1985 poll found that nearly half of those questioned thought that infection with the virus could be acquired by casual contact. Public health authorities and other experts seemed unable to reassure people that many of their fears had little or no basis in fact. It was little wonder that the reaction to AIDS reports sometimes became bigger news than the reports themselves.

Some responses to the AIDS epidemic, while controversial, were perhaps understandable, like New York City's closing of gay bathhouses where promiscuous sex acts were common or the Screen Actors Guild's pronouncement that actors must be notified in advance of scenes that require open-mouth kissing. Whether such steps would actually have any effect in halting the spread of AIDS was widely questioned.

In other cases, responses seemed almost entirely rooted in fear: prospective jury members asked to be dismissed from a case where the defendant had AIDS, a county ended the use of prison road gangs to avoid the spread of AIDS, a proposal was made to quarantine people with AIDS on an island off Cape Cod, and workers demanded that a male homosexual employee be restricted from using the company cafeteria.

Picketing and parent-organized student boycotts occurred at some schools where AIDS children were to attend regular classes if their health permitted. Policies in response to these protests varied widely: some cities announced they would make their decisions on a case-by-case basis, sometimes concealing the identity of the affected child and isolating children only when it seemed they might present a danger to others. Elsewhere, children were barred from school and given separate instruction.

There were, however, a few encouraging signs in 1985 that a more reasoned reaction was setting in. At a junior high school in Swansea, Mass., a student with AIDS attended classes with other pupils, with the full support of his schoolmates (who knew his identity) and without any community protests. In November, NBC televised a two-hour drama about a young lawyer with AIDS; the network followed the program with a special news report about the disease and undertook a national educational campaign as well. Benefit galas were staged in Hollywood and at the Metropolitan Opera in New York by entertainment industry stars to raise funds for AIDS-related causes, and in August the Los Angeles City Council, responding to the epidemic of fear, unanimously passed a regulation barring discrimination against homosexuals in jobs, housing, and healthcare.

A Need for Research—and Perspective

Some of the public reaction to AIDS seemed to represent not ignorance so much as a just-in-case attitude: "Just in case the experts are wrong, I will avoid certain people, places, or activities." Indeed, it would not be truthful for public health officials to assure the public of absolute safety, but this is so whether the question at hand is one of avoiding AIDS, preventing polio with polio vaccine, or preventing lung cancer by not smoking cigarettes. Adding to public confusion and uncertainty is the fact that, because AIDS was first described just a few years ago, many questions about how the virus and the disorder behave remain unanswered; experts may differ with each other on sometimes crucial points.

Clearly, more AIDS research is needed. Connected with this obvious fact is yet another AIDS-related controversy: whether the U.S. goverment is giving the proper priority to AIDS funding. Some have questioned whether the federal research effort to understand and combat the disease, as well as an all-important public education campaign aimed at preventing its spread, is adequately organized and funded. The Reagan administration has been accused of dragging its feet. Congress has increased AIDS funding over administration requests every year since 1982. It approved $244 million for the 1986 fiscal year, more than twice the amount spent the previous year. (The 1986 figure was expected to be cut by several million dollars because of federal deficit reduction action.)

Money is needed not only to fund research; providing medical and hospital care for AIDS patients is enormously expensive. Researchers have estimated that expenditures for hospitalization and economic losses from disability and premature death for the first 10,000 patients with AIDS in the United States total $6.3 billion. Decisions will have to be made as to how the continuing costs can best be met. □

SOURCES OF FURTHER INFORMATION

Centers for Disease Control toll-free hot line, (800) 342-AIDS; in Atlanta, (404) 329-3534.

AIDS Action Council, Federation of AIDS-Related Organizations, 729 Eighth Street, S.E., Washington, D.C. 20003; (202) 547-3101.

AIDS Committee of Toronto, P.O. Box 55, Station F, Toronto, Ont. M4Y 2L4, Canada; (416) 926-1626

SUGGESTIONS FOR FURTHER READING

AIDS: The Emerging Ethical Dilemmas. Hastings-on Hudson, N.Y., Hastings Center, 1985.

GONG, VICTOR, ed. *Understanding AIDS: A Comprehensive Guide.* New Brunswick, N.J., Rutgers University Press, 1985.

LANGONE, JOHN. "AIDS." *Discover,* December 1985, pp. 28-53.

LAURENCE, JEFFREY. "The Immune System in AIDS." *Scientific American,* December 1985, pp. 84-93.

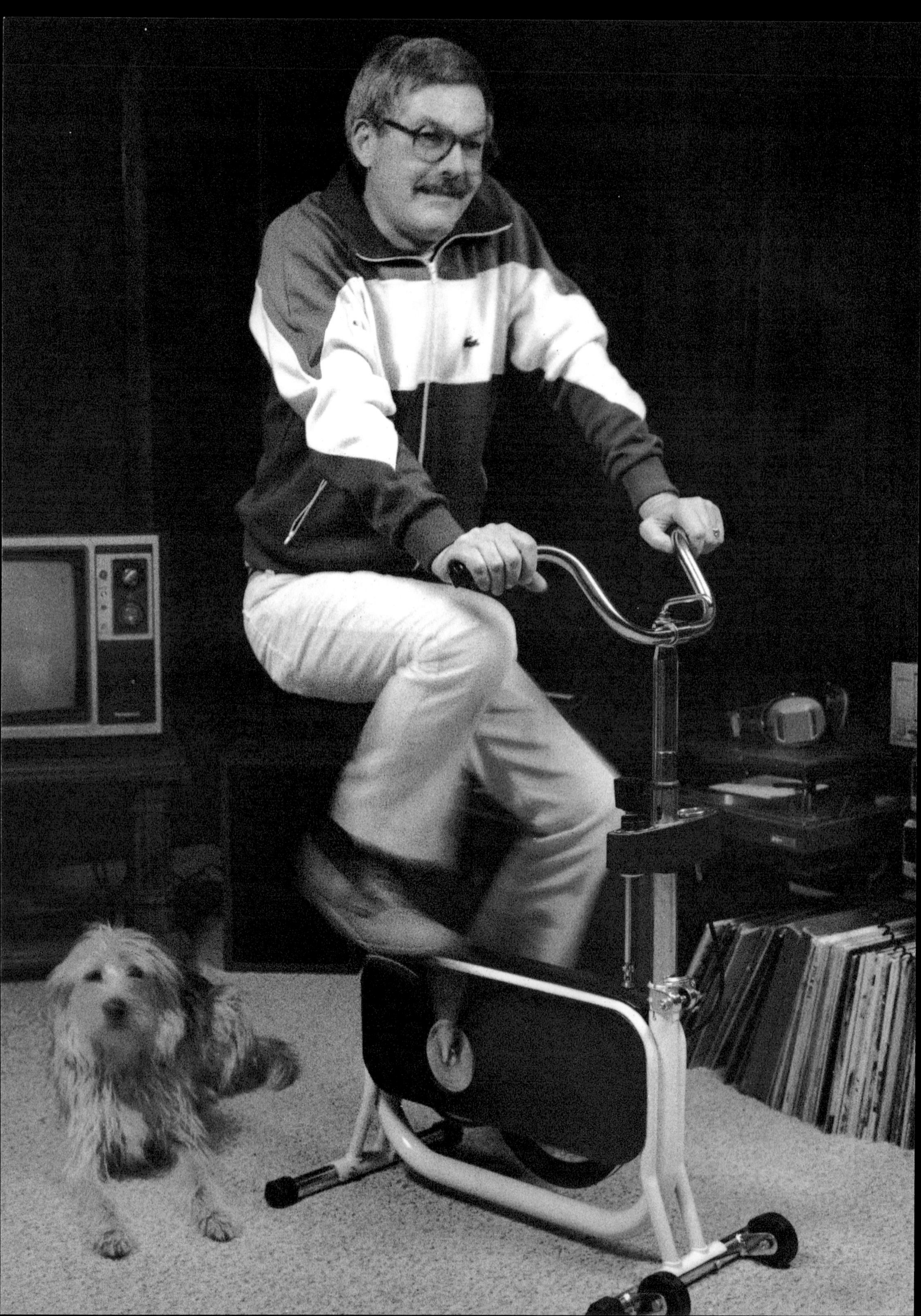

Exercising at Home

What You Need to Know

Martha G. Wiseman

The day is cold and rainy, and you simply don't want to jog. The last time you went to your health club, you had to wait over half an hour to use your favorite machine. The last time you swam in the pool, you were caught in a head-to-toe traffic jam and barely escaped with your life. Or perhaps you haven't been able to afford to join a club in the first place—many are very pricey—or you don't want to plunk down all those dollars annually. Maybe you can't find a club or a Y that's convenient anyway. And maybe your last aerobic dance instructor harangued you right out of class with a pulled ligament. Of course, if you want to get fit, stay fit, and fit into the smaller sized clothes in your closet, you must fit fitness into your life and life-style. How to do it? Go home—but don't give up.

High-tech or low-budget, with elaborate equipment or without, exercise at home is now the choice of many people. Instructors are being replaced by videos, records, tapes, books, and TV gurus. There are even personal trainers who make house calls for an hourly fee. For some, exercising has become a family event; for others, quiet, solitude, and a chance to concentrate are primary reasons for choosing to work out in the privacy of their own living rooms or ad hoc gyms.

How should you decide what exercise or combination of exercises is best for you? (There is probably no one form of exercise that is the right ticket for all of us.) What are the advantages and disadvantages, the benefits and risks, of making home base your fitness center? There is an overwhelming array of exercise equipment for home use—what type will best suit your individual needs, and how can you get the best value?

Before You Start

Before you begin a fitness regimen, you must first know what your exercise goals are and recognize the constraints imposed by your physical limitations, by limitations on your time, space, and finances—and by your tastes. How much you enjoy doing something is a very good gauge of the likelihood of your persisting with a program of exercise after the initial flush of enthusiasm.

There are some drawbacks to the home-based workout, and this waning of enthusiasm is one of them. Without a set, externally imposed schedule, without the supervision of an instructor or the motivation that other people exercising around you can inspire, self-discipline may falter. Too many days when you "just don't feel like it" can throw off your program, which can be a problem since consistency is tremendously important if you are to derive the maximum benefit from your workout (this does not necessarily mean exercising every day).

You'll have to decide for yourself just how much the absence of supervision will affect you and how much you need a social aspect to your program—you may find yourself lonely and bored at home. Some find that exercise equipment itself can provide motivation: its presence may spur its use. Others depend on the taped voice of a Jane Fonda or a Richard Simmons to get them going.

You must also keep in mind, however, that with no one making sure you are doing exercises or using machines correctly, you can run the risk of injury. Many people may assume that because no actual teacher is goading them on, they are unlikely to work hard enough to make exercising worthwhile. But partly because of this assumption, you may be tempted to overcompensate and push yourself too hard. Especially if you are out of shape and unused to exercise, you must start off your exercise program slowly and gradually increase the length and strenuousness of your workout to the suggested or desired level. See the accompanying box for some other cautionary notes.

Some Medical Precautions

1. Smokers, people who are extremely overweight, and people who have heart or respiratory disease, high blood pressure, diabetes, high blood cholesterol, or a family history of heart disease should seek the advice of a physician before beginning any exercise program.
2. People over 35 (some doctors say 40) should have a checkup and possibly a stress test before taking up vigorous exercise.
3. Individuals who have suffered a muscle or joint injury should get medical advice on which forms of exercise are safe for them.
4. See your doctor if your exercise program causes you to experience lightheadedness, pain or pressure in the chest area, irregular or fluttering heartbeat, nausea, dizziness, trembling, hot or cold flashes, chronic fatigue, or numbness or pain in your neck, jaw, shoulders, or arms.

What Are Your Goals?

There are two basic types of fitness activities: aerobic and anaerobic. Aerobic exercise increases the body's intake and use of oxygen and conditions the heart and lungs to work more efficiently. This conditioning, which may lower the risk of certain types of heart disease, has become a common goal of exercisers. Running, walking, and swimming are the activities most often thought of as aerobic, but for the home, many kinds of equipment now available—rowing machines, stationary bikes, treadmills, cross-country ski machines, even jump ropes—can, if used properly, provide excellent aerobic conditioning.

Since aerobic exercise uses up calories rapidly, it is a highly effective means of losing or controlling weight—another common goal of exercisers. Regular activity means that you will be less likely to gain weight even if you eat more than you did previously. But you may find that you eat less. It has been shown that moderate exercise can often reduce appetite by increasing the efficiency of the body's appetite control mechanism—the amount of food desired is better matched to the amount required.

Even if you don't actually lose weight, you may develop a leaner, firmer body from a regular exercise program. Muscle tone can be improved by a wide range of activities, from aerobics to weight lifting to calisthenics that require virtually no equipment. The home exercise programs featured in various books, videotapes, and cassettes are useful primarily for improving muscle tone and agility. (Though many have an aerobic component, it is often not extensive enough to ensure real aerobic conditioning.)

Another goal of an exercise program can be relaxation. Any moderate exercise will probably be an effective tension reducer if performed accurately and not overdone. And since you're working out at home, you're not bound by a health club's hours: you can wind down at midnight if you choose.

Suppose building muscle size or strength is your primary goal. You are interested then in some kind of anaerobic activity, like weight lifting. In anaerobic activities, the muscles use energy that is already stored in the body. Because they do not involve the intake and use of large amounts of oxygen, anaerobic exercises do not promote cardiovascular fitness.

If you are primarily interested in strengthening and firming up your muscles, you should train with relatively light weights but do many repetitions of each exercise. If you want to significantly increase muscle size as well as build strength, you should use heavier weights but do each activity fewer times.

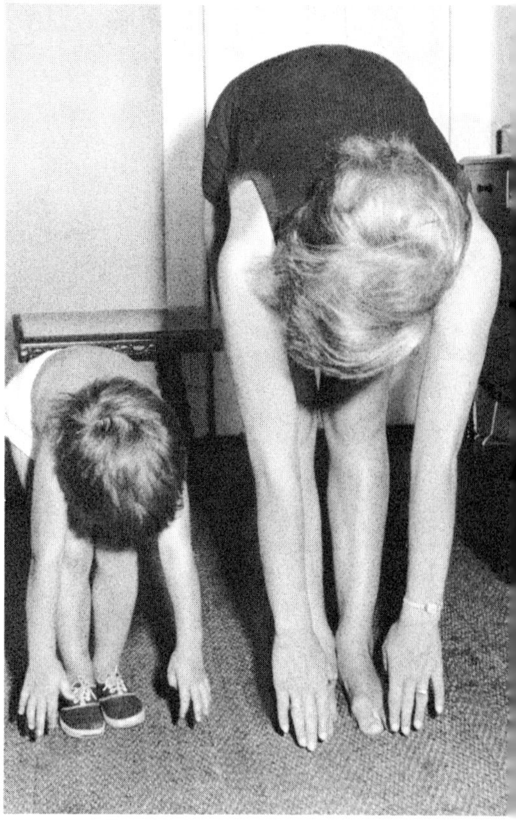

Making fitness a family affair can provide an added incentive.

To Equip or Not?

Whether or not you use equipment at home depends in part on some practical matters. How much space do you have? Some equipment can be at least partially folded up and is readily storable—but will it merely collect dust if it is not immediately handy? And some home gyms require a rather large area they can call their own.

Another consideration is financial. How much can you afford to spend? The price range for home exercise equipment is enormous—from a few dollars for a mat or a jump rope to $5,000 for a top-of-the-line, state-of-the-art minigym. To get quality equipment, particularly of the more elaborate kind, you will have to spend some money. If the cheapest machine is all you think you can afford, you may be better off forgoing it altogether and opting instead for a well-planned program of calisthenics at home or membership in a Y with good equipment.

A Few Ground Rules

There are some basic, generally agreed upon guidelines for exercising to best advantage. First, of course, learn as much as possible about the proper technique required for your chosen form of exercise. Some instruction or supervision, a book or two, and well-formed questions put to knowledgeable people should help get you started. Realize that no matter what exercise program you decide to follow, pain should not be part of it. Do not try to make your body do something it clearly resists.

Martha G. Wiseman is a writer and editor.

Pain does not mean gain. Know your limitations.

To achieve the potential benefits to your cardiovascular system from aerobic exercise, you should work out for a minimum of 30 minutes at least three times a week. The activity must be rhythmic and continuous—no starting and stopping during the exercise session. Your heart should be working at about 70 to 85 percent of its capacity. This is known as your individual target zone, which is linked to your age. To find your target zone, subtract your age from 220 and multiply the resulting figure by 0.70 and by 0.85. Your target zone—the range within which your heartbeat rate per minute should be during exercise—lies between the two numbers. In order to find out your heart rate, take your pulse for ten seconds after you've been working out for about 15 or 20 minutes, then multiply the beats you counted by six.

Many new exercise machines of different types have computers that will determine your heart rate for you and give you a readout. Also available for a few hundred dollars is a heart-monitoring minicomputer, worn on the wrist like a watch, into which you program your target zone. If you exercise beyond or below the programmed range, an alarm will sound.

It is essential to frame your minimum 30 minutes of activity with a warm-up period and a cool-down period. They get your muscles, heart, and lungs ready for vigorous exercise and let them gradually return to their normal state after they've been used hard. All experts warn that if you skip the warm-up and cool-down, you are courting injury and doing your heart no favors.

Warm-ups limber muscles and—possibly more important—increase blood flow to the muscles. If you stop exercising abruptly, your heart rate and blood pressure drop rapidly, and blood pools up in the vessels of the muscles; this means that not enough blood is circulating to the brain, heart, and other vital organs, which can cause dizziness, nausea, fainting, and irregular heartbeat. A cool-down session will prevent these problems by slowly returning your blood flow to its usual state. Five to ten minutes of low-intensity stretches are often recommended for both warming up and cooling down.

Starting Weight Training

Certain people—those with heart problems and bad backs, for instance—should not work out with weights without a doctor's approval, but even the healthiest individual must be aware of other risks of unsupervised weight training. Instruction is really a must to help you avoid lifting, pressing, and pulling in the wrong way, which can strain or tear muscles and ligaments. You should use light weights at first and work up very gradually.

Aim for a minimum of 20 minutes of weight lifting two to three times a week. To increase endurance, add calisthenics like push-ups, pull-ups, and sit-ups to your weight training. Remember to warm up and cool down before each session; this is as important in anaerobic activity as it is in aerobic exercise.

You can work toward your ideal strong self either by lifting what are known as free weights—such as barbells, sets of dumbbells, and smaller wrist or hand weights—or by exercising on the newest sleek weight training machines, which allow you to push or pull against some form of resistance. These machines, once found only in health clubs and corporate fitness centers, have entered the home market with a vengeance.

Both free weights and weight training machines have their advocates and critics. Some say that machines let the stronger side of the body assume most of the work burden, thus increasing any disparity between the two sides; machines may also overisolate and thus overdevelop particular muscle groups. Free weights, according to this point of view, can provide a more balanced workout. But barbells and dumbbells have their drawbacks, too. To get the maximum benefit, you should both raise the weight slowly (during which you encounter positive resistance, which contracts the muscle) and lower it slowly (during which negative resistance stretches the muscle). Lowering slowly, however, is not easy to do with free weights; people have a tendency to let the weight down too quickly, missing some of the potential benefit of the exercise—and also possibly risking an injury. To avoid this problem, the weight machines are designed to ensure a constant amount of resistance during both lifting and lowering, or pushing and recovering. Many experts recommend a combination of free weights and machines for a well-rounded workout.

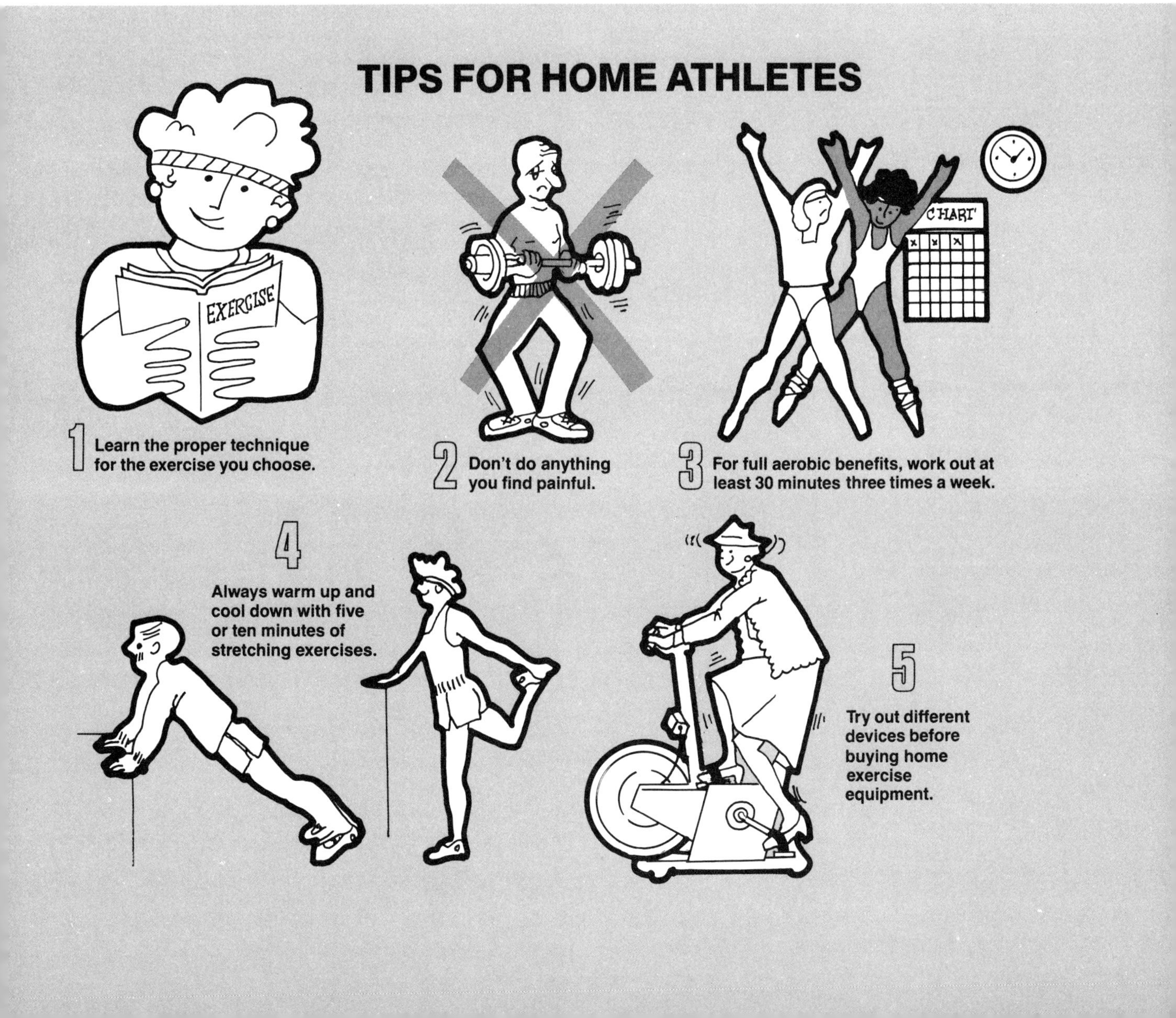

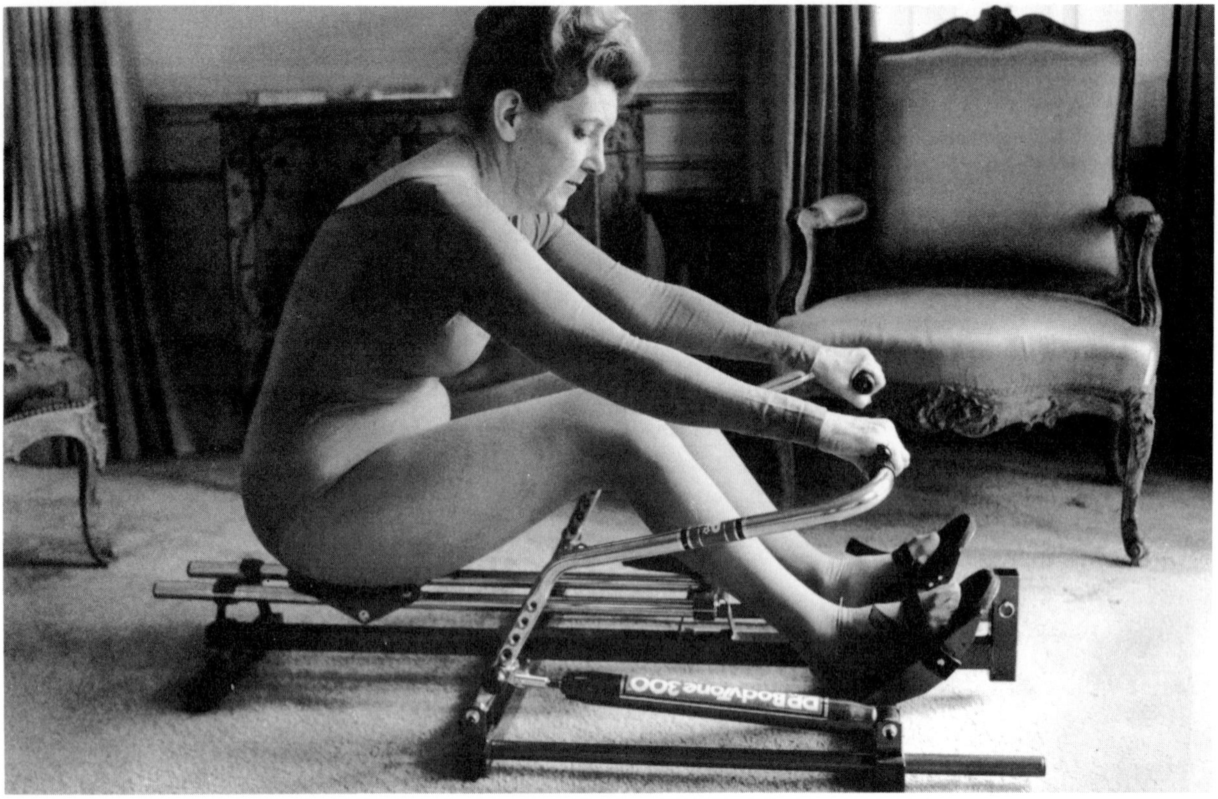

How Do the Machines Rate?

Before you invest in home exercise equipment, research it by shopping around and trying out various devices in the store. Look for a machine with solid construction and smoothness of operation. Discuss all your questions with a knowledgeable salesperson, and make sure the equipment comes with a manual that offers guidelines on proper use and care.

Rowing and cross-country ski machines. Among the aerobic exercise devices, rowing machines and cross-country ski machines are generally acknowledged to give the most thorough workout. In addition to working the heart and lungs, a rowing machine builds both upper-body and leg muscles. The seat moves backward and your legs extend as you pull back on the oars, and the seat moves forward and your knees bend as the oars move forward. Some people develop lower back pain from rowing, but this can be avoided if proper technique is used. An already bad back, however, is generally not helped by the rowing action. Rowing machines cost anywhere from $150 to nearly $600 for a rower with an electronic display of calories being burned.

With your feet strapped to "skis" that slide back and forth, and your hands pulling grips attached to a cable with pulleys or grasping "ski poles" that move back and forth along a rail, you can ski in your living room for about $450 to $600. Ski simulators are rated high for strengthening the upper and lower body and providing aerobic conditioning.

Stationary bicycles. Stationary bicycles generally work only the lower body while providing aerobic fitness, although some models have movable

Equipped To Be Fit

Rowing machines (left) and cross-country skiing machines (right) condition your heart and lungs and also give both upper body and leg muscles a thorough workout.

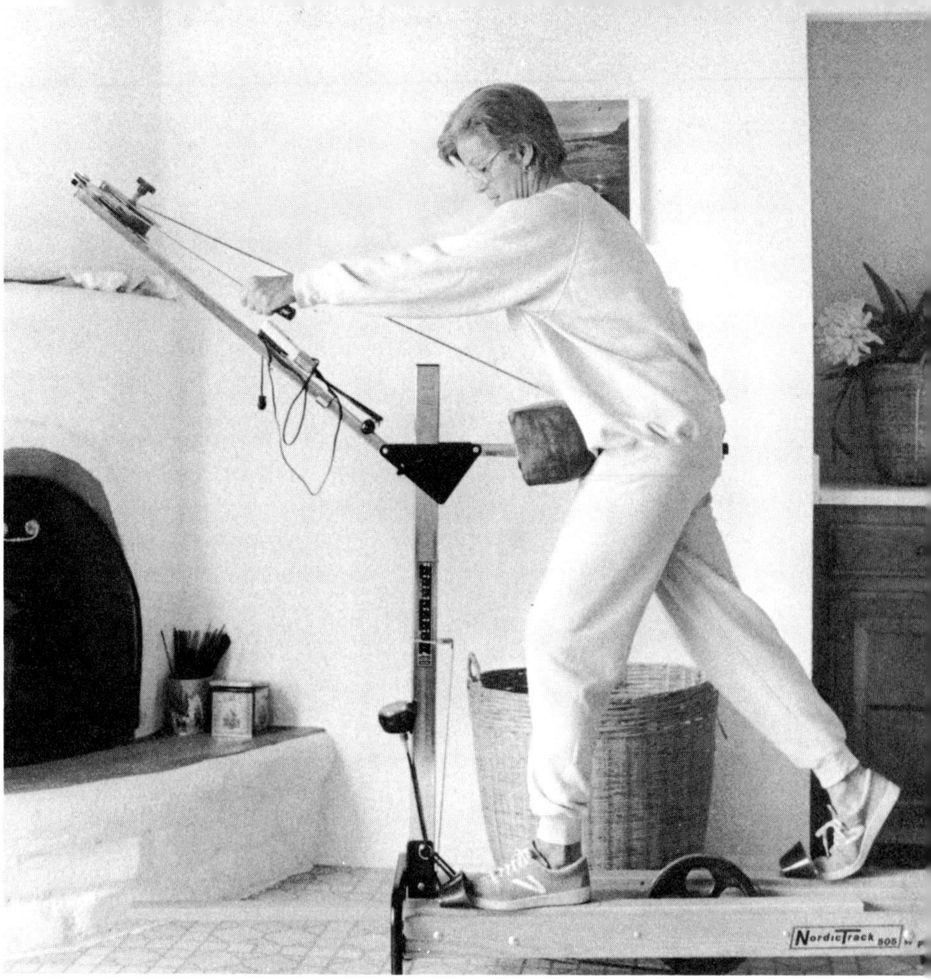

handlebars for exercising the arms. Otherwise, if you want to balance your increasing leg strength with a strong upper body, use hand weights or add some calisthenics to your bicycling regimen. Some people find the time spent on the bike boring; you can prevent boredom by reading (there are bikes with magazine holders), watching television, or listening to music. There is even an hour-long video, peddled by Cycle Vision Tours Inc., that takes you through Yellowstone Park as you pedal; other companies market similar escapist fare.

Prices of bikes vary widely: no-frills versions cost as little as $100, while bikes with adjustable pedal pressure are available for $200 to $500. Other models are equipped with more sophisticated technology: computers programmed to adjust the pedal pressure to simulate uphill grinds and downhill flying, or computers that show heart rate, calories burned, and so on. These models can cost from $600 to $1,000. Bikes made of steel, with a nylon strap (not cotton or rubber) around the flywheel, hold up best. Make sure the seat is solid, comfortable, and sturdy.

It is important to know how fast you are cycling and how much resistance you are pedaling against, so be sure to look for a bike with both a speedometer and adjustable pedal pressure. To get aerobic benefits, you must maintain a speed of more than 10 miles per hour. Set pedal pressure at a level that works your legs but does not strain them. You can also alternate between greater and less pressure in order to build strength without strain.

Treadmills. Treadmills, both motorized and nonmotorized, allow you—at some expense—to walk or jog at home. The action of walking causes the belt on a nonmotorized treadmill to move; a motorized treadmill moves its belt automatically at speeds and at simulated inclines that can be adjusted. For dedicated walkers or for those whose health limits them to walking, treadmills provide good exercise and sound cardiovascular benefits. They do, however, take up a good deal of room, and they cost from $800 to $5,000. The nonmotorized types are probably just as beneficial as the more expensive motorized models.

Jump ropes. Jump ropes are among the cheapest alternatives in terms of equipment for home use. You don't even have to buy a rope designed for jumping—you can use heavy wash line or cord instead, although some experts do recommend a durable leather jump rope. You can also buy a weighted rope, to increase the strenuousness of the activity and build upper-body strength. One new model, an 8-foot length of rubber tubing filled with silica, is available in weights from 2 to 6 pounds and sells for about $30.

Jumping rope can be either your regular form of exercise or a supplement or substitute, say, in inclement weather. To protect yourself from injury, don't jump on a concrete floor, and wear shoes that give adequate support and cushioning. If you've already had a foot, hip, or knee injury, it would probably be wise not to skip rope.

Rebounders. Small rebounders, or trampolines, are available at prices from about $50 to $150. It is not altogether clear that using a rebounder aids in aerobic conditioning. Simply bouncing on the device is probably not enough to increase the heart rate sufficiently; even if you do recommended exercises as you bounce, you still do not have to work as hard as you would on a rower or a bike. Advocates suggest that using hand weights while jumping will increase aerobic benefits. Experts advise buying a sturdy square or rectangular rebounder rather than a round one. A round surface may rotate the feet inward, throwing the legs out of alignment and creating pressure on leg joints and the back.

Inversion devices. Advocates of inversion devices like gravity boots and bars, which enable you to hang upside down, claim that this activity is relaxing, can help strengthen a bad back, and is good for your circulation. Actually, according to many experts, it can be dangerous and should be attempted with caution if at all. According to many physicians, inversion devices can actually hurt the back and can raise blood pressure substantially, which is especially dangerous for anyone with glaucoma or hypertension.

Weight training machines. Perhaps the best way to find out which sort of machine you want for weight training is to work on one under supervision in a club or a sports training facility. A large variety of minigyms are now available. There are the elaborate multistation machines, on which you can exercise various sets of muscles, and there are machines made specifically for individual muscle groups—abdominals, upper body, thighs, and arms. Costs range from $500 to $5,000. Resistance is provided by stacks of weights on cables, by springs, by rubber straps, or by hydraulic systems (these are the most expensive).

Free weights. Free weights are inexpensive by comparison with machines. Hand-held weights of various kinds are available for $10 to $30 a pair. Steel weights are often recommended (they can't break like vinyl-covered cement ones), but they cost a little more, perhaps $40 to $50 for a

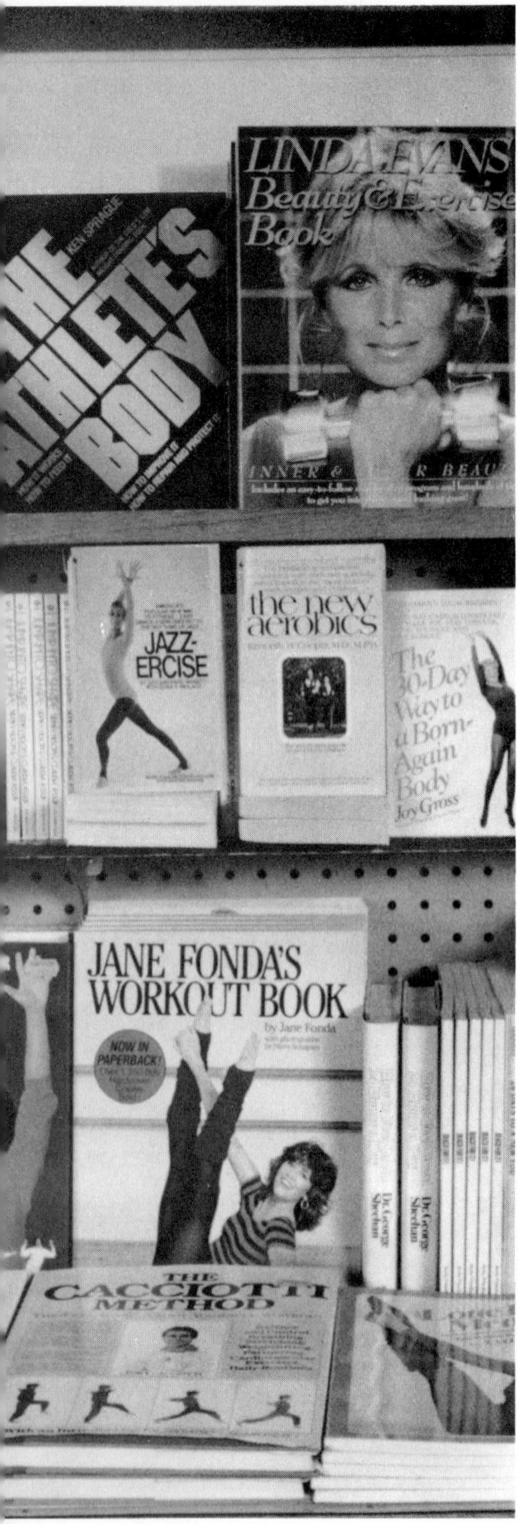

Celebrities may inspire you, but beware of unrealistic goals.

pair of dumbbells, or twice that for a dumbbell set with attachable weights of different sizes. A barbell set might cost $200 to $300, and you can purchase a bench from which to lift your weights for $50 to $200.

At Home With the Stars

The promise of a leaner, healthier body is frequently implied by the books, cassettes, records, and videos on home exercise programs—presumably a body like that of the celebrity/author/instructor. The encouraging voice and the image of the in-shape star may serve to motivate some at-homers. However, orthopedists and sports medicine experts advise caution in following these programs.

First, some of the recommended exercises may be questionable—carrying a fairly high risk of injury. Second, the programs tend to encourage people to push themselves beyond safe limits. According to doctors, Jane Fonda's exhortation to "go for the burn" is simply bad advice and should not be heeded. Patient records of orthopedists are filled with instances of injuries caused by home workouts. Warm-ups and cool-downs often tend to get short shrift, and people are urged to plunge into vigorous exercises too quickly.

Choose your program wisely, start slowly, and work steadily.

On the other hand, though most of these programs cannot offer a thoroughgoing fitness workout, they may be very helpful in improving flexibility and imparting a greater sense of physical well-being, particularly for those who want to exercise indoors but have limited space and money. Most of these programs are amalgams of basic calisthenics, dance training stretches, and yoga exercises. Some also use hand-held weights. Make sure, if your choose one of these programs, that exercises and positions are well explained and easy to understand and follow.

There are several more pointers to help you avoid injury while following an exercise routine at home. Don't bounce in any position; this can tear ligaments and does nothing for your stretch. Don't hold your breath. And if any exercise or position hurts, don't do it. Remember that many of the instructors featured in these programs are not experts; what works for them may not work for you. You may discover, though, that you can adapt exercises to your own abilities. □

SUGGESTIONS FOR FURTHER READING

ALTER, JUDY. *Surviving Exercise.* Boston, Houghton Mifflin, 1983.

ANDERSON, BOB. *Stretching.* Bolinas, Calif., Shelter Publications, 1980.

CANNELL, MICHAEL T. *The At-Home Gym: Stationary Bicycles.* New York, Villard Books, 1985.

KUNTZLEMAN, CHARLES H. *Home Gym Fitness: Free Weight Workouts.* Chicago, Contemporary Books, 1983.

LAFAVORE, MICHAEL. *The Home Gym: A Guide to Fitness Equipment.* New York, Avon, 1984.

NETTER, PATRICK. *Patrick Netter's High-Tech Fitness.* New York, Workman Publishing, 1984.

ZIMMER, JUDITH. *The At-Home Gym: Weight Machines.* New York, Villard Books, 1985.

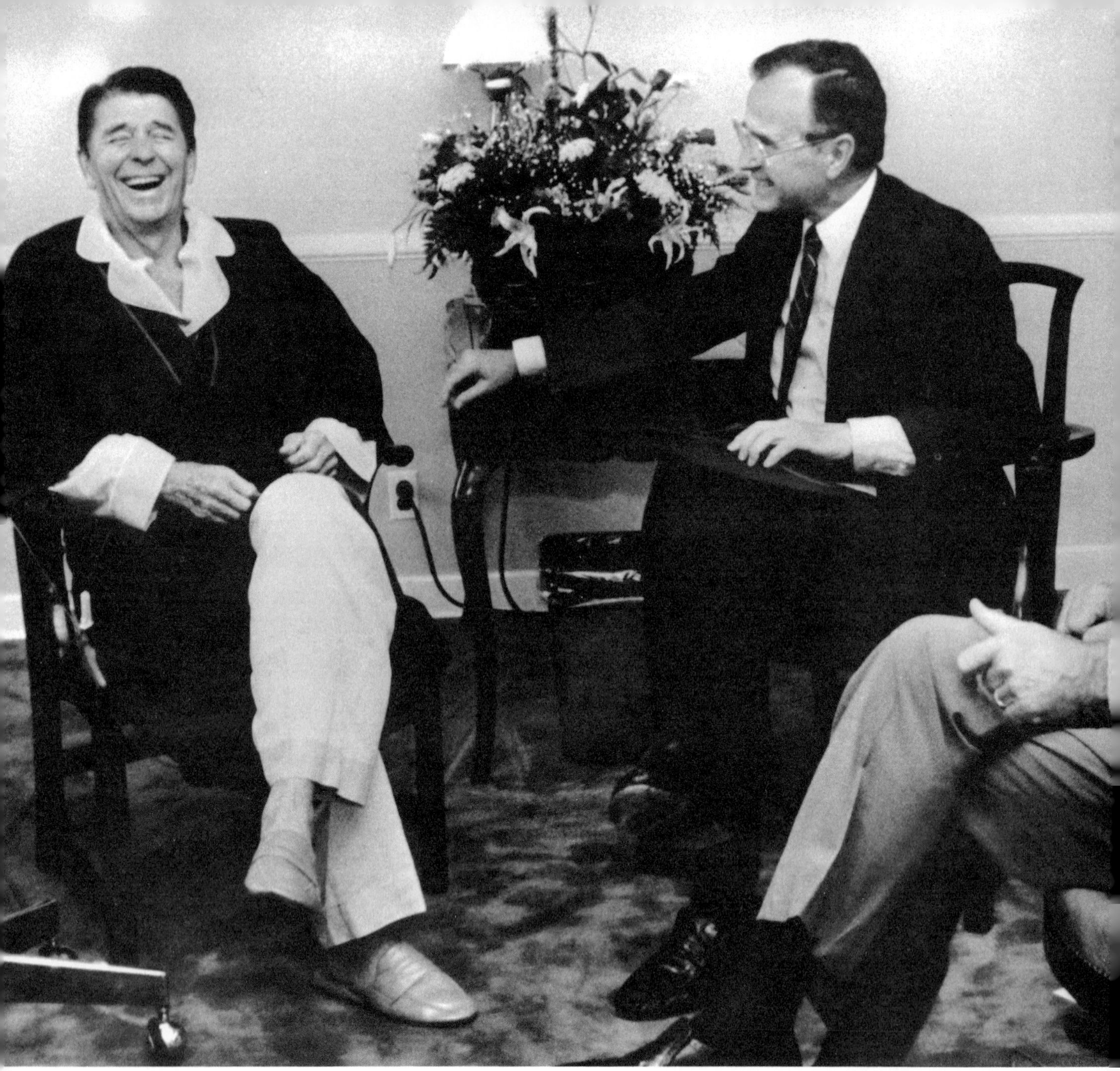

Colon Cancer

Prevention and Treatment

Daniel Pelot, M.D.

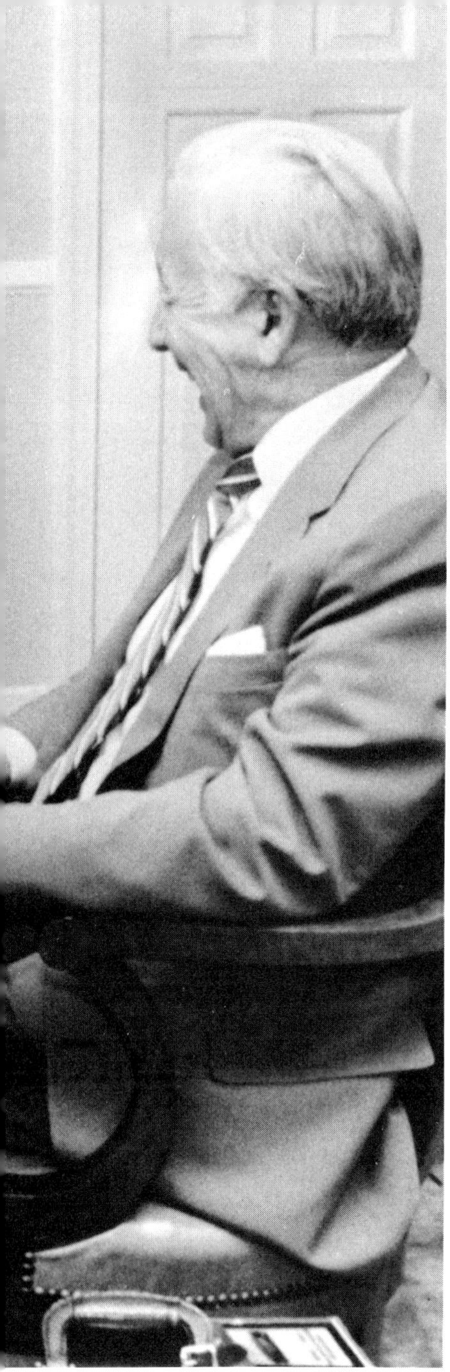

President Ronald Reagan—shown in the hospital with Vice-President George Bush (center) and White House Chief of Staff Donald Regan (right)—underwent surgery for colon cancer in 1985.

Colorectal cancer—cancer of the large intestine—causes more deaths in the United States and Canada than any other type of malignancy except lung cancer. The American Cancer Society estimated that in 1985, 138,000 new cases of colorectal cancer would be diagnosed in the United States and 60,000 people would die from the disease. According to the Canadian Cancer Society, 10,380 new cases and 5,220 deaths were expected in Canada. The diagnosis of colon cancer in President Ronald Reagan in mid-1985 drew widespread public attention to the disease—which is extremely important since early detection and treatment can literally mean the difference between life and death.

The large intestine is the final loop for food passing through the digestive system. Its principal parts are the colon and, in its last few inches, the rectum. Shorter but wider than the small intestine, the large intestine absorbs fluids and essential chemical substances from undigestible food residues and stores semisolid wastes. Unfortunately, it is subject to many disorders, of which colorectal cancer is one of the most serious.

Who Is at Risk?

In general, colorectal cancer is far more common in developed than underdeveloped countries. Its incidence is high in North America and Europe and low in South America, Africa, and Asia; the United States has one of the highest rates in the world. Although Japan is a developed country, it has a low incidence.

These incidence rates appear to be related to dietary habits. Japanese immigrants to Hawaii and the U.S. mainland have a higher incidence of the disease than Japanese living in Japan, apparently because they adopt the U.S. diet, high in fat and animal protein (particularly from beef). In the traditional Japanese diet, key protein sources are fish and vegetables, both of which are low in fat. It has been suggested that the Western diet leads to the presence of certain types of bacteria in the colon that are able to convert foods or intestinal secretions into potential cancer-causing substances (carcinogens).

Dietary factors other than meat or fat have also been implicated in the development of colorectal cancer. In some African populations with low incidences of this cancer, the typical diet contains more fiber and fewer refined carbohydrates than the diet in more developed areas. (Typical refined carbohydrates are processed cereals and white flour, from which the outer coating, or bran, of the grain has been removed.) High-fiber diets cause waste to move rapidly through the intestinal tract, so that carcinogens may be in contact with the lining of the colon for a shorter time. Also, various components of fiber may combine with carcinogens or may increase the bulk inside the colon, thereby diluting the strength of cancer-causing substances.

Apart from diet, there are other factors that place individuals at a greater than average risk for colorectal cancer. These include age above

40 years (at 50 the risk increases sharply, with continuing marked increases in subsequent decades until a peak is reached at 75 to 80), a personal history of prior colorectal growths called polyps or of colorectal cancer, a family history of colorectal cancer, long-standing ulcerative colitis (a severe inflammation of the colon), and hereditary colon polyposis syndromes (inherited conditions resulting in multiple polyps in the intestines).

Polyps and Colorectal Cancer

Polyps are growths of new tissue on the lining of the intestine. They are often benign, but they are important because of their suspected role in the development of colorectal cancer. Polpys are classified as either hyperplastic (an increased number of normal cells) or neoplastic (a growth of abnormal cells); hyperplastic growths are benign, but neoplastic growths may be benign or malignant. A small hyperplastic polyp was found in and removed from President Reagan's colon in May 1984. The next year, a routine checkup revealed a second benign polyp. Eventually, further tests showed a much larger growth, which was surgically removed and ultimately found to be malignant.

Polyps are also classified by shape. The most common polyp is the adenoma, which occurs as one of three distinct types: a tubular adenoma (sometimes called an adenomatous polyp), the most common, which looks grapelike and usually has a smooth surface; a villous adenoma, which is irregular in shape and has fingerlike surface projections; and a tubulovillous adenoma, with features of the first two types. Villous adenomas have a marked tendency to become malignant; up to 50 percent of these growths removed from the colon show evidence of cancer. By contrast, only about 5 percent of adenomatous polyps display evidence of cancer. Tubulovillous growths are intermediate in risk. Since people who have polyps seem to be at an increased risk of developing colorectal cancer, the detection and removal of polyps can significantly decrease the incidence of the disease.

Colorectal cancer affects thousands of Americans annually.

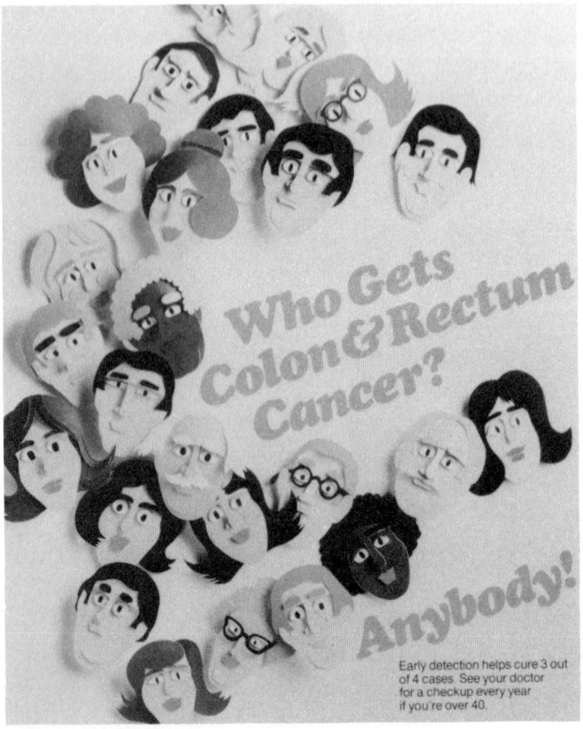

Warning Signs

Warning signs that colorectal cancer has developed may include changes in bowel habits and visible blood in the stool. Whether such symptoms occur is determined to a great extent by the location and function of the segment of the intestine in which the tumor is located. Cancers in the right (ascending) colon tend to be large and without obvious symptoms; although they are accompanied by anemia due to bleeding, often the blood is "occult" (not visible to the naked eye) in the stool. Cancers in the left (descending) colon and in the rectum cause obstructive symptoms at an earlier stage; there is usually gradual but progressive constipation or smaller-diameter stools and bright red blood in the stool.

Prevention and Early Detection

Dietary changes to increase fiber and decrease fat intake have been advocated by the U.S. National Cancer Institute to decrease the risk of colorectal cancer (although there is no conclusive evidence that a low-fat, high-fiber diet is effective in preventing the disease). In the United States and Canada the average person consumes under 20 grams of dietary fiber a day. There is no "official" recommended dietary allowance for fiber, but 30 to 40 grams a day has been suggested as a moderate, healthful level. Even if high-fiber foods do not prevent colorectal cancer, they are

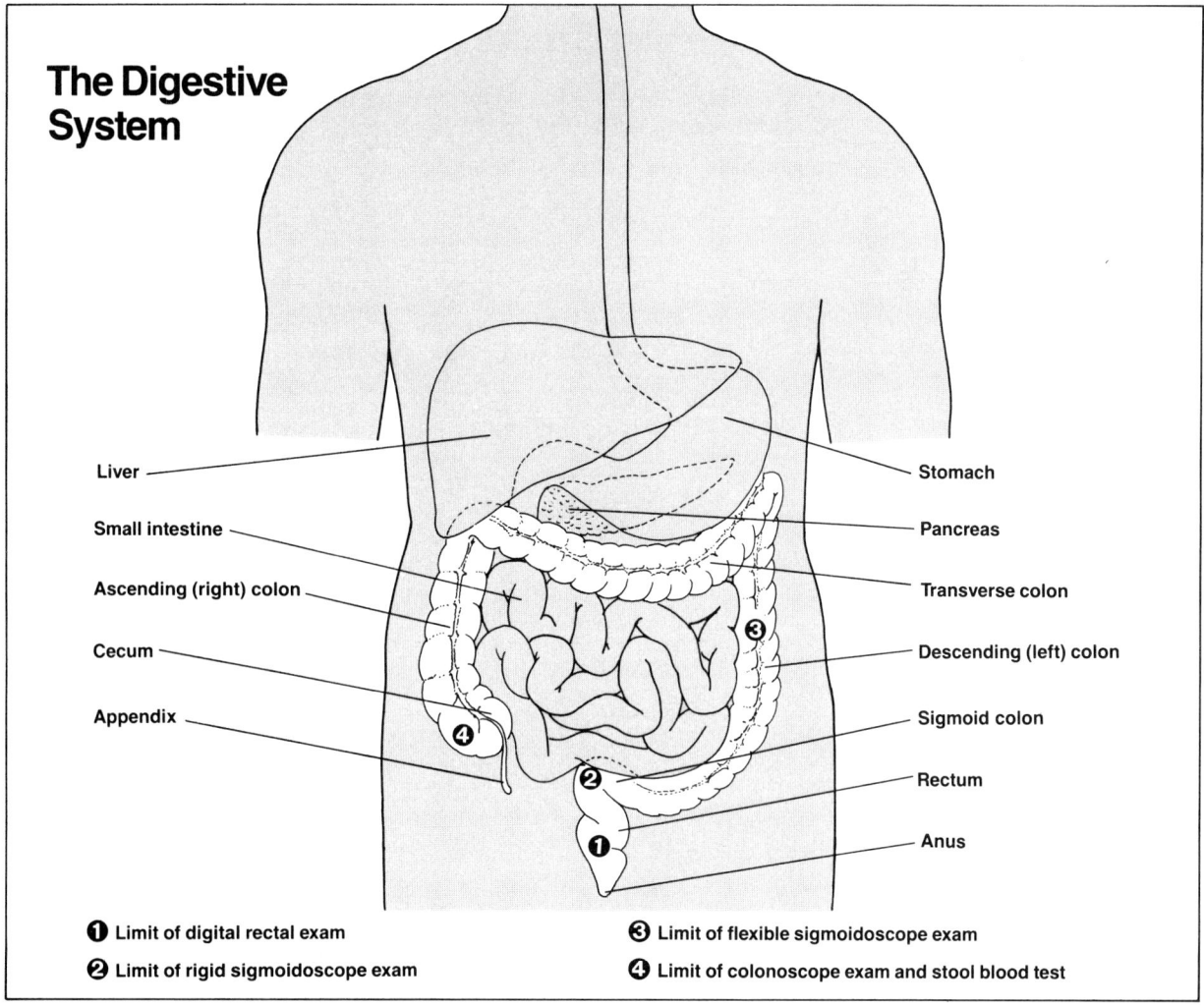

The Digestive System

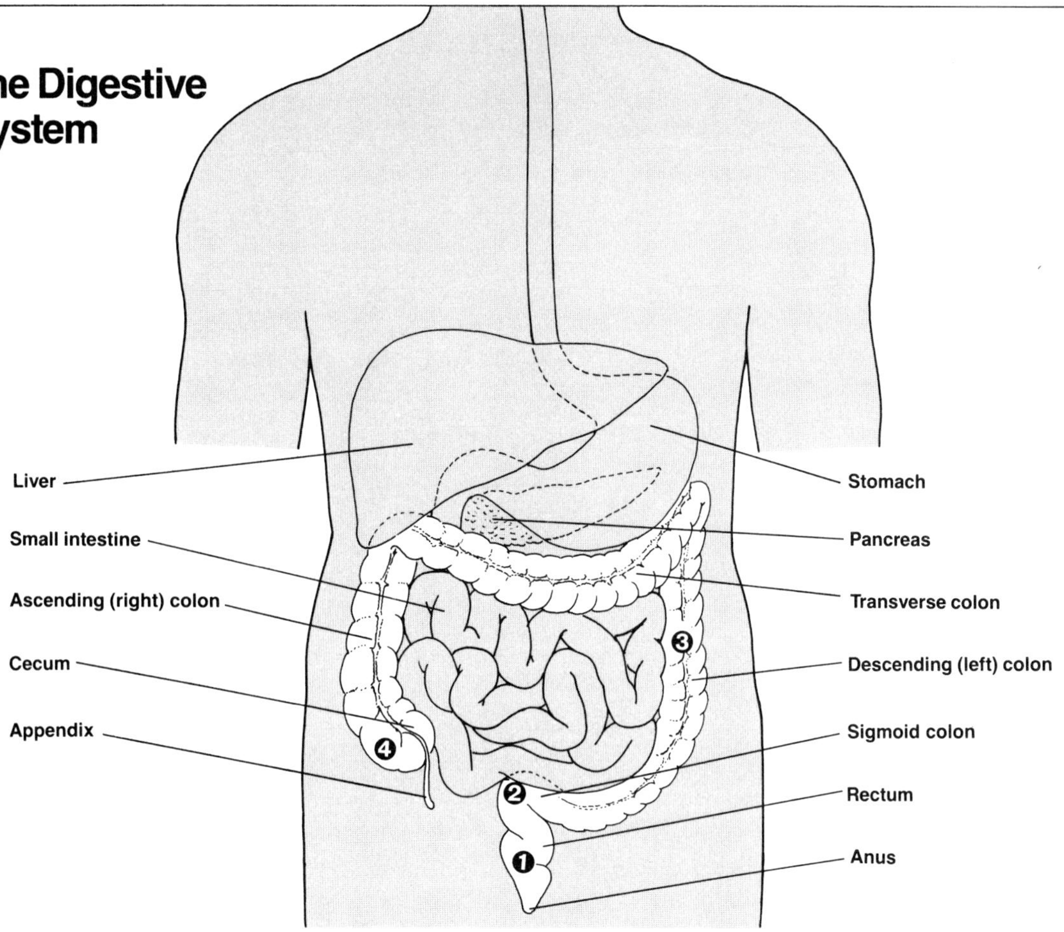

❶ Limit of digital rectal exam
❷ Limit of rigid sigmoidoscope exam
❸ Limit of flexible sigmoidoscope exam
❹ Limit of colonoscope exam and stool blood test

certainly a wholesome substitute for fatty foods, which cause a number of health problems. Some doctors recommend an increase in calcium intake as well; recent studies show that calcium may help decrease the risk of colorectal cancer.

Another line of defense is the detection and removal of colorectal cancers early enough to achieve cure of the disease, as well as the detection and removal of polyps before they can perhaps develop into cancers. People considered to be at risk should be screened for such growths even if they are without symptoms.

Screening Tests

Because of late diagnosis, at present only about 50 percent of patients with colorectal cancer survive for five years or longer after the disease is found. If the disease is diagnosed early, however, the five-year survival rate is greater than 75 percent. It is obvious that detection of colorectal cancer before symptoms appear is all-important. Several screening and diagnostic techniques are helpful in early detection.

Digital rectal examination. This quick, simple, and inexpensive office procedure allows the doctor to feel some rectal tumors without the use of instruments. It detects about 10 percent of all colorectal cancers. The American Cancer Society recommends an annual digital rectal examination for all persons 40 years of age or over.

Testing for occult blood. Occult blood in the stool can be detected by testing the stool with certain chemicals. The test most commonly used by physicians, the Hemoccult slide test, is performed on stool obtained from bowel movements on three consecutive days and is most effective when the

---

Daniel Pelot is Associate Clinical Professor in the Division of Gastroenterology, Department of Medicine, University of California at Irvine.

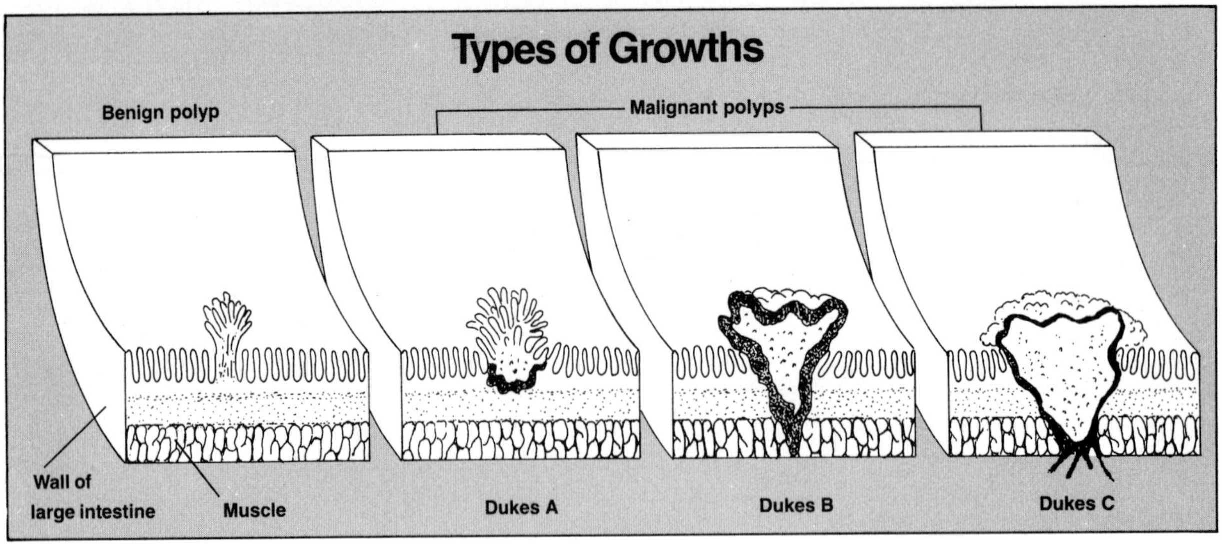

patient has been on a diet that is high in fiber and free of red meat for the preceding several days. A person who tests positive while on a normal diet should switch to the restricted diet and repeat the test.

In 1983 the U.S. Food and Drug Administration approved for over-the-counter sale the Fleet Detecatest, which yields results without laboratory analysis and can therefore be performed at home. The test requires smearing two samples of stool a day for three consecutive days onto a paper slide containing the chemical guaiac. Several drops of another chemical are then added to the slide. The appearance or absence of a blue color indicates the presence or absence, respectively, of hidden blood. Other over-the-counter tests to detect occult blood in the stool are also now available in the United States and Canada.

Although the home tests are essentially the same as the Hemoccult test used by many doctors and can be helpful in diagnosis, doctors have voiced concern that without professional supervision, some people may misinterpret the results. Some people with negative test results may conclude that they are healthy and do not need to see a doctor. But a negative result means only that no blood was detected, not that there is no serious condition. Many tumors do not bleed or bleed sporadically.

Similarly, a positive result does not necessarily mean a person has cancer, since it can reflect the existence of blood in the digestive tract from a variety of causes: a nosebleed that occurred a day or two before the test, bleeding peptic ulcers, bleeding hemorrhoids, or even bleeding gums. Eating rare meat or taking vitamin C or aspirin may also cause a positive result. Of those people with positive tests, about half have either a benign growth or a cancer; the rest have some other condition or no disorder at all. It is important, therefore, that a person with a positive result undergo other, more definitive tests—for example, barium enema X rays (in which X-ray films are made after a barium liquid is inserted through the rectum into the colon), sigmoidoscopy, or colonoscopy.

The American Cancer Society recommends that persons over 50 years of age be tested annually for the presence of blood in the stool. The test may also be used to screen younger people who are at high risk for developing colorectal cancer.

Sigmoidoscopy. Another method of detecting colorectal cancer before symptoms appear is conventional proctosigmoidoscopy, in which the physician is able to see into the rectum and lower colon (the location of about half of all colon cancers) by means of a hollow, rigid tube containing a light source. The American Cancer Society recommends that persons over 50 have two initial proctosigmoidoscopies, a year apart, with the examination repeated every three to five years thereafter if the two initial exams are negative. Because of the discomfort involved, many people avoid this procedure. The proctosigmoidoscope can examine only the lower 10 inches of the large intestine.

Several years ago, a flexible fiber-optic sigmoidoscope was developed that is less uncomfortable for the patient and permits the doctor to examine the lower 25 inches of the large intestine. Many more lower colon abnormalities are detected with this instrument than with the rigid sigmoidoscope. At present, its use is limited because it is more expensive and requires greater skill on the part of the physician.

Colonoscopy. The colonoscope, a fully flexible instrument capable of examining the entire large intestine, was introduced in the early 1970's and has since come into wide use. (It was with this instrument that President Reagan's doctors, on July 12, 1985, removed his second polyp and found the larger growth that they took out surgically the next day.) In making possible direct examination of the entire large intestine, the colonoscope has added greatly to the capability for early detection of colorectal cancer. Besides being considerably more accurate than barium X rays in detecting colon abnormalities, the colonoscope has the added advantage of permitting nonsurgical removal of certain growths by means of a radio-frequency current passed through to a remotely controlled wire snare at the far end of the scope. Colonoscopy is not intended as a routine screening procedure; it can take 1½ hours, and the patient must be given a sedative. Rather, it is performed on persons with occult blood in the stool or an abnormality detected in a barium X ray and used for screening high-risk patients.

Stages of Colorectal Cancer

Once a malignant growth has been detected, doctors find it helpful to "stage" (classify) the tumor before deciding on a course of treatment. The staging systems used in colorectal cancer are based on a system devised by Cuthbert Dukes, a British pathologist, in 1932 (see the accompanying diagram). Dukes demonstrated that long-term survival is related to the degree to which the tumor has penetrated various layers of the intestinal wall and the extent of lymph node involvement near the tumor. Generally, Dukes stage A tumors have invaded only the inner lining of the intestine. Stage B tumors have invaded the muscles in the intestinal wall, and stage C growths have penetrated through the wall and into the lymph nodes. Five-year survival rates following removal of the tumor are 80 to 90 percent for patients with a Dukes A growth, 70 to 80 percent for Dukes B, and 30 to 50 percent for Dukes C. The cancer removed from President Reagan's colon in July 1985 was classified as a Dukes stage B tumor.

The term Dukes stage D is occasionally used for cancers that have spread to the liver or other organs. In general, the greater the spread of the disease beyond its original site to other parts of the body, through the lymph system or bloodstream, the less likely it becomes that the patient can be cured.

Treatment

Surgical removal of the tumor is the primary and most effective method of treating colorectal cancer. The location of the cancer within the colon and its Dukes stage determine the type of operation performed. President Reagan's cancer was located in the cecum, where the small intestine joins the large intestine. As is usual for cancers in this location, the segment of right colon containing the cancer was removed and the healthy end attached directly to the nearby small intestine without the need for a colostomy—surgical creation of an opening from the large intestine to the surface of the abdominal wall, for the elimination of waste. For cancers in the left colon, the cancerous part of the large intestine is removed and the remaining healthy parts reconnected. If the cancer is in the transverse colon, that part of the colon is removed along with the right colon; the left colon is then connected to the small intestine. And if the cancer is in the sigmoid colon (just above the rectum) or in the rectal area, a colostomy is probably necessary following removal of the cancerous region.

Nonsurgical forms of treatment, including chemotherapy and radiation therapy, also play a role. The goal of such treatment is to prevent recurrence following surgical removal of the tumor or to offer relief of symptoms if the tumor cannot be removed surgically or when the cancer has spread. □

SUGGESTIONS FOR FURTHER READING

HECHT, ANNABEL. "The Colon Goes Up, Over, Down and Out." *FDA Consumer*, June 1984, pp. 28-32.

"What Everyone Should Know About Colorectal Cancer" and "Colorectal Cancer: Go for Early Detection," free brochures available from the American Cancer Society.

SOURCES OF FURTHER INFORMATION

American Cancer Society, 90 Park Avenue, New York, N.Y. 10016.

Canadian Cancer Society, 77 Bloor Street West, Suite 401, Toronto, Ontario M5S 2V7.

National Cancer Institute, 9000 Wisconsin Avenue, Bethesda, Md. 20205.

WHAT IS GENETIC

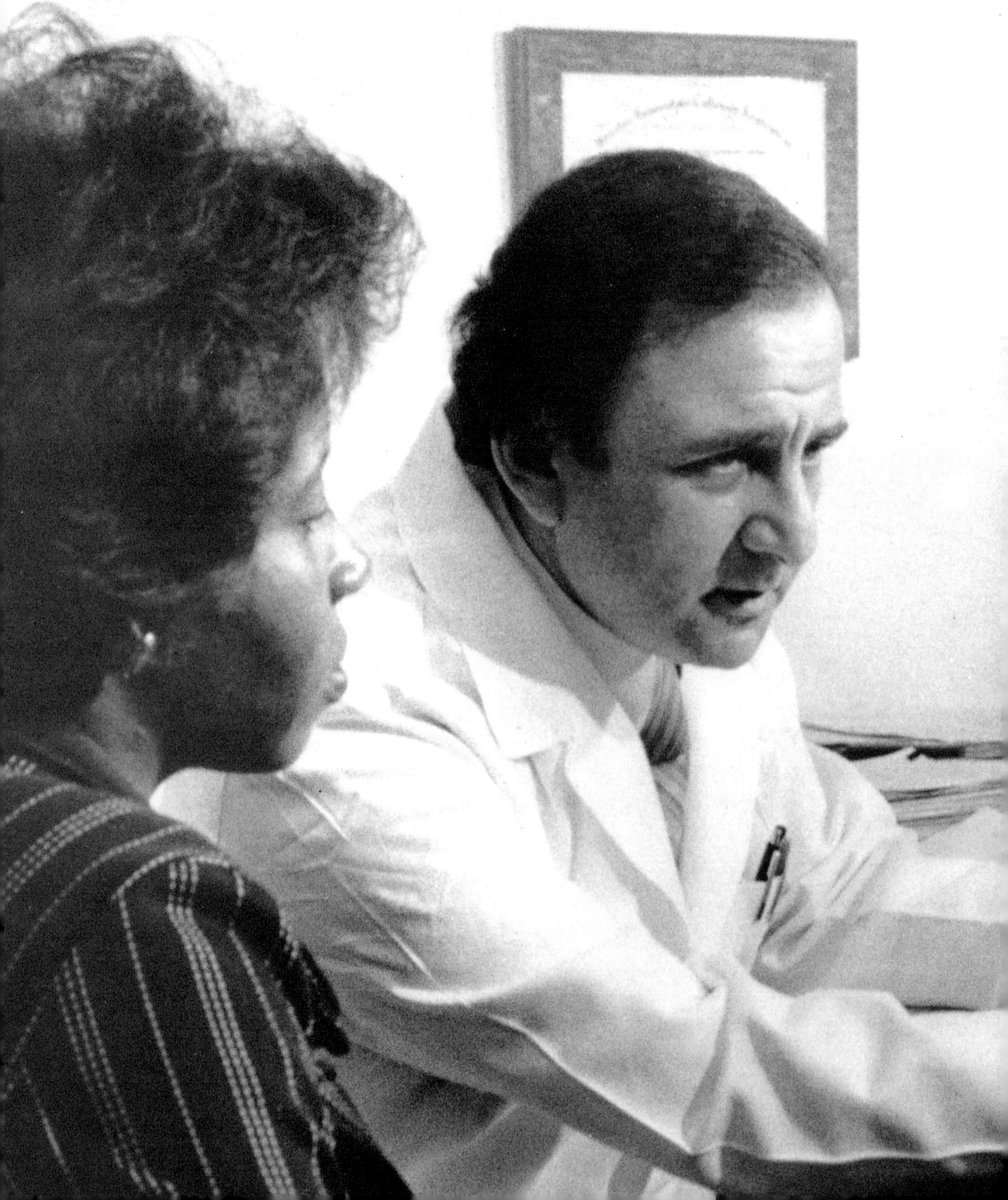

COUNSELING ?

Diane J. Rosenthal

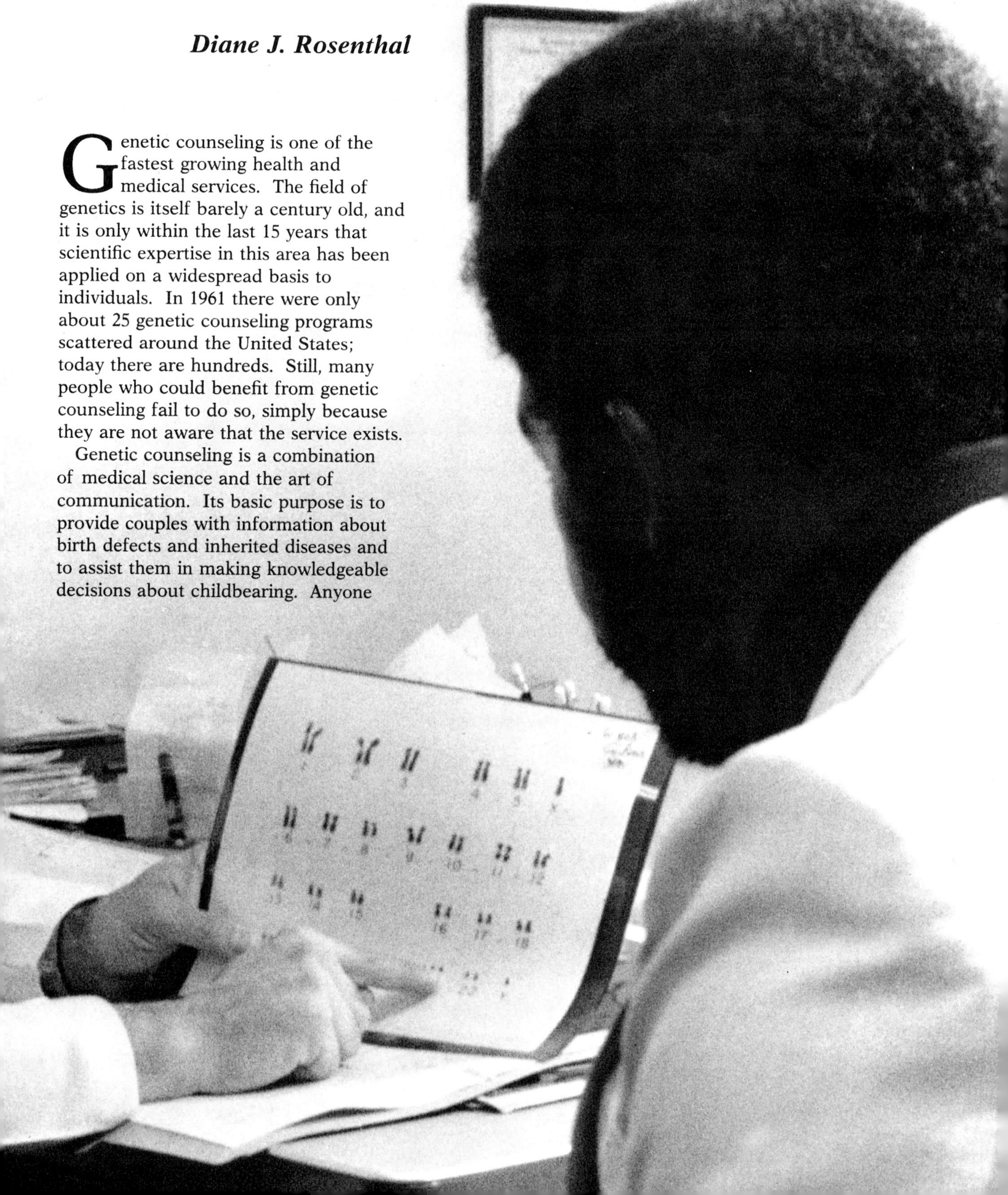

Genetic counseling is one of the fastest growing health and medical services. The field of genetics is itself barely a century old, and it is only within the last 15 years that scientific expertise in this area has been applied on a widespread basis to individuals. In 1961 there were only about 25 genetic counseling programs scattered around the United States; today there are hundreds. Still, many people who could benefit from genetic counseling fail to do so, simply because they are not aware that the service exists.

Genetic counseling is a combination of medical science and the art of communication. Its basic purpose is to provide couples with information about birth defects and inherited diseases and to assist them in making knowledgeable decisions about childbearing. Anyone who suspects that he or she is at greater than normal risk of having a child with a birth defect is a candidate for genetic counseling. This includes pregnant women age 35 or older, couples who have already had a child with a birth defect, couples with a family history of a birth defect or inherited disease, and members of ethnic groups in which certain genetic disorders are most prevalent.

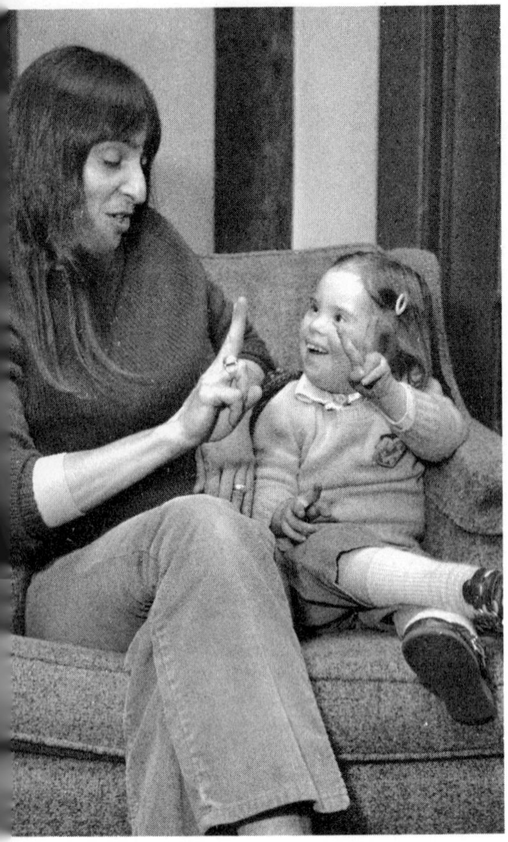

This child has Down's syndrome, one of the most common genetic disorders; its incidence increases with the age of the mother.

In a few cases genetic counseling may lead directly to the detection and treatment of defects that would otherwise leave a newborn seriously impaired. More often, the benefits of genetic counseling are educational, providing a couple with a clearer picture of the odds of having a child with a birth defect, a better understanding of what such defects may entail, and a careful assessment of the available options.

Often the outcome is reassuring: many couples discover that the potential dangers are much less than they had thought. On the other hand, some couples may find themselves faced with extremely difficult decisions regarding a current pregnancy or the prospect of future childbearing. The genetic counselor's role then becomes one of helping them choose a course that best accords with their individual beliefs and needs. Genetic counselors do not advocate a given position or attempt to influence a couple's decision; rather, they provide factual information and seek to encourage an honest discussion of the situation.

Although genetic counseling may be provided by a family physician or obstetrician, most people seeking counseling are referred to university medical centers that offer specialized programs in the field. In the past, the counseling was almost always done by physicians with expertise in genetics; recently, however, specially trained genetic counselors with a master's degree in medical genetics and counseling are providing the service. In addition, some counselors are nurses or social workers with training in both genetics and counseling techniques.

Genes and Chromosomes

All of our inherited traits and characteristics are determined by genes, the basic biochemical units of heredity. Each of us has approximately 50,000 gene pairs (one set supplied by each parent) that regulate the growth and function of our cells, tissues, and organs. This genetic material is contained in tightly coiled structures called chromosomes, housed in the nuclei of our cells. In humans, each cell nucleus contains 23 pairs of chromosomes, or 46 in all; the only exceptions are the reproductive cells—the sperm and the egg—each of which contains just 23 single chromosomes. At fertilization, the 23 chromosomes from the sperm match up with the 23 from the egg to form the full complement of 46: the blueprint for a new and unique individual.

Human reproduction is such a complex process that it is remarkable that genetic abnormalities are so infrequent. As it is, an estimated 2 to 3 percent of babies in the United States are born with major genetic defects, and another 5 to 10 percent may have less serious or minor (sometimes barely noticeable) abnormalities. In addition, another 4 to 5 percent of

---

Diane J. Rosenthal is a free-lance medical writer and editor.

babies have genetic-related susceptibilities that may eventually show up in later life in disorders such as diabetes, heart disease, and certain types of cancer and mental illness.

Genetic Defects

There are three basic types of genetically inherited disorders: chromosomal abnormalities, single-gene defects, and multifactorial defects.

Chromosomal abnormalities. These are defects in the structure or number of chromosomes, usually caused by an error of development in

The Risk of Abnormalities

The risk of Down's syndrome and other chromosomal abnormalities increases with the mother's age.

Maternal Age	Down's Syndrome Risk	Risk of Any Significant Chromosomal Abnormality
15 or under	1:1,000	1:455
18	1:1,429	1:526
21	1:1,429–1:2,000	1:526
24	1:1,111–1:1,429	1:476
27	1:1,000–1:1,250	1:455
30	1:833–1:1,111	1:385
32	1:667–1:909	1:323
34	1:417–1:526	1:244
35	1:256–1:400	1:179
36	1:200–1:313	1:149
37	1:156–1:244	1:123
38	1:123–1:192	1:105
39	1:95–1:152	1:81
40	1:73–1:118	1:63
41	1:56–1:93	1:49
42	1:43–1:72	1:39
43	1:33–1:57	1:31
44	1:25–1:44	1:24
45	1:19–1:35	1:18
46	1:15–1:27	1:15
47	1:11–1:21	1:11
48	1:9–1:17	1:9
49	1:6–1:13	1:7

Reprinted with permission from Ernest B. Hook, M.D., and The American College of Obstetricians and Gynecologists. (*Obstetrics and Gynecology*, Vol. 58, No. 3, 1981, pp. 282-285.)

the sperm or egg. The most common example is Down's syndrome, once called mongolism, in which the fetal cells contain one chromosome too many (specifically, an extra copy of chromosome number 21). Children with Down's syndrome tend to have characteristic facial features and generally short stature, are mentally retarded, and may be born with heart disease. Other, less common, chromosomal abnormalities usually produce more severe mental retardation and physical defects than are found in Down's syndrome. The risk of chromosomal abnormalities increases markedly with the mother's age (see the table on page 73).

Single-gene defects. All of us receive a few improperly functioning genes from our parents, but in the great majority of cases, no functional defects result. This is because genes work in pairs, and a malfunctioning gene from one parent is usually compensated for by a properly functioning gene from the other parent. In such cases the trait controlled by the malfunctioning gene is said to be "recessive"—the trait does not show up in the baby—and the characteristic controlled by its normally functioning partner is "dominant"—the trait does appear. Sometimes, however, the improperly functioning gene is dominant, and a child receiving this gene will be born with a defect. This is the case in Huntington's disease (a progressive neurological disease), achondroplasia (a form of dwarfism), and polydactyly (extra fingers or toes).

Blood tests can show prospective parents if they are carriers of some inherited diseases.

Inherited disorders can also occur if both parents pass on an improperly functioning recessive gene for a given trait. Included among the approximately 1,200 recessively inherited disorders are a number of diseases largely confined to certain ethnic groups, such as Tay-Sachs disease, a progressive, ultimately fatal childhood neurological disorder that primarily affects descendants of Eastern European Jews. In sickle-cell anemia, a disease most prevalent among blacks, red blood cells are abnormally shaped and cannot circulate easily; hence the body does not receive the oxygen it needs to function. The various forms of thalassemia, most common among people of Mediterranean ancestry, also affect the red blood cells.

A third group of single-gene disorders are those that follow a sex-linked pattern of inheritance. The malfunctioning gene is located on the X chromosome, one of the chromosomes that determines a child's sex. (Normal females have two X chromosomes, and normal males have one X and one Y.) Typically these disorders are carried by the mother on one of her X chromosomes, but they affect only her male offspring. Examples include color blindness, hemophilia, and some forms of muscular dystrophy. When a carrier mother and a normal father conceive, there is a 50 percent chance that a male child will have the disorder and a 50 percent chance that a female child will be a carrier.

Multifactorial defects. These disorders are probably the most common and least understood of all genetic disorders. They result from the interaction of several different genes or from the effects of the environment on certain susceptible genes. Examples include spina bifida and anencephaly (severe disorders in which the fetal spine and brain, respectively, do not develop properly), cleft palate, diabetes, and most congenital heart defects. If a couple has already had one child with a multifactorial genetic problem, the chances of recurrence in a future child are approximately 1 to 5 percent.

HOW GENETIC DEFECTS ARE INHERITED

Dominant Inheritance

One parent, who has the condition, has a faulty gene (**D**) that is dominant – it dominates the normal gene (**n**). The other parent has two normal genes. Each child has a 50 percent chance of inheriting the condition.

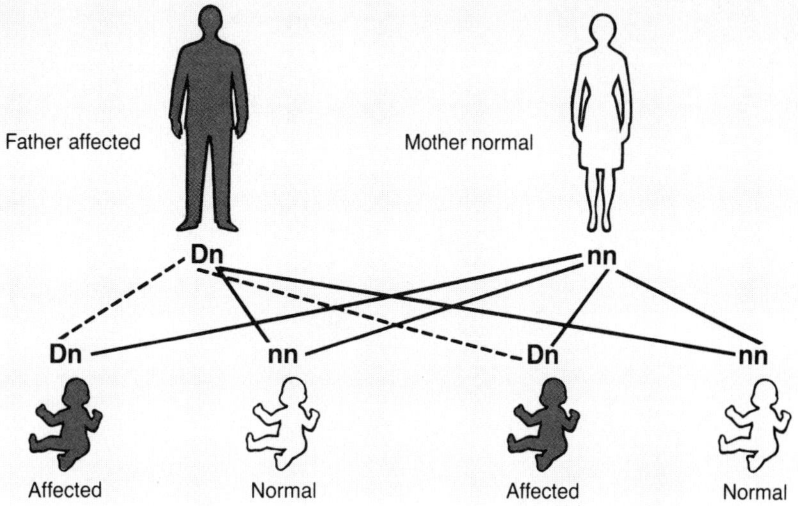

Recessive Inheritance

Both parents are carriers of the condition: each has a normal dominant gene (**N**) and a faulty recessive gene (**r**). Each child has a 25 percent chance of inheriting the condition.

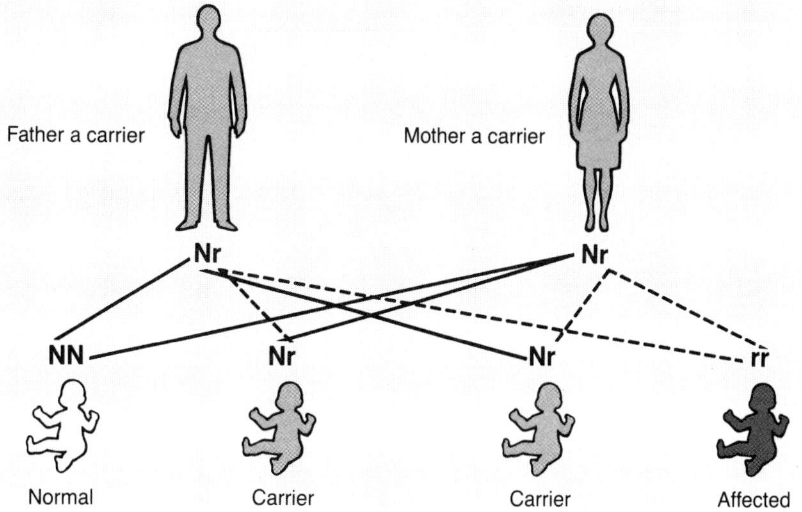

X-Linked Inheritance

One of the mother's sex chromosomes carries a faulty gene (**X**) while her other sex chromosome is normal (**x**). The father's sex chromosomes (**x** and **y**) are both normal. Each male child has a 50 percent chance of inheriting the condition.

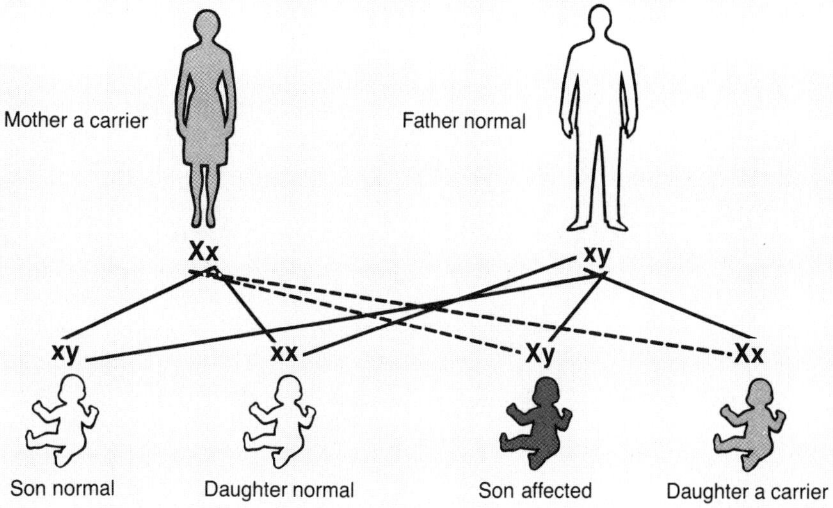

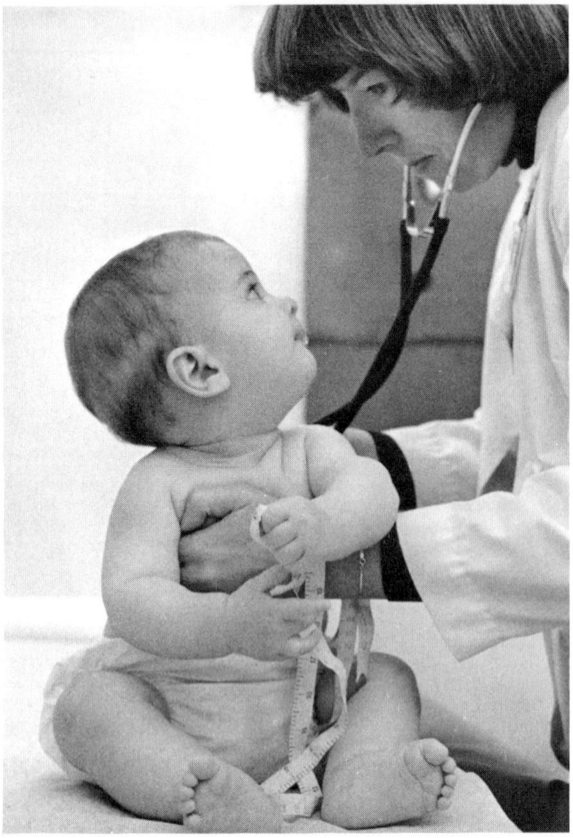

When Conditions Appear

Some genetic diseases and defects are apparent at birth, but others do not show themselves until months or even years later. Among late-appearing genetic diseases, with the age at which symptoms often are noticed, are:

- **Cystic fibrosis** at birth or during the first years of life
- **Hemophilia** early childhood
- **Huntington's disease** from late 30's on
- **Muscular dystrophy (Duchenne form)** 2 to 4 years
- **Sickle-cell anemia** from 6 months on
- **Tay-Sachs disease** 6 to 12 months

Note: The age at which symptoms appear and diagnosis is made may vary widely from case to case.

The Counseling Process

For genetic counselors, the main task is to evaluate a couple's risk of transmitting a genetic defect, to explain the situation in terms the couple can understand, and to help the couple cope with this information. To do this job properly, the genetic counselor needs a great deal of information.

One of the most valuable tools in genetic counseling is the "family pedigree"—a kind of genealogical "tree," or diagram, showing known and suspected disorders in blood relatives on both sides of the family. The more thorough the family pedigree, the more accurate the assessment that can be made. It is therefore the couple's responsibility to spend some time and effort on researching their family medical history.

Couples may also be asked to undergo certain tests, usually giving samples of blood that can be analyzed for biochemical or chromosomal abnormalities. If the couple has had a previous child with a birth defect, in some cases it may be essential that the child (and sometimes his or her healthy siblings and the parents) receive a complete medical examination to help determine the cause and extent of the problem, to ensure accurate genetic counseling.

Once all the information is gathered and evaluated, the genetic counselor can work up a statistical estimate of risk. Statistics, however, are easily misunderstood; the "counseling" aspect of genetic counseling involves helping the couple to grasp the significance of the numbers. A one-in-four chance of transmitting a disease does *not* mean that three of four youngsters in the family have guaranteed bills of health, but rather that in each pregnancy there is a 25 percent risk of the child inheriting the disorder. A detailed explanation is also given of the severity of a given defect and of the kind of care that a child having this defect may require. If a couple decides that the risk of passing on a genetic disorder is higher than they are willing to accept, the genetic counselor may suggest other options, such as artificial insemination or adoption.

Scientific and Social Trends

Two factors are primarily responsible for genetic counseling's recent rise in popularity. First, great advances have occurred in the scientific understanding of genetics and in the technological capacity for detecting disorders—before conception, during pregnancy, and after birth. Simple blood tests are now available for screening, before conception, carriers of several inherited diseases—including Tay-Sachs, sickle-cell anemia, and thalassemia—so that couples can decide whether to attempt a pregnancy at all. Prenatal diagnostic techniques, such as ultrasound, amniocentesis, and—rarely—fetoscopy (examination of the fetus with a fiber-optic viewing device), can identify hundreds of different fetal defects before the baby is born. And in most of the United States and Canada, newborns are now routinely tested for several potentially severe but treatable genetic disorders. If babies are found to have phenylketonuria (PKU), which can cause mental retardation, they can be fed a special diet to correct the problem. Hypothyroidism, which can also cause mental retardation, can be treated with medication.

The second factor is the growing trend toward delayed childbearing. Because the risk of chromosomal defects increases with the mother's age, so does the need for genetic counseling. Amniocentesis is recommended for all pregnant women who at the time of delivery will be at or over age 35 (the age at which the risk of chromosomal defects first exceeds the risks of the amniocentesis procedure). Anyone undergoing this procedure should first have a genetic counselor explain how the test is done, what its potential complications are, and how results are interpreted.

In a new technique called chorionic villus sampling, doctors remove samples of one of the membranes surrounding the embryo to test for genetic disorders.

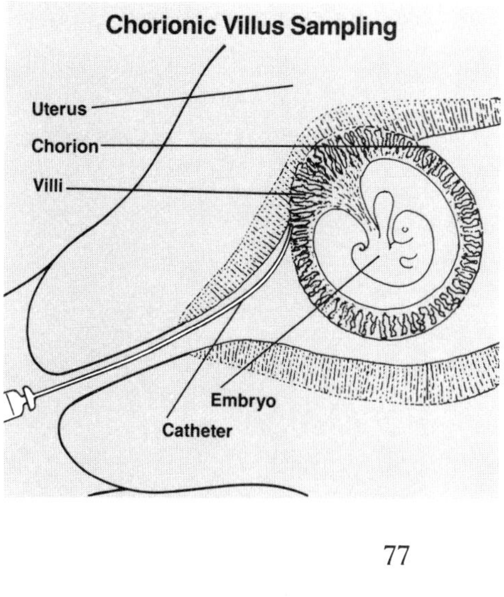

Prenatal Diagnosis

Amniocentesis is usually performed around the 16th week of pregnancy, when there is enough amniotic fluid surrounding the fetus and sufficient fetal cells in the fluid for analysis. It consists of inserting a long, thin needle through the mother's abdomen into the uterus and withdrawing a sampling of amniotic fluid. (Ultrasound images are taken just prior to the procedure to help determine exactly where to place the needle.) The fetal cells from the sample are then grown in the laboratory for another three to four weeks, at which point they are ready for analysis. Usually, tests for Down's syndrome and other chromosomal abnormalities and for neural tube defects (spina bifida and anencephaly) are the only ones performed. If, however, the couple's personal or family medical history suggests additional risk, tests for many other genetic disorders may be carried out.

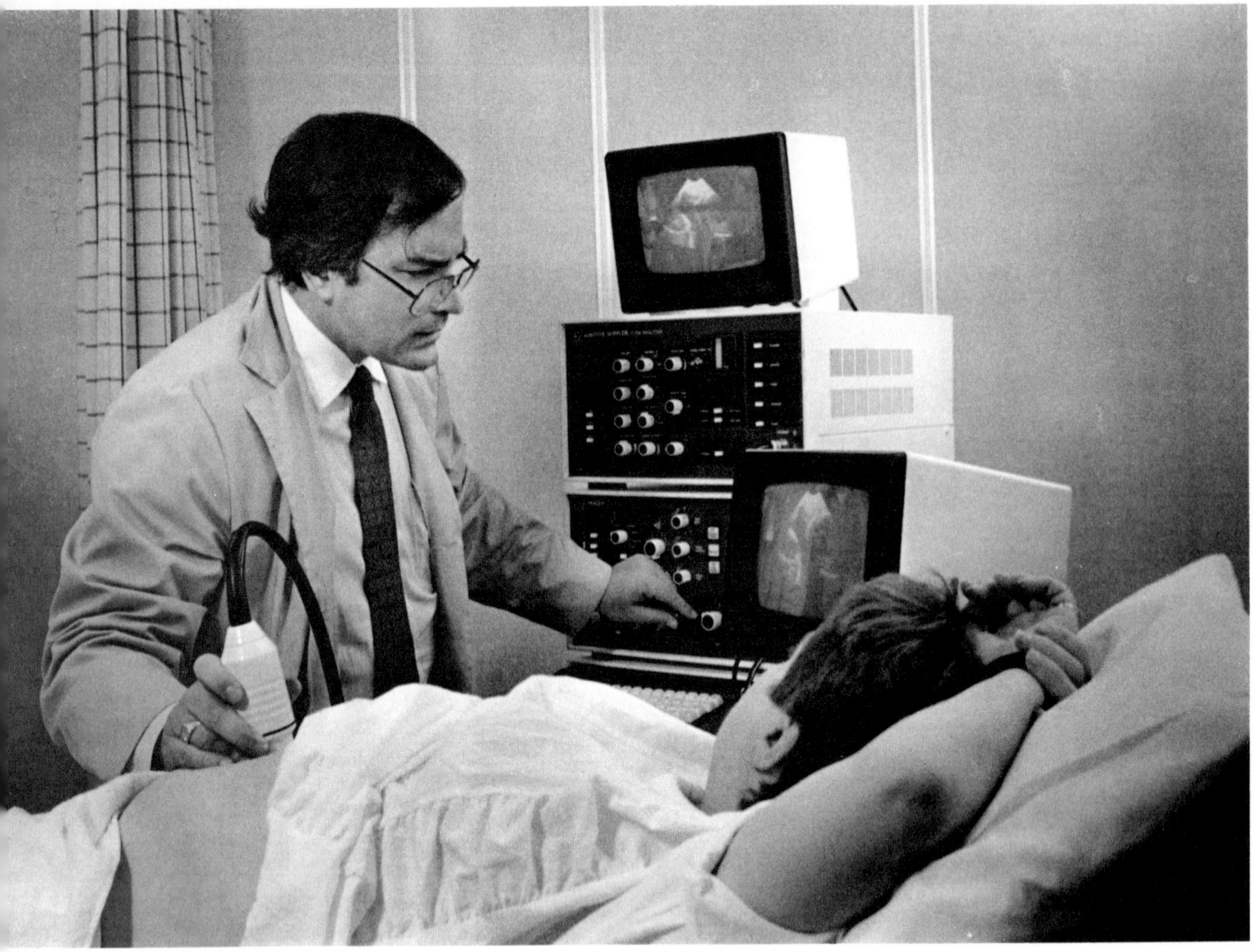

Ultrasound images guide the doctor in performing amniocentesis.

Amniocentesis is considered a very reliable procedure. Nevertheless, a major drawback is that amniocentesis is performed relatively late in pregnancy, with results sometimes not available until the 20th week or later—by which time the fetus is five months old. Occasionally complications occur in the cell culturing process. These "artifacts"—unusual findings such as an apparent structural abnormality in a chromosome—may not reflect the fetal chromosomes. To be certain, however, additional fetal cells and sometimes parental chromosomes must be studied. This may cause additional anxiety for the couple.

A new alternative to amniocentesis, called chorionic villus biopsy, or CV sampling, has stirred considerable interest. CV sampling—in which a long, thin catheter is used to take samples of the fingerlike projections (villi) of the chorion, one of the membranes that surround the embryo—is performed as early as the seventh or eighth week of pregnancy. Some results may be available within a few days. CV sampling can be used to detect such disorders as Down's syndrome, sickle-cell anemia, and Tay-Sachs, but it cannot diagnose the neural tube defects. Also, the risks of CV sampling have not yet been fully established. Currently, approximately

50 medical centers around the world, including some in the United States and Canada, are performing CV sampling. They are participating in an international registry to monitor the outcomes of the pregnancies and any problems that may arise. Researchers are also working on other methods of prenatal diagnosis that may provide even faster results.

Current and Future Problems

Advances in medical genetics have enhanced the ability to detect many genetic disorders during pregnancy and soon after birth. Genetic counseling and screening has also enabled medical geneticists to identify some couples who are at risk for having a child with a genetic disorder. As a result, for some couples the information gleaned from genetic counseling and testing creates special problems. A couple may learn that they are at risk for having a child with a genetic abnormality, but the disorder may not be detectable before birth, even with amniocentesis and other prenatal diagnostic procedures. Or they may find that they are at risk for having a child with a disorder that can be detected during pregnancy but cannot be corrected, such as Down's syndrome. Once the woman is already pregnant, a couple has but two choices: continue the pregnancy or terminate it, sometimes without knowing for sure if the fetus is actually affected. On the positive side, by offering realistic assessments and accurate prenatal diagnosis, genetic counseling helps many couples to decide to proceed with a wanted pregnancy.

Hundreds of defects can be detected in the fetus through prenatal tests.

New treatment methods are being developed. Already some genetic disorders, if diagnosed prenatally, can be treated immediately after birth. Attempts have been made to correct certain physical defects while the fetus is still in the uterus, and medical geneticists are exploring the possibilities of gene therapy—replacing defective genes with normal ones produced in the laboratory. While it will probably be years before these treatments become widely used, researchers say the potential seems virtually limitless.

But as new techniques become available, ethical problems will certainly arise: with new knowledge will come a potential for questionable applications. For instance, the danger increases of genetic information or gene therapy being abused by some individuals as a form of eugenics, an attempt to ensure the "perfection" or desired sex of their children. Mastering the genetic mechanism may well solve many serious medical problems—but it could generate almost as many ethical questions. Society might be well advised to begin now exploring ways to resolve such ethical dilemmas before they actually arise. □

SOURCES OF FURTHER INFORMATION

March of Dimes Birth Defects Foundation, 1275 Mamaroneck Avenue, White Plains, N.Y. 10605.

National Genetics Foundation, 555 West 57 Street, New York, N.Y. 10019.

National Center for Education in Maternal and Child Health, 38th and R Street, N.W., Washington, D.C. 20057.

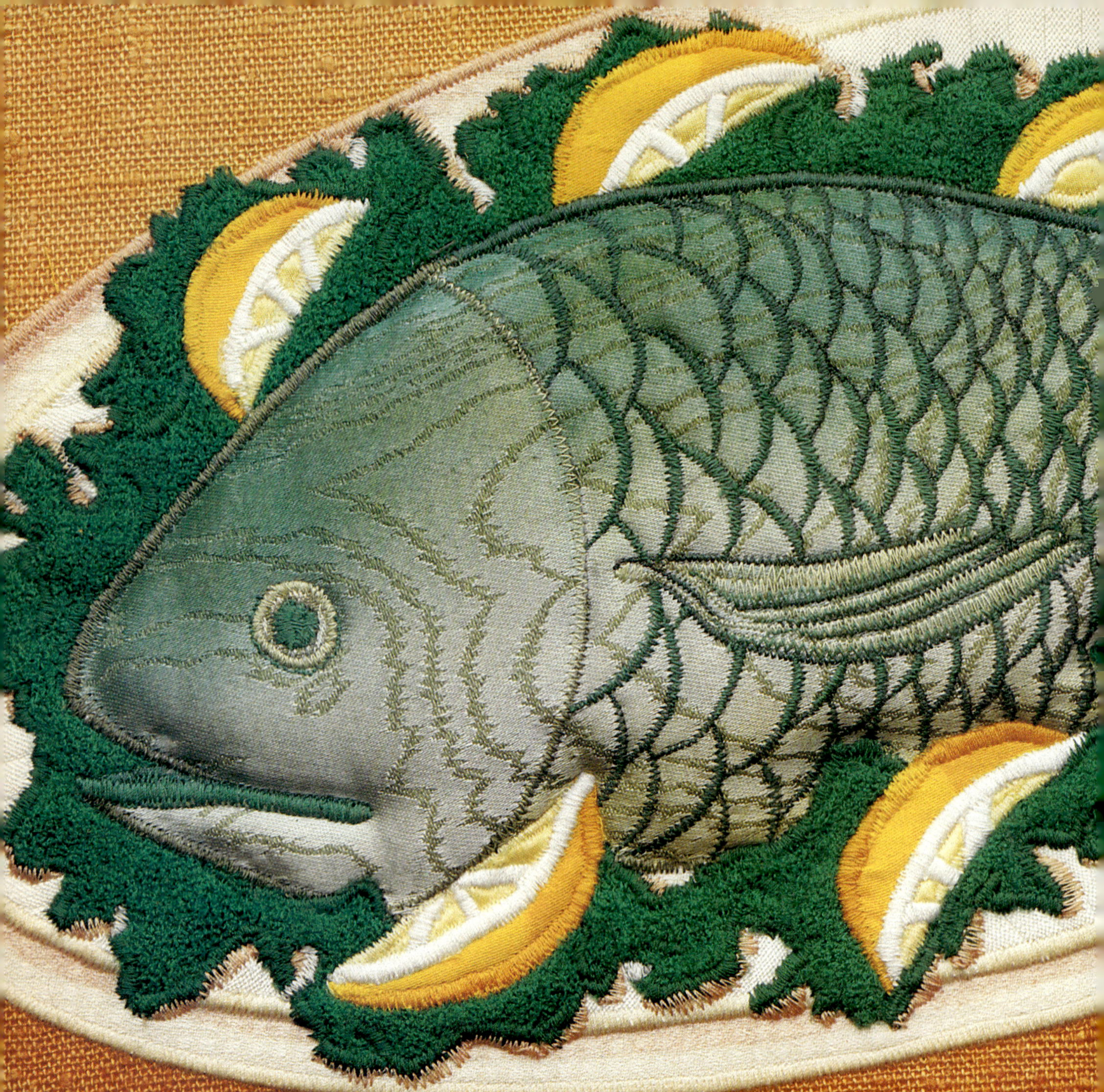

Fish in the Diet

Eleanor R. Williams, Ph.D.

ARTWORK BY MARGARET CUSACK

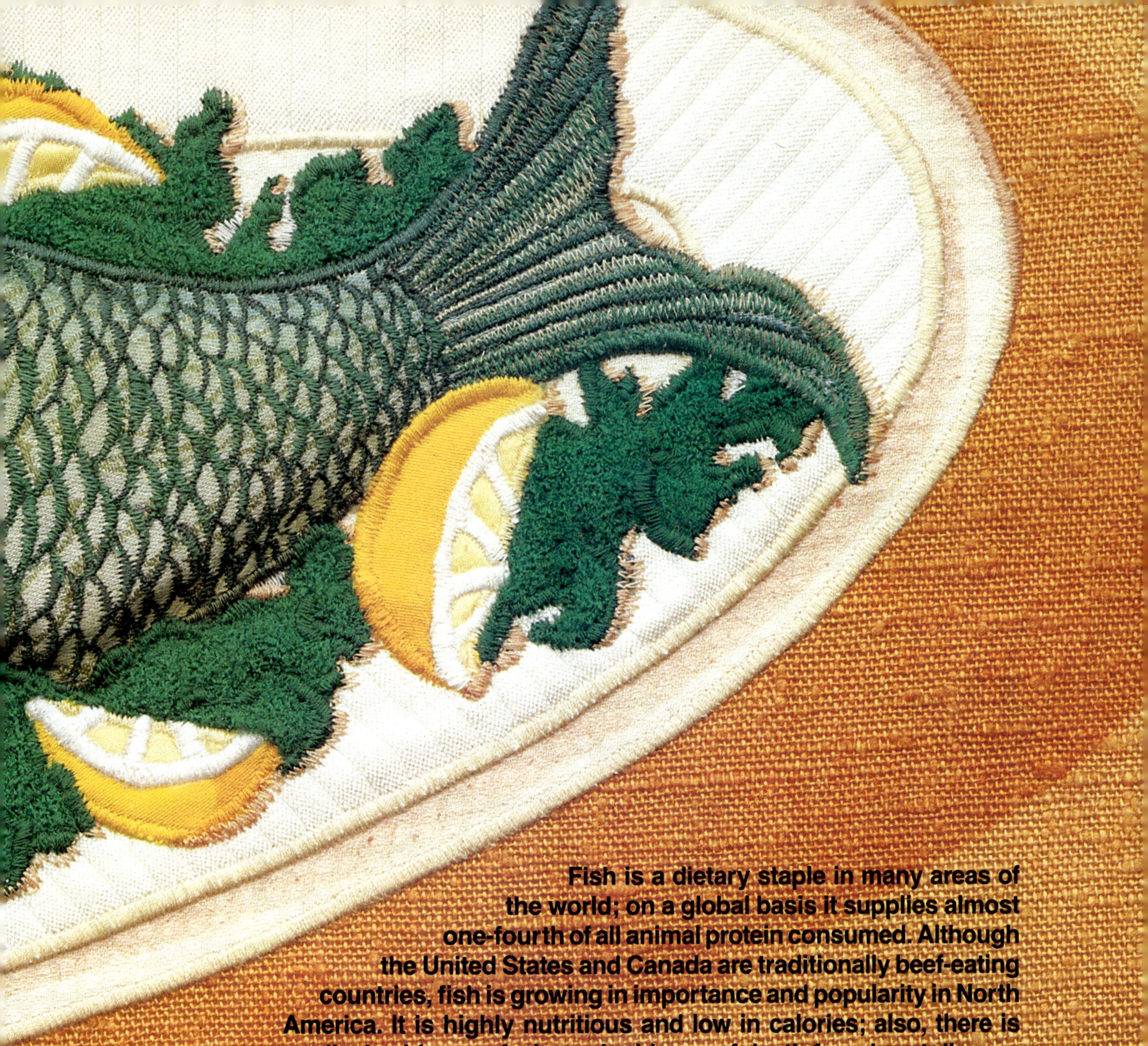

Fish is a dietary staple in many areas of the world; on a global basis it supplies almost one-fourth of all animal protein consumed. Although the United States and Canada are traditionally beef-eating countries, fish is growing in importance and popularity in North America. It is highly nutritious and low in calories; also, there is medical evidence of a lower incidence of death from heart disease among regular fish eaters.

Many questions can be asked about fish. Why does fish play a larger role in the diet of some countries than others? Are all types of fish equally nutritious? Are all ways of preparing fish equally healthful? Are there any dangers in eating certain fish (aside from choking on bones)?

The answer to the first question is easy. Economic realities have forced certain nations, such as Japan, Portugal, and the Philippines, to become major fish consumers. In Japan, a mountainous country with long coastlines, the limited land resources are of necessity devoted to rice production. The Soviet Union, after suffering considerable problems with livestock raising in the 1950's and 1960's, began expanding its fisheries, sending out fleets of ship factories that could catch, freeze, and process fish in distant waters. Soviet fish consumption is about twice that of of the United States. Fish consumption in the United States and

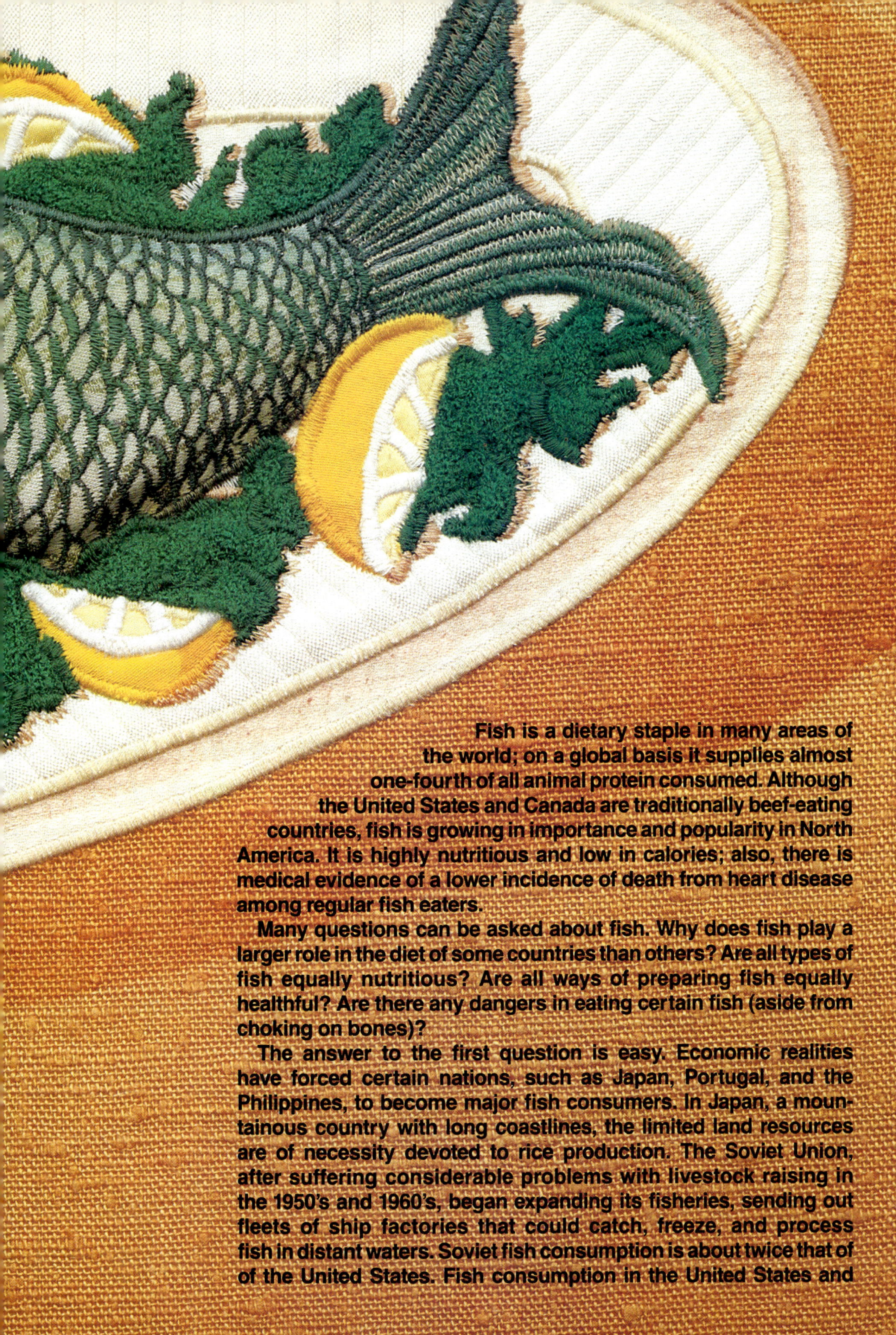

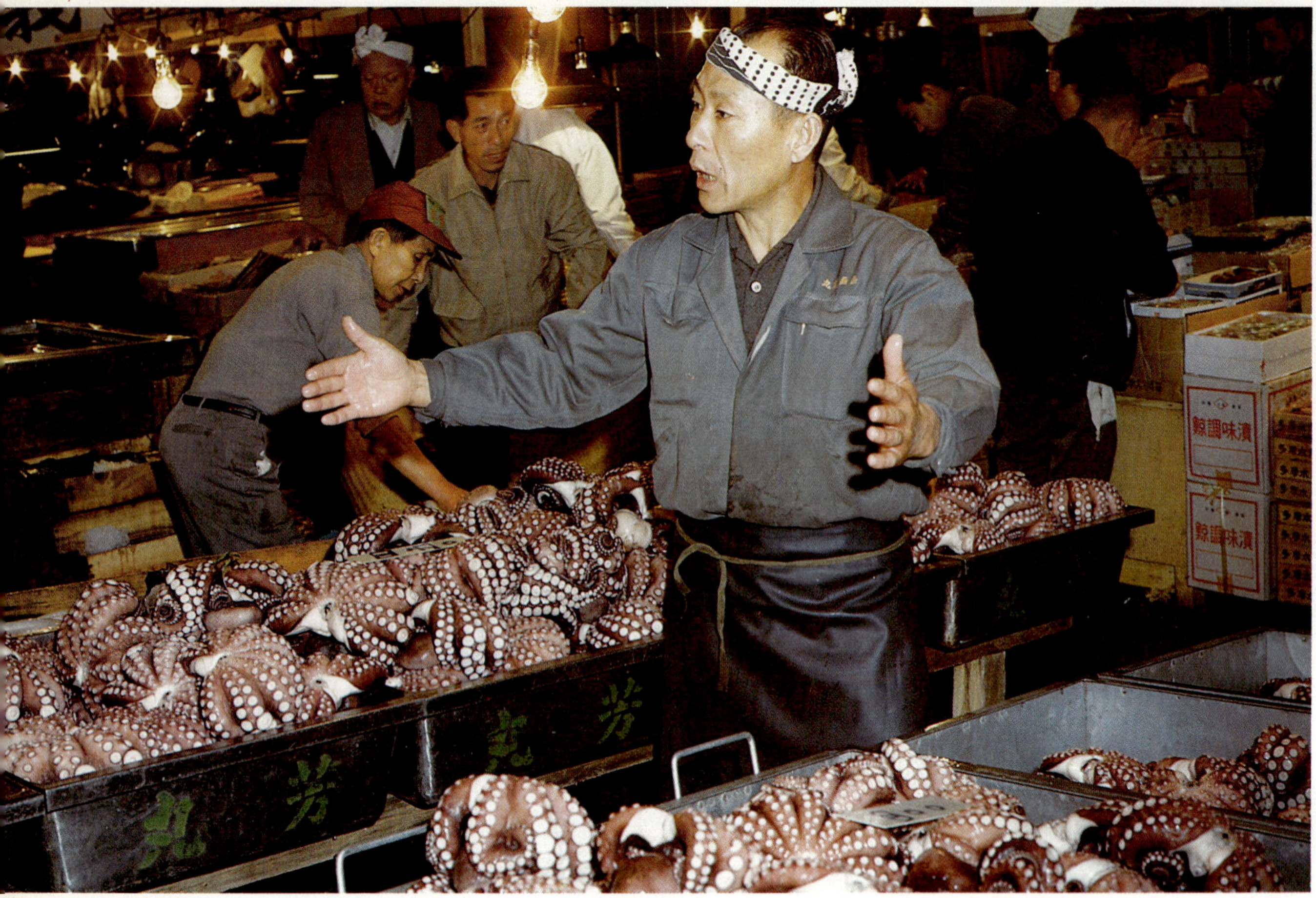

A Tokyo fish wholesaler displays bins of bright pink and white octopus. Fish in all varieties are a staple of the Japanese diet.

Canada is relatively low—under 20 pounds per person annually from both commercially caught fish and recreationally caught fish.

Countries vary not only in the amount of fish consumed but in the type of fish preferred. Tuna is by far the favorite in the United States; more than one-third of the entire world tuna catch is eaten by Americans. Spain, Italy, Portugal, and Japan consume most of the squid, a fish viewed with disfavor by many Americans.

Nutritive Values

Both finfish (vertebrates having gills and fins) and shellfish (invertebrates with shells) are highly nutritious, as nutritious as meat in many respects. They contribute valuable amounts of protein, vitamins, and minerals to the diet; like most meats, they contain little, if any, carbohydrates. Fish tends to be low in fat, although species vary in the amount of fat they contain. The Fish Facts table on page 83 compares the number of calories, percentage of protein, and percentage of fat in different types of

---

Eleanor R. Williams is an associate professor in the Department of Food, Nutrition and Institution Administration at the University of Maryland.

finfish and shellfish. The table is arranged in descending order by amount of fat; the fattiest fish head the list.

Protein is a primary nutrient in fish just as it is in meats. The amount varies in finfish species from about 15 to 25 percent and in shellfish species from about 8 to 18 percent. Fish protein is highly digestible and contains in the correct proportions all of the essential amino acids that must be in the diet because the body cannot make them. In addition, fish

FISH FACTS

	Calories (for 3½ ounces*)	% Protein	% Fat
Finfish			
Salmon, Atlantic	217	22.5	13.4
Mackerel, Atlantic	191	19.0	12.2
Herring, Atlantic	176	17.3	11.3
Lake trout	168	18.3	10.0
Sardines, Pacific	160	19.2	8.6
Mackerel, Pacific	159	21.9	7.3
Tuna, bluefin	145	25.2	4.1
Swordfish	118	19.2	4.0
Catfish	103	17.6	3.1
Herring, Pacific	98	17.5	2.6
Halibut, Atlantic and Pacific	100	20.9	1.2
Ocean perch	88	18.0	1.2
Flounder, sole	79	16.7	0.8
Cod	78	17.6	0.3
Haddock	79	18.3	0.1
Shellfish			
Mussels (8 or 9)	95	14.4	2.2
Oysters, Pacific and Western (7 or 8 medium)	91	10.6	2.2
Crab, steamed	93	17.3	1.9
Lobster	91	16.9	1.9
Clams (6 or 7)	82	14.0	1.9
Oysters, Eastern (7 or 8 medium)	66	8.4	1.8
Shrimp (17 large)	91	18.1	0.8
Scallops	81	15.3	0.2

* Figures are for uncooked finfish and shellfish, except for steamed crab.

Source: Bernice K. Watt and Annabel L. Merrill, *Composition of Foods.* Agriculture Handbook No. 8, U.S. Department of Agriculture, Washington, D.C., 1963.

Fish provides protein as well as many important vitamins and minerals.

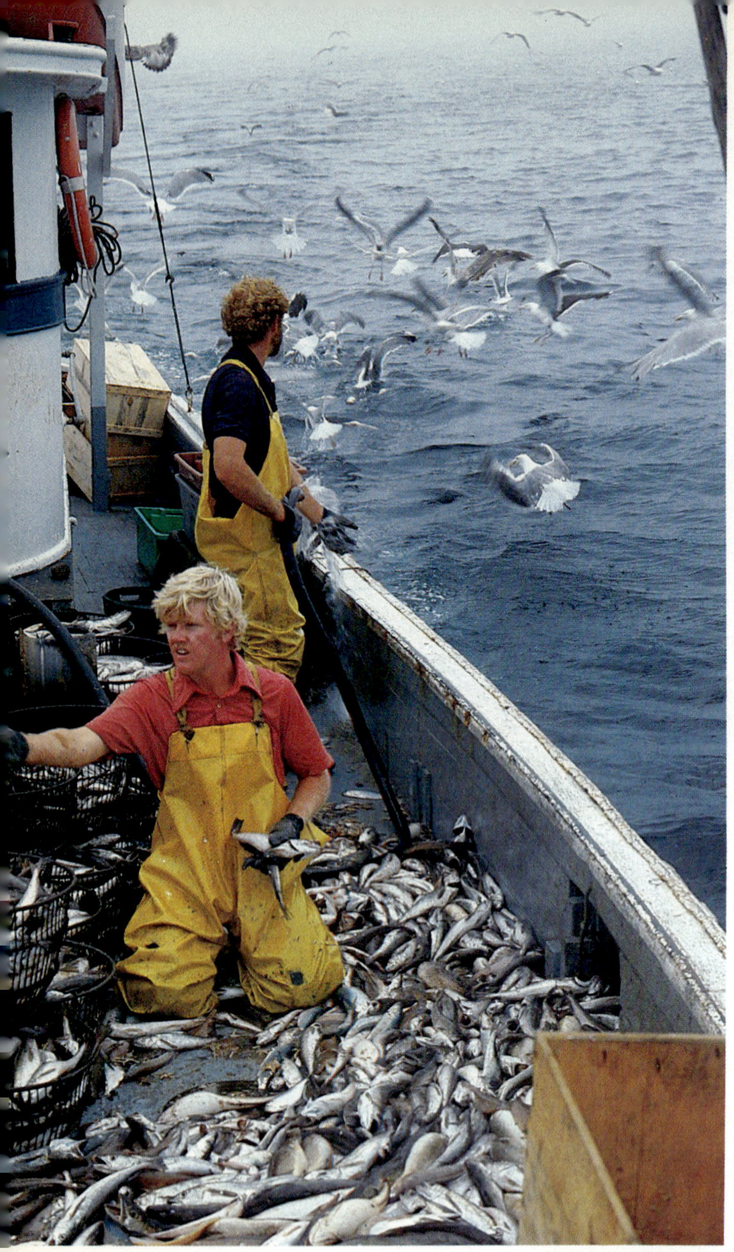

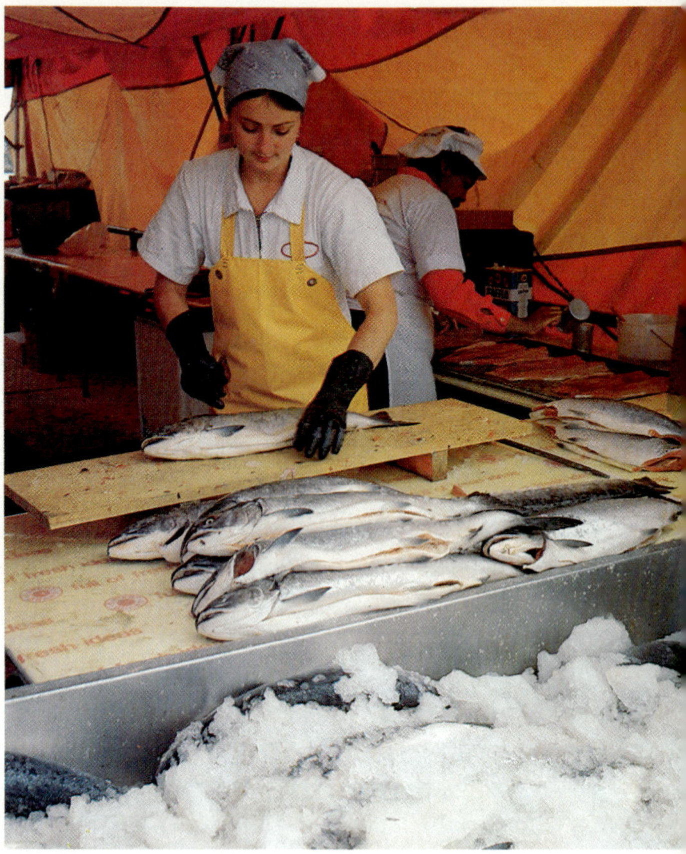

Massachusetts fishermen (left) rush their abundant catch to market with seagulls in hot pursuit. Above, with only a quick cleaning and slicing, salmon can go straight from ice to griddle for a simple gourmet treat. Even city dwellers (right) can choose from a great variety of fresh fish, crabs, clams, and mussels at an open air market.

contain those amino acids that are low in cereal grains (such as millet, rice, and corn), peanuts, and cassava (a root that is a dietary staple in many African countries). Combining fish with these foods greatly enhances their protein value. Even small amounts of fish in diets in which these plants are staples can make the difference between nutritionally adequate and nutritionally deficient diets—an important consideration in many developing countries, where the protein intake is relatively low.

Lowering the Risk of Heart Disease

Fish currently makes a relatively small contribution to the total protein in the American diet—about 4 percent. Yet interest in fish consumption is increasing as more is learned about its contribution to good health.

Scientists have long realized that high levels of cholesterol in the blood increase the chances of developing coronary heart disease. Deposits of cholesterol (and other fatty substances) build up along artery walls, where they harden and narrow the arteries, in the condition called

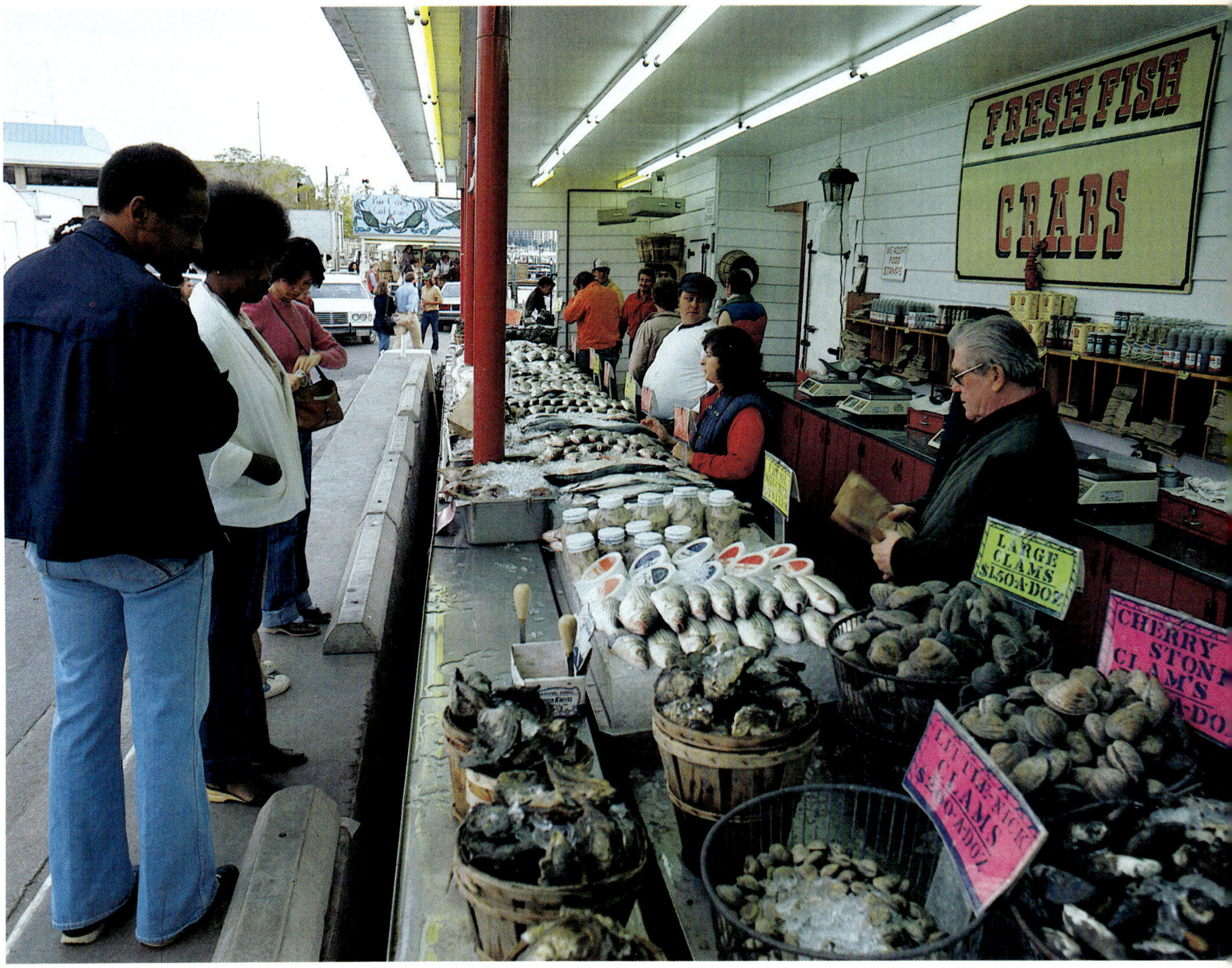

atherosclerosis. If a blood clot forms and gets stuck in an area where there is such narrowing, it can block off the artery. When this happens in a blood vessel supplying the heart, the result is a heart attack. Many years of research have shown that diets high in saturated fat and cholesterol increase blood cholesterol. Diets high in polyunsaturated fat and low in saturated fat and cholesterol lower blood cholesterol levels, diminishing the risk of heart attack.

For several reasons, fish is recommended as part of a diet designed to reduce or keep down blood cholesterol levels. One reason is that fish tends to be lower in saturated fat than beef, pork, or lamb. The fat in fish is mostly polyunsaturated, so that fish has a higher ratio than meat of polyunsaturated to saturated fat. This is called the P/S ratio. A P/S ratio of 1 or more is considered desirable in a diet to lower blood cholesterol. A 3½-ounce serving of lean beef has a P/S ratio of 0.12; the same serving of lamb has a P/S ratio of 0.13. In contrast, a 3½-ounce serving of salmon, one of the fattiest fish, has a P/S ratio of 1.3. A lean fish such as haddock, with little of each type of fat, has a highly desirable P/S ratio of 2.0.

Besides being lower in saturated fat than meat, most types of fish are lower in cholesterol than either meat or chicken. New methods of analysis have shown that even shrimp, which was once thought to be fairly high in cholesterol at 150 milligrams a serving, actually has only 50 milligrams. A serving of pork and a hamburger each contain about 90 milligrams of cholesterol.

Studies in Japan and among the Eskimos of Greenland show that low death rates from coronary heart disease are associated with high fish consumption. Recently, a 20-year study in the Netherlands found that the death rate from coronary heart disease was more than 50 percent lower among middle-aged men who ate at least 1 ounce of fish a day than among those who ate no fish. On the basis of this study, the researchers recommended eating one or two fish dishes a week to help prevent coronary heart disease.

The Dutch researchers suggested a third possible reason, besides being low in saturated fat and cholesterol, why fish has a protective effect: fish contains specific polyunsaturated fatty acids (a fatty acid is a component of fat), called omega-3's, that are not found in meat or even in polyunsaturated vegetable oils. One of these substances is eicosapentaenoic acid (EPA). To study the role of EPA or similar fatty acids in lowering the incidence of heart disease, researchers fed fish oils containing EPA to volunteers. They found that fish oils not only lowered blood cholesterol levels but also slowed down the formation of blood clots that can clog arteries, leading to heart attacks. In addition, EPA and perhaps other fish oils appeared to prevent roughening of the inner lining of the arteries, which is the first stage of atherosclerosis.

It is premature to jump to the conclusion that people should consume fish oils to prevent heart disease—these oils have drawbacks. One is that EPA and other fish oils prolong the time required for blood to clot, and unwanted and harmful bleeding can result from a large intake of fish oils. In the near future, scientists may be able to establish the extent to which fish oils actually are responsible for the lower incidence of heart disease in fish-consuming populations. Meanwhile, it makes sense for people to eat fish, but not fish oils, as part of a balanced diet.

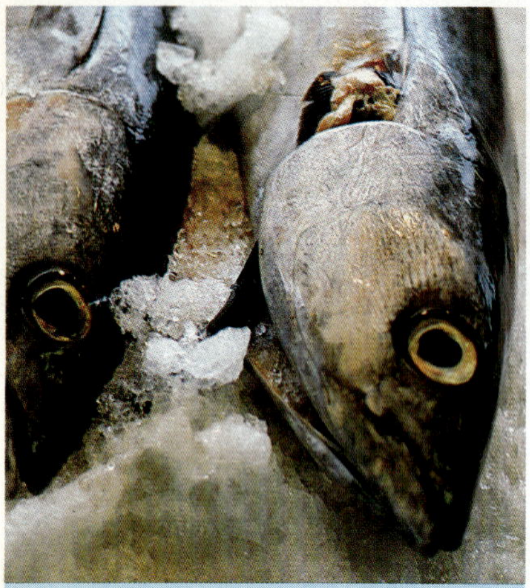

Selecting Fresh Fish

The best fish for taste and nutrition is fresh fish. To be sure fish is fresh, follow these guidelines for shopping:

- White fillets should be glossy with no brown around the edges. Pink fillets, such as salmon, should also have a sheen and should not be darkening to a red or brown color.
- Juices should not be leaking from the fillets.
- Whole fish should have shiny skin, bulging and transparent eyes, and flesh that feels firm to the touch.
- The shells of clams, mussels, and oysters should be closed.
- The most important test is smell. Fresh fish does not have a pungent odor.

Vitamins and Minerals

Fish and fish products supply significant amounts of some vitamins and minerals. Fish liver oils are excellent sources of vitamins A and D. (At one time pharmaceutical companies obtained these vitamins from fish liver oils, although today vitamin supplements contain synthetic equivalents.) More than a teaspoon of cod liver oil a day can be harmful, though, because of the toxic effects of too much vitamin A and D. The flesh of most fish is low in vitamin A, but swordfish and whitefish are exceptions; among shellfish, crabs are good vitamin A sources. The flesh of fatty fish, such as salmon, mackerel, sardines, and some tuna, is a good vitamin D source.

Most fish are good sources of niacin, vitamin B_6, biotin, and vitamin B_{12}. Salmon is also rich in riboflavin and pantothenic acid. Generally, fish is only a fair source of riboflavin and a poor source of folic acid and vitamin C.

With regard to minerals, canned salmon and sardines are good sources of calcium because the fish bones are softened enough to be palatable; otherwise, fish supplies little calcium. Canned salmon and sardines also contain fluoride, which accumulates in the bones of ocean fish. Finfish and shellfish are excellent sources of phosphorus, iron, selenium, and zinc. Oysters are particularly high in zinc; all shellfish are excellent sources of copper. Ocean fish, but not freshwater fish, are good iodine sources.

Low-Cal Fish

If people look beyond fish and chips or fried fish on a bun, fish can play a significant role in controlling one's weight or losing excess pounds. Prepared in the right way, many species of finfish and all types of shellfish are relatively low in calories and fat. Since fat furnishes more than twice as many calories by weight as do carbohydrates or protein, a sensible way to cut down on calories is to lower fat intake. Maintaining normal body weight and lowering fat intake are considered to be good strategies for decreasing the chances of developing various diseases, including certain cancers.

A species of fish is classified as lean, or low in fat, if the flesh is less than 5 percent fat, and as fat if it is higher. Cod, haddock, flounder, ocean perch, halibut, catfish, and most species of tuna are lean, while most species of mackerel, herring, and salmon are fat. To keep dietary fat intake low, primarily low-fat fish should be chosen (see the Fish Facts table) and prepared by baking, broiling, or poaching or by stir-frying the fish in a little oil. Avoid cooking or serving methods that use breading or

Get rid of the breading and deep fryer and fish is the perfect food to help you control your weight.

A tin of sardines packs in a significant amount of calcium from the edible bones, along with the other nutrients commonly found in fish.

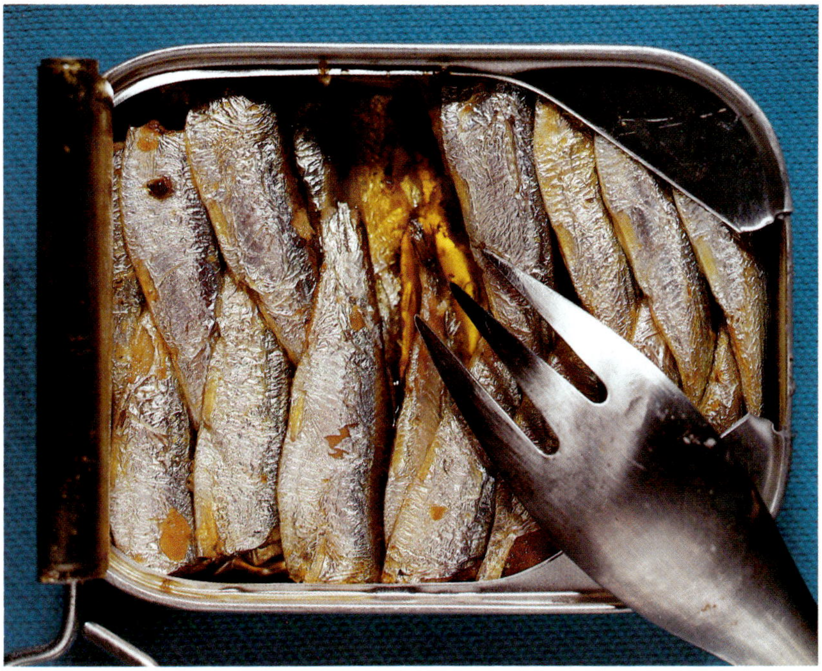

more than a minimum of margarine, butter, oil, cream, or mayonnaise. These ingredients markedly increase the calories in a fish dish. For example, a 3½-ounce serving of plain ocean perch has 88 calories, only 1.2 percent of which come from fat. The same sized piece of breaded, fried perch has 319 calories, with 53 percent coming from fat. Despite these restrictions, virtuous fish dishes do not have to be dull. Tempting, imaginative fish dishes can be prepared by using onion, garlic, julienned vegetables, herbs, fish stock, lemon, or small amounts of wine.

When buying canned fish, such as tuna and sardines, select products packed in water or tomato sauce, not oil. The oil adds needless calories.

Fish dishes served in fast-food restaurants rarely meet the needs of diet-conscious diners. Fish fillets are breaded or dipped in batter and fried, and shrimp and tuna salads are made with high-calorie dressings. The fried fillets served in most fast-food restaurants provide about 430 calories a serving, 50 percent of which come from fat. Recently, however, one fast-food chain began serving baked fish with only 150 calories per serving, 12 percent from fat, and another chain now offers shrimp salad with dressing on the side. The salad itself has only 115 calories, 8 percent from fat, and the customer can keep the calories low by adding a small amount of dressing or using only lemon juice.

Buying for Freshness, Cooking for Flavor

Fish are highly perishable, and fresh fish must be kept on ice or refrigerated from the time they are caught until they are cooked. Otherwise, bacteria readily break down a compound in fish flesh to produce the characteristic odor of "bad fish."

Choose a market where the fish are handled in a sanitary way. To test the freshness of a whole fish, notice whether the eyes are bulging (sunken eyes indicate lack of freshness), and press the flesh with your finger. It should feel firm and spring back when pressure is released. Fish fillets should have a uniform, glossy white or pink color and should not be leaking juices. The shells of clams, mussels, and the like should be closed tightly, which means that the fish are still alive. There should be no offensive odor from any type of fish.

Finfish and shellfish are easily toughened by intense or prolonged heat. For a tender finished product, *simmer*—never boil—fish or shellfish, if cooking in a liquid. To test for doneness of baked or broiled fish, use a thin knife to separate the meat in its thickest part. If the flesh is no longer translucent and flakes apart readily, the fish is done.

Enjoying Fish at Home

To get the most flavor and nutrition out of fish, without adding calories, practice these simple culinary tips:

- Use the fish you buy as soon as possible.
- Avoid cooking or serving methods that use breading or a good deal of butter, margarine, oil, or mayonnaise.
- Baking, broiling, and poaching in fish stock or other low-calorie liquids are better cooking methods than frying.
- To test for doneness, follow what is known as the Canadian method: bake or broil the fish ten minutes for each inch of thickness.
- For flavor, add onion, garlic, celery, herbs, lemon, fish stock, or small amounts of wine.

The Safety of Fish

Raw fish is a delicacy in many parts of the world and is now frequently offered in restaurants in North America. If raw fish is to be consumed safely, it must be obtained from uncontaminated waters and handled in a strictly sanitary manner before it is eaten. Raw fish otherwise may be contaminated with bacteria or other organisms. (Cooking destroys these organisms.) Raw clams and oysters have been linked to hepatitis and to a virus called the Norwalk virus, which causes nausea, vomiting, and diarrhea; other disease agents are also thought to contaminate shellfish.

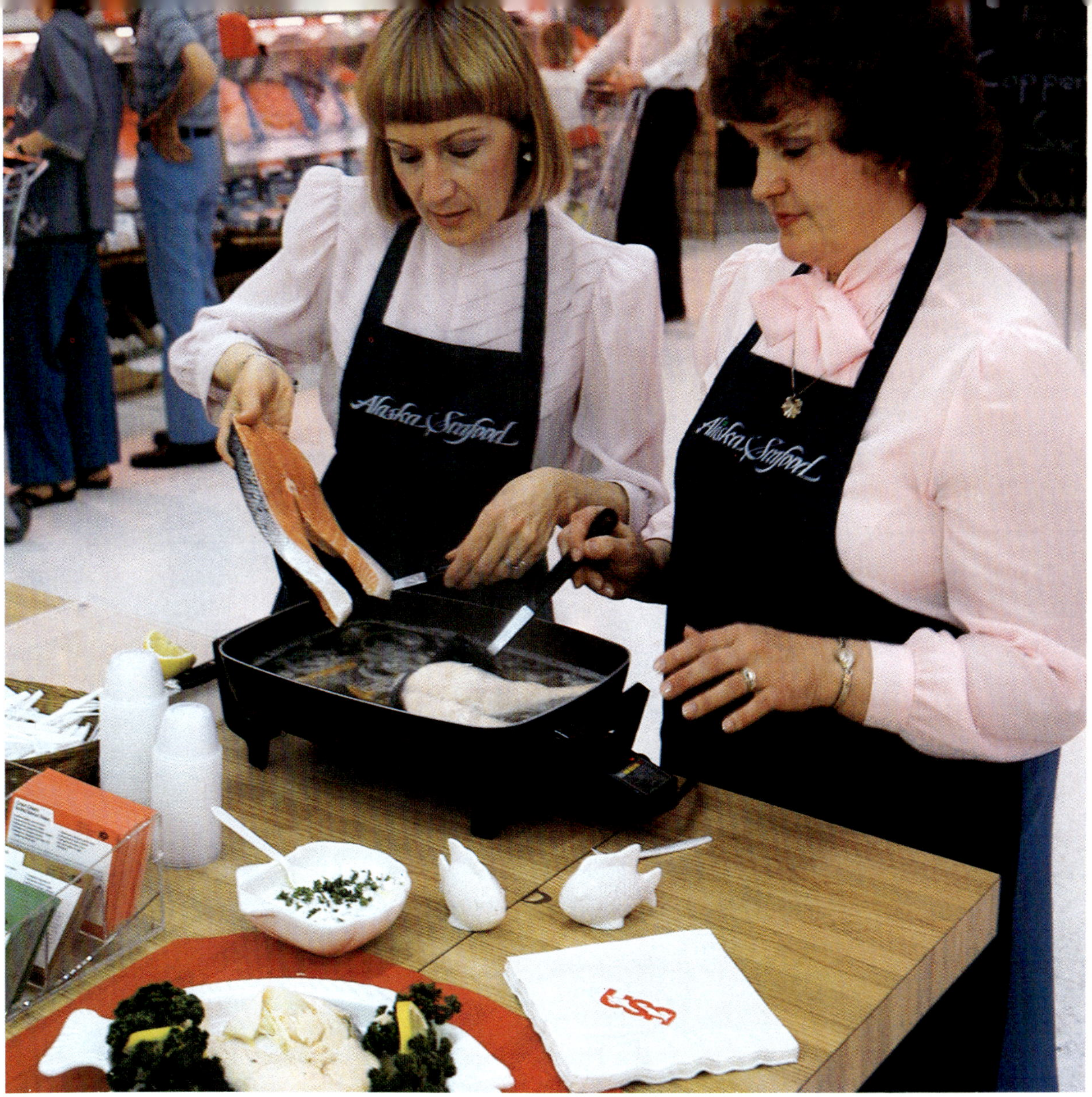

A successful team of fish "consultants" demonstrate to supermarket shoppers the simplest ways to cook perfect fish.

As a result, some health officials believe people—especially those with liver disease, immune system disorders, and certain other conditions—should not eat raw shellfish. They recommend that shellfish, if steamed, be cooked at least four to six minutes.

Smoking and salting have been used to preserve fish in the past, but freezing is used more frequently today. In 1982 a report from the National Research Council of the U.S. National Academy of Sciences voiced concern about salted and smoked foods because of their possible cancer risk. Some methods of pickling and smoking foods appear to produce compounds that cause cancer in animals, and, in fact, the incidence of cancer of the esophagus and stomach is unusually high in parts of China, Japan, and Iceland where large amounts of salt-cured (including salt-pickled) and smoked fish are consumed. Occasional consumption of fish such as smoked salmon, finnan haddie, and dried, salted cod is probably not harmful, but they should not be a major part of the diet.

Canned fish can provide ideal conditions for the growth of spores of the bacterium *Clostridium botulinum*, which produces one of the most lethal toxins known. During the canning process, the fish must be subjected to

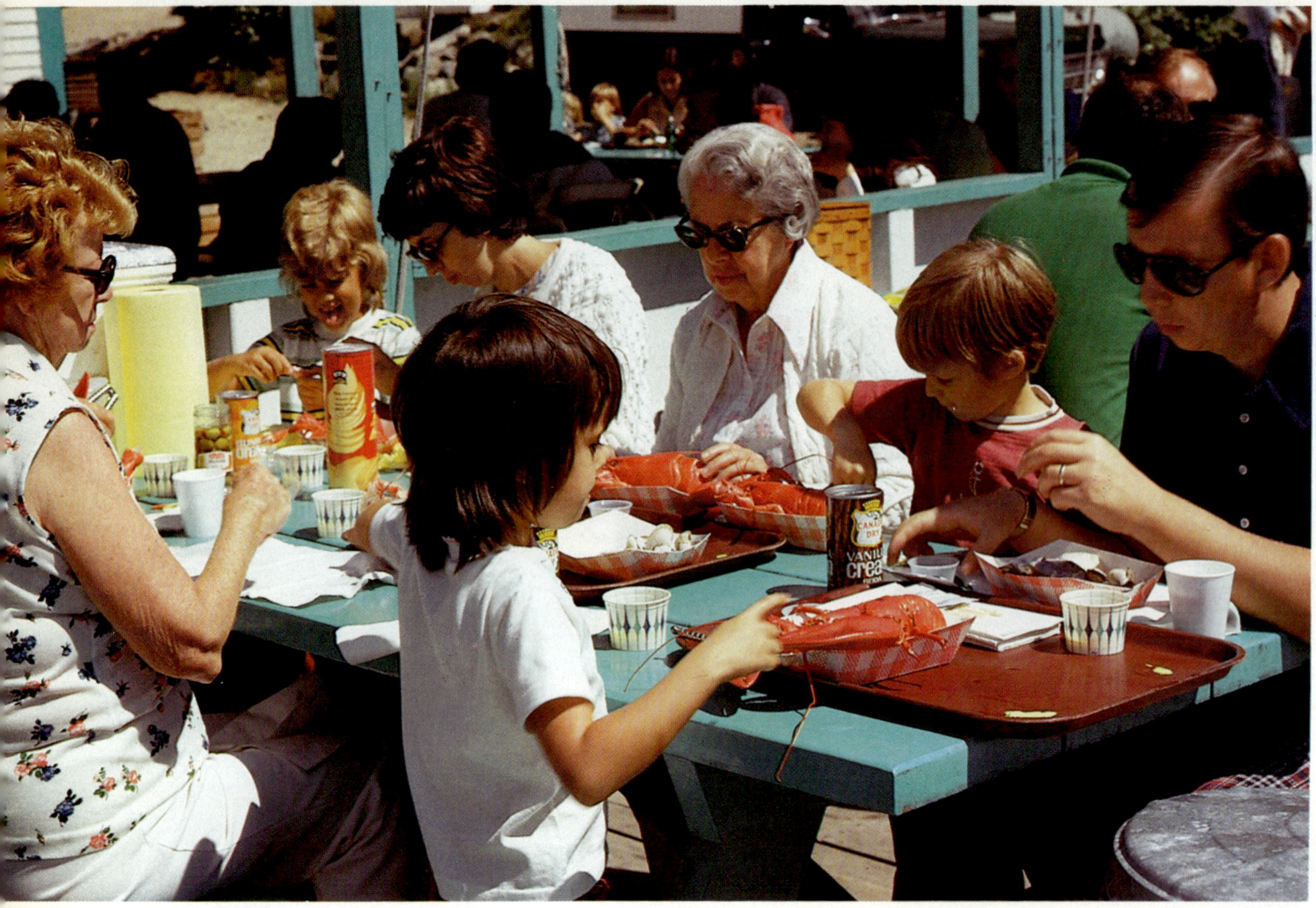

Cracking steamed lobsters at a sunny picnic table can be a family treat.

temperatures considerably above 212°F for several minutes to ensure destruction of the spores. Commercial canners make great efforts to be sure that their products are safe; botulism poisoning from one of their products can not only cost lives but also ruin a company's reputation.

Fish may become contaminated with industrial wastes that enter the food chain. The process begins when wastes are dumped or leak from landfills into lakes, streams, or coastal waters and contaminate plankton. Small fish eat the plankton, and larger fish eat the smaller ones, so that wastes may become highly concentrated in fish flesh, as well as widely distributed among different types of fish. The fish are unable to break down the chemicals in their bodies or eliminate them. Although the production of some toxic chemicals, such as PCB's (polychlorinated biphenyls) and PBB's (polybrominated biphenyls), is now banned, chemicals can linger in the environment. Since some industrial chemicals can cause cancer or other serious disorders, public health warnings should be issued when fish are known to be polluted with these substances. A number of state governments now monitor the fish in specific bodies of water and do issue such warnings.

Mercury poisoning of fish by wastes from a plastics factory in Japan in the 1950's caused the deaths of over 40 people who had eaten the contaminated fish. Since that time, the discharge of mercury into the environment has been restricted, but consumers need to maintain vigilance about protecting their environment and food supply from possible contaminants.

Natural Poisons

Parts of some types of puffer fish, which include blowfish, globefish, and fugu fish, are intrinsically poisonous, and eating only small amounts of the poisonous portions can be lethal. (Cooking will not affect the poison—the fish remains dangerous.) The Japanese and Chinese are fond of the most poisonous species of puffer fish, and the Japanese government licenses specialists who skillfully remove the poisonous visceral organs without contaminating the flesh.

Finfish and shellfish may become poisoned by consuming toxic algae. The "red tide" that periodically is reported along the North American Atlantic or Pacific coasts is caused by an accumulation of toxic algae that gives the water a reddish-brown color and poisons fish living there. Some species of finfish and shellfish die from ingesting the toxic algae, but others survive and give no signs of having the poison. People who eat the poisoned finfish and shellfish may become seriously ill or die. Toxic algae flourish when certain temperature and environmental conditions coincide. Government agencies periodically check for fish poisoning and warn the public of any danger. As in the case of puffer fish, the red tide toxin is not affected by cooking.

Checks on fisheries by public health officials and regulations for canning are important in ensuring the safety of fish products.

In general, fish are not more apt to cause health problems than are other foods. Proper sanitary practices from the time fish are caught until they reach the table and the vigilance of public health authorities help to ensure the public of a safe fish supply.

Eat More Fish

Should Americans consume more fish? The answer is yes. One of the tenets of good dietary planning is to include a wide variety of foods to increase the probability of getting all the nutrients needed. Eating more fish increases the varieties of animal protein sources in the diet and increases the intake of the beneficial fatty acids found only in fish. Choosing mostly low-fat fish to replace some meat in the diet is recommended by the American Heart Association as one way to aid in lowering blood cholesterol levels.

The health benefits of fish aside, the many types of fish available to home cooks and restaurant-goers offer numerous opportunities for tempting fare. □

SUGGESTIONS FOR FURTHER READING

"Benefits of Eating Fish." *Tufts University Diet & Nutrition Letter,* July 1985, pp. 1-3.

HAGER, TOM. "Food for the Heart." *American Health,* April 1985, pp. 50-55.

SILBERNER, JOANNE. "Heart Disease: Let Them Eat Fish." *Science News,* May 11, 1985, p. 295.

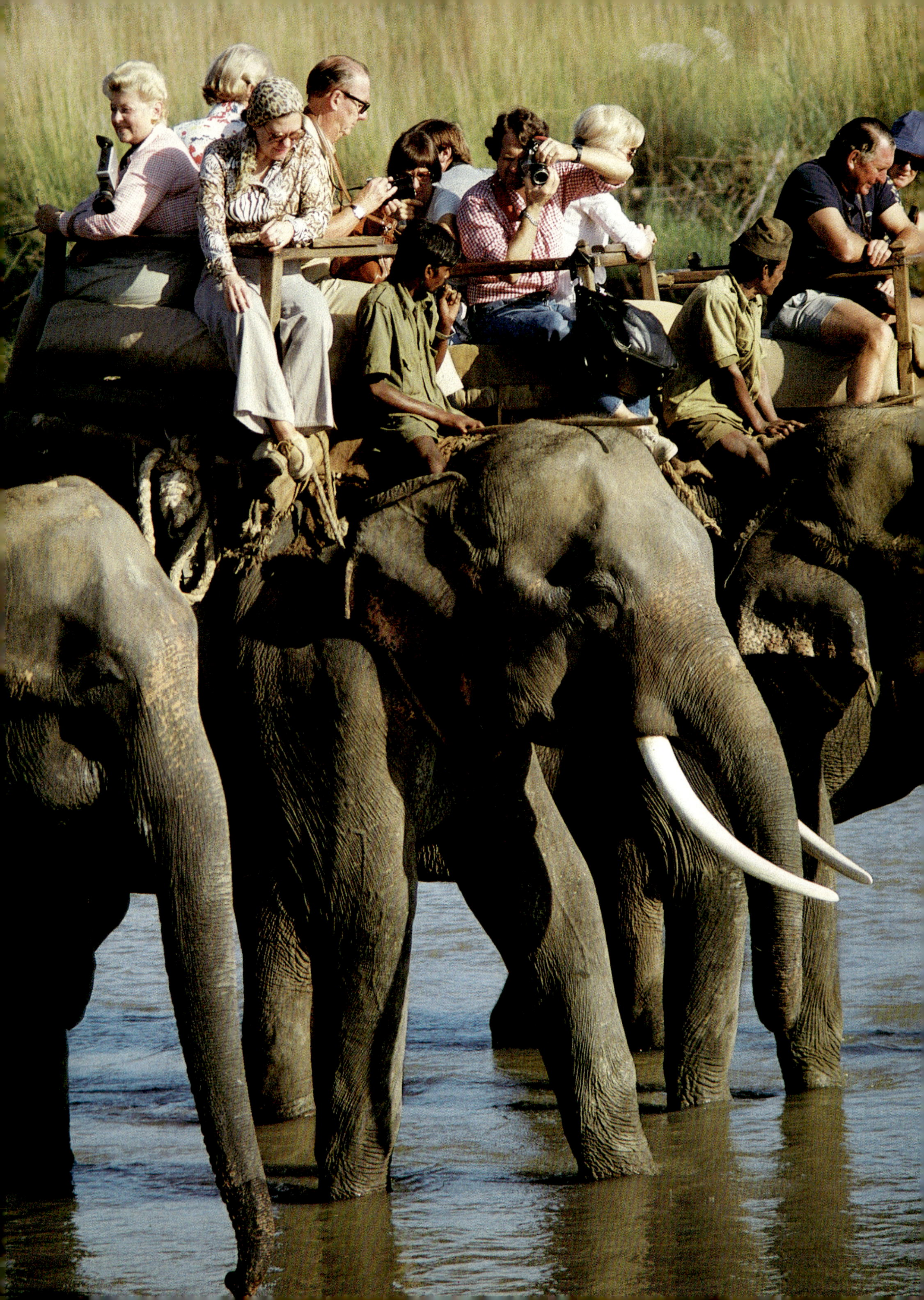

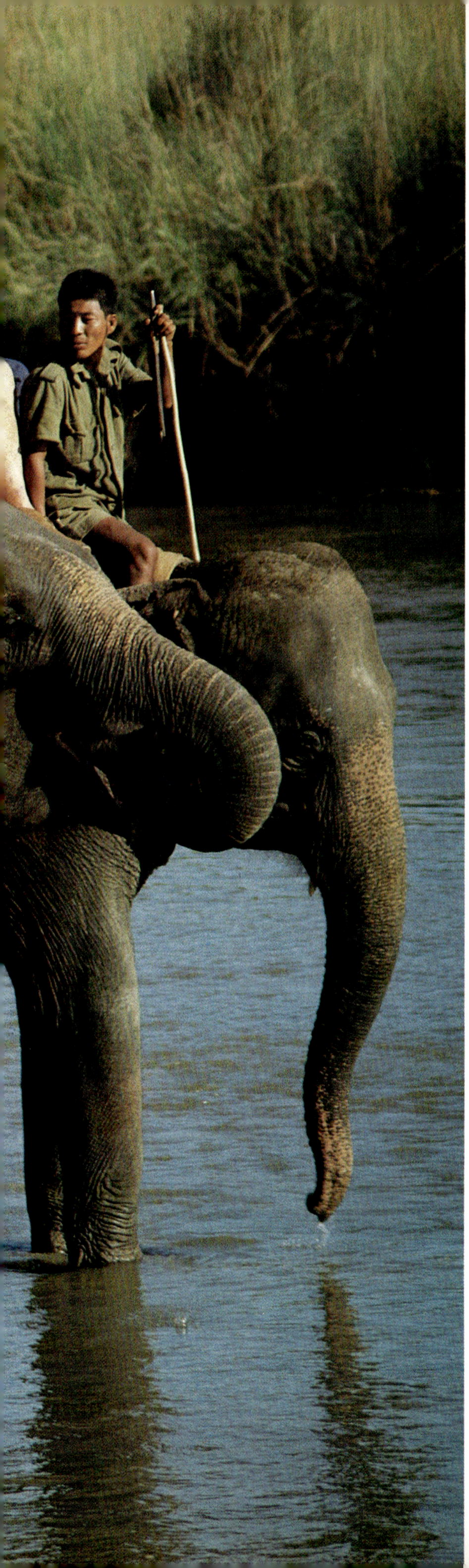

STAYING HEALTHY WHEN TRAVELING

James Chin, M.D.,
and Leonard Davis, M.D.

Every year millions of Americans travel away from their homes for work or pleasure. Trips within the United States, Canada, or other industrialized countries basically carry no greater risk to health than the traveler would meet at home. Most of the problems might be minor annoyances like motion sickness and diarrhea, which are often preventable through simple measures. Increasing numbers of people, however, are journeying to more remote areas—whether drawn by the lure of the exotic or by the excitement of a safari in East Africa, mountain climbing in Nepal, or rafting down the headwaters of the Amazon. Such adventurers need to take more precautions, since travel to the less developed countries of the world can be associated with significant health risks—some, like malaria, potentially very serious.

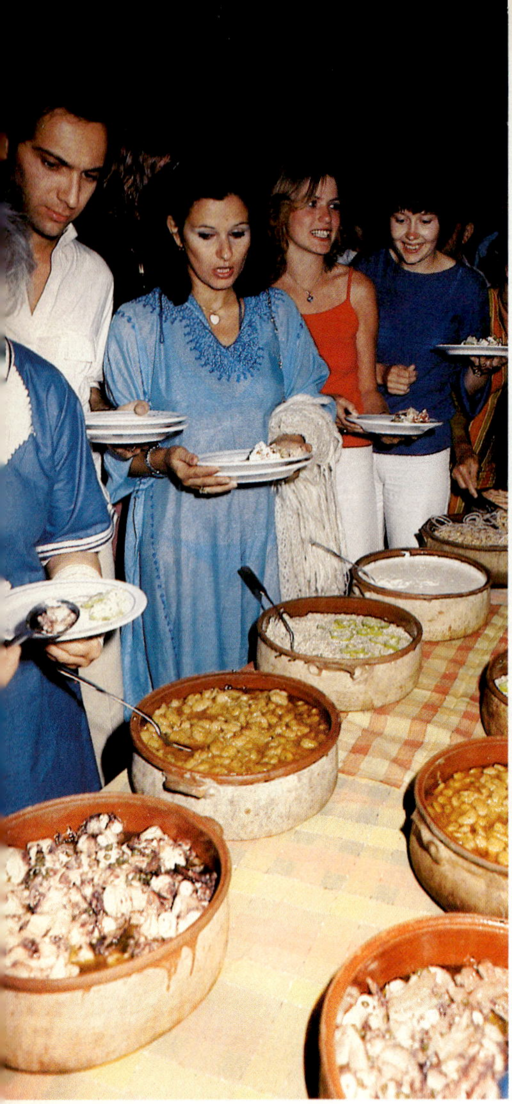

One of the delights of traveling is tasting new and unfamiliar foods—but stomach upset can result.

Traveling in Developed Countries

While there are no serious health problems associated with travel within most industrialized countries, some knowledge of health matters can make for a safer and more comfortable trip.

Travelers going abroad should inquire about the availability of any medications they regularly use, including such items as birth control pills. It is safest to take an adequate supply from home; this is also good advice if you are going to a remote region of your own country.

A first aid kit—as well as a first aid manual, such as the one published by the American Red Cross—is an essential on certain trips. The kit should be taken along on any lengthy journey by car, especially if you will be spending a fair amount of time in areas where professional medical help may not be readily available—as on a camping or hiking trip. If you are going abroad but won't be traveling extensively by car, a first aid kit is probably not necessary, unless, again, you will be in areas where the availability of professional medical care is uncertain.

First aid kits, in varying sizes to meet specific needs, can be bought in most large drugstores and many camping-supply stores. For those who wish to make up their own kit, a few different sizes of Band-Aids will take care of minor cuts and scratches. To control the bleeding of more serious wounds, carry some 4-inch gauze pads, adhesive pads like Telfa (featuring a film that keeps the bandage from sticking to the wound), a selection of Kerlex or Kling bandages in rolls 1, 2, and 3 inches wide, and some paper adhesive tape. The kit can also contain a mild over-the-counter eye-washing solution and some commonly used nonprescription medications, such as an antacid, an antihistamine, and a painkiller like aspirin or acetaminophen (one common brand is Tylenol). It is probably not necessary to include a disinfectant, since wounds can be cleaned well enough by washing them thoroughly with ordinary soap and water.

Even in some major cities abroad it may not be easy to quickly find a doctor who can speak English. A world directory of English-speaking physicians is offered by the International Association for Medical Assistance to Travellers (736 Center Street, Lewiston, N.Y. 14092; in Canada, 188 Nicklin Road, Guelph, Ont. N1H 7L5). IAMAT can also provide detailed health information for international travel.

Digestive Upsets and Motion Sickness

Diarrhea and other digestive troubles are a common experience when traveling. In industrialized countries diarrhea is usually not caused by a microorganism; it is more likely the result of changed eating patterns. Diarrhea and other gastrointestinal problems can thus be minimized by

---

James Chin heads the Infectious Disease Branch of the California Department of Health Services and is clinical professor of epidemiology at the University of California at Berkeley. Leonard Davis is in private practice and is the chairman of the Alameda-Contra Costa Medical Society's Occupational Health Committee.

eating regularly, avoiding too much coffee and alcohol, getting adequate rest, and as far as possible duplicating the way of life followed at home. The prescription drug diphenoxylate (sold under such brand names as Lomotil) can be of help in cases of simple diarrhea that do not respond to these measures. (Although many over-the-counter drugs are promoted for the treatment of diarrhea, their effectiveness is doubtful.) If the diarrhea is accompanied by blood in the stools, a high temperature, or severe exhaustion or collapse, diphenoxylate should not be used, and professional medical advice must be obtained.

The traditional travel experience of leaning over the rail of a ship at sea and emphatically not looking at the fish is still with us today. Motion sickness with its nausea and vomiting is particularly likely to affect people traveling on small commercial aircraft, on coastal ferry boats, on oceangoing ships, or by car on mountain roads. Dimenhydrinate (sold under various brand names, including Dramamine), which is available without a prescription, is an effective medication for the control of this problem. It may, however, cause drowsiness and should not be used by the driver of a car. Moreover, it should not be used, except on the advice of a physician, by people with asthma, glaucoma, or enlargement of the prostate gland, by children under the age of two, by pregnant women and nursing mothers, and by those who are taking certain antibiotics.

The new scopolamine ear patches (sold as Transderm Scōp), which are applied on the skin behind one ear, are effective against motion sickness for three days. But they have potentially more serious side effects than Dramamine and should be used only on the advice of a physician.

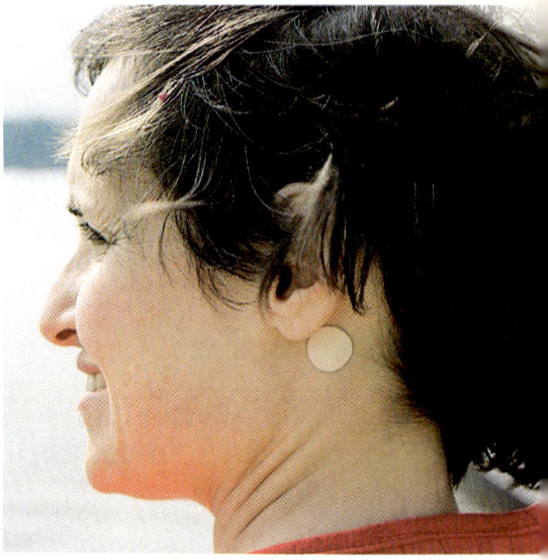

An excursion in a small boat can bring exhilaration and also seasickness; there are, however, over-the-counter and prescription drugs for motion sickness. A new popular type of medication comes in the form of a small patch that is applied behind the ear (above).

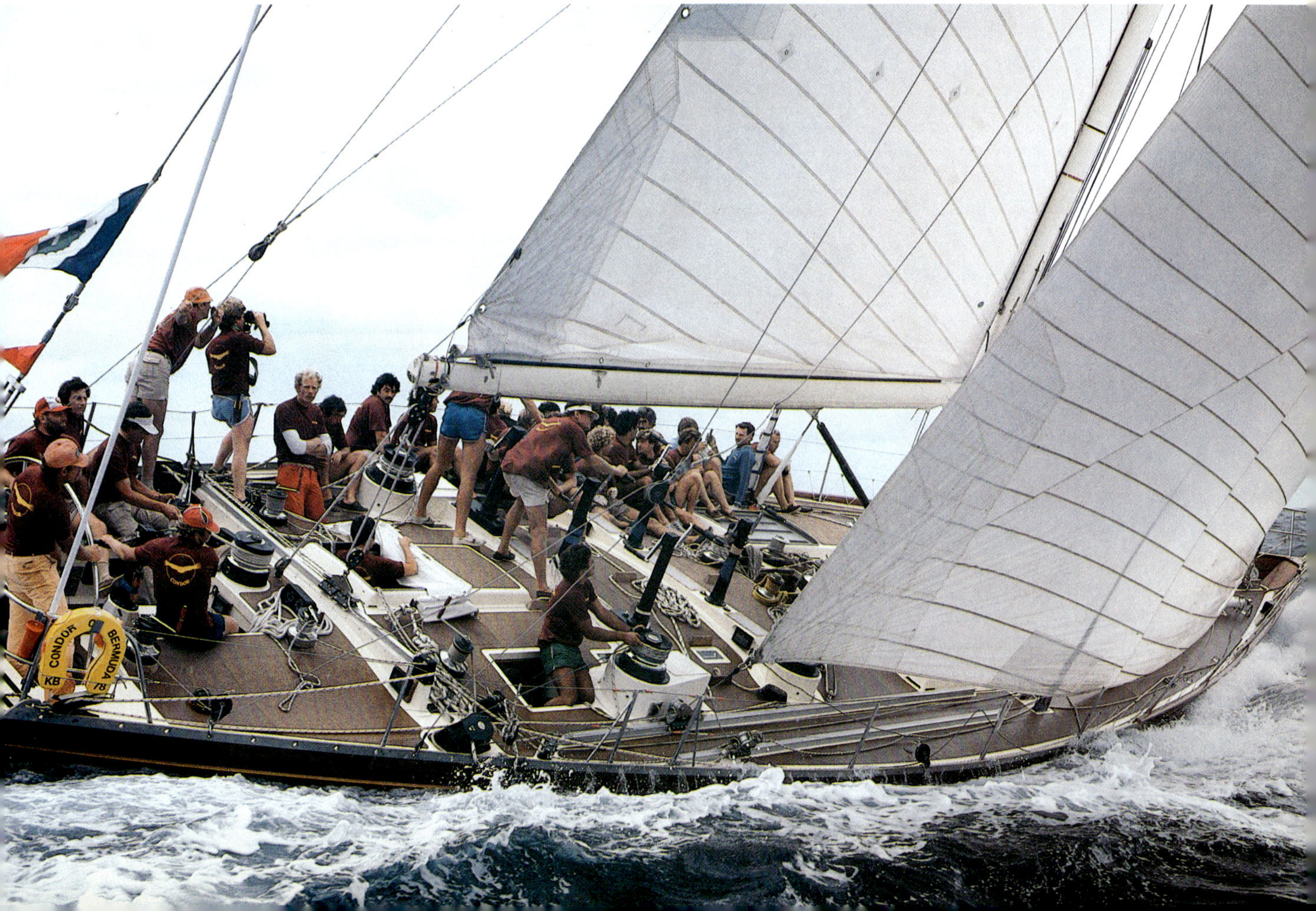

What About Flying?

The rickety flying machines that daring young men and women once flew have become safe, stable behemoths. Travel in a modern commercial jet is generally a quite comfortable experience, but there are a few possible medical problems.

Air-pressure changes within the aircraft cabin may cause some difficulty, particularly for infants and young children. Especially during descent, gases trapped in the sinuses and middle ear may produce ear and sinus pain. The problem can be compounded by congestion from a respiratory infection or allergy. People with congestion who cannot avoid flying may find over-the-counter decongestants helpful, either a nasal spray or a syrup or tablet such as Sudafed (pseudoephedrine), which is taken one hour before flying and every three to four hours during flight. During descent, the passenger who is bothered by pressure changes should frequently perform the so-called Valsalva maneuver—holding the nose and forcing air into the ears by trying to exhale with the mouth closed.

It can take several days for the body's "internal clock" to overcome the effects of jet lag.

Prolonged immobilization in an airplane seat (or on a car, bus, or train trip) can cause swelling of the ankles and make blood clots more likely to form in the legs. To prevent such problems, passengers should contract the muscles of their legs frequently while seated and get up and move around when possible.

Scuba divers should plan to allow 12 to 24 hours between their last dive and boarding a commercial airplane, because the possibility of getting the bends, or decompression sickness, is aggravated by the relatively low air pressure in an aircraft.

People who suffer from severe anxiety at the thought of flying may wish to ask their physician for a prescription for diazepam (commonly sold under the brand name Valium) or another mild sedative. Pregnant women should consult their doctor before flying, as should people with significant

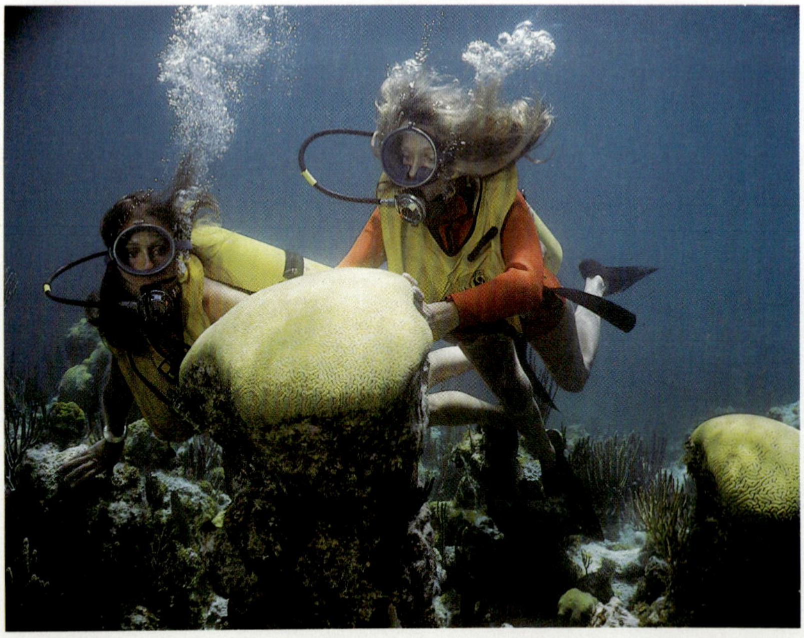

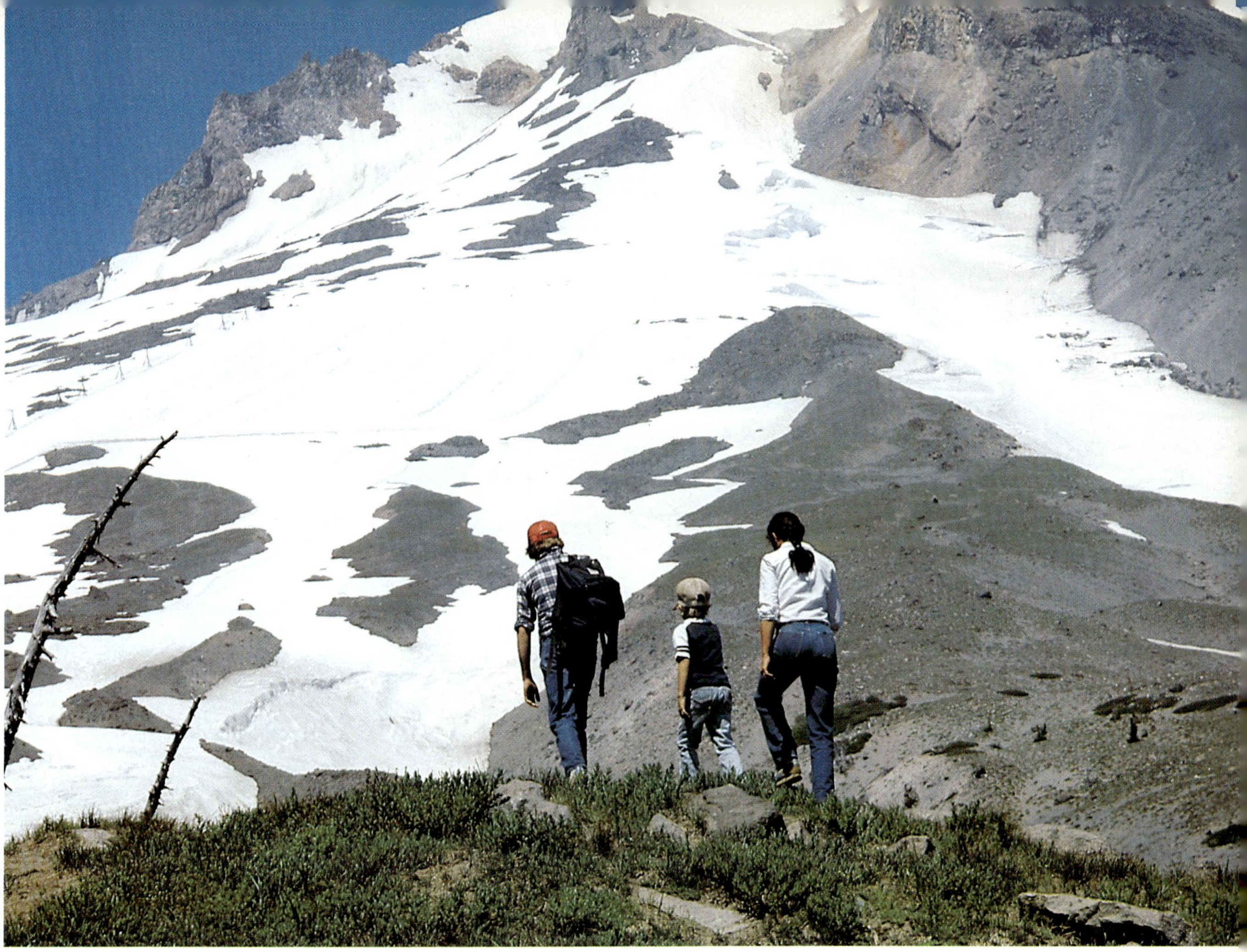

respiratory, cardiovascular, ear, nose, or throat ailments. Others who should see a physician before flying include people who have recently had severe gastrointestinal problems; who suffer from anemia, hernias, poorly controlled seizures, or psychiatric problems manifested by poorly controlled behavior; or who have recently undergone chest or bowel surgery.

Sports enthusiasts should take special health precautions. It is important for scuba divers (facing page) to leave sufficient time between going for a last underwater dive and boarding a plane. Mountain hikers (above) should prepare for the rare atmosphere of high altitudes.

Jet Lag

Travelers who fly across many time zones may arrive at their destination quite exhausted, only to find that it is still early in the day by local time and everybody is up and bustling around. It can take the body's "internal clock" several days to adjust to this drastic change in the day-to-day cycle. To minimize the effects of jet lag, it is a good idea to spend the first day relaxing around the hotel and to get an early dinner and a good night's sleep before tackling an ambitious schedule.

Mountain Sickness

Being on top of the world doesn't always make you feel on top of things. The high altitudes sometimes reached by skiers, mountain climbers, and other visitors to ranges like the Alps may be dangerous for some. Victims of mountain sickness suffer headaches, nausea, and a flulike malaise, symptoms which usually disappear after a few days. A more serious

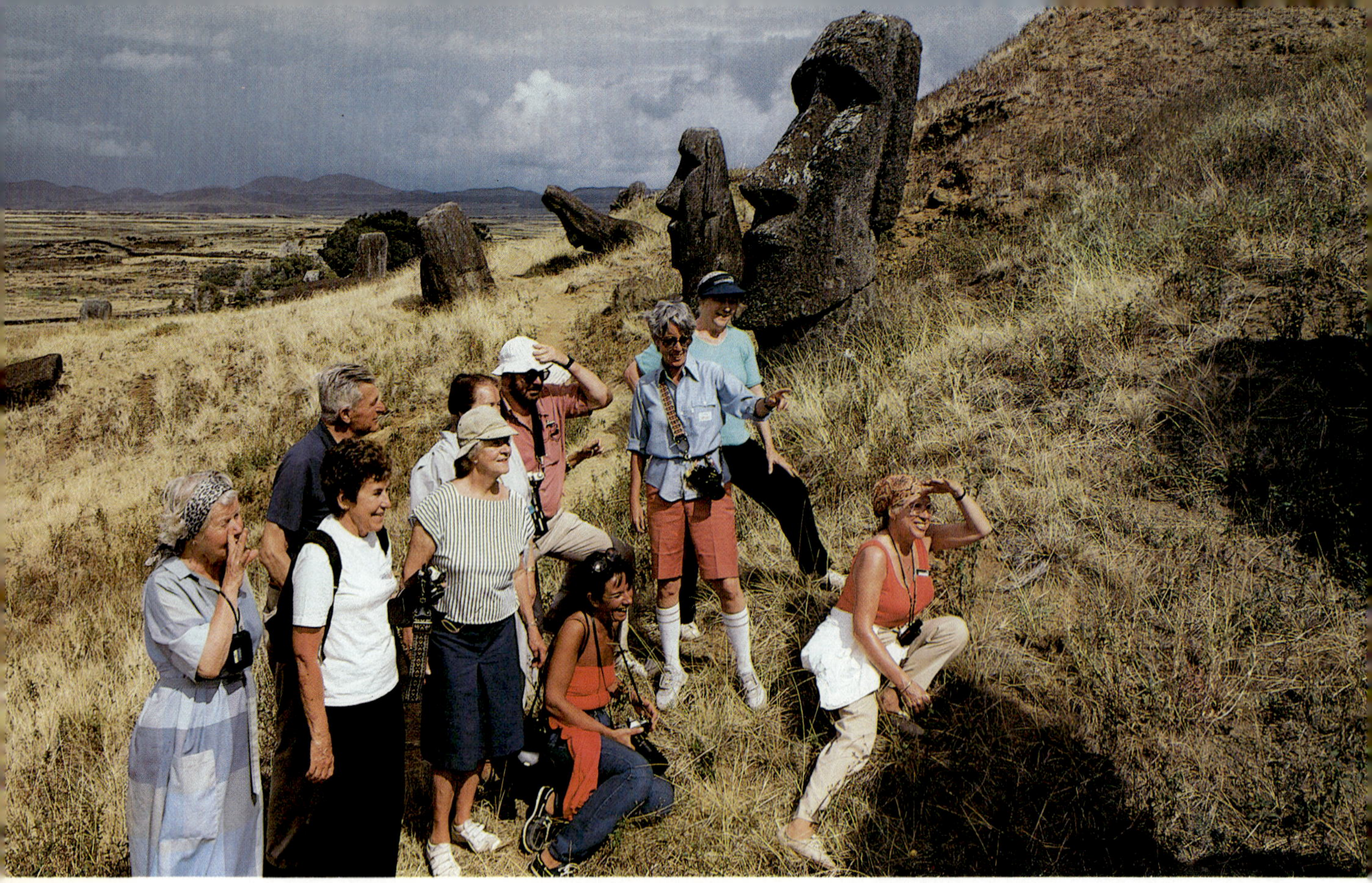

It is sensible to wear a hat and take other precautions against the sun when sightseeing.

problem is high-altitude pulmonary edema, or fluid in the lungs, which can occur even in healthy young people and can be fatal. It may result from ascending too rapidly, sleeping at high altitudes, and overexerting oneself. The drug acetazolamide (Diamox) has been shown by at least one study to lessen the symptoms of altitude sickness. All travelers to high altitudes, and especially those who will be sleeping above 8,000 feet, should consult a physician before departure.

Heat and Sunshine

When you get to that sun-drenched tropical beach you've been dreaming about all year, use a little care. Travelers to very hot climates may be risking medical problems that include heat exhaustion, skin disorders, and severe sunburn. Physical fitness and getting used to high temperatures gradually are important for avoiding such problems. Travelers to tropical or subtropical areas need to drink plenty of fluids to avoid dehydration—but not too much alcohol, which can increase sensitivity to heat. Some medications, including diphenoxylate for the control of diarrhea, also decrease tolerance to heat.

To reduce the chances of getting fungal infections and other skin problems, travelers in hot, humid areas should wash frequently and practice scrupulous skin hygiene. They should dust an antifungal powder such as Desenex between the toes and in other sweaty skin places after each bath or shower.

Those who expect to spend a great deal of time in the sun should take along a sunscreen containing the substance called PABA, which provides good protection against sunburn.

Traveling in Developing Countries

You may want to visit a developing country because you are interested in learning about other cultures, because you enjoy the excitement of exploring out-of-the-way places, or because it means an inexpensive week in the sun. Whatever the reason, it is important to keep in mind that you may encounter disease-bearing insects, parasites of various kinds, and a host of infectious diseases that are rare or nonexistent in the developed countries.

Besides the basic health cautions already noted for travel in the industrialized world, if you are going to a developing country, you may have to take special precautions. You may need shots against various diseases, recorded on a properly validated international certificate of vaccination. You may also require medications for the prevention of malaria, as well as medical advice about other potential problems. The extra precautions may apply even to trips to such familiar places as parts of the Caribbean and Mexico. Because some immunizations require weeks to be effective, at least a month should be allowed before departure for making inquiries about health needs and getting shots.

Immunizations against several diseases are often necessary for travel to developing countries.

State, county, or local health departments in the United States—and in Canada, local practitioners or the federal agency Health and Welfare Canada—are usually good sources of information on what shots are needed for a particular journey and whether there are any additional health recommendations. They may be able to supply the names of physicians in your area who specialize in taking care of travelers. The local medical society office may also have a list of such physicians, and they may be listed in the telephone book.

Health centers authorized to administer yellow fever vaccine are often located near shipping facilities in large ports, at airport medical clinics, or in large urban areas. These centers normally can provide the immunizations that may be required for overseas travel, and most can officially validate international health certificates.

Before and After

You probably do not need a medical checkup before departure if you are in good health, are going to a developing country for just a short period of time, will be staying in normal tourist facilities, and do not plan to engage in unusually strenuous activities, such as mountain climbing. However, people with known medical problems or those who are planning to spend a long time in remote areas should have a checkup, as should those who intend to take up residence and work in a developing country.

It would be prudent to take on your trip a written summary of any medical problems. In order to avoid any customs difficulties, personal medications should be in separate, well-marked containers and should be accompanied by a letter from your physician stating what drugs have been prescribed for what purpose and the dosage. It might be wise to schedule a regular visit to the dentist before leaving, especially if your trip will be longer than a few weeks. If you wear glasses or contact lenses, an extra pair and the prescription should be taken along.

Travelers returning from prolonged residence in developing countries should again have a medical checkup, including laboratory tests for intestinal parasites.

Food and Water

That vegetable salad may be beautiful, the skewered meat grilling on the street corner may smell irresistible after a long day of sightseeing—but you'd probably better not. In areas of the world where sanitation is poor, food should be selected with care to avoid illness. Contaminated foods can be a source of diarrhea, food poisoning, hepatitis, various intestinal parasites, and a host of other health problems. Only pasteurized milk and milk products should be consumed, and even these may not be safe unless they have been boiled or are canned. Rare meat and raw fish may carry disease-causing parasites, and raw shellfish can give you hepatitis. Raw vegetables in salads may also be a source of disease. Follow the adage, If you can't boil it, cook it, or peel it, forget it. These rules hold true in people's homes, as well as in hotels and restaurants, however well selected.

In areas of poor sanitation water that is not chlorinated may not be safe to drink; only adequately chlorinated or boiled water offers significant protection against disease. Better hotels and restaurants frequented by tourists from industrialized countries will usually provide safe bottled drinking water. However, the ice used in drinks, the water you brush your teeth with, and water remaining on the outside of cans and bottles cooled in ice may also be a potential source of disease. Normally safe are soft drinks, beer, wine, canned or bottled water, and beverages like tea or

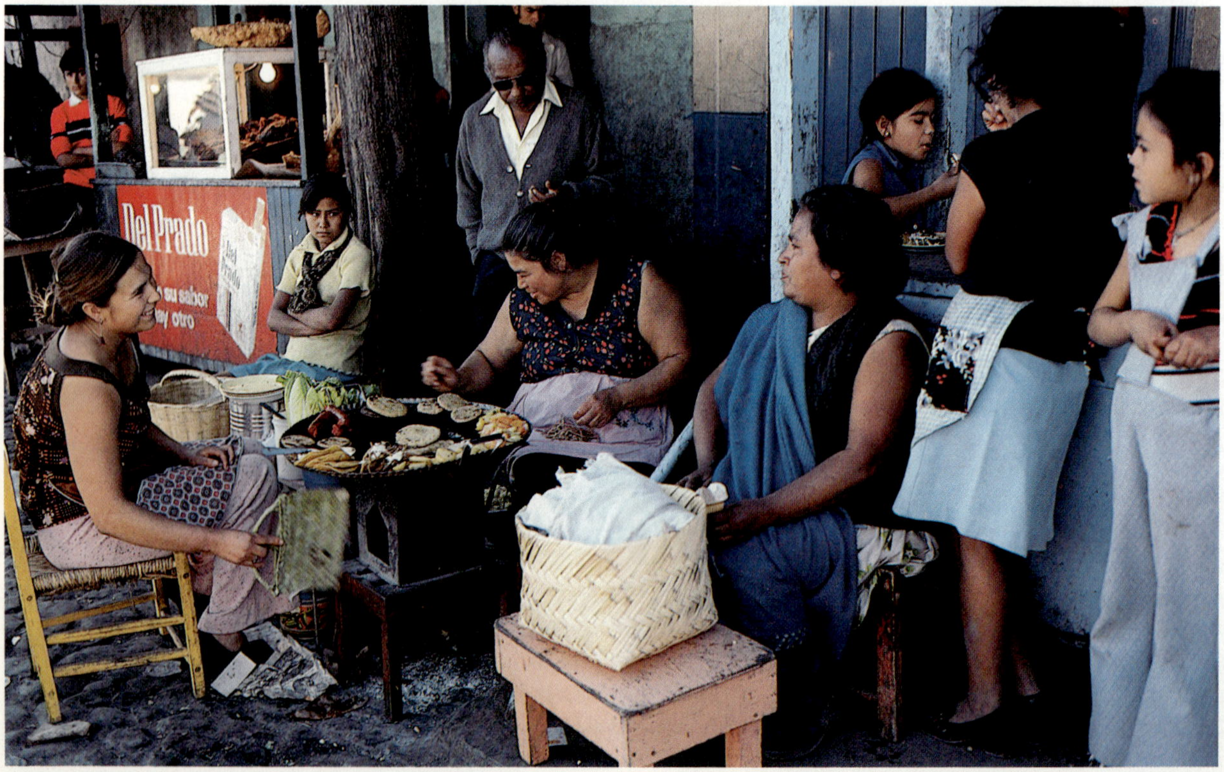

An exotic fast-food snack may be tempting, but travelers in developing areas, where sanitary standards are not rigorous, should select food carefully.

coffee that are made with boiled water. Travelers to truly remote areas may need to carry chemicals such as iodine tablets to purify the water they drink.

Schistosomiasis (a serious disease caused by infection with parasites called blood flukes) and the liver disorder hepatitis can be contracted by swimming in contaminated water. In some localities it may be prudent to make careful inquiries about the safety of swimming areas.

Diarrhea

Probably the most common result of carelessness about food and drink is traveler's diarrhea. Usually a mild illness and frequently caused by a microorganism, it affects a large portion of travelers to countries where sanitation is less than advanced.

There have been many attempts to develop safe and effective drugs for the prevention of traveler's diarrhea. Even though some drugs have been reported to be partially effective, there is no medical consensus that drugs, including antibiotics, should be used routinely. Entero-Vioform (iodochlorhydroxyquin) and similar medications promoted in some countries for the prevention or treatment of diarrhea are harmful and should be avoided.

Some experts recommend that travelers carry a prescription drug, usually a tetracycline or sulfa compound, for use in case diarrhea develops. An advantage of this approach over using a preventive drug is that medication is taken only if it becomes necessary. Prompt use of such medications when symptoms appear can often reduce the duration and severity of the diarrhea. If your doctor prescribes such a drug, be sure to follow closely all instructions regarding its use.

Traveler's diarrhea is the most common result of carelessness about food and drink.

Malaria

In many parts of the world, mosquito bites are not just an annoyance that can ruin a summer evening. The mosquitoes may transmit malaria, a very serious and occasionally fatal disease that is the most significant threat to the health of travelers in many developing countries. The risk of catching it can be reduced by taking precautions to avoid mosquito bites and by the use of preventive drugs.

Malaria occurs in parts of Africa, Asia, Mexico, Central and South America, the Middle East, the Indian subcontinent, the Caribbean, Oceania (the islands of the central and south Pacific), and other subtropical and tropical areas. It is caused by several species of a single-celled organism called plasmodium, which is transmitted to humans by the bite of the anopheles mosquito. In most types of malaria these infecting organisms go through a latent, or incubation, stage in the liver. When they are released into the bloodstream, they cause fever and chills. In some cases relapses may occur months or years after the initial infection.

The anopheles mosquito is active primarily between dusk and dawn. Travelers can reduce the risk of getting malaria by remaining in well-screened areas during these hours and by sleeping in air-conditioned rooms free of mosquitoes or under mosquito netting. Exposure to mosquitoes outdoors can be reduced by wearing clothing that adequately

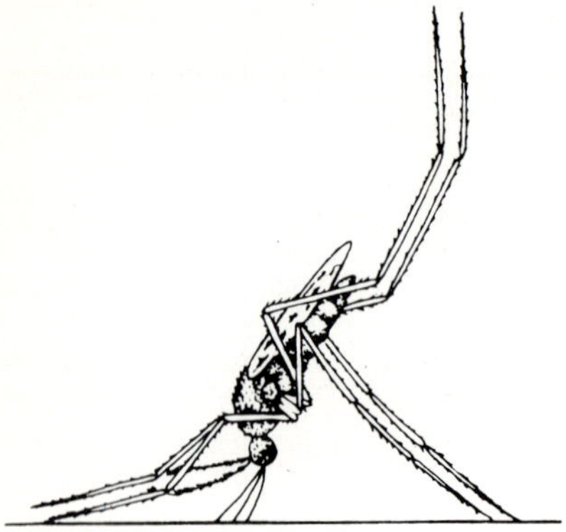

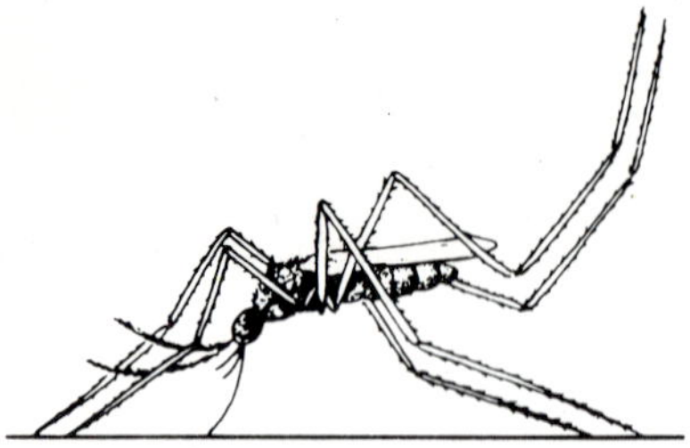

Malaria is transmitted by the bite of the anopheles mosquito (top), compared here with the more common and safe culex mosquito (bottom). Below, a stamp highlights the regions of the world where malaria occurs.

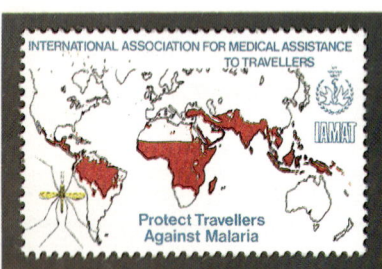

covers the arms and legs and by applying mosquito repellent to thin clothing and exposed skin. The most effective insect repellents contain a substance known as DEET (for NN diethyl-meta-toluamide). Prolonged and extensive use should be avoided.

The official recommendations of the U.S. Centers for Disease Control for preventing malaria in travelers were changed in early 1985. The new recommendations call for the use of preventive medication only in areas and situations where the risk of malaria is considered moderate to high. (Before the guidelines were revised, medication was recommended even in low-risk areas.)

Travel to some areas of Africa and Oceania—whether urban or rural—presents a high risk. In such areas weekly doses of a drug called chloroquine, as well as the medication pyrimethamine-sulfadoxine (Fansidar) for strains of malaria resistant to chloroquine, may be advised. For the Indian subcontinent, chloroquine alone is recommended. Travel to many other regions is considered to be of low malarial risk, and no preventive drugs are advised unless you will be visiting rural areas between dusk and dawn.

People going to areas where malaria is prevalent will need to consult a knowledgeable physician who has access to the most up-to-date information on prevention so that a careful assessment can be made of the risks involved and a decision made about what medications, if any, are to be used.

Immunizations

No immunizations are required of persons entering the United States or Canada. Some countries, however, require entering travelers to have a properly validated international certificate of vaccination as proof of current immunization against cholera and/or yellow fever. A shot affording protection against hepatitis A is a good idea for most everyone going to a developing country. Vaccination against various other diseases, such as typhoid fever or rabies, may also be advisable, depending on your destination, types of activities, and length of stay.

Routine immunizations. All travelers should be up to date on those immunizations normally given residents of their own country. For Americans this means that adults should have received an adult diphtheria-tetanus booster within the past ten years, while children should have had all the recommended vaccinations (including the appropriate boosters) for diphtheria, tetanus, whooping cough, mumps, measles, and rubella. The risk of acquiring most of these diseases is greater in developing countries than in the industrialized world.

In addition, children and adults who have already had a complete series of doses of oral polio vaccine and who are going to a developing country should receive an additional dose. (They require no further boosters thereafter.) Adults who believe they have never had the oral polio vaccine should consult their physician.

Cholera. The risk to the average traveler of contracting cholera is so low that the benefits of cholera vaccine are questionable. The vaccine is not very effective, and minor side effects such as fever and an aching arm are common. In some parts of the world, however, failure to produce documented evidence of cholera vaccination may lead to on-the-spot immunization, often with a needle of doubtful sterility, followed by some form of quarantine for up to five days. Consequently, vaccination is often recommended to protect the traveler from immunization policies, rather than from cholera itself. Normally, a single dose of vaccine is sufficient to satisfy local requirements, but with the threat or occurrence of a cholera epidemic some countries may require evidence of a completed series of two doses taken at least a week apart. Validation of cholera immunization is good for only six months.

Yellow fever. A greater danger is presented by yellow fever. The risk of contracting this potentially fatal disease is present in both urban and rural areas in Africa in a zone from 15 degrees north of the equator to 15 degrees south, and in South America from 15 degrees north to as far as 30 degrees south. Cases of the disease are often not reported, so the fact that a locality is not officially an area of risk does not necessarily mean it is safe. All people going to these zones, especially those who will be in rural areas, ought to be immunized with yellow fever vaccine. Some countries may require evidence of immunization from all entering travelers.

Certain people should not receive yellow fever vaccine. These include individuals who are clearly allergic to eggs, infants less than six months of age, and, normally, pregnant women.

Hepatitis. Travelers to developing countries run a greatly increased risk of contracting hepatitis A, which is spread primarily by food or water contaminated by human waste. All such travelers should ordinarily receive an injection of immune globulin (a concentration of antibodies against the hepatitis A virus made from human blood plasma), which offers at least partial protection against the disease. Those spending a prolonged period in developing countries can receive a shot every five to six months. Before leaving home they should have their blood tested to make sure they are not already immune because of once having had a hepatitis A infection.

Typhoid fever. Vaccination against typhoid fever is not required for international travel but is generally recommended for those going to areas with poor sanitation. Two doses of vaccine should be given, preferably four or more weeks apart; a booster dose can follow every three years. □

Tips for Travelers

- Before departure, make sure your routine immunizations are up to date, and find out whether you need any other immunizations or preventive medication.
- Don't change your day-to-day habits too quickly or too drastically.
- Take your time in adjusting to new conditions such as hot weather or high altitude.
- In areas where sanitation is suspect:

  Do not eat prepared food purchased from street vendors.

  Avoid raw fruits and vegetables—including salads—that you have not peeled and sliced yourself.

  Try to eat in restaurants that practice good sanitation. (In many countries you can look in the kitchen to see if it's clean.)

  Eat only dairy products that have been pasteurized and properly refrigerated.

  Drink bottled water, carbonated water, soda, beer, or wine, never tap water (unless boiled).

  Wash your hands often, and practice good hygiene.

SUGGESTIONS FOR FURTHER READING

DuPont, Herbert, and Margaret DuPont. *Travel With Health.* East Norwalk, Conn., Appleton-Century-Crofts, 1981.

Harkonen, W. Scott. *Traveling Well: The Comprehensive Health Guide for Every Traveler.* New York, Dodd, Mead, 1984.

Health Information for International Travel. Annual publication of the Centers for Disease Control, Atlanta.

Scotti, Angelo T., and Thomas A. Moore. *The Traveler's Medical Manual.* New York, Berkley, 1985.

Vaccination Certificate Requirements for International Travel and Health Advice to Travelers. Annual publication of the World Health Organization, Geneva, Switzerland.

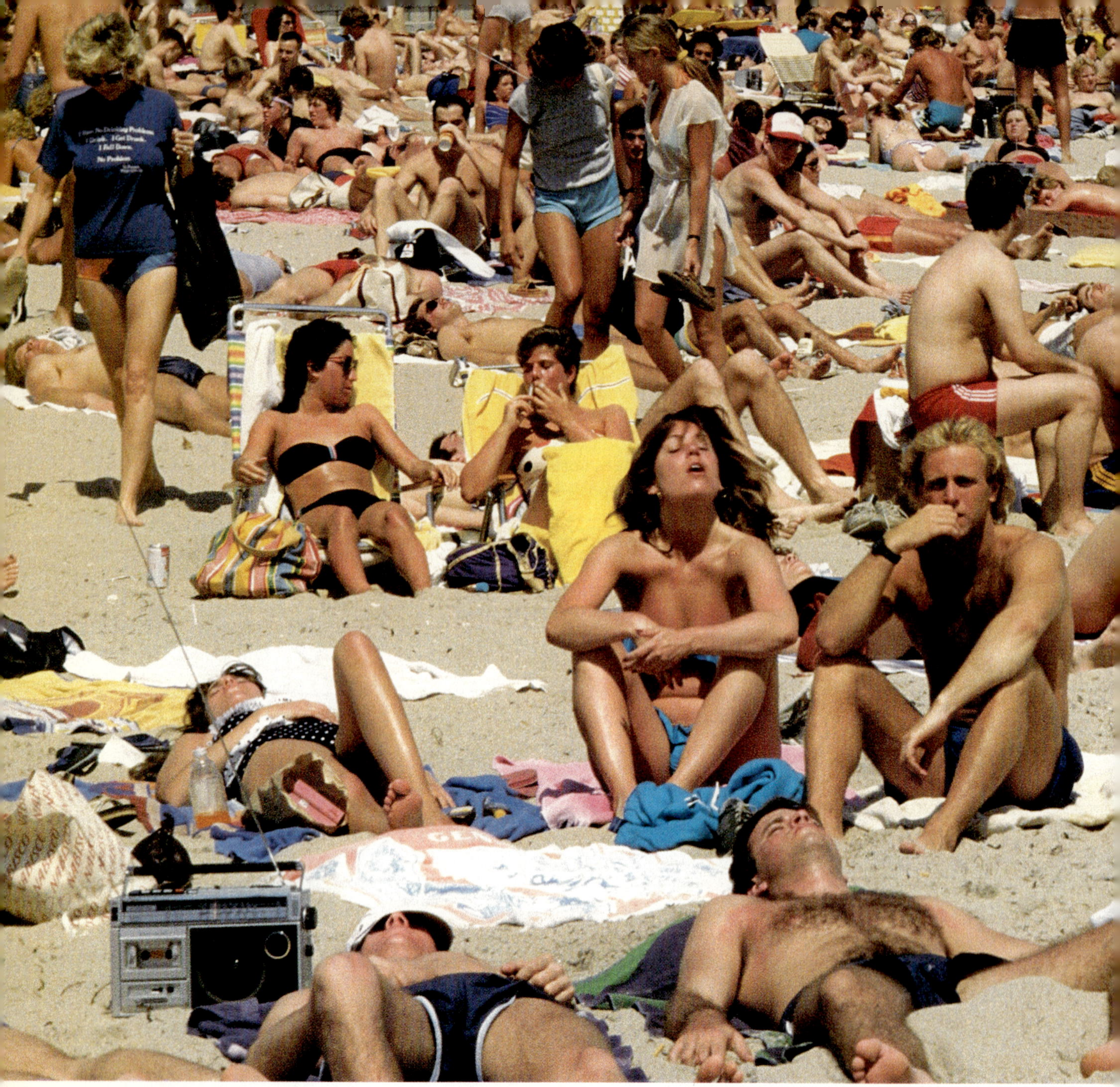

THE SKIN

A Vital Organ

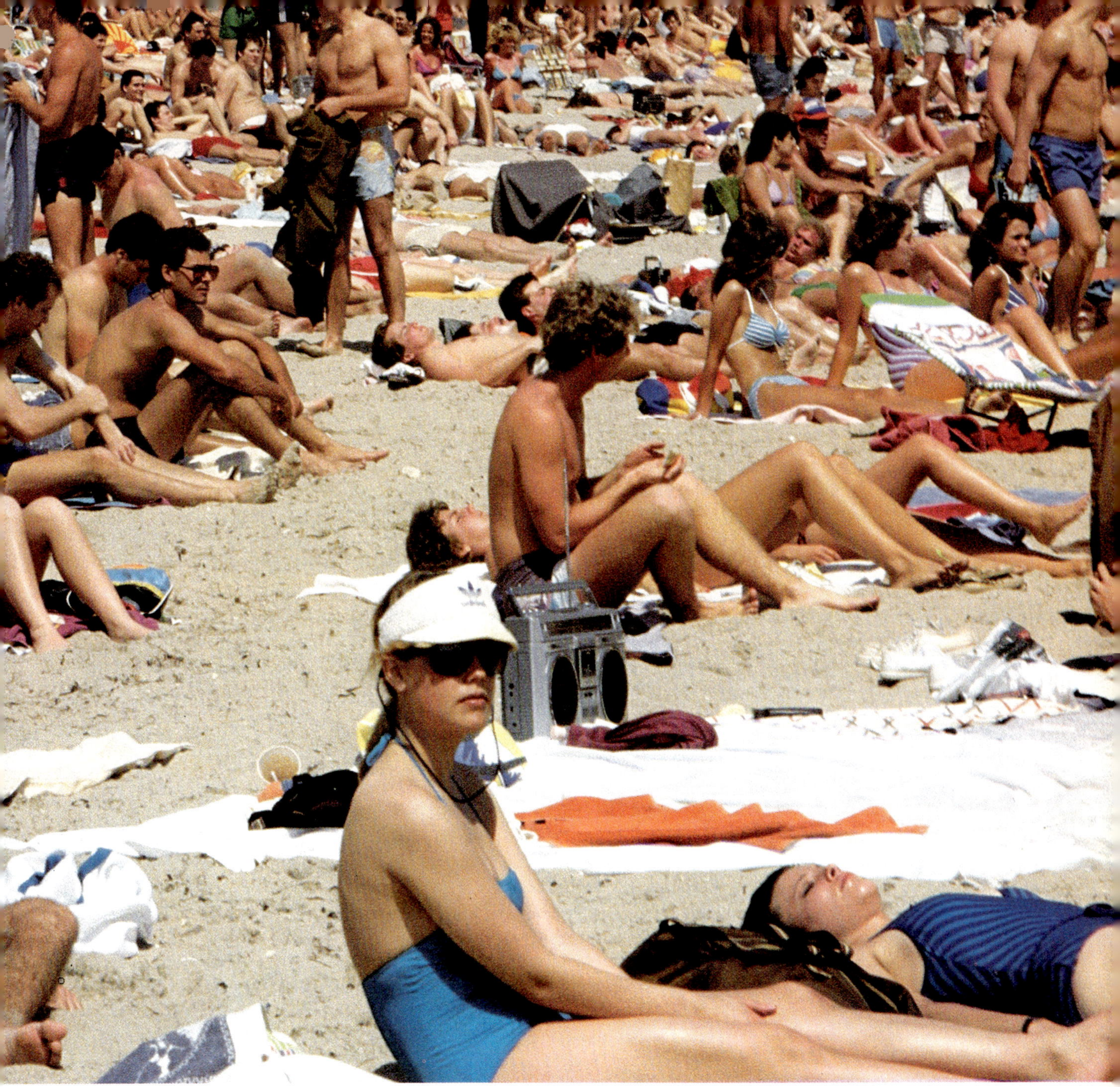

Edward E. Bondi, M.D.

The skin is, in many ways, the most maligned part of the body. Such common expressions as "skin deep," "skinflint," and "thin-skinned" all have a derogatory meaning. When the body's exceptional features are enumerated, the unique qualities of skin are frequently overlooked.

The skin is the largest organ in the body—and one of the most versatile, dynamic, and interesting. It functions as a vital protective shield against infection and wounds, pollutants and cosmetics, and extremes of heat and cold; serves as a "container" for the body's contents; and plays a major role in the body's temperature-regulation, immune, and sensory systems. The skin is also the "garb" in which the world sees us. Although the skin may seem a rather fragile fabric, ill-suited to its many tasks, close inspection reveals an extremely complex, resilient organ that continuously renews itself and is ingeniously designed to perform its varied functions.

Virtually no one goes through life without developing some disorders of the skin. The total number known to exist is enormous. Although these diseases rarely endanger the skin's basic structure or keep it from carrying out its principal functions, they can produce effects that extend from the unsightly or uncomfortable to serious health problems. The diagnosis and treatment of skin disorders is the subject of the field of dermatology.

The Skin's Structure

The skin is composed of three basic layers: the epidermis, the dermis, and the subcutaneous tissue. Each contains specialized structures for carrying out essential functions.

The three layers of the skin act as barrier, sense organ, and thermal insulator.

The epidermis is the outermost layer. At its base is the basal-cell layer, composed of self-duplicating cells that proliferate to provide the cells (keratinocytes) making up almost the entire epidermis. As new epidermal cells move from the basal-cell layer toward the skin surface, each cell matures and produces large quantities of a durable fibrous protein called keratin. At the surface, the epidermal cells die. These interlocking dead cells, composed mainly of keratin, are like the shingles on a roof. Forming what is known as the horny layer, they constitute the major barrier between the body and the outside world.

Below the epidermis lies the dermis, consisting mostly of sturdy fibers of collagen, a kind of protein. An intricate weave of these fibers forms the main structural framework of the skin: when we pinch or touch skin, what we feel is largely this middle fibrous layer. Within the dermis is a rich network of blood vessels, providing nourishment to the epidermis above, as well as an abundance of nerves. In conjunction with a variety of specialized sensory receptor cells, these nerves enable the skin to act as a major sensory organ. Our ability to distinguish pain, temperature, and touch depends greatly on this sensory function of the skin.

The subcutaneous (literally, under the skin) tissue, the third and deepest of the skin's principal layers, is composed mostly of large fat-containing cells. This layer functions as a physical cushion and thermal insulator. It also constitutes the body's major reserve of energy, stored in the form of fat that can be mobilized when needed to provide nourishment elsewhere in the body.

In addition to the epidermis, dermis, and subcutaneous tissue, skin has on or within it various structures technically known as appendages. These include the hair, nails, sebaceous glands (secreting the oily substance called sebum), and sweat glands.

A Dynamic Organ

The skin and its appendages function as a dynamic organ, at all times able to adjust and readjust to changes inside the body and in the surrounding

---

Edward E. Bondi is associate professor of dermatology at the University of Pennsylvania.

environment. It is this ability to respond to change that makes the seemingly delicate skin a flexible, versatile, and yet durable shield against the environment. In response to cuts and bruises, the rate at which the epidermis's basal cells multiply increases to one of the highest levels of cell multiplication in the human body. This stepped-up supply of epidermal cells enables the skin to repair minor damage rapidly with healthy new skin. If the injury is superficial, penetrating no deeper than the epidermis, repair is complete and no scar will form. For a deeper skin injury a rapid replacement of collagen fibers in the dermis is required for healing, and a fibrous scar usually results.

The skin's response to an increase in body temperature offers another example of its dynamic quality. If the body's temperature rises, more of the blood supply to the skin is directed through the network of blood vessels close to the skin's surface, making it easier for heat to leave the body. At the same time the sweat glands receive a signal from the central

Structure of the Skin

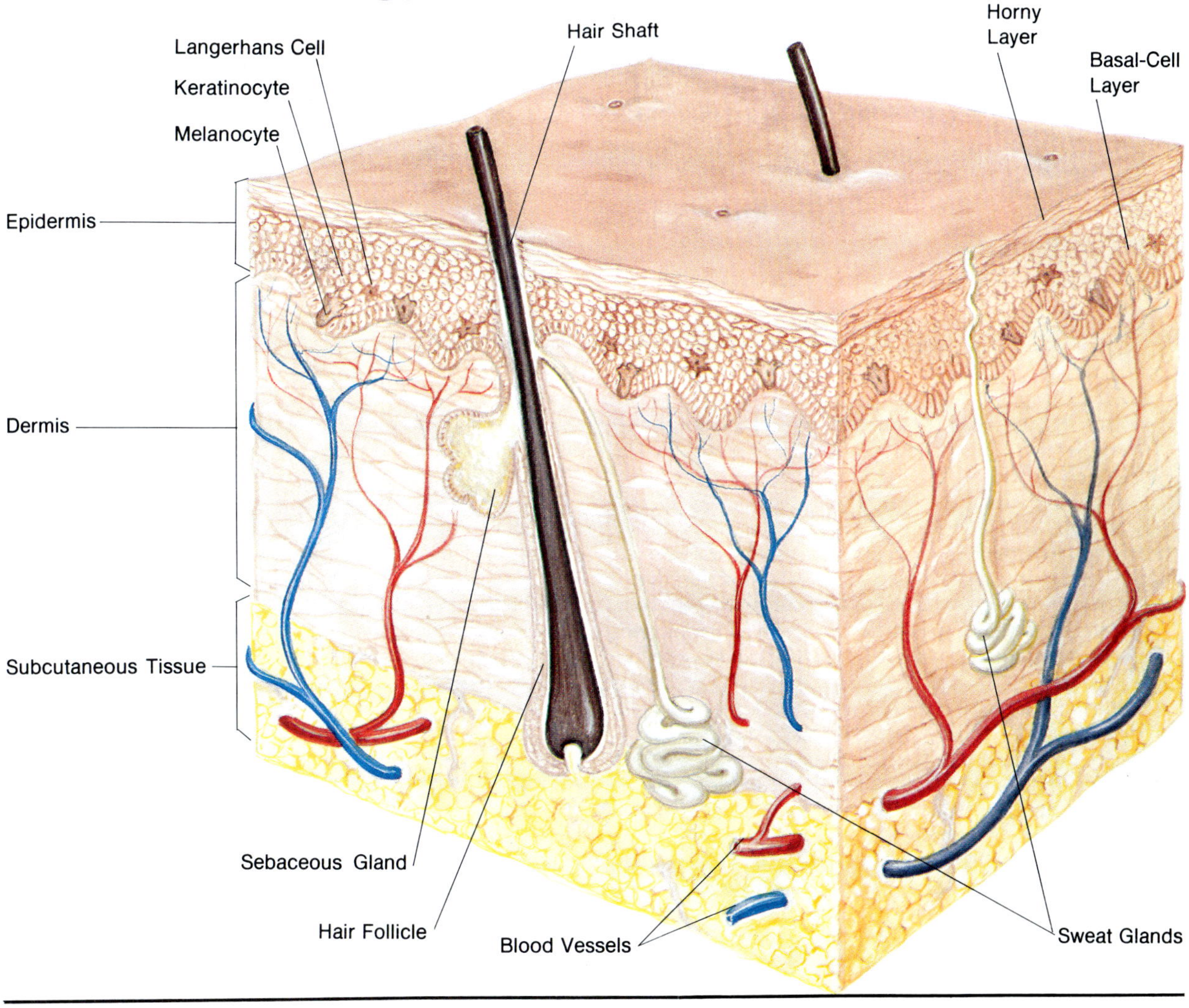

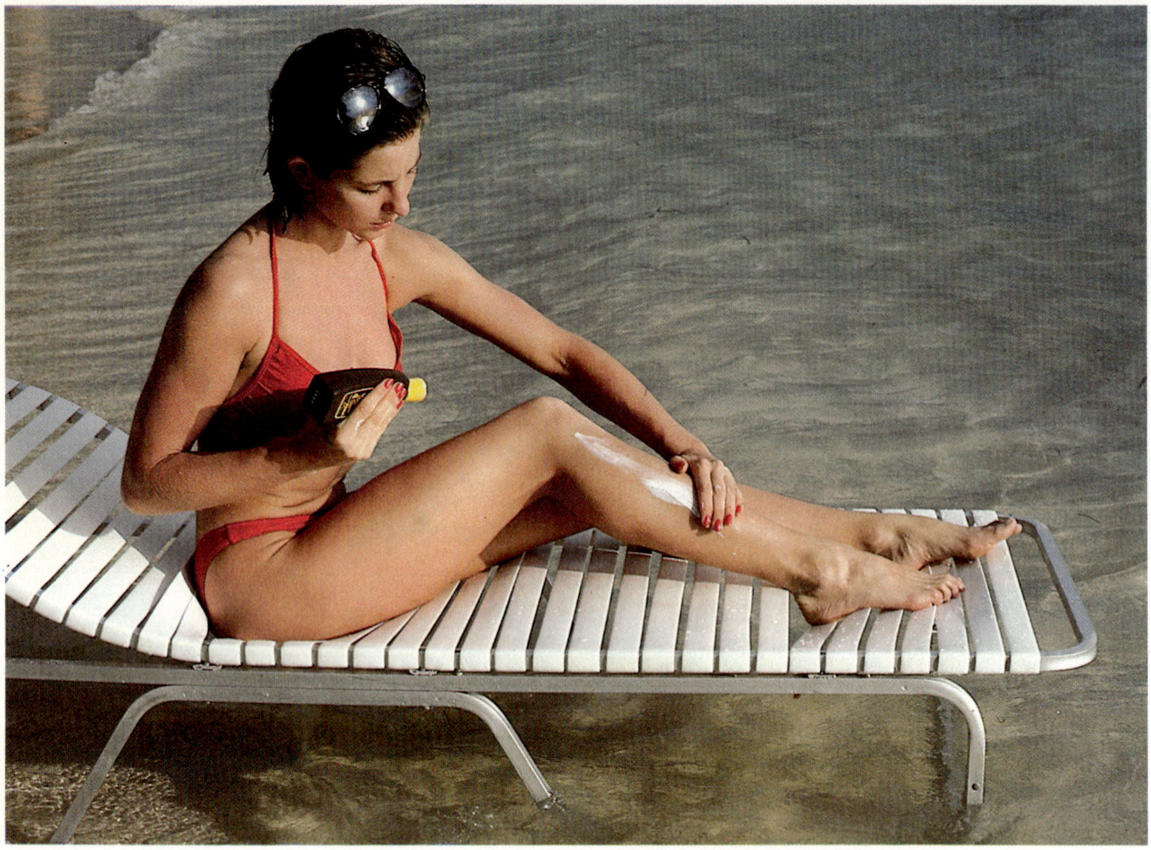

Sunscreens and SPF's

Sunscreens are combinations of chemicals that, when spread on skin, either reflect or absorb the sun's harmful ultraviolet rays. Zinc oxide, in the form of a thick, white paste (often used by lifeguards to protect the nose), is an example of a sunscreen that reflects sunlight. Para-aminobenzoic acid, or PABA, is the most commonly used chemical in sunscreen products that absorb ultraviolet radiation. Since it absorbs the kinds of rays most harmful to the skin, PABA can provide significant protection both against sunburn and against skin cancer and the accelerated aging of the skin caused by years of exposure to too much sun.

When buying a sunscreen, it may be difficult to choose from the multitude of different products available, each adorned with seductive summer images and accompanied by spectacular marketing claims. The decision is made easier by the Skin Protection Factor, or SPF, a standardized measure of relative effectiveness that should be clearly displayed on each package. The SPF number (usually in the range of 1 to 15, although products with higher numbers are beginning to appear) indicates the amount of sun exposure required to produce a given degree of redness with and without the sunscreen. For example, if the SPF is 15, it would take 15 hours of sun exposure with the sunscreen to cause the same sunburn that would result from one hour of exposure without it. The higher the SPF number, the greater the protection, but it is important to remember that no sunscreen completely blocks the sun's ultraviolet rays. The Skin Cancer Foundation in New York City recommends the regular use of sunscreens with an SPF of 15 or greater.

To obtain maximum benefits from sunscreens, sunbathers should reapply the product after swimming or vigorously perspiring, since most sunscreens lose at least part of their effectiveness after exposure to water or moisture. Caution should be exercised while a bather is actually in the water as well, because the sun's ultraviolet rays that burn the skin penetrate water. A sunscreen should be used even on hazy days, since ultraviolet radiation also penetrates cloud cover, and when skiing, because the combination of high altitude and reflection of the sun's rays off the surface of the snow may intensify the sun's effect. Since sunscreens slow down but do not prevent sunburn, sun lovers who use them still need to wear protective clothing and to place a judicious limit on the amount of time they spend in the sun.

nervous system to bathe the skin surface with sweat, which—through evaporation—causes the skin surface to cool. What at first glance may seem like an inconsequential blush on the face of an exercising athlete actually represents an ingenious skin-cooling mechanism. Conversely, in a cold environment the body seeks to preserve warmth: sweating lessens, and the blood circulates mostly through vessels deeper in the body.

Effects of Sun

Sunlight endangers a healthy skin in a variety of ways. The sun's ultraviolet rays have the ability to severely injure body cells by damaging the genetic information stored in the cell nuclei. Usually the cells can repair the damage, but sometimes it results in cell death or irreversible alterations of genetic information that may later evolve into cancer. The skin defends itself against this ultraviolet challenge through a complex interaction of special cells (melanocytes) with other cells in the epidermis. The melanocytes produce melanin, a black pigment that absorbs the energy of ultraviolet light, in little "packets" called melanosomes. These packets move to the surrounding epidermal cells, where they form a kind of cap over the nuclei. Like a parasol, they protect the cells' genetic information from the ultraviolet light.

This interaction between melanocytes and other epidermal cells is a dynamic one, able to respond to changing environmental conditions. When the skin is exposed to the sun, melanocytes become activated, producing more melanin. The resulting increase of melanin in the epidermal cells—visible as a suntan—provides the skin with a greater tolerance for ultraviolet light.

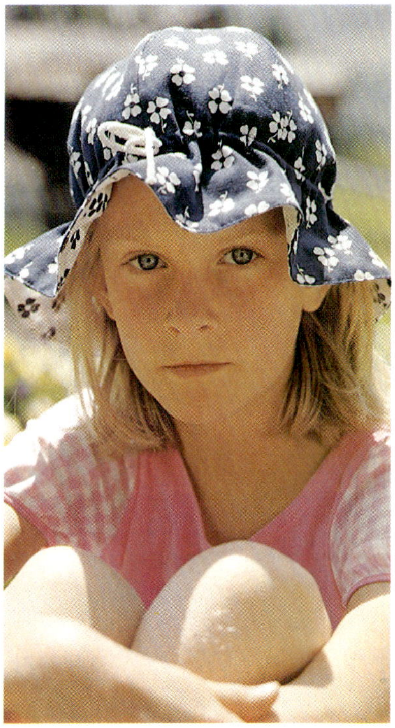

Sun shading by bonnet, hat, or beach umbrella should begin young, especially for those with fair skin.

Unfortunately, melanin affords only partial protection from the sun, and some ultraviolet radiation always penetrates the skin. Fair-skinned individuals are particularly vulnerable, since they produce relatively little melanin, providing only limited natural protection from the damage of ultraviolet light. In the short term, skin exposed to larger amounts of ultraviolet light than it can safely tolerate acquires a painful sunburn; over a long period, too much sun causes the skin to age more quickly—and can lead to cancer.

Skin subjected to years of exposure to the sun becomes dry, thickened, leathery, and wrinkled. All parts of the skin are damaged by long-term bombardment with solar energy, but the most noticeable effect is that the elastic tissue in the upper portion of the dermis that keeps skin looking firm breaks down, leading to premature wrinkling. Most of this sun-induced skin damage, including wrinkles, can be avoided by the use of protective clothing and sunscreens (see facing page).

The widely held notion, fostered by the cosmetic industry, that skin moisturizers can prevent wrinkles is a misconception. It is true that moisturizing creams can counteract the dry scaliness of sun-damaged skin, but this effect is temporary. While moisturizers may briefly make such skin look better, in no way do they eliminate the wrinkles and other effects of sun damage. With the exception of such procedures as facelifts and repeated collagen or silicone injections, the only answer to premature wrinkles is to prevent them by limiting sun exposure. It is ironic that often the same individuals who most strongly desire a deep, dark tan in

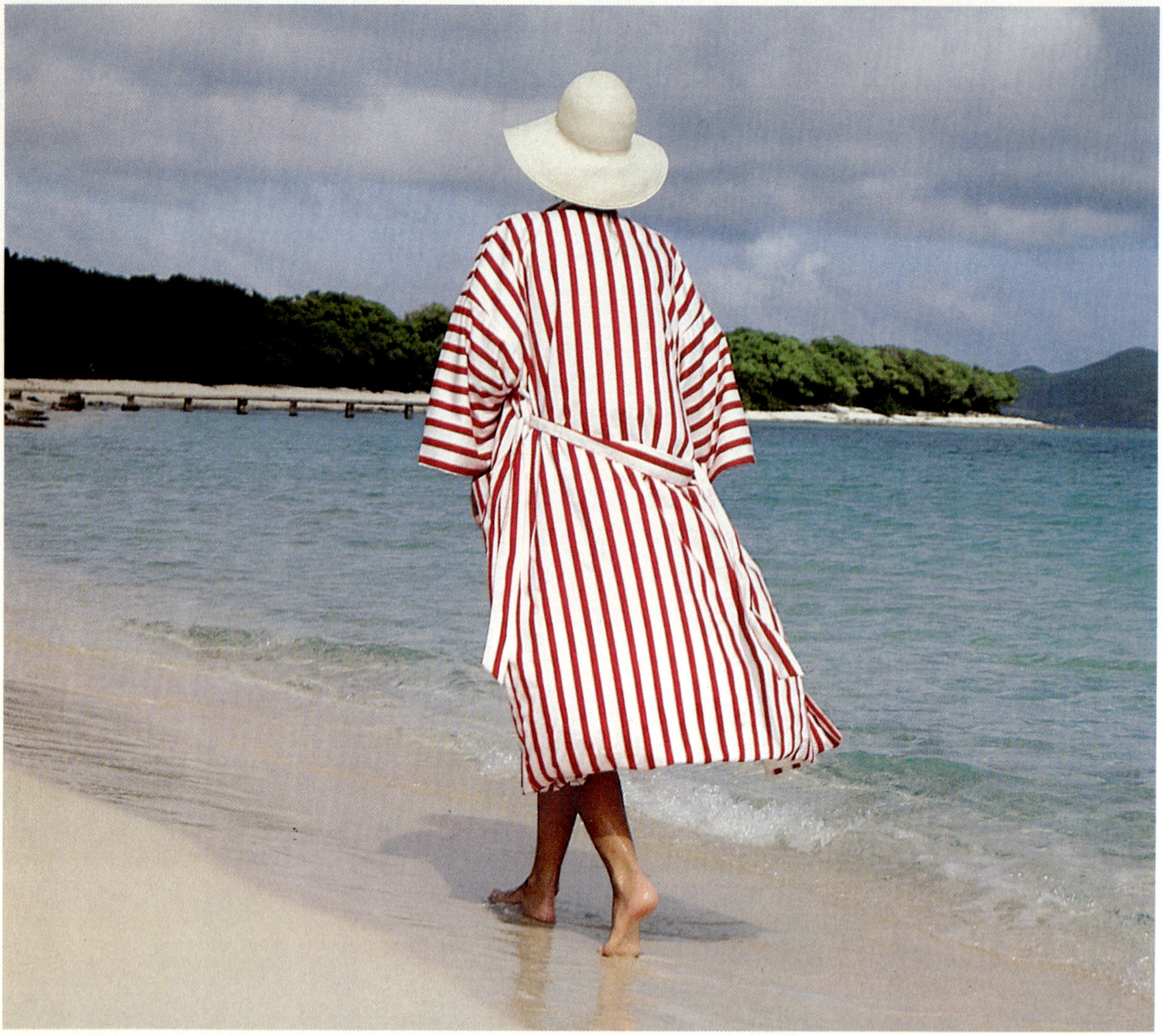

When the sun is strong, colorful protective clothing can make a virtue of a necessity.

their teens and 20's are those who are most horrified by the accelerated aging of the skin that occurs later.

Three Types of Skin Cancer

There are three principal types of skin cancer, with basal-cell carcinoma the most common. Its name reflects the fact that the tumor cells have many characteristics in common with the basal cells of the epidermis. The malignant cells appear to originate in the epidermis but then slowly invade the dermis. The cancer begins as a flesh-colored or translucent bump on the skin, often displaying small blood vessels on its surface. In time the bump is likely to develop a central sore, or ulceration, and may bleed. Fortunately, this kind of skin cancer has little tendency to metastasize, or spread to other areas of the body, and rarely represents a threat to life. But because it can invade neighboring tissue if left untreated, it can be markedly disfiguring. The cancer cells removed from President Ronald Reagan's nose in 1985 were basal-cell carcinoma.

Squamous-cell carcinoma, arising among the flat, scalelike (or "squamous") cells lying above the basal cells, is the second most common type of skin cancer. Because of its greater tendency to spread, it is more dangerous. It develops as a flesh-colored tumorous mass on the skin that, like basal-cell carcinoma, may bleed spontaneously. Although it usually occurs in chronically sun-damaged skin, squamous-cell carcinoma may also appear in areas of the skin that have suffered chronic irritation or infection or have been damaged by X rays. If it is diagnosed while still limited to the skin, it can be easily cured. However, once it spreads—to nearby lymph nodes or throughout the body—it has the potential to kill.

Too much sun doesn't just give you a sunburn—it can lead to early wrinkles and even skin cancer.

The third skin cancer, malignant melanoma, occurs least often but is by far the most lethal. Composed of pigment-forming malignant cells derived from melanocytes, the tumor almost always spreads if left untreated. Fortunately, in most cases melanoma occurs in a recognizable form, permitting it to be readily detected and cured before it spreads. With increased public awareness, melanoma cases are more often being diagnosed and treated at an early stage; consequently, the cure rate in the United States has been improving dramatically. But the news is not all good. The total number of cases has been growing at a disturbingly high rate, with the incidence of melanoma in the United States more than doubling between 1971 and 1983, the last year for which solid figures are available. Estimates suggest the trend is continuing. (The American Cancer Society predicted that 1986 would see 23,000 cases, compared with 22,000 in 1985.) As a result, the overall number of deaths from this skin cancer has continued to rise.

Recognizing Melanoma

Early diagnosis and surgical removal of a melanoma tumor are the most important factors in achieving a cure. Because the tumor is composed of pigment-forming cells, it usually has a distinctive appearance. It begins as an expanding black spot, in about half the cases as a new spot on the skin; in the other half it evolves from a preexisting mole. The tumor often grows asymmetrically, producing an irregular border.

At some point after a tumor begins to develop, the body's immune system recognizes it as "foreign." Inflammation results, generally producing a variety of coloration within the tumor that makes it look even more bizarre. Some areas appear black, from large numbers of pigment-forming tumor cells; some areas may be pink because of the inflammation; some areas are white because the immune system has destroyed cells within the tumor; and still other areas show variations of these colors. The result is an irregularly shaped, enlarging, pigmented structure with a variety of shades of black, brown, red, blue, and white.

A convenient device when checking for signs of early melanoma is to look for the "ABCD's" of the tumor: A for asymmetrical shape, B for borders that are irregular, C for variable coloration, and D for a diameter that is larger than about one-quarter of an inch.

There has been a major advance in identifying people who run a high risk of developing melanoma. Most people have at least a few pigmented spots, called moles or nevi, on their skin. Investigators have now found that one type of mole appears to be a warning sign for high-risk individuals. Known as a dysplastic nevus, it usually develops on the skin, often on covered areas such as the breast or buttocks, about the time of puberty. It is typically flat with irregular, poorly defined borders and is black, pink, tan, or brown in color. Although dysplastic nevi generally remain benign, individuals having these nevi, especially if they belong to a melanoma-prone family, are more likely to develop melanoma in later life. Identifying such people and monitoring them carefully throughout life should improve the chances of making an early diagnosis and successfully treating melanoma should it in fact occur.

Preventing Skin Cancer

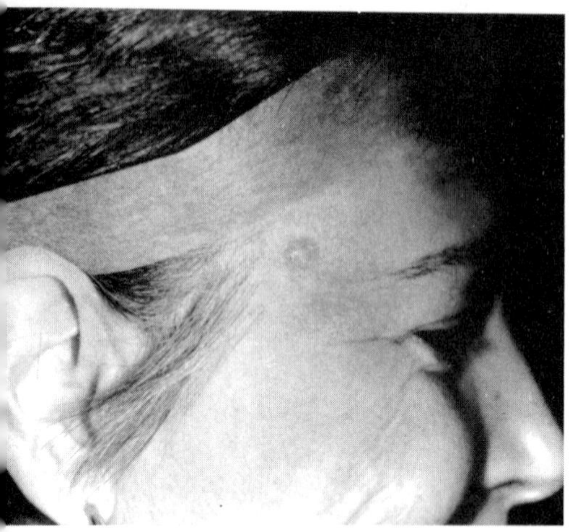

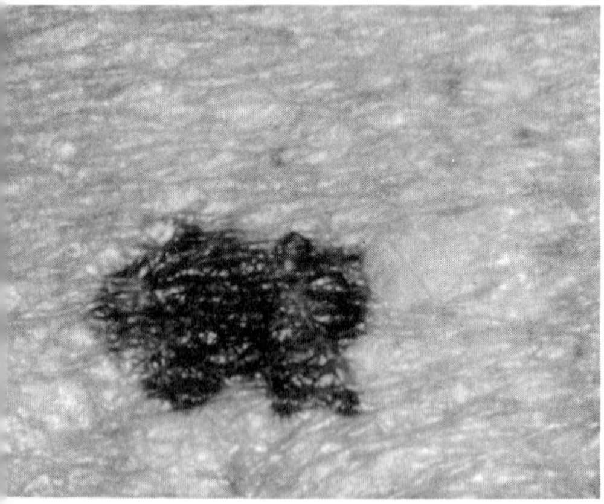

Both basal-cell carcinoma (top), the most common type of skin cancer, and malignant melanoma (bottom), the most lethal type, can usually be cured if detected in their early stages.

There is no question but that chronic exposure to the sun is the major cause of skin cancer. Repeated studies of large groups of people have shown that the incidence of basal-cell and squamous-cell cancers is directly proportional to the amount of sun exposure. Sun exposure is also an important factor in causing melanoma, although the relationship is less strong. People who live close to the equator, where the intensity of sunlight is greatest, have a higher incidence of all types of skin cancer. At greatest risk are fair-skinned, blue-eyed, freckle-faced individuals. The surest way for such people to reduce their chances of developing skin cancer is for them to limit their exposure to sunlight.

When skin cancer does occur, it can be easily cured if it is recognized early and treated aggressively. Any newly developed, unexplained growth or sore on the skin should be evaluated promptly by a doctor. If it turns out to be cancer, early surgical treatment, radiation therapy, or cryotherapy (freezing) will usually provide a cure, with only modest scarring.

Like the accelerated aging of the skin, the increased risk of cancer from too much sun can often be lessened by the judicious use of clothing and sunscreens. These precautions allow even the fairest-skinned individuals to enjoy outdoor activities, free from the pain of acute sunburn and relatively well protected from the cancer-causing effects of chronic sun exposure.

Acne

Humans are social animals; they naturally want to look attractive. Since the skin is our "face" to the outside world, a minor rash that in no way impairs the skin's other functions can tragically alter a person's appearance, causing devastating psychological damage.

Acne is perhaps the best example of this. Even severe acne has no significant effect on how the skin performs its basic functions, but it unquestionably affects the victim's appearance. Usually occurring during adolescence, severe acne can lead to social withdrawal and emotional wounds, sometimes leaving a damaged self-image that persists long after the disease has disappeared. It provides an excellent example of how the major "site" of injury from skin disease is often one's self-image, rather than the skin itself.

Acne is an inflammatory disease of the sebaceous glands and the associated hair follicles (sheathlike structures enclosing the root of a shaft of hair). The oily sebum secreted by a sebaceous gland is carried to the surface of the skin by the adjoining hair follicle. If the upper portion of the follicle becomes blocked, sebum will accumulate, swelling the follicle. The plug of sebum and dead cells clogging the opening is called a comedo. If this plug pops out of the follicle opening, the blemish left on the skin is a blackhead (it darkens because of exposure to the air); if it stays below the skin surface, it is a whitehead. The comedo represents the initial stage of acne. The subsequent growth of bacteria on the comedones, and the inflammation that occurs in and around them, produces the red pimples that are the scourge of adolescent life and that in severe cases can cause disfigurement and lasting scars. Hormonal changes associated with puberty are known to increase the amount of sebum produced during the teenage years, but the precise cause of acne—why the follicles become blocked—is not known.

Traditionally, there have been three approaches to the treatment of acne. Antibiotics, such as tetracycline, can be used to reduce or eliminate bacterial growth. Keratinolytics (substances that dissolve keratin), like salicylic acid or retinoic acid, may be employed in an attempt to remove the "plug" of sebum blocking the hair follicle. Finally, in rare cases hormones and X rays are used to reduce the amount of sebum production. In the past, acne could usually be controlled by a combination of these approaches, but flare-ups generally occurred after

Acne doesn't interfere with the skin's ability to function but may significantly damage self-esteem.

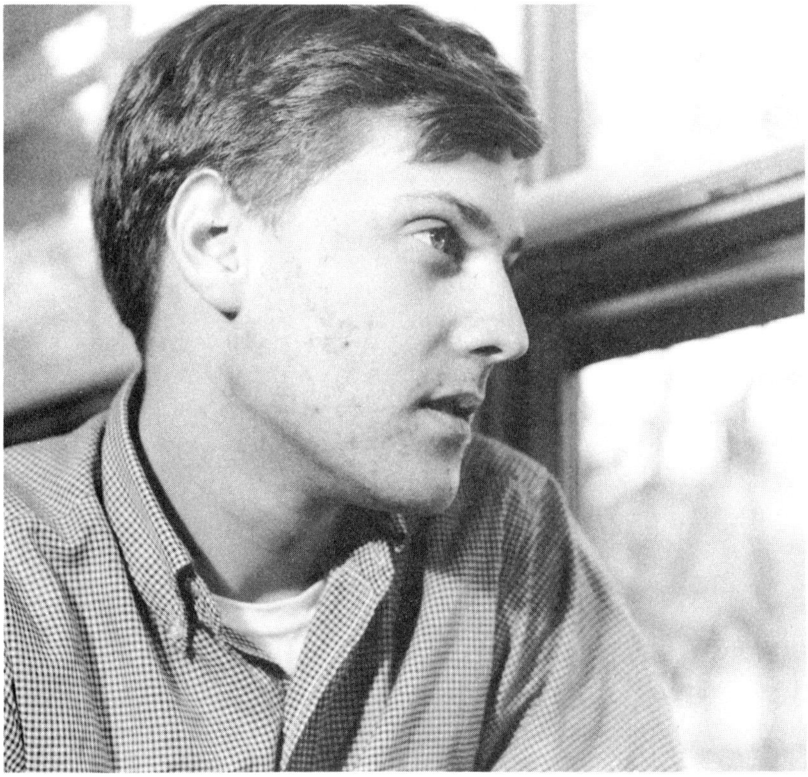

treatment was discontinued. Now, however, a compound is available that offers a more effective, longer acting, and simpler means of acne treatment; it is part of a group called the retinoids, substances related to vitamin A.

The retinoid 13-cis-retinoic acid is proving spectacularly effective in treating severe, inflammatory forms of acne. This vitamin A derivative, available by prescription in the United States and Canada as the drug isotretinoin, causes a rapid reduction in sebaceous gland activity, a decrease in the number of bacteria, and an alteration in keratin formation by the epidermis, helping to prevent blocked pores. Thus, almost miraculously, a single drug seems able to combine all three conventional treatments. Most exciting of all, isotretinoin not only produces great improvement (or even elimination) of severe acne during the typical five-month course of treatment, but after use of the drug has been stopped, recurrences seem far less frequent. However, because of serious concern about side effects of isotretinoin and other retinoids, particularly their role in causing birth defects in infants born to women who take the drug during or shortly before pregnancy, the drug is used only for the most severe cases of acne.

Tanning Shortcuts?

The perpetual quest for a "safe" golden tan has led to the marketing of numerous products that at best are ineffective and at worst may actually be harmful. For years various dyes have been incorporated into tanning products that are applied directly on the skin and that claim to give a "tan without the sun." More recently, the chemical canthaxanthin has been sold in Europe and Canada in the form of a "tanning pill." This chemical is actually a food dye that, when taken in large quantities, imparts a darker color to the skin.

Whether the dyes are applied to the skin or taken internally, they often give the skin a sickly yellow-orange tint rather than the desired golden tan. Furthermore, this coloring effect does not protect the skin from the harmful rays of the sun to the same degree that a normal tan does. Finally, questions have been raised about the safety of canthaxanthin. Tanning pills containing it are illegal in the United States. Health concerns center on complaints that night vision is impaired with use of the pills, and on documented reports of abnormal crystal deposits in the eyes of canthaxanthin users. Moderate exposure to sunlight combined with the correct use of sunscreens remains the safest road to tanning.

The Immune System

In the past few years researchers have found that the skin performs an important role in the body's immune system. Within the skin, high up in the epidermis and just below the horny layer, is a network of cells known as the Langerhans cells (named after the 19th-century German anatomist Paul Langerhans, who also discovered, during his first year of medical school, the insulin-producing cells of the pancreas). The function of these specialized epidermal cells was long unknown, but it now appears that they have the ability to engulf substances that come in contact with the skin. After ingesting the foreign material, the Langerhans cells communicate with other elements of the body's immune system—which can lead to an inflammation reaction. The inflammation reaction sets off a process by which the foreign substance and any tissue that may have been damaged are eliminated. In this way the skin is able to "recognize" substances as foreign and to make an appropriate defensive response.

Langerhans cells have been found to play an essential role in skin allergy reactions like poison ivy rash. The same processes are probably at work when the immune system identifies precancerous and cancerous skin growths as dangerous and rapidly responds in order to minimize the threat to the individual.

It has been found that such immune system elements in the skin as the Langerhans cells are adversely affected by sunlight; even a modest sunburn will temporarily deactivate Langerhans cells. Research in the new field of photoimmunology—the study of normal and abnormal interactions between the body's immune system and ultraviolet light—should provide an understanding of such effects, particularly in relation to skin cancer.

Another discovery is that keratinocytes seem to show striking similarities to cells of the thymus gland, an immune system organ. Moreover, substantial numbers of T cells—white blood cells important in the immune system that mature in the thymus gland—have been found in skin, and malignant T cells involved in several kinds of cancer, including some leukemias, seem to have an affinity for skin. The exact nature and importance of these relationships remain to be worked out.

An Extreme Drug Reaction

The skin is frequently a major site of allergic reactions in the body. Most allergic reactions to drugs are identified only because they cause a dramatic eruption—a sudden rash, for example—on the skin. In this way the skin serves as an important alarm system for indicating that something is wrong, and the patient can be taken off the drug before more severe consequences are suffered. There is a wide variation in the symptoms of drug reactions, from simple redness and itching to hives to a severe blistering that causes the loss of large quantities of skin. This blistering, the severest form of drug reaction, is called toxic epidermal necrolysis. It illustrates how a condition that interferes with the skin's ability to function can result in death.

Special skin cells serve the body's immune system by defending against foreign substances.

Toxic epidermal necrolysis may begin innocently with redness and itching of the skin. But within hours it usually progresses to a diffuse redness and swelling, accompanied by large areas of blistering and separation of the epidermis from the dermis. The epidermis can be easily peeled off, almost in sheets, leaving an open, oozing, ulcerated surface. The affected area may closely resemble severely burned skin.

Stripped of its protective epidermis, the skin is totally unable to carry out its basic functions. With no barrier against fluid loss from within, large quantities of clear fluid—blood plasma—ooze from the open wounds, rapidly depleting the body's supply of fluids, salts, nutrients, and other substances that are necessary to maintain life. Because the protective epidermis has been destroyed, substances placed on the skin can rapidly penetrate the body. Even such ordinarily harmless substances as antibiotic ointments now become dangerous, since they can enter the bloodstream, possibly giving rise to lethal kidney or liver damage. Even when such problems are controlled, the patient is left with the affected area of the body unprotected by its skin shield and thus vulnerable to infection. Ultimately the growth of bacteria on the open wounds can lead to blood-borne infection and death.

Treatment of toxic epidermal necrolysis consists mainly of discontinuing the drug that caused the allergic reaction while giving the patient steroid drugs such as intravenous hydrocortisone or prednisone. Steroids are used because their anti-inflammatory effect limits the extent of skin destruction by the allergic reaction. In spite of vigorous treatment with such modern medications, the death rate from toxic epidermal necrolysis continues to be a disappointing 30 percent. However, recent developments in treating burn victims may someday help victims of severe drug reactions as well. Techniques now exist to grow "test-tube" skin from tiny patches of the burn victim's own healthy epidermal cells. The laboratory-grown skin is grafted onto the open burn wounds, thus quickly restoring the epidermal barrier. This approach should reduce the death rate from toxic epidermal necrolysis and other severe skin diseases that, like burns, cause the destruction of large quantities of skin. □

HYPOCHONDRIA

Bruce Shapiro, M.D.
ILLUSTRATIONS BY ROBERT SHORE

Convinced that his health was failing, the French novelist Marcel Proust was transformed from a man-about-town into a hypochondriac—a virtual invalid who spent his days in bed, living and working in a cork-lined, dust-proof room. While in hypochondriacal isolation, Proust proceeded to write his long masterpiece, *À la recherche du temps perdu (Remembrance of Things Past).* Other illustrious and productive hypochondriacs include the poet Percy Bysshe Shelley and the naturalist Charles Darwin.

Unfortunately, not all hypochondriacs can make peace with their condition. For many, the illness means a disrupted life, crippling fear, and considerable emotional pain. It is not always possible to overcome hypochondria, but therapy can help many sufferers lead happier and more productive lives.

A Preoccupation With Disease

Hypochondria (technically, hypochondriasis or hypochondriacal neurosis) is a condition in which a person interprets physical signs and sensations—a quickened heartbeat, a small sore, or an occasional cough—in an unrealistic way, believing them to be symptoms of a serious illness. Hypochondriacs become preoccupied with disease and are often so fretful about their health that they cannot lead a normal work or family life.

The American Psychiatric Association (APA) defines hypochondria as a psychiatric illness with four major characteristics: physical symptoms that

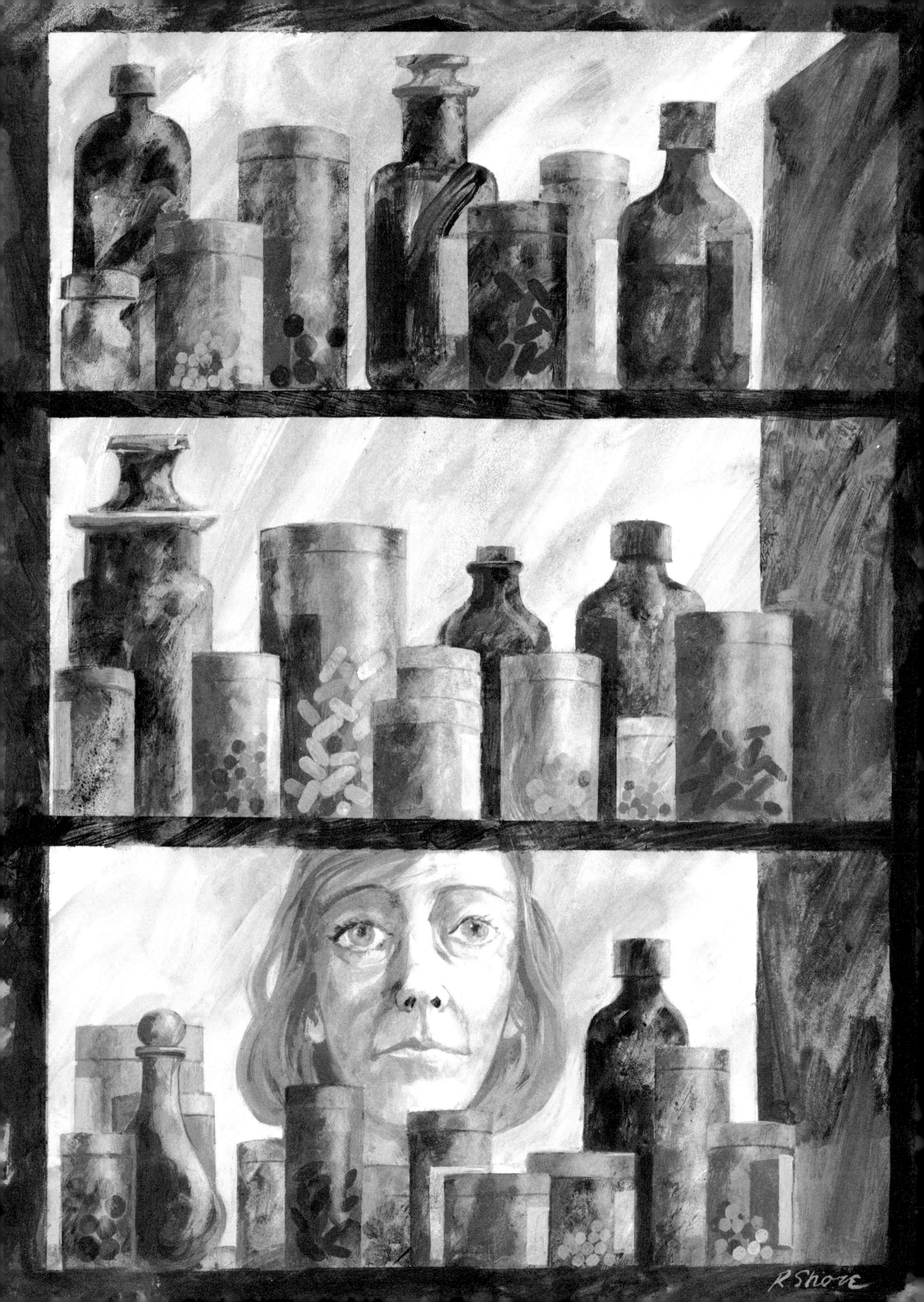
R Shore

are disproportionate to any actual physical disease that can be found; a fear of disease and the conviction that one is sick; a preoccupation with one's body; and the persistent and unsatisfying pursuit of medical care. The condition is usually chronic, with a waxing and waning of symptoms.

Although the statistical prevalence of hypochondria is not known, it is an extremely common disorder, accounting for many of the physical complaints brought to family physicians, internists, and other doctors. Studies of primary care physicians show that a significant proportion of the patients coming to them complaining of symptoms do not have serious physical diseases; in fact, the most common diagnosis general practitioners make is that the patient has no physical illness at all. At the same time it is estimated that between 15 and 20 percent of the population has a diagnosable mental or emotional disorder, and thus it seems logical to assume that some of the patients found to be without a physical disorder may actually be more appropriately in need of mental health care. Most general practitioners and family physicians will state that hypochondriacal complaints account for a significant percentage of their consultations.

Although there are often stereotypes of hypochondriacal women, the problem is equally common among men and women. Also in contrast to common belief, hypochondria usually arises either in adolescence or between the ages of 30 and 50—not in old age. Older people with hypochondria have usually developed their initial fears when they were younger.

It must be remembered that concerns about the body and hypochondriacal fears occur from time to time in many people under stress or after the media, or personal experience, focus attention on a

Hypochondriacs monitor every flush of the skin, every rapid heartbeat—fearing the worst.

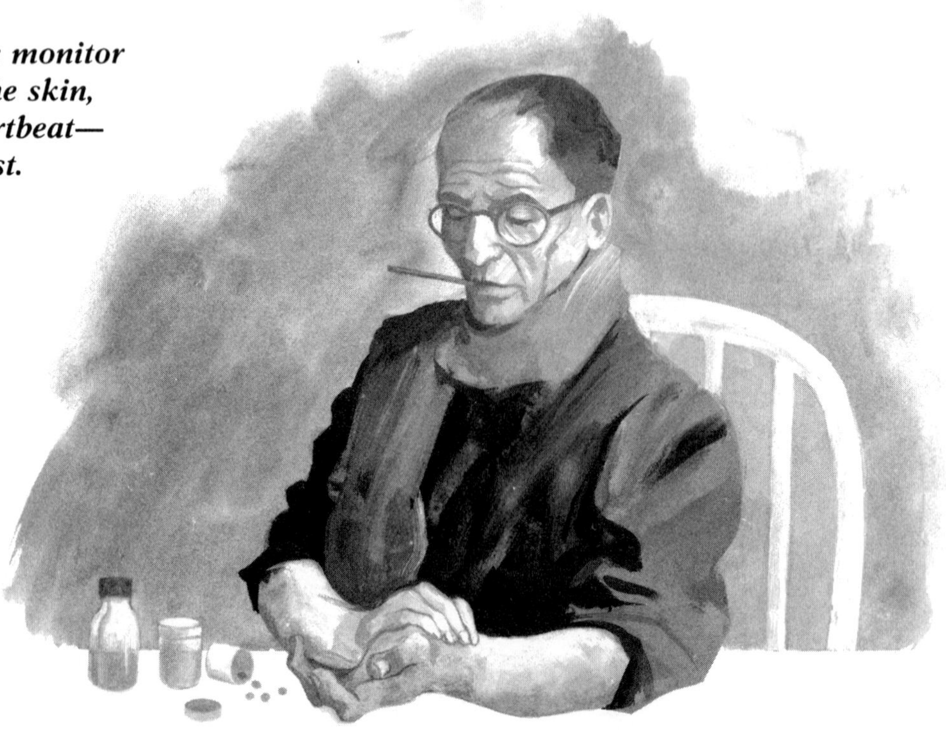

particular disease. Many feared that they had colon cancer after President Ronald Reagan's 1985 surgery for the disease, and hypochondriacal fears often are found among medical students and young physicians. It is not uncommon for doctors in training to fear that they have the disorder about which they are currently learning or the disease of one of their patients. This has been happening for hundreds of years. A 17th-century textbook on melancholy states: "Some young physicians, that studying to cure diseases, catch them themselves, will be sick, and appropriate all symptoms they find related to others to their own persons." These brief, limited experiences, however, do not have the intensity or duration of true hypochondria.

Theories About Hypochondria

Hypochondria has always been a puzzling disorder for physicians, and many theories have been formulated about why it develops. Some theories relate hypochondria to other psychiatric problems, while other theories see it as caused by actual experiences of the patient. Of course, no one theory need explain every case of hypochondria. Different cases may have entirely different causes, and at times a combination of factors may come into play. A determination of the cause or likely cause of each patient's hypochondria affects a doctor's choice of treatment and the possibility of a cure.

The APA's current diagnostic manual states that past experience with a real illness in the patient or a member of the patient's family may well be a contributing factor to the development of hypochondria; a great deal of psychological or social stress may also play a role. Some psychiatrists feel that hypochondriacal fears are usually brought to the surface or made worse by severe anxiety or underlying depression; thus, hypochondria is often a symptom of a treatable underlying psychiatric problem, such as depression or an anxiety disorder (like phobias or panic attacks).

Alternatively, hypochondria is seen as arising from unconscious emotional forces. Freud felt that hypochondria was a result of blocked aggressive or sexual impulses, which, because of societal pressures, the person unconsciously transformed into bodily sensations and concerns about the body. Similar to this is the theory that hypochondriacal symptoms result from past rejections or disappointments, which lead to feelings of anger that are transformed into physical complaints. Other observers have focused on emotional dependency as the central cause of hypochondria. According to this theory, the true wish on the part of hypochondriacs is to receive support, reassurance, nurturing, sympathy, and physical contact. In seeking treatment for the feared physical illness, they receive this caring and attention.

Still another view is that the cause of hypochondria lies in an unresolved, unconscious sense of "badness." Physical suffering may function as atonement or deserved punishment for a vague sense of

---

Bruce Shapiro is psychiatrist-in-chief of the Department of Psychiatry, The Stamford Hospital, Stamford, Conn., and associate professor of clinical psychiatry at New York Medical College in Valhalla, N.Y.

wrongdoing that has persistently plagued an individual. Or hypochondria may serve an "ego-defense" purpose—that is, it is more tolerable for hypochondriacs to feel that they have physical illnesses than that they are incapable or deficient in any way. The psychological views of hypochondria also include the theory that hypochondria may result from identification with a close friend or relative who had been physically ill or had successfully used physical illnesses to manipulate others.

Hypochondria also may be related to a "perceptual abnormality." In this view, certain individuals tend to amplify and misinterpret normal bodily sensations and thus, for example, will experience normal chest tightness as chest pain. Another theory is that certain individuals (called alexithymic) are unable to experience their true emotions in their thoughts but rather experience strong emotions in bodily symptoms.

The Patient's Symptoms

The symptoms hypochondriacs complain of are often vague and variable pains in many parts of the body, though at times the complaints are specific. The gastrointestinal, cardiac, respiratory, musculoskeletal, and central nervous systems are most commonly involved. Some patients will perform what physicians have come to call an organ recital—in listing their symptoms they go methodically through the body's major organ systems. Patients are highly anxious about their symptoms and are absorbed in their suffering or their bodily sensations.

Most hypochondriacal patients will feel well for a while and then—sometimes related to stress—will become hypochondriacal again. Some individuals will have only one hypochondriacal episode (which can last for months), while others will continue to worsen until they are bedridden and live as invalids.

Hypochondriacs are often seen as egocentric, unduly sensitive to criticism, conscientious, or rigid. Not surprisingly, they seem to want to focus their interest and energy on themselves and their bodies rather than on other people and the world around them.

Yet hypochondriacs should not be dismissed as self-absorbed complainers. The dread of a serious disease can create alarming anxiety in these people. The fear that they will suffer a heart attack or that they have signs of cancer can be paralyzing, and in many cases it is fear that motivates them to continually seek medical attention. The treatment of hypochondria must ultimately deal with these fears and anxieties.

Differentiating Hypochondria

Although hypochondria can be a means to manipulate people, it is not the same as malingering. Malingerers intentionally make up or induce symptoms to obtain a goal—to avoid work, get financial compensation, or obtain drugs. In contrast, hypochondriacs sincerely believe themselves to be ill and have no conscious desire either to be in pain or to have the symptoms from which they truly suffer emotionally.

Hypochondria should also be differentiated from what is called somatic delusion. In somatic delusion patients have a fixed false belief that they have a feared, often deadly, disease. People with somatic delusions are

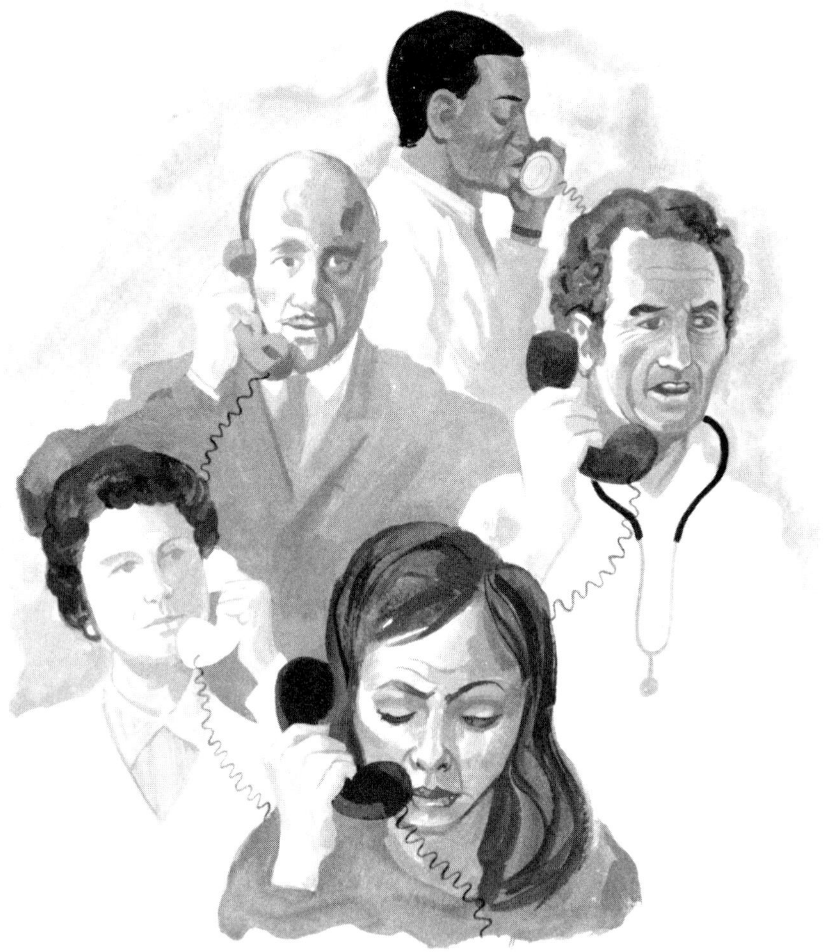

The true hypochondriac seeks out one doctor after another, looking for the one with a cure for a variety of ailments.

psychotic (out of touch with reality) and refuse all attempts to reason with them about the possibility that they are not ill. Hypochondriacs will at least entertain the possibility that they are not ill. Patients with somatic delusions are absolutely rigid in their thinking about their health; hypochondriacs are more flexible.

It should be stated that hypochondria is not a psychosomatic illness. According to current thinking, psychosomatic disorders are real physical illnesses—asthma, ulcers, skin conditions—that are often exacerbated by psychological stress. But in hypochondria the patients' complaints cannot be attributed to any physical disease.

Doctor Shopping

An integral part of the pattern of hypochondria is "doctor shopping": the patient consults with physician after physician, while no physical or laboratory abnormalities are found that might account for the individual's symptoms. Meanwhile, the patient's condition remains unchanged. Hypochondriacs engage in doctor shopping in an attempt to quiet their anxiety by finding a doctor who will diagnose and treat the physical illness they "know" they have. During their quest they often receive multiple tests, treatments, and medications—usually to no avail. When the latest doctor reassures them that nothing is wrong, they usually are relieved for a short time. But then they begin to believe that the physical problem is there but was missed by the doctor, leading them to seek yet another doctor who can help them.

Of course, in true hypochondria no doctor can successfully treat the suspected bodily disease since the patients' complaints stem from emotional problems. The patients may wind up with long lists of doctors who have "failed" to help them. Hypochondria thus often becomes a relentless search for the right doctor, the right diagnosis, the right treatment, and a cure.

Even hypochondriacs—or suspected ones—need a thorough examination to rule out true physical illness.

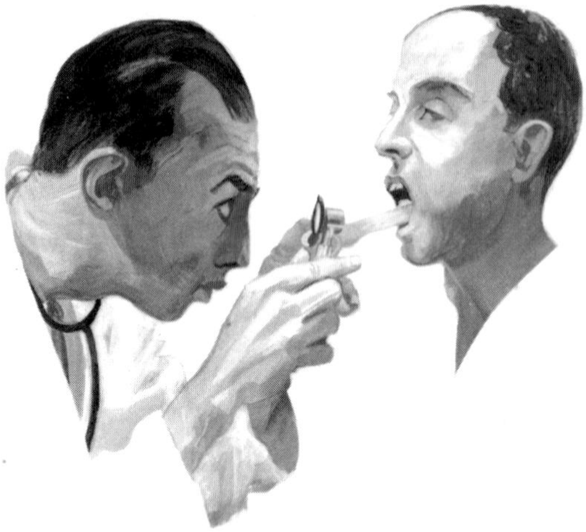

Making the Diagnosis

Hypochondriacs are a troubling puzzle for the family physician, who faces the problem of assessing their complaints and would probably like to refer such patients to a psychiatrist. Indeed, such a referral would be a wise move: psychiatrists are uniquely qualified to treat hypochondriacal patients. Only a psychiatrist combines the psychological and medical training that it takes to effectively relate to such individuals and understand their concerns. Unfortunately, however, most hypochondriacs refuse to see a psychiatrist. They do not think they have an emotional problem, and they often view a psychiatric referral as a rejection on the part of their family physician.

Before physicians can make a diagnosis of hypochondria, all other possibilities must be ruled out. First and foremost is the presence of actual physical disease, including those illnesses (multiple sclerosis, for example) that in their early stages have vague or difficult to diagnose patterns. Also, even the physical complaints of patients who have previously been diagnosed as hypochondriacs need to be taken seriously. These patients may have since developed a true physical disorder.

The physician must also watch for the signs and symptoms of depression, psychoses (such as schizophrenia or psychotic depression), or anxiety disorders.

Arriving at a Cure

The type of treatment used for hypochondria varies from case to case, depending on what is considered to be the cause of the disorder in each individual. (Treatment can also be given if the true cause is not known.) For hypochondria related to an underlying disorder, a combination of treatments may be used. If it is a symptom of an underlying depression, both psychotherapy and antidepressant medications may well be in order. If it is related to an anxiety disorder, the judicious use of antianxiety medications (minor tranquilizers) may be appropriate. And if it is connected to a psychosis, then the treatment of the psychosis (with medication, psychotherapy, or perhaps electroconvulsive treatment) is the first order of business. Treating these patients with drugs alone is rarely recommended; some form of psychotherapy should be combined with medication. However, it should also be remembered that with many, if not most, hypochondriacs, their hypochondria is not related to another psychiatric disorder. Moreover, some hypochondriacs will not be able to tolerate the side effects of psychiatric medication and may develop additional fears after feeling the side effects.

For most hypochondriacs, psychotherapy without medication may be the best treatment. The choice of which type of psychotherapy (individual, group, family, psychoanalytic, behavioral, or cognitive) is best made after a careful psychiatric evaluation. Certainly hypochondriacal patients need support and understanding from someone who is familiar with both their physical and their psychological status. The psychiatrist should be able to understand the patient's condition; allow the individual to talk about medical anxieties, physical examinations, and relationships with other doctors; and also help the patient uncover the underlying anxieties that have generated the hypochondriacal preoccupations.

An important aspect of treatment is the work that should be done with the patients' relatives. The families have often endured significant disruption of their lives. They may have been frightened by the continuing possibility that the patient has a serious illness. If family members realize that the patient has no physical illness, they may become frustrated and angry with the hypochondriac. Family members need to be informed about the nature of hypochondria. They must be reassured that there is no cause for concern about serious medical illness, and yet they also must be made to understand that the patient is not malingering but is truly suffering. The family of the hypochondriac often needs assistance in overcoming anger toward the patient, who may have been quite demanding.

Mental and Monetary Costs

Finally, it is important to understand the emotional and financial costs of hypochondria. To individual sufferers and their beleaguered families, the emotional costs are inestimable: the preoccupying emotional pain of hypochondriacs may be unbearable and may disrupt the lives of all the people close to them. Experts have estimated that the financial cost of "the worried well" to society runs into billions of dollars. Of course, it is important that people get periodic checkups and practice good preventive medicine. But because of hypochondria, a large portion of physician and hospital time and laboratory effort is fruitlessly consumed in searches for diagnoses. Further research is needed into the diagnosis and effective treatment of hypochondria to help quiet the fears of these patients and allow them to lead fulfilling lives away from the doctor's office. □

SUGGESTIONS FOR FURTHER READING

EHRLICH, RICHARD. *The Healthy Hypochondriac.* Philadelphia, Saunders, 1980.

MEISTER, ROBERT. *Hypochondria: Toward a Better Understanding.* New York, Taplinger, 1980.

Heart Attacks
Reducing Deaths

John F. Schneider, M.D.

Heart attacks continue to plague most industrialized societies, where they remain the number one cause of disability and death in people over the age of 40. Each year about half a million people in the United States and close to 50,000 in Canada die from heart attacks. Nevertheless, there has been a steady decline since the 1950's in the death rate from coronary heart disease—that is, disease of the blood vessels nourishing the heart, whose blockage can trigger a heart attack. The exact reasons for the decline are not clear, but it is probably related to a reduction in factors that make heart attacks more likely: cigarette smoking, high blood pressure, and excessive cholesterol and saturated fat in the diet. Moreover, there have been great advances in the treatment of coronary heart disease, including new drugs and better hospital monitoring, as well as treatment of heartbeat irregularities in patients who have had heart attacks. Ways of improving blood flow to the heart muscle, either before or after a heart attack, have also played a role in the reduced number of deaths.

This article will examine some of the major advances that have occurred in the past several years in understanding how and why heart attacks happen and the factors that help to reduce their occurrence. It will also review the important new treatments for patients in the early hours of a severe heart attack that show great promise in reducing deaths and disability.

What Is a Heart Attack?

The ominous symptoms of a heart attack—including sometimes extreme chest discomfort, difficulty in breathing, sweating, and nausea—have been recognized as danger signs for centuries. But doctors did not learn until the early part of this century that they were caused by a shortage of blood supply to the heart.

Paramedics give emergency treatment to a heart attack victim.

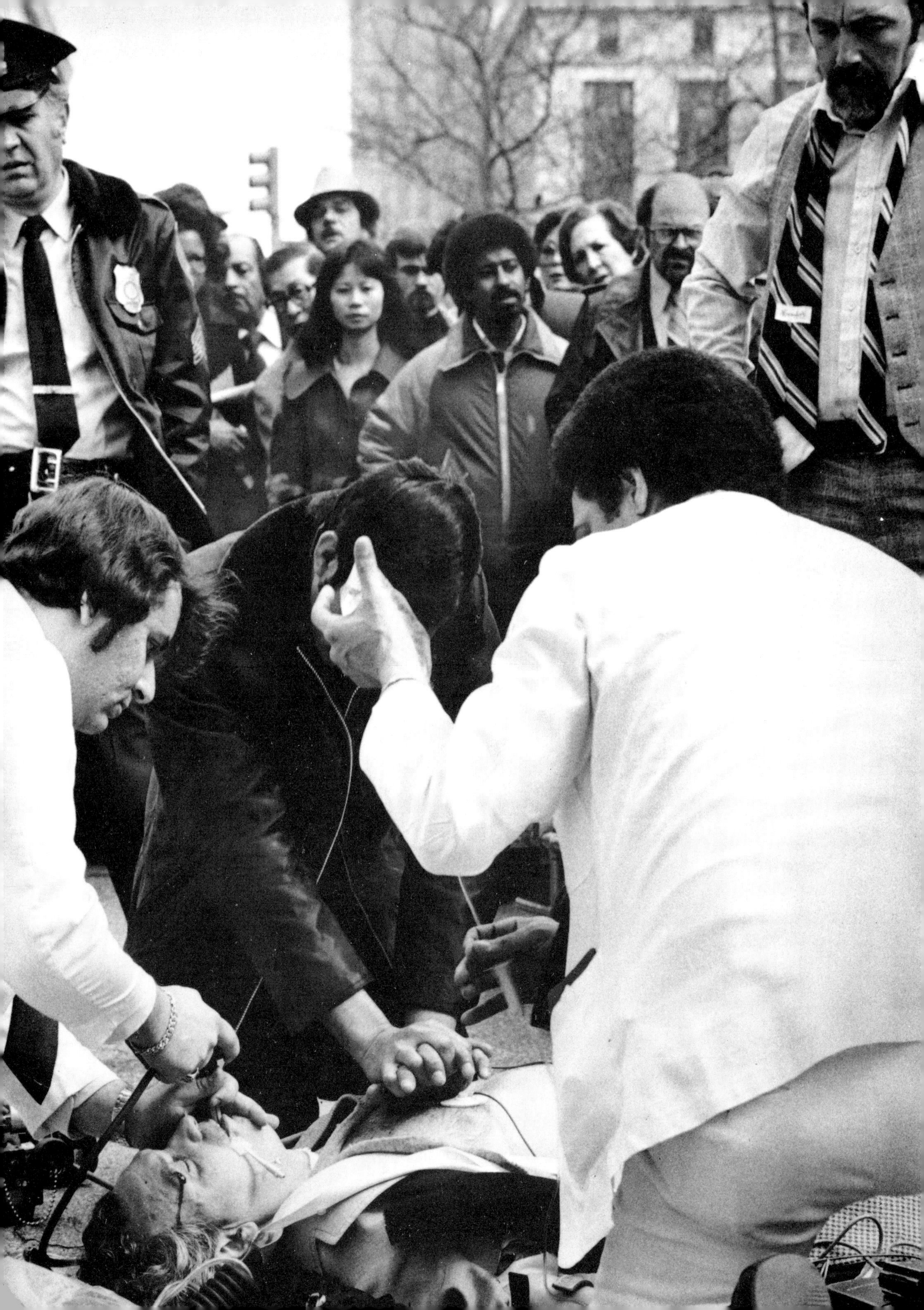

The gradual buildup of plaque in the coronary arteries can keep the heart from getting enough blood—and cause a heart attack.

The heart, responsible for pumping all the blood the body needs, requires a substantial blood supply of its own to do its work. This is delivered through blood vessels called coronary arteries. In many people, the coronary blood vessels are subject to a gradual process known as atherosclerosis. In this process, fats, cholesterol, and other substances, such as calcium and fibrous tissue, build up on the inner lining of the blood vessels and form what are known as plaques. With time, plaque material accumulates to the point where it narrows the opening through which blood flows—much as rust and corrosion can narrow plumbing pipes. When this narrowing reaches a critical point—usually when it has reduced the opening within the vessel by 70 to 75 percent—the heart's need for blood cannot always be met, particularly during exertion or stress, when the heart must work harder than usual. When a shortage of blood supply develops—a condition called myocardial ischemia—it is usually accompanied by an uncomfortable or painful sensation in the chest region, a sensation known as angina pectoris. After the exertion or stress eases, the blood supply and the heart's demand for blood usually come into balance again, and the discomfort ceases. The condition is called stable angina pectoris if predictable amounts of exertion or stress bring it on, if it is not becoming more frequent, severe, long lasting, or easy to provoke, and if it does not occur without provocation.

A different condition, called unstable angina pectoris, is diagnosed if angina has recently developed and occurs during rest or minimal activity, or if a previously stable angina pattern changes to become more frequent, more easily provoked, or more severe. Recognizing unstable angina is important because in the days, weeks, and months after it develops, the patient is at a higher risk of going on to have a full-blown heart attack.

A heart attack begins when a critically narrowed coronary artery becomes completely blocked—say, by a blood clot. The attack can actually go on for some hours. The portion of the heart muscle the blocked blood vessel supplies usually dies for lack of blood supply, a process known as myocardial infarction. The actual time from the moment the artery is blocked until there is irreversible damage to the heart muscle it supplies probably varies among individuals, but most of the muscle involved is irreparably damaged within four hours. Because heart muscle death is gradual, the amount of heart muscle that can be saved by reestablishing a blood supply through the obstructed coronary artery or alternate blood vessels will be largely determined by the time that has elapsed: the shorter the time since the blockage, the greater the amount of salvage.

Why Heart Attacks Kill

People die from myocardial infarction in two main ways. First, especially in the early minutes and hours of a heart attack, the electrical impulses of the heart, which are responsible for "sparking" and controlling the

---

John F. Schneider is associate professor of clinical medicine at the University of Cincinnati Medical Center and director of the cardiac catheterization laboratory at University Hospital.

heartbeat, can become extremely irregular and unstable. States of rapid, chaotic electrical activity known as ventricular tachycardia and fibrillation can occur. The heart muscle cannot beat effectively, and death usually occurs within minutes. Such fatal heartbeat irregularity happens most frequently in the early hours of a coronary blockage; it is over ten times more likely to occur in the first hour than 12 to 24 hours later.

Sudden loss of the heart's pumping function demands prompt treatment. This need for immediate action, plus the fact that the problem tends to arise soon after a heart attack begins, accounts for the fact that as many as one-third to one-half of heart attack deaths occur before the victims get to the hospital. In the 1960's techniques were developed for reversing ventricular tachycardia and fibrillation by applying an electric current to the heart with a device called a defribrillator. In addition, drugs to prevent fibrillation and the establishment of specialized monitoring areas in hospitals to provide rapid warning of electrical instability became routine. With these procedures, death because of electrical instability after the patient was hospitalized became far less common, although the number of such deaths before the heart attack sufferer reaches the hospital has remained disturbingly high. Mobile coronary care units, highly trained paramedic squads, and more people trained in cardiopulmonary resuscitation (CPR) have helped somewhat.

The second way that heart attacks cause death and disability is by actually destroying heart muscle, which impairs the pumping capacity of the heart. The extent of impairment is directly related to the amount of heart muscle damaged. If only 10 to 20 percent of the left ventricle—the heart's main pumping chamber, and the area most commonly affected—is injured, the consequences are relatively moderate; the remaining healthy heart muscle can usually take over the work load of the affected muscle. But if more of the left ventricle—20 to 35 percent—is damaged, the remaining muscle can no longer completely compensate. The heart usually functions well enough to keep the person alive, but it is no longer able to pump the desirable amount of blood, particularly during exertion; fatigue, shortness of breath, and leg swelling usually develop. And if more than 35 to 40 percent of the left ventricle is damaged, the heart is usually so impaired that it cannot pump enough blood to sustain life, a condition known as cardiogenic shock. The victim usually dies shortly after the heart attack.

Prevention Can Help

Certain steps can be taken by everyone to reduce the risk of a heart attack. Such primary prevention includes reducing the level of cholesterol in the diet, lowering high blood pressure, not smoking, and getting enough exercise. Aggressive prevention may become the most effective means of lowering the toll exacted by coronary heart disease.

Controlling cholesterol. Cholesterol—a fatty substance that is both produced by the liver and consumed in the diet, especially in meat and dairy products—is essential to many bodily functions. But it is also a major risk factor in heart disease. Since the 1920's and 1930's it has been recognized that the vast majority of people who die from heart attacks have severe coronary atherosclerosis—a buildup of cholesterol and other

How to Tell If You're Having a Heart Attack

Recognizing the signs of a heart attack early—and getting to the nearest hospital emergency room without delay—could save your life.

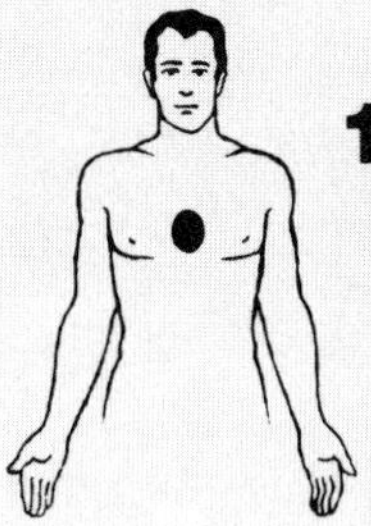

1. Pain or pressure in the center of the chest is usually the first sign.

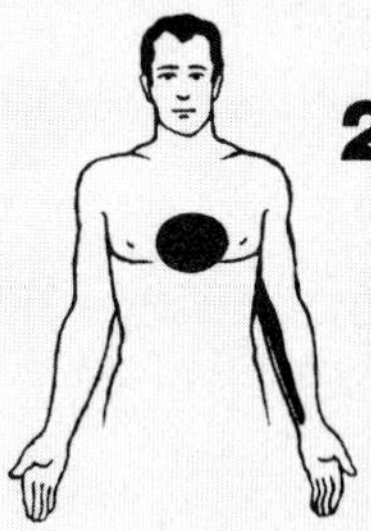

2. The discomfort may become severe and viselike or may seem more like indigestion. The pain can spread across the chest and down the left arm.

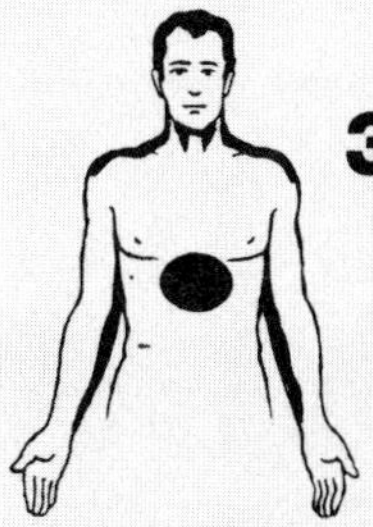

3. The pain, which can go away and then return, may radiate to both arms, shoulders, neck, or jaw.

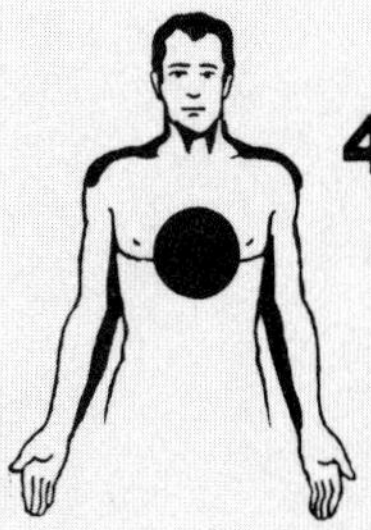

4. Sweating, nausea, vomiting, or shortness of breath may also occur.

REDUCING THE RISK OF A HEART ATTACK

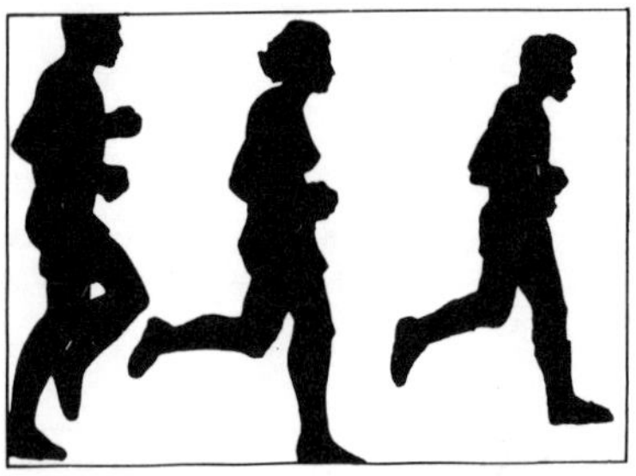

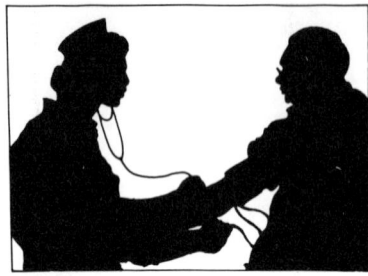

DO get enough exercise. Regular exercise conditions the heart and circulatory system.

DO have your blood pressure checked regularly, and take steps to reduce high blood pressure.

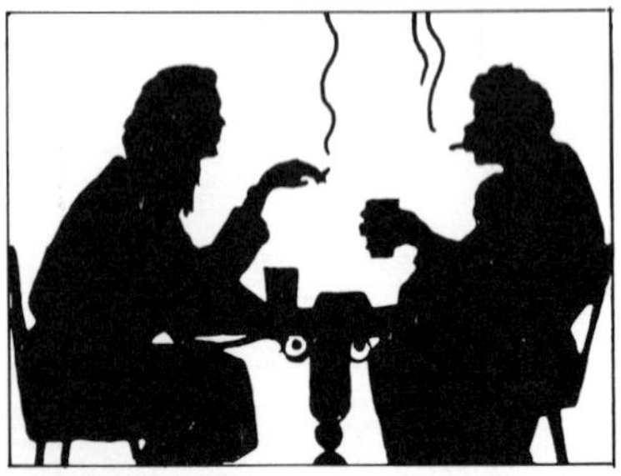

DON'T smoke. The more you smoke, the greater the risk.

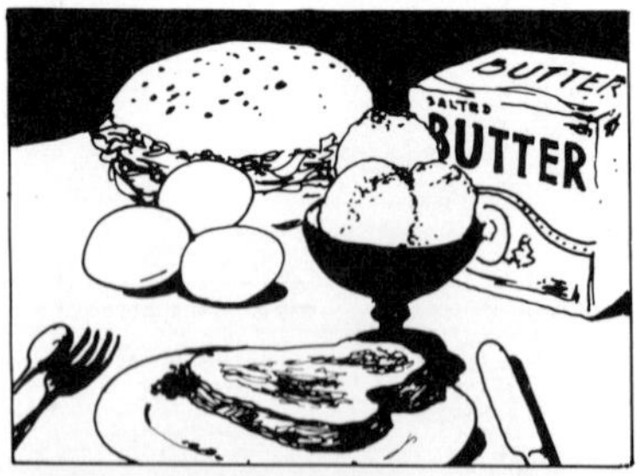

DON'T eat too many foods high in cholesterol and saturated fat.

fatty substances in the artery walls that greatly narrows the size of the channels through which blood can flow to the heart. Many scientific studies carried out over the past four decades have clearly shown that the higher the level of cholesterol in the blood, the more likely a heart attack will occur. Many doctors have thus reasoned that lowering the blood cholesterol level would reduce the risk of a heart attack. Until recently, this belief had not been proved. But a large-scale study begun in the 1970's by the U.S. National Institutes of Health and recently completed has conclusively shown that lowering blood cholesterol through a combination of diet and a cholesterol-lowering drug does effectively reduce the risk of heart attack in men who had high cholesterol levels when the study began.

It is reasonable to assume that some reduction of risk can also be achieved if similar measures are taken by women with high cholesterol levels and by men and women with less severely elevated cholesterol levels. The mechanism by which lowering cholesterol reduces the risk of heart attack almost certainly involves slowing the narrowing of coronary arteries caused by atherosclerosis. This slowing has been documented by using the diagnostic technique called coronary angiography on treated and untreated patients with high cholesterol levels. (Coronary angiography is a procedure for examining the coronary arteries in which a thin tube, or catheter, is inserted into a groin or arm artery and then snaked along to the coronary arteries. A special dye that shows up on X rays is injected via the catheter and circulates to the heart, allowing doctors to observe any coronary blood vessel obstructions.)

There is as yet no proof that attempting to lower blood cholesterol through dietary changes alone will reduce the risk of heart disease, but reducing dietary consumption of cholesterol and saturated fats does appear to reduce the level of cholesterol in the blood. It is reasonable to suppose that this has a beneficial effect in slowing atherosclerosis. On the basis of the evidence so far, the U.S. National Heart, Lung, and Blood Institute has recommended that people cut down on their consumption of cholesterol and fat—particularly saturated fat, the type found in meat and dairy products. This would require eating less red meat and more fish and poultry, drinking low-fat or skim milk, and consuming less butter, egg yolks, and fatty sauces and dressings.

Reducing high blood pressure. Hypertension, or high blood pressure, is another factor that strongly increases the risk of heart attacks, as well as the risk of heart failure, stroke, kidney failure, and other health problems. Although some earlier studies on hypertension and heart attacks were inconclusive, recent research has clearly shown that aggressive and sustained treatment to lower even mild high blood pressure significantly reduces the risk of heart attacks. The greatest reduction in risk appears to be achieved in those people who do not yet show signs of damage to any vital organs, which suggests that the earlier high blood pressure is lowered, the more the risk of a heart attack is reduced.

Hypertension generally has no symptoms; it can be detected only by a simple blood pressure test that is part of a basic checkup. It hypertension is diagnosed, a patient should carefully follow the doctor's advice, which may involve losing weight, quitting smoking, taking medication, and making changes in the diet (cutting down on salt, for instance).

Quitting smoking. Doctors have long urged that people not smoke, for various health reasons. It has been known for years that cigarette smokers run an unusually high risk of heart attacks, but a recent study showed that if they quit the habit, the risk almost disappears. Researchers at Boston University studied the habits of over 1,800 men hospitalized with heart attacks with the habits of almost 2,800 men hospitalized for other reasons. They discovered that smokers were three times more likely to suffer heart attacks than nonsmokers, but the risk declines rapidly when they quit.

Getting enough exercise. Part of the credit for reduction in heart attack deaths in recent years has been attributed to the increasing trend toward regular exercise. There is no rock-solid scientific evidence that exercise reduces the risk of coronary heart disease, but there is considerable indirect evidence suggesting that this is so. Moreover, exercise does promote weight loss and improve the efficiency of the heart and blood vessels, and it appears to raise the level of a type of cholesterol—called high-density lipoprotein—that, unlike other types of cholesterol, seems to have a protective effect against atherosclerosis.

On the other hand, there is little evidence to suggest that beginning an exercise program following a heart attack protects against further attacks. And suddenly beginning a strenuous exercise program can be dangerous for certain groups of people. Such a program can actually cause a heart attack or bring on chest pain and other angina-like symptoms in those who have undetected atherosclerosis. In general, while regular exercise is probably a good idea for healthy people, those at risk for coronary artery disease (like smokers or people with high blood pressure) and individuals over the age of 30 should not begin a strenuous exercise program without the advice of a physician.

When a heart attack strikes, speed is the key to preventing death; the sooner the victim is rushed to the hospital, the better the chances of survival.

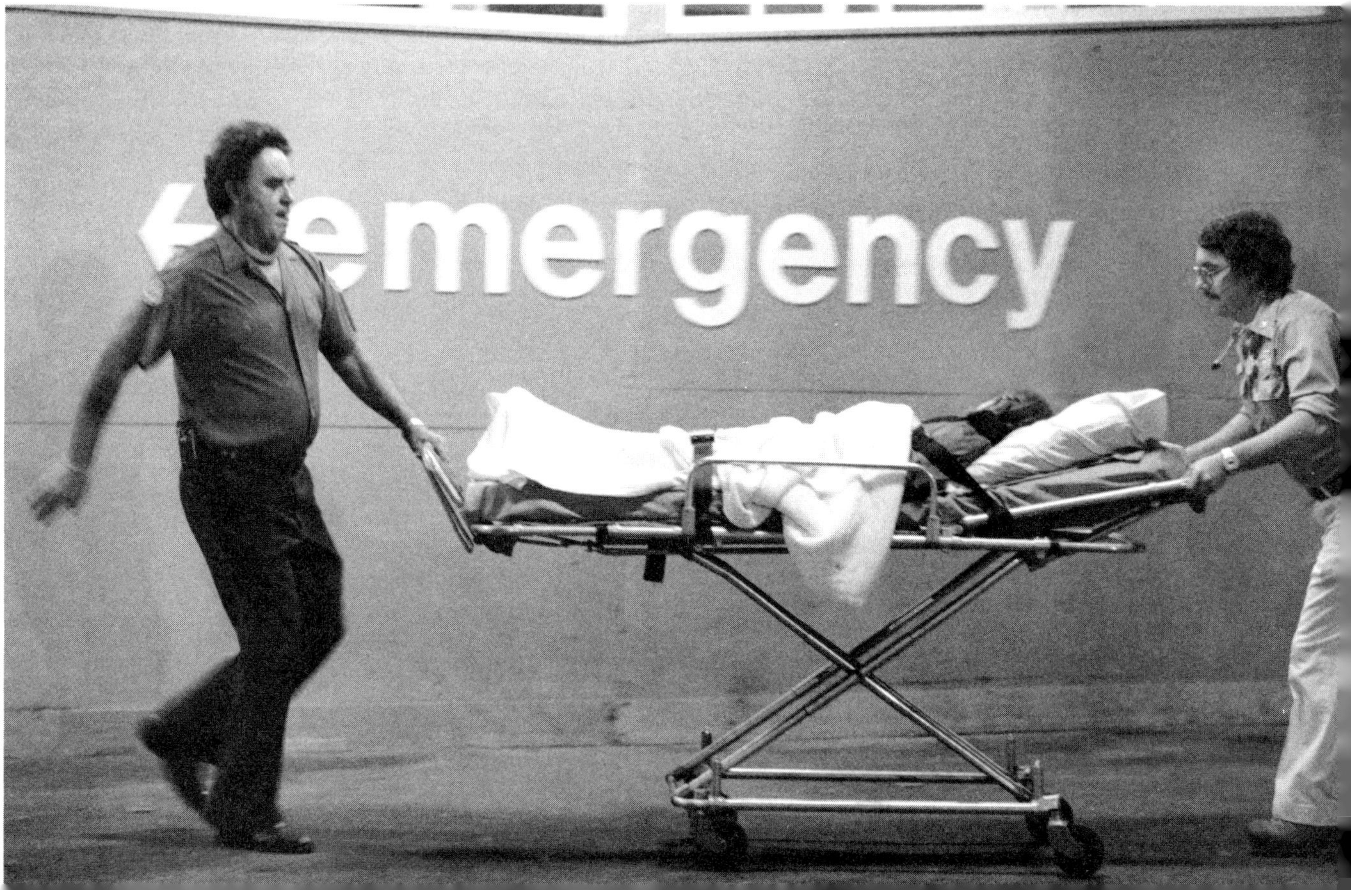

The Dangers of Unstable Angina

People who develop unstable angina are at greatly increased risk of suffering a full-blown heart attack shortly afterward. This has been known for years, based on studies carried out in the 1950's, before many of the drugs and procedures now used to treat the condition were available. Such early research demonstrated that one-third of patients hospitalized with unstable angina who had previously had stable angina and who had episodes of pain while resting in the hospital, together with abnormal readings on an electrocardiogram (which measures the heart's electrical impulses), suffered a myocardial infarction within three months. One-fourth of this group of unstable angina patients died within that period. Today, one-half to two-thirds of the individuals who suffer heart attacks have shown symptoms of unstable angina in the preceding days and weeks. Thus, prompt recognition and treatment of unstable angina may be one of the most effective means of preventing heart damage. Recent advances in understanding the development of unstable angina have led to great strides in this area.

People with stable or with unstable angina usually have seriously narrowed coronary arteries. Yet angiograms of the coronary arteries of the two groups do not reveal obvious differences in the extent of coronary narrowing. Recent studies on a series of coronary angiograms do suggest, however, that patients with unstable angina are more likely than those with stable angina to have had a sudden worsening of coronary narrowing brought about by a change in the shape of a coronary plaque. The sudden narrowing makes further changes, such as blood clot formation, slowed blood flow, or a spasm of the artery, more probable, and these changes can lead to total vessel blockage—which explains why unstable angina is likely to lead to a heart attack. Stabilizing coronary narrowing or mechanically relieving the narrowing can reduce the risk of heart attacks for patients with unstable angina.

An aspirin a day can help prevent blood clots in patients with unstable angina.

Preventing Blood Clots

Studies of areas of severe coronary narrowing and blockage indicate the presence of a large concentration of the blood particles called platelets. Thus it can be assumed that platelets, which play an important role in blood clotting, are involved in the events that lead to unstable angina and often to a severe heart attack.

Simple aspirin has a very powerful action on blood platelets: low doses of aspirin decrease the "stickiness" of platelets, making them less capable of helping to form blood clots at the site of a plaque buildup. Aspirin also reduces the production and release by platelets of a substance that powerfully stimulates blood vessel constriction.

In a study to test whether aspirin could help to reduce the risk of heart attacks in patients with unstable angina, the U.S. Veterans Administration divided more than 1,200 men hospitalized with unstable angina into one group that received the equivalent of one buffered aspirin tablet daily and one group that received an inactive substance, or placebo. The two groups were comparable in the factors known to influence the risk of heart attack and in the other drugs they received for their condition, so

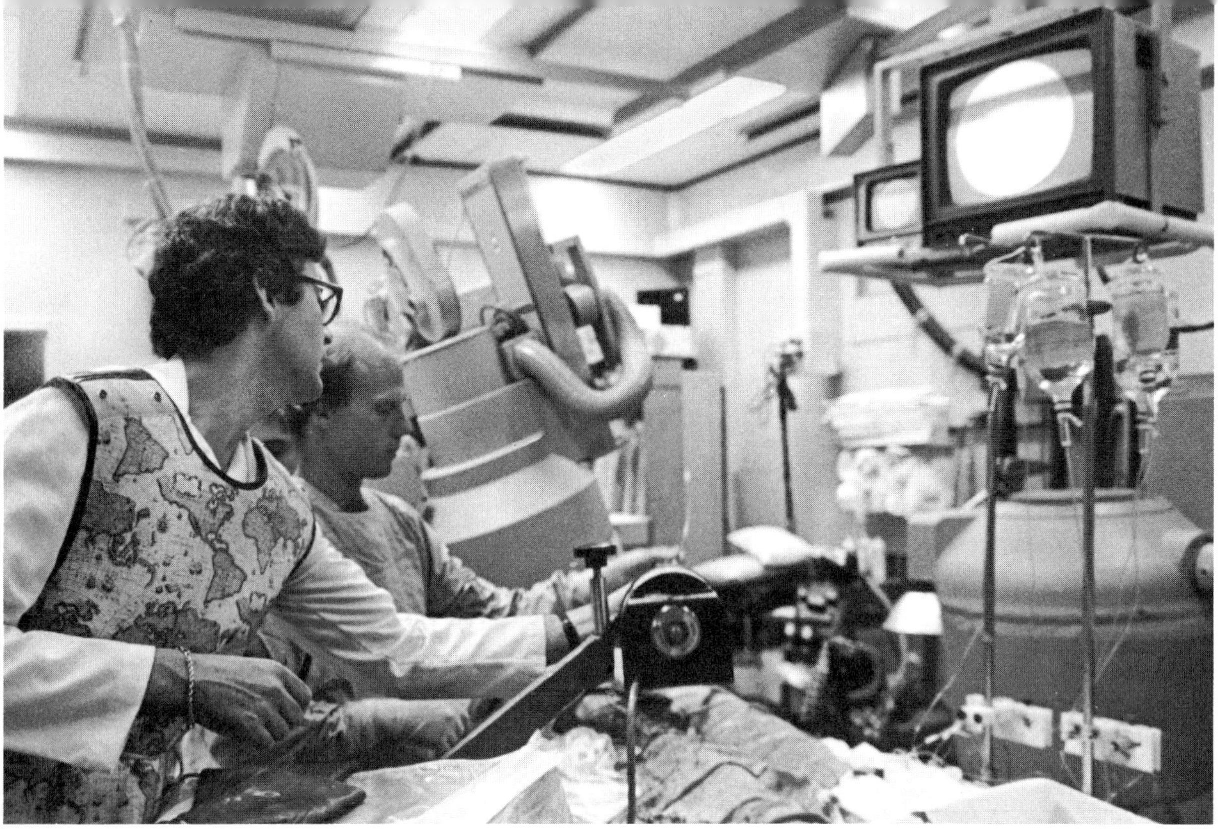

Many patients who would have had to undergo bypass operations can now be treated with balloon angioplasty, a nonsurgical technique in which clogged arteries are widened.

that differences in outcome between the two groups could be attributed to the aspirin therapy. After 12 weeks, the number of deaths and acute heart attacks was 51 percent lower in the group that received aspirin. It is almost certain that aspirin lowers the risk of heart attacks by interfering with the platelets' role in making coronary artery narrowing progress to a total blockage. Wide use of this aspirin-a-day treatment, which is simple and has few side effects, should lead to a substantial reduction in heart attack frequency in unstable angina patients. In October 1985 the U.S. Food and Drug Administration approved new labeling for aspirin noting that one tablet a day could help prevent heart attacks in patients with unstable angina and could prevent a recurrence of heart attacks in those who have already had one. The evidence that aspirin prevents a recurrence of heart attacks is, however, much less conclusive than the evidence for its usefulness in treating unstable angina patients.

Another blood clot-inhibiting drug, known as heparin, has also recently been shown to reduce the frequency of heart attacks in patients with unstable angina. Heparin interferes with blood clotting by inhibiting certain proteins vitally involved in the process. The drug can be given only by intravenous injection. During a one-week period in one study, unstable angina patients in a group not receiving heparin were almost six times more likely to have a heart attack than those in a comparable group receiving heparin. It is not known whether further benefits could be attained by combining heparin and aspirin, but too much interference with blood clotting could lead to bleeding complications; this possibility limits the potential of such a combination.

Opening Clogged Arteries

The underlying problem that makes coronary artery blockage by a blood clot a danger to patients with unstable angina is the presence of at least one very severely narrowed coronary artery. While the anticlotting effects of aspirin and heparin may protect the patient from a blockage in the short term, the persistence of a severe narrowing means there is a continued risk of blockage and a likelihood of continuing angina. Since the late 1960's surgeons have been able to improve blood flow to the heart by means of a coronary bypass, a major, open-heart operation in which the narrowed area is literally "bypassed"; segments of artery or vein taken from other parts of the body are connected to the affected coronary artery beyond the narrowed area, creating an alternative blood route. Coronary bypass has been shown to be effective for relieving the pain of angina and for prolonging life in certain groups of angina patients.

In 1977 another technique, balloon angioplasty (technically called percutaneous transluminal coronary angioplasty), was first used. In this procedure a catheter is inserted into an artery in the leg and threaded up into the narrowed coronary artery. A small balloon at the end of the catheter is then inflated and deflated several times, compressing the fatty deposit and greatly widening the channel through which the blood can flow. All this is done without the need for open-heart surgery. The technique is not suitable for all patients, but up to 40 percent of those who would once have had a bypass operation can benefit from nonsurgical angioplasty instead. Angioplasty is not without problems: a few patients (less than 1 percent) die while undergoing the procedure. Furthermore, about one-fourth of blood vessels opened by this means become narrowed again within six months, necessitating either repeat angioplasty or bypass surgery.

However, a recent study in the Netherlands showed far fewer heart attacks than would otherwise be expected in a group of hospitalized unstable angina patients who underwent successful angioplasty. Thus, it

A new, aggressive strategy is to halt a heart attack in its first hours by administering streptokinase, an enzyme which activates the body's own clot-dissolving mechanism.

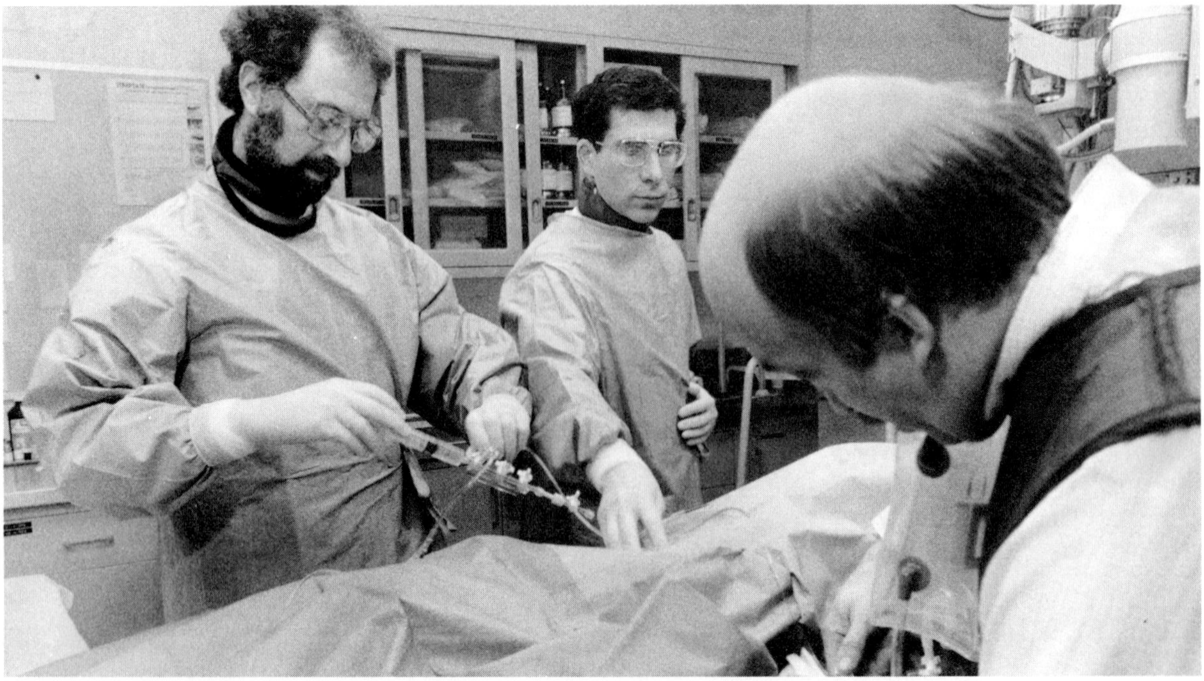

appears that, if appropriate, angioplasty can play a vital role in reducing death and heart attack rates in patients with unstable angina, especially when their condition cannot be stabilized with medication alone.

Recently, some doctors have begun experimenting with using laser beams for opening clogged coronary arteries. The technique remains highly experimental.

Halting an Attack in Process

Dramatic breakthroughs have enabled doctors to treat heart attacks more aggressively and effectively—in some cases, while the attack is actually still going on. This capability represents a remarkable change in approach to heart attacks. Early in this century, treatment dealt merely with complications as they arose, such as pain, heart irregularities, and heart failure. Little was or could be done about the underlying problem of a blocked blood vessel and a cutoff of blood to the heart. But in the late 1970's a new strategy emerged when it was shown that most patients in the early hours of a heart attack had evidence of a clot totally blocking the involved artery. Intensive effort has since focused on salvaging jeopardized heart muscle by opening the obstructed artery to reestablish blood flow. Efforts to open arteries in heart attack patients have taken two forms: injection of clot-dissolving enzymes and direct mechanical improvement of coronary blood flow through angioplasty.

The body has a mechanism for breaking up unwanted blood clots, and certain proteins can be administered to activate it. Two such agents are streptokinase (sold as Streptase and Kabikinase) and urokinase (Abbokinase). The most serious drawback of these substances is that they activate the clot-dissolving system throughout the body, and, by preventing necessary blood clotting, can lead to serious bleeding problems.

Doctors, using catheters inserted into blood vessels in the leg and then snaked up to the heart, have begun administering streptokinase directly into the coronary arteries of heart attack victims within the first several hours of the attack. When this is done within the first six hours after heart attack symptoms begin, streptokinase dissolves the clot and reestablishes blood flow in 70 to 80 percent of cases. Since a considerable delay is involved in bringing the patient to special laboratories where facilities for this procedure are available, treatment has often been delayed beyond the time during which substantial salvage of heart muscle can be achieved. Nevertheless, one large, carefully controlled study strongly suggested that successfully opening an obstructed artery by this method, even within the first 12 hours, could lead to a significant reduction in deaths during the first year after the attack in patients who suffered damage to a large area of heart muscle on the front wall of the heart.

The quest for faster therapy that could potentially save more heart muscle has led many doctors to inject large doses of streptokinase into a vein rather than into the coronary artery. Special laboratories are not needed, and medical personnel do not need special training. While results have varied, most studies show that only 40 to 50 percent of obstructed arteries can be opened with this intravenous injection of streptokinase. Furthermore, the larger doses of streptokinase used in the intravenous injections lead to a higher potential for serious bleeding. (Despite these

Arteries Become Blocked

In the process known as atherosclerosis, fatty material builds up on the inner lining of the coronary arteries.

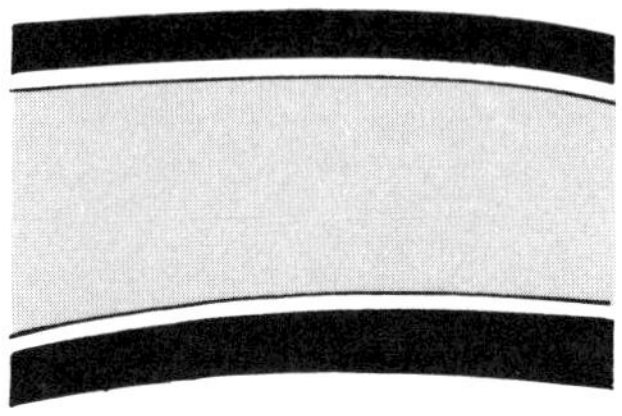

Normal blood vessel.

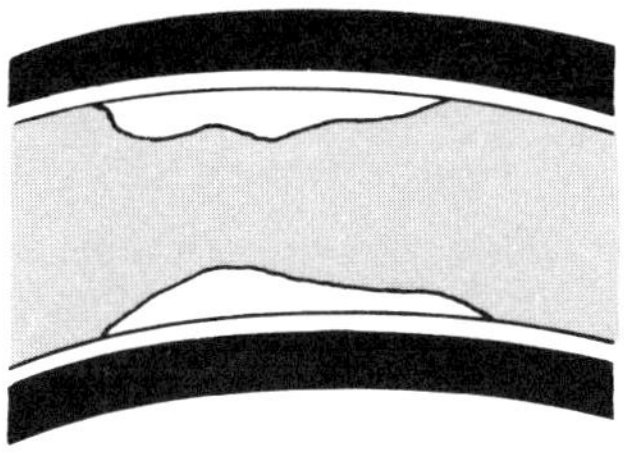

Small amount of fatty buildup.

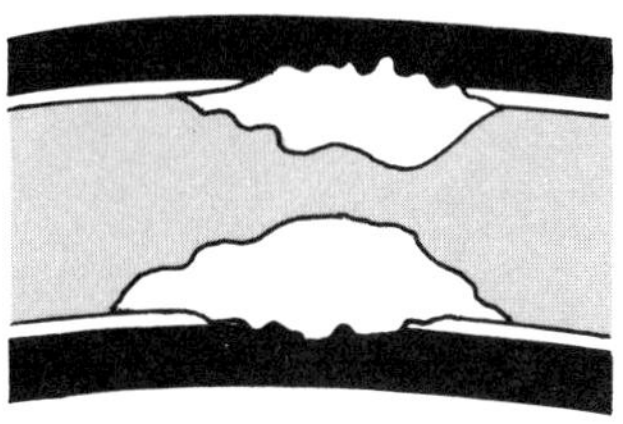

Larger fatty deposit significantly narrows vessel opening.

problems, a recently completed Italian study of over 12,000 heart attack victims showed that when given within the first three hours of the onset of an attack, intravenous streptokinase led to a 20 percent reduction in deaths soon after the attack.)

The need for a more effective clot-dissolving substance, with less risk of bleeding, has led to tests of a substance called tissue plasminogen activator. TPA is actually a naturally occurring substance that acts to dissolve clots only after it has firmly bound to the clot itself. It therefore has a more concentrated effect on the large blood clot the doctor is trying to dissolve and less of a tendency to cause bleeding elsewhere in the body. Recent genetic engineering advances have made TPA more widely available for experimental use. A study that compared intravenous injection of TPA to intravenous injection of streptokinase in patients in the early hours of an acute heart attack showed that TPA was more successful in reopening blocked arteries (a 66 percent success rate) than was streptokinase (36 percent). If further studies confirm TPA to be safe and effective, giving it to heart attack victims within one or two hours after the appearance of symptoms may result in the greatest possible salvage of jeopardized heart muscle. Additional studies are also needed to confirm the long-term benefits of TPA treatment, to help identify those most likely to benefit from it, and to determine what kind of care should follow.

Beta blockers, which slow the heart rate, have become standard treatment for high-risk heart attack survivors.

One of the major difficulties with clot-dissolving treatment, whether given intravenously or directly into the coronary artery, is that after the clot has dissolved, the patient often still has severe narrowing in the artery that had been blocked. The patient thus remains at risk of another blockage. For this reason, many researchers have tried to improve blood flow through the narrowed arteries of a heart attack victim by performing balloon angioplasty either at the time of or shortly following streptokinase injection. Others have begun doing angioplasty without first administering streptokinase, by pushing the balloon catheter past the obstruction and compressing both the clot and the plaque material in the obstructed artery. This technique has several potential advantages over clot-dissolving therapy alone. First, one can usually open the artery more quickly than the 30 to 45 minutes required for the clot-dissolving treatment to take effect. Second, immediate angioplasty relieves the underlying atherosclerotic narrowing more completely, potentially reducing the risk of later, repeated obstruction. And third, if angioplasty is successful, the patient can be spared the bleeding problems possible with clot-dissolving treatment.

In a study of more than 50 acute heart attack victims, doctors at the University of Michigan found that patients who got balloon angioplasty as their first treatment had better recovery of function in the damaged heart muscle and fewer cases of repeated obstruction in the affected artery than did patients treated with streptokinase alone. Researchers in Kansas City and elsewhere have shown that immediate angioplasty for patients who have the shocklike symptoms of a massive heart attack may reduce their expected in-hospital mortality from 80–90 percent to 30–40 percent.

There are, however, drawbacks to such an approach. Time is required to transport the patient to the laboratory where angioplasty is done, during which time tissue destruction continues. Furthermore, facilities and skilled people to perform the procedure are not available everywhere.

Finally, early reclosure of the artery by remaining clot material occurs frequently, requiring repeat angioplasty and clot-dissolving drugs.

Because of these problems, the eventual standard treatment for a massive heart attack will likely become immediate intravenous injection of a clot-dissolving substance like TPA, followed by rapid transport to a regional medical center for coronary angiography; if the X rays show severe remaining coronary narrowings, angioplasty will be done.

Long-term Treatment for Heart Attack Survivors

Patients who survive a heart attack and are discharged from the hospital continue to be at increased risk of heart attacks and death from heart disease. Approximately 10 percent of heart attack survivors under the age of 70 will die within a year, with the highest proportion of deaths occurring within the first three months. High and low risk groups can be determined on the basis of the amount of heart muscle damaged, the regularity of the heart's electrical impulses, and the extent to which still living heart muscle is jeopardized by inadequate blood flow. Treatment of irregularities in heartbeat rhythm and efforts to improve blood flow to the heart, either by angioplasty or by coronary bypass surgery, probably improve the outlook for selected patients.

Studies have shown that a certain class of heart drugs called beta blockers—which block nerve impulses that stimulate the heart, thus slowing its rate and decreasing the force of its contractions—can significantly reduce deaths among heart attack survivors over at least a three-year period. A Norwegian study of heart attack victims showed a 39 percent reduction in deaths and a 34 percent reduction in nonfatal heart attacks in patients taking the beta blocker timolol (sold under various brand names), compared to comparable patients given a placebo. In a larger U.S. study of heart attack survivors, mortality was 26 percent lower and nonfatal heart attack 16 percent less frequent in those receiving the beta-blocking drug propranolol (sold as Inderal and Inderide) than in a comparable group getting a placebo. In both studies, the beneficial effects of the beta blockers were most prominent among those at highest risk. Beta blockers have become routine treatment for high-risk heart attack survivors and will undoubtedly give them an improved prognosis.

When doctors finally understand fully the causes of atherosclerosis, heart attacks may become a curiosity of the past.

Future Directions

While the next decade will undoubtedly see further refinement of many of the new drugs and techniques used to treat heart attack victims, a truly dramatic reduction in the toll exacted by coronary heart disease will come only when doctors have learned how to prevent or substantially slow atherosclerosis and its harmful effects on the coronary arteries. This will require breakthroughs in basic understanding of how atherosclerosis develops and the factors that convert a stable plaque into an unstable one, leading to arterial obstruction and heart muscle damage. With continued support of basic research into the underlying causes of heart disease, the day may arrive when heart attacks are looked upon as poliomyelitis is today—as a curious medical phenomenon of the past, very rarely producing death or disability in those in the prime of life. □

HOW LONG CAN WE LIVE?

William R. Hazzard, M.D., and Matthew Tayback, Sc.D.

People have always wondered how long they could expect to live. The Bible talks of extraordinary longevity, spanning centuries: "Thus all the days of Methuselah were nine hundred and sixty-nine years; and he died" (Genesis). Yet for some, fate seemed to promise a sum of years not too different from our lot today: "The years of our life are threescore and ten," it says in Psalms. In biblical times, and for centuries afterward, what was known about longevity was a mixture of legend and haphazard observation.

The past 200 years have seen enormous advances in knowledge about human longevity. Statistical methods have been developed for determining how long the average person can expect to live and for estimating how long people lived in earlier eras. Progress in

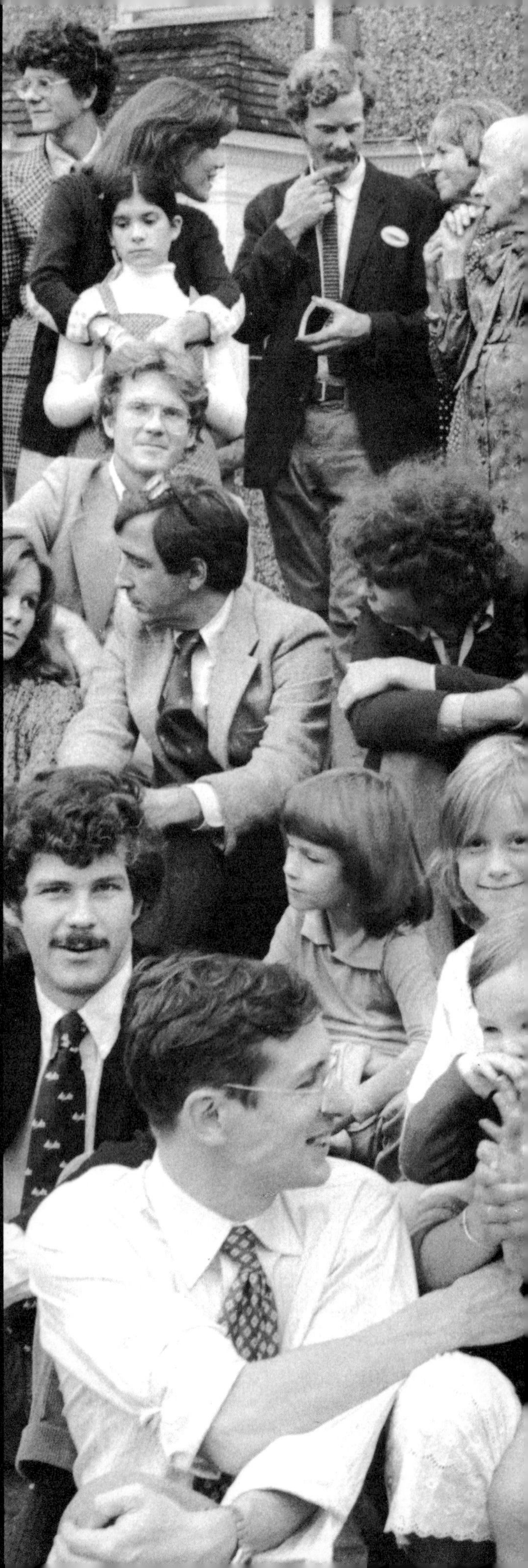

Four generations of a New York family gather at a 90th birthday celebration.

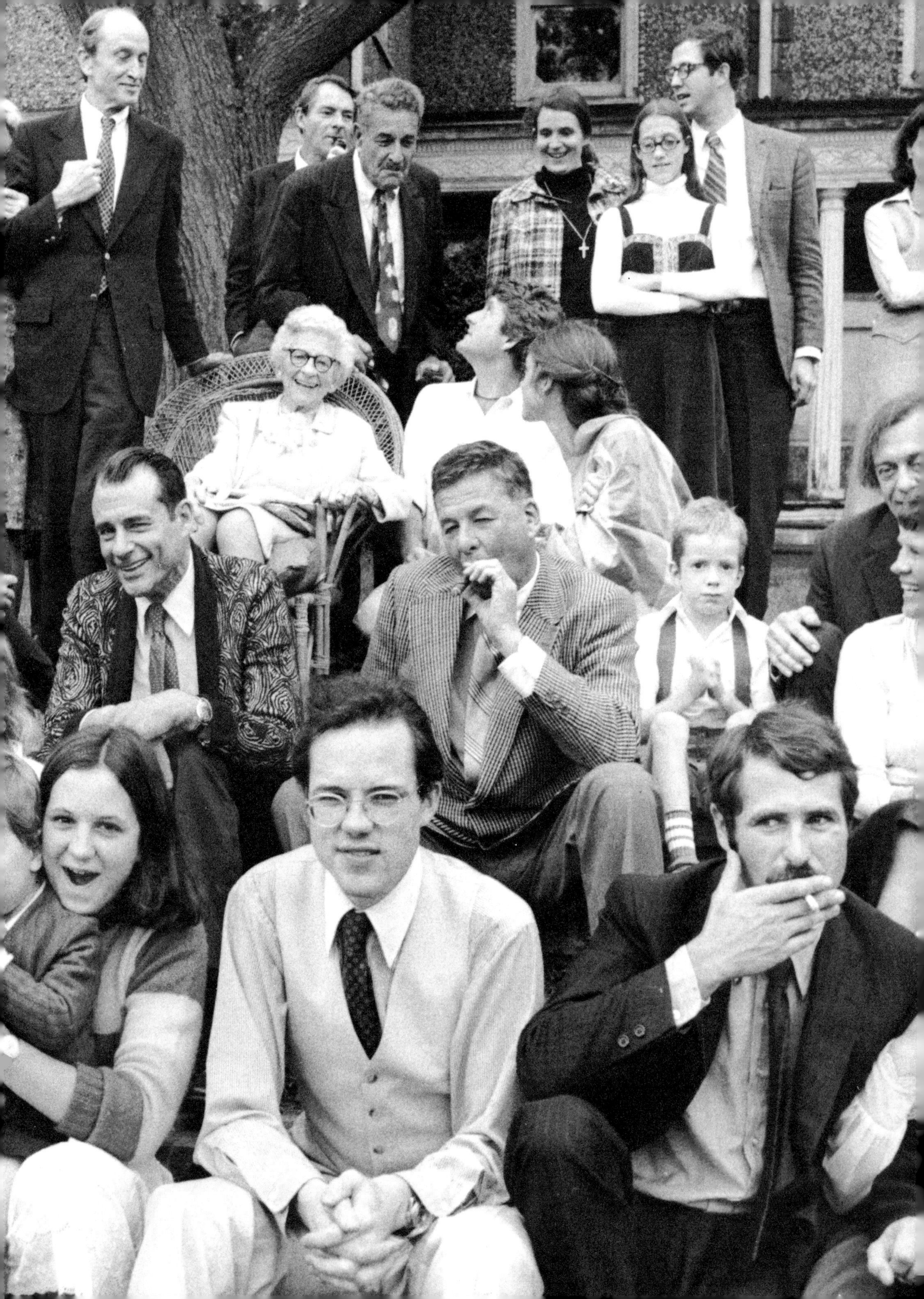

medical research, in public health and sanitation measures, and in treatment of disease have increased the average lifetime dramatically, especially in the industrialized world. Scientists have also sought to learn why people age and eventually die. There is as yet no definite answer to this question, but a number of intriguing theories have been proposed.

Averages and Extremes

The newborn baby who dies at birth has lived 0 years, and the centenarian, 100 years. The difference is enormous. How, then, to describe the length of the average lifetime?

The psalmist's threescore and ten was, no doubt, meant as the age adults were likely to reach before death. It was clearly not the maximum number of years a person could live. Nor could it be, for that era, an expression of the average length of life from birth. It was probably based on the frequency with which death was observed to occur at about 70. It certainly did not take into account the considerable loss of life that took place among infants and children.

A common way of describing average lifetime today is life expectancy at birth. This figure is obtained by constructing a "life table," reflecting the number of years lived by each member of a group. Typically, the group would consist of 100,000 people, all considered to be born at the same time. Life expectancy at birth is determined by adding up the group members' ages at death and then dividing by 100,000.

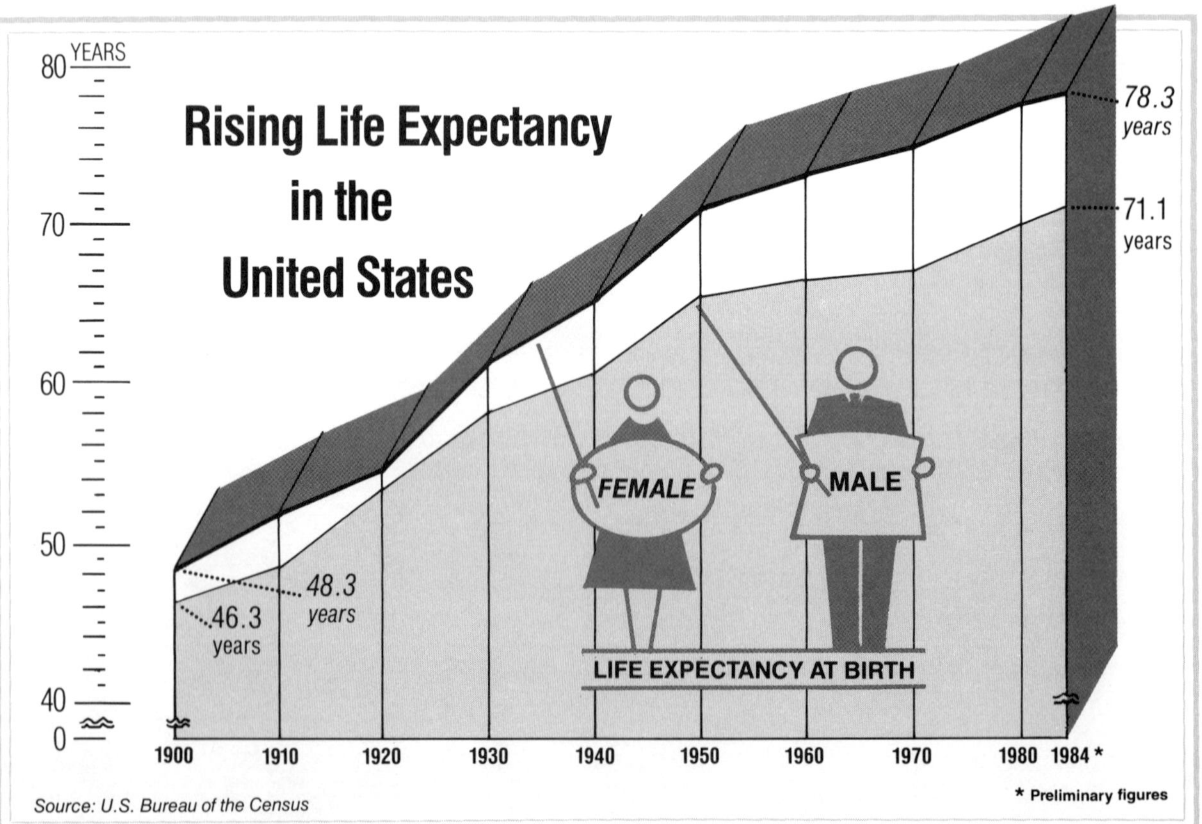

Source: U.S. Bureau of the Census

Another measure used in talking about longevity is the remaining lifetime at a specified age, such as 65. Unlike life expectancy at birth, this measure describes not the total life experience of all 100,000 people, but the average number of years subsequently lived by those who reach the age of 65. Life expectancy at 65 is an expression of the vitality, as a group, of those who attain old age.

In contrast to life expectancy, the concept of life span is concerned not with averages but with the longest possible individual existence—a maximum determined in practice by the oldest reliably reported age of death, a subject about which there is much dispute.

The notion that there is a limit to the possible length of human life is actually present even in the reference in Genesis to Methuselah. Written about 1000 B.C., the story reflected oral tales that had been passed down from one generation to another over several centuries. It is not uncommon in folklore to attribute very long life to heroic individuals. But according to the biblical scholar Walter Brueggemann, accounts of longevity are more restrained in Genesis than in other writings of that time, such as Sumerian king lists: "By keeping the ages under 1,000 years, it seems that the Old Testament is saying there is a limit to one's life expectancy, and the fantastic, mythological figures for the ages of royal figures in pagan cultures are not valid."

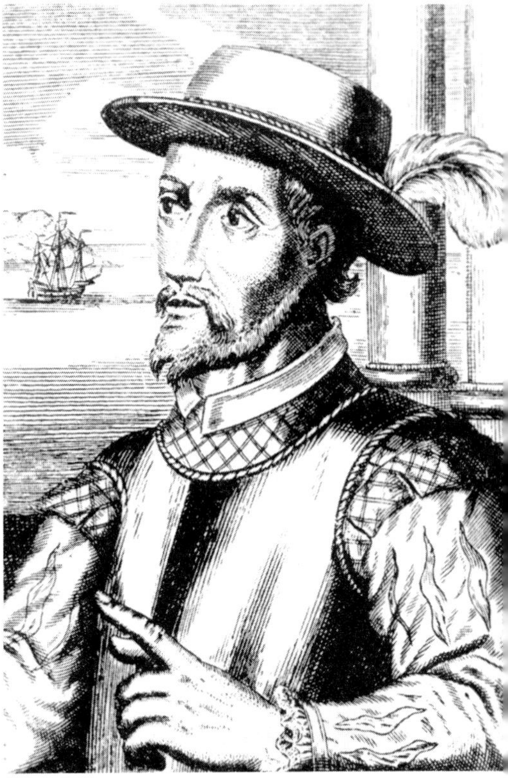

The Spanish explorer Juan Ponce de León searched in the New World for the Fountain of Youth, which, according to Indian legend, rejuvenated all who bathed in it.

Life Expectancy Through the Ages

Scientists today have somewhat more precise knowledge about longevity in ancient times—largely because of a remarkable set of studies undertaken by the British statisticians Karl Pearson and W. R. Macdonell from 1900 to 1910. Using the ages recorded on mummy cases in Egypt and the age at death recorded for Roman citizens in the first two centuries after Christ, they were able to estimate, for the areas studied, how many years people of various ages could expect to live. Pearson and Macdonell's conclusions still had built-in limitations: they were based on the ages at death of selected individuals and required certain assumptions about the birthrate and the effects of migration. Nevertheless, they establish, with a fair degree of certainty, 20 years as the life expectancy at birth around the time of Christ, with the life expectancy at 65 being about 10 years.

A major early contribution to knowledge about longevity was made by someone better known for predicting a comet's return: the English astronomer Edmund Halley. Halley compiled a life table based on the record of births and deaths that existed for the city of Breslau (now Wroclaw in Poland). Commonly believed to be the first life table prepared by a competent scientist and based on current data, it was published in 1693. The expected lifetime at birth that Halley obtained was 33.5 years, while life expectancy at 65 was 9.73 years.

Accurate data for Western European countries became increasingly

---

William R. Hazzard and Matthew Tayback are the director and coordinator, respectively, of the Center on Aging of the Johns Hopkins Medical Institutions in Baltimore, Md.

available from the mid-19th century onward. For the United States, life expectancy at birth and at 65 has been calculated since 1900 for the three-year period around the start of each decade.

The U.S. figures show considerable improvement in life expectancy at birth, rising from 47.3 years in 1900 to 74.7 in 1984. Canadian data are similar, with life expectancy increasing from 61 in 1931 (the earliest figure available) to 75.4 in 1981. The same trend has been seen in other industrialized countries, with several countries—such as Iceland and Japan (where the average life expectancy at birth is 77)—outperforming the United States and Canada in this regard. Even many poorer countries have made great advances, though some lag far behind; according to the latest available estimates, Afghanistan has a life expectancy at birth of only about 37, Gambia 35, and North Yemen 44.

Methuselah may not have lived to 969, but some reasonably ripe old ages have been documented.

Life expectancy at 65 has also shown improvement, rising from 12 years in the United States in 1900 to 16.7 years in 1981. In Canada in 1981 it was 16.9 years.

Looking back over the past 2,000 years, we can draw at least two broad conclusions from the available information: for people in some countries today, the life expectancy at birth is nearly four times the 20 years that the ancient Romans could expect to live, and the average remaining lifetime at 65 years of age has nearly doubled.

The Longest Livers

Methuselah may be just a legend, but some reasonably ripe old ages have been documented. Among the ancient Greeks, the rhetorician and educator Isocrates was said to have died at the age of 98 years. This appears to be the longest recorded lifetime for a leading figure of the Greco-Roman era. A Dane named Christian Jacobsen Drakenberg is supposed to have lived from 1626 till 1772, a total of 146 years—a claim most authorities doubt. In 1985, Shigechiyo Izumi of Japan, at the time widely considered the world's oldest living human, reportedly celebrated his 120th birthday. (He died in early 1986.)

According to the historian of the U.S. Social Security Administration, the longest-lived person in the agency's official records was Charlie Smith, who died October 7, 1979, at the apparent age of 137. Another Social Security recipient, William E. Davis, died in 1960, apparently at the age of 122. The determination of age in these cases was based not on birth certificates but on early records of marriages and on what the individuals in question could recall of their own lives, so these ages cannot be regarded as 100 percent reliable. Of the approximately 31,500 males who became eligible for old-age insurance benefits in 1940 and whose ages at that time could be accepted as 65-67 years, all have since passed away, the two longest-lived dying at 107 and 108 years of age.

A careful weighing of all the available data leads to the conclusion that the human life span—the longest a person can expect to live—probably falls within the range of 105 to 125 years. There is no satisfactory evidence that over the past 2,000 years the life span has undergone a change like that of life expectancy at birth or at 65 years of age. Some researchers even believe that the human life span has remained virtually unchanged for hundreds of thousands of years.

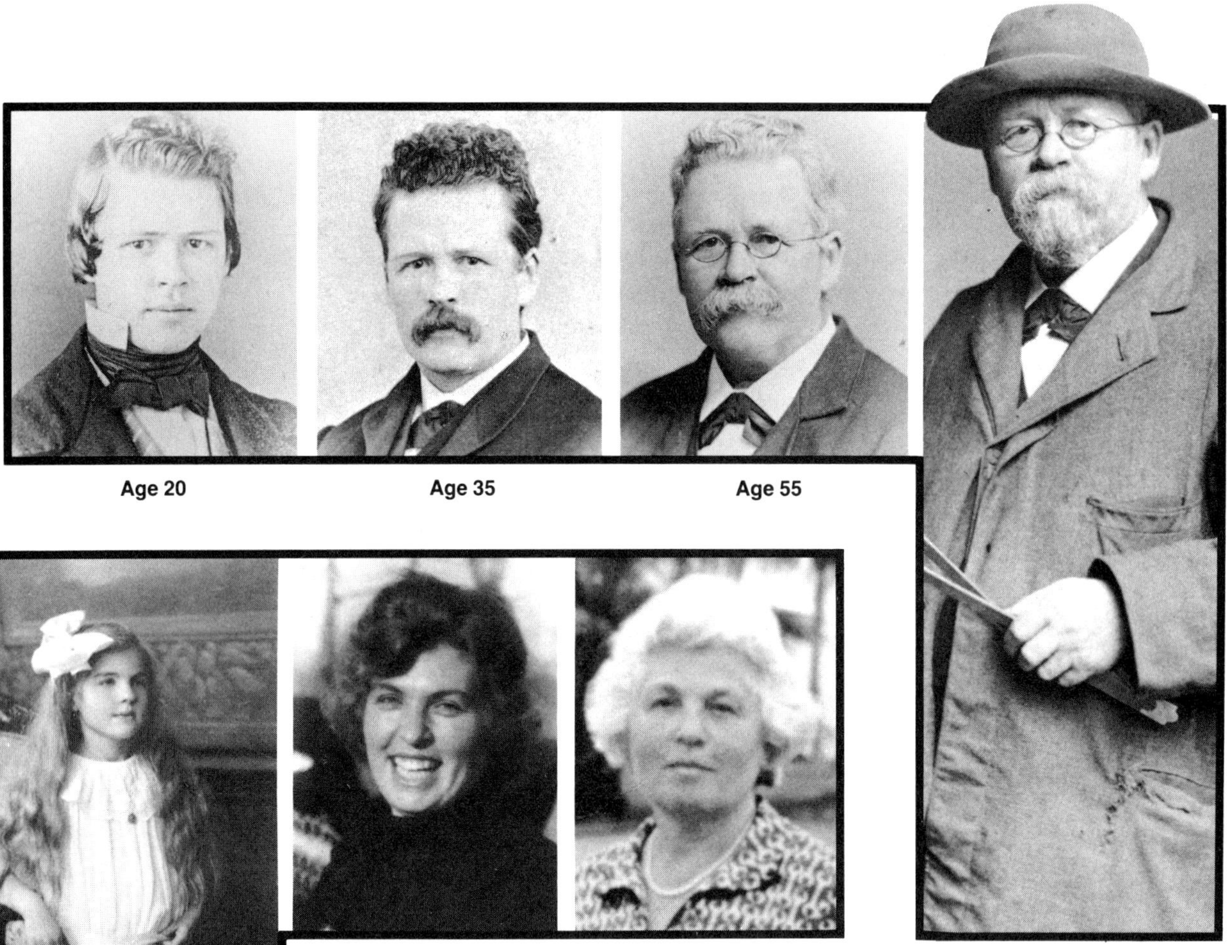

Age 20 Age 35 Age 55 Age 75

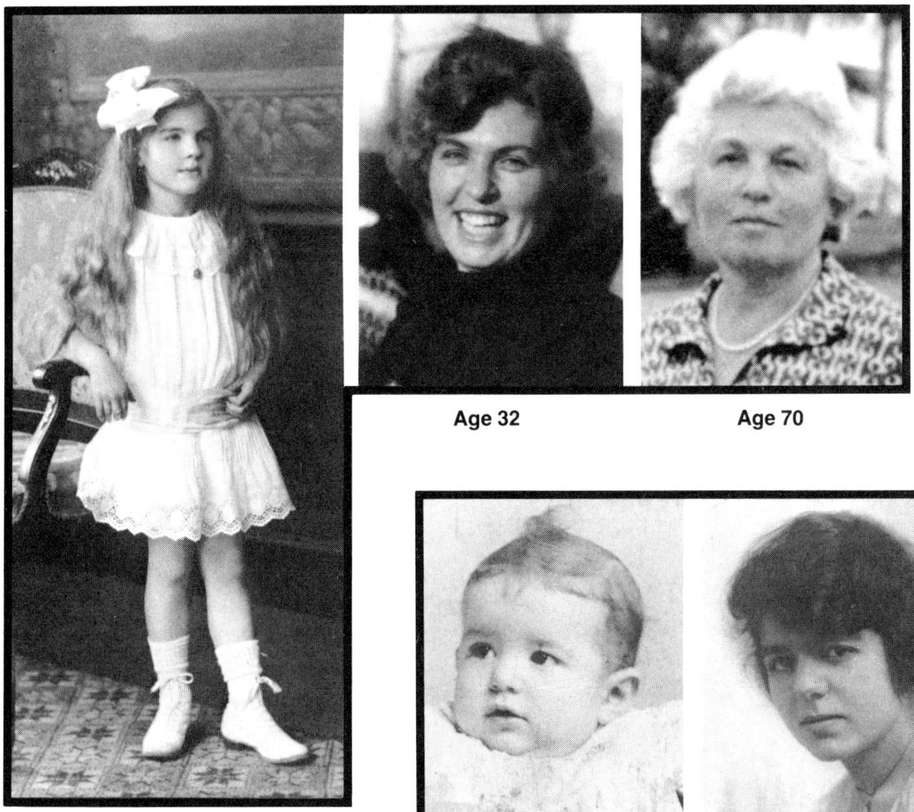

Age 7 Age 32 Age 70

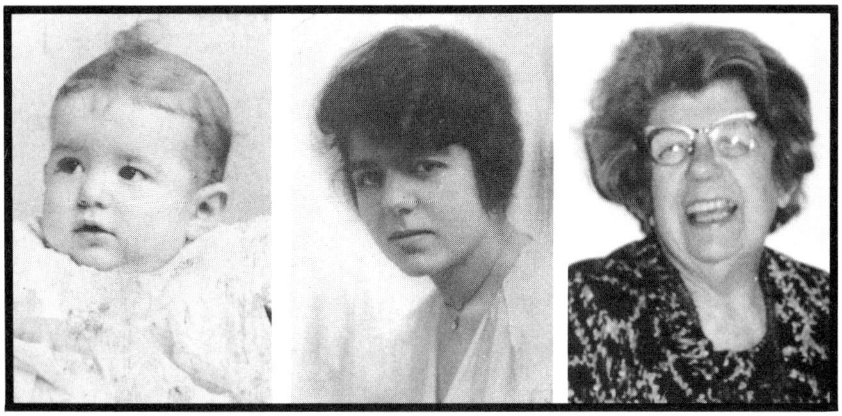

Age 1 Age 24 Age 80

Shown here, three individuals and how they aged.

Press reports of whole villages where nearly everyone seems to live to a great age, and where the oldest inhabitant is in the 15th or 16th decade of life, must be treated with skepticism. Three instances often cited are villagers in some areas of the Caucasus in the Soviet Union, the Hunzukuts of Nepal, and the people of Vilcabamba, a village in the Ecuadoran Andes. Generally speaking there is no documentation for the advanced ages claimed in these cases. Birth certificates offered by some of the Caucasians have turned out to belong to a father or older brother or to be forgeries meant to prove their holders were too old for conscription in World War I. It may well be that the inhabitants of these communities are quite long-lived, but the unsupported claims made for them are no basis for raising the estimate for maximum human life span.

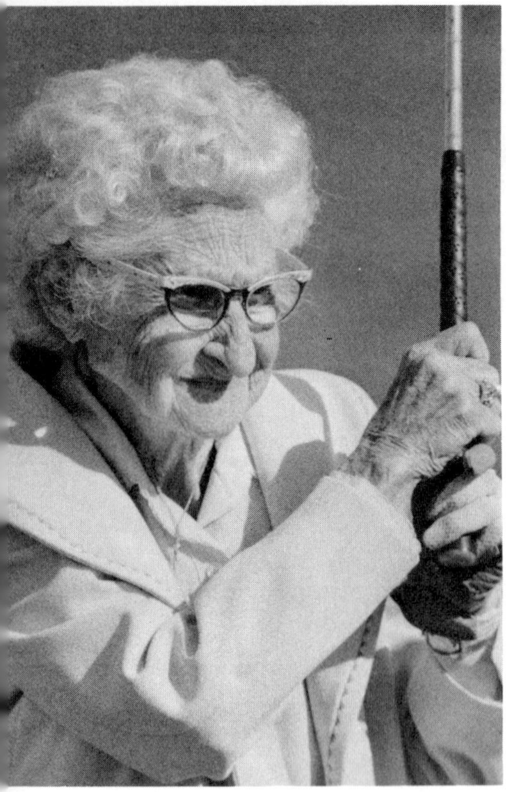

Active life need not end as one grows older. This 100-year-old golfer pursues a sport she took up at age 8.

Why People Are Living Longer

The striking improvement in life expectancy at birth over the centuries, and especially in more recent times in the developed nations, can be attributed to five major factors.

First, the availability of abundant clean water for food preparation and personal hygiene has dramatically reduced deaths among infants and children because of diarrhea—a major killer of children where sanitation is poor.

Second, common communicable diseases take the lives of far fewer children than they once did, thanks to the use of vaccines.

Tuberculosis and pneumonia have also been brought under much better control, first by widespread socioeconomic improvements and then by the discovery of new and effective medications, including antibiotics.

Fourth, adult loss of life because of cardiovascular disease and other serious diseases has been delayed—at least in some countries—by improved treatment and by changes in the life-style (including diet) of many people.

Fifth, improved medical knowledge and care have sharply reduced the number of women who die in childbirth.

Over the past century life expectancy at 65 has not changed by as many years as that at birth. Nonetheless, the improvement has been substantial and is probably due to three major factors: reduction in deaths from pneumonia in old age, because of better medical care and more effective drugs; increased availability of medical care for the control of major chronic diseases afflicting the elderly, such as heart disease, diabetes, and high blood pressure; and the improved social and economic circumstances of the elderly that have resulted from greatly expanded social welfare programs.

The Gulf Between the Sexes

There is a major difference in longevity between the sexes: in 1984 the life expectancy at birth in the United States was 71.1 years for men and 78.3 years for women. (Comparable Canadian figures for 1981 were 71.9 and 79 years, respectively.) What is more, the gap is much wider than it once was; the difference in the United States in 1920 was only one year.

There is no real consensus on the reasons for this striking disparity. Clearly the tendency of men to develop heart disease earlier accounts for a major portion of the difference, but the underlying causes remain a matter of dispute. It has been suggested that women are simply hardier in genetic makeup, or that female hormones—determined, of course, by heredity—have a protective effect. Other researchers contend that higher rates of smoking by men explain much of the difference (it is generally conceded that men's smoking does account for some of the gap). Like many other questions in the study of longevity, the reasons for this "gender gap" require more research.

Reducing Premature Death

Since the upper limit of the human life span seems to lie between 105 and 125 years, many researchers are concentrating their attention on understanding and counteracting the factors that limit average longevity to roughly two-thirds of that maximum. Ways are being sought to reduce the gap between average and maximum longevity by preventing premature death, whether caused by disease (including such widespread killers as heart disease and cancer) or other factors. The focus of medical efforts to increase longevity has shifted, over the years, from causes of death in infancy and childhood, such as infantile diarrhea and malnutrition, to medical problems of young adulthood (notably, for women, complications of childbearing) to the predominant chronic diseases of middle and old age.

The most common cause of death in the United States today is cardiovascular disease attributable to atherosclerosis—a degenerative condition of the arteries. Cardiovascular diseases include coronary heart disease (heart attack and heart failure), stroke, and vascular diseases affecting the kidneys and circulation in the limbs. As with other chronic diseases of later life, atherosclerosis has many causes, and the likelihood of its onset increases with time.

Certain risk factors that appear to be at least somewhat controllable increase the odds for developing atherosclerosis. These include, in roughly descending order of importance, a low level in the blood of the type of cholesterol called high-density lipoprotein (HDL), a high level of low-density lipoprotein (LDL) cholesterol, high blood pressure, cigarette smoking, and diabetes. There is some evidence that regular exercise can help decrease LDL levels and increase HDL levels.

Some other notable risk factors cannot be modified, such as advanced age and male gender. While aging as such may contribute to atherosclerosis, age appears to influence the process mostly because it means that other risk factors have been present longer. Gender acts at least in part by directly affecting other risk factors: estrogens (female hormones) increase levels of HDL, and androgens (male hormones) decrease them; estrogens decrease LDL, and androgens increase it.

The role of excess weight in heart disease and other disorders has come under intensive study. Being overweight may or may not accelerate atherosclerosis directly. Overweight is clearly associated with increased LDL and total cholesterol, decreased HDL,

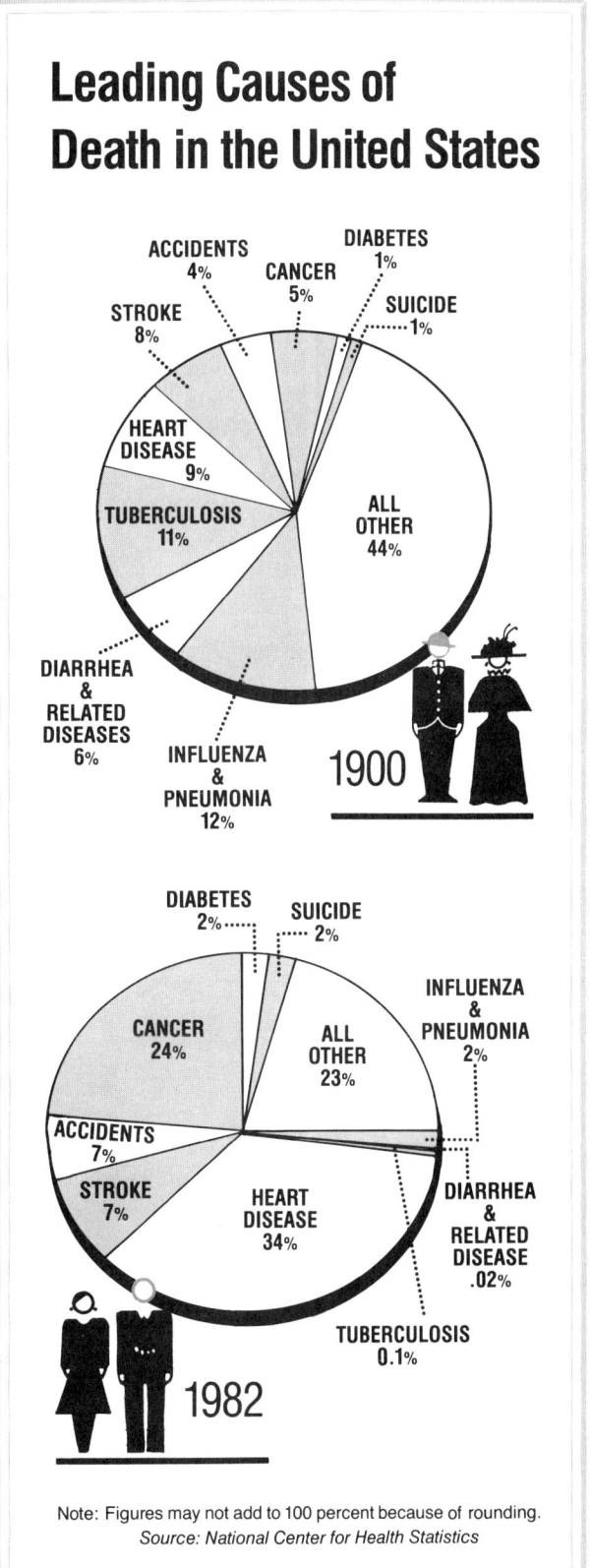

Leading Causes of Death in the United States

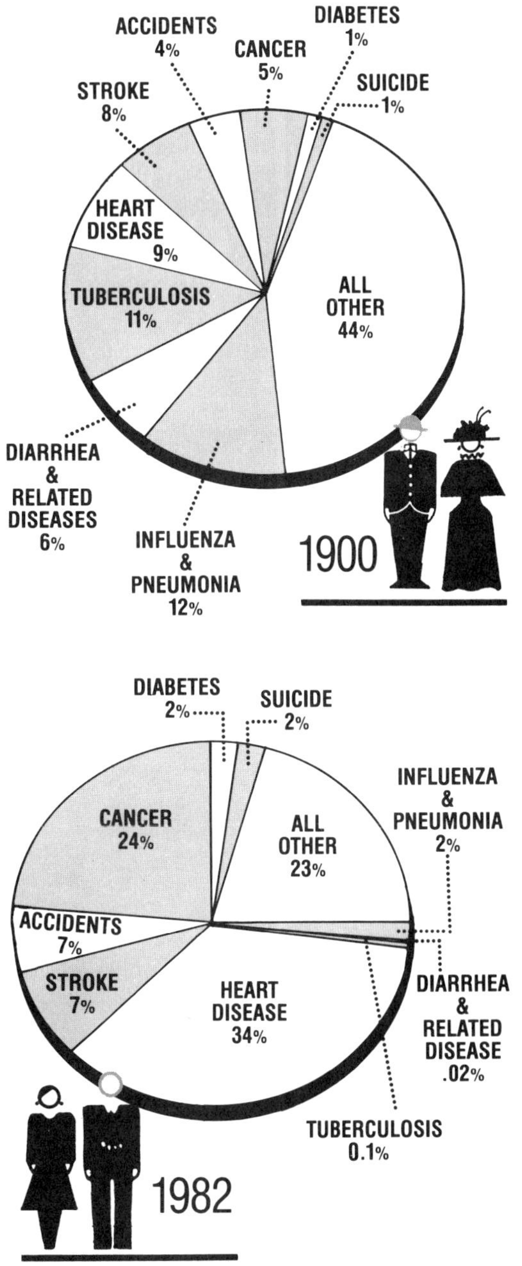

Note: Figures may not add to 100 percent because of rounding.
Source: National Center for Health Statistics

increased blood pressure, and a greater likelihood of diabetes. This suggests that regulating weight may be a way of reducing multiple risks to an individual. On the other hand, moderate overweight does not appear to curtail overall longevity, particularly beyond mid-life. Researchers are seeking overweight-related factors that might even increase longevity, such as a decrease in the rate of osteoporosis (a condition in which bones become thin and brittle) and of hip and spine fractures in postmenopausal women.

Research aimed at increasing longevity by retarding atherosclerosis is gaining momentum. There are clear findings of a decrease in coronary heart disease associated with the reduction of blood cholesterol levels in middle-aged men. Also, there is evidence that the continuing decrease in coronary heart disease in recent years in the United States is linked with several factors: the consumption of less saturated fat and cholesterol (primarily through decreased intake of animal fats), the consumption of more unsaturated vegetable fats, decreased cigarette smoking among middle-aged and older people, and better control of high blood pressure in the population.

Theories of Aging

What causes people to age and eventually die? No one has any final answers yet, but scientists are exploring a number of possibilities.

A Built-In Timer
Our heredity contains preprogrammed instructions that cause our cells to stop reproducing at a certain point and ultimately to die.

Free Radicals
Unstable molecules called free radicals cause damage to the body's tissues that builds up over time.

Crumbling Defenses
The immune system, the body's defense against disease, deteriorates as the years go by, leaving people more open to infection, cancer, and disorders of the immune system itself.

Damage to DNA
Errors caused by radiation or chemical damage gradually accumulate in DNA—the body's genetic blueprint—until they overwhelm its capacity to function.

Failing Central Regulation
The interactions between the brain and nervous system and the hormone-producing glands that regulate our bodily functions become disordered with age.

Genetic Factors in Short and Long Lives

As life-style changes reduce premature atherosclerosis, genetic factors become more important as causes of the gap between life expectancy and life span. Genetically determined conditions contributing to atherosclerosis appear to be the major inherited cause of shortened life in humans. Among such conditions identified so far are disorders in which high levels of LDL or low levels of HDL seem to be inherited. However, since even relatively rare genetic disorders that promote atherosclerosis appear to be affected by dietary and other life-style factors, the average age at which coronary disease develops in those afflicted with such disorders is likely to increase with improved habits.

The search for genes that may increase longevity has not proved too fruitful. Not surprisingly, inherited causes of increased HDL or decreased LDL have been found to be more common in people who have lived to 80 or 90 than in the general population. These factors have been dubbed longevity syndromes. Identifying such inherited causes of longevity is a very difficult task, complicated by the need to account for the difference in longevity between the sexes while at the same time trying to separate the influence of environmental and time-related factors from the role of inheritance.

A Genetic Limit to Life Span?

The reasons for the gap between average and maximum longevity are not the only central concern of current research. Many scientists are focusing on the basic biological reasons why people grow old and die. One widely held view is that longevity is basically determined by the genetic blueprint, or code, carried by the substance DNA (deoxyribonucleic acid) in each cell of the body. This code is unique to each individual and, more generally, to each species. One reason for the belief in a genetically determined age limit is that each animal species appears to have its own relatively fixed

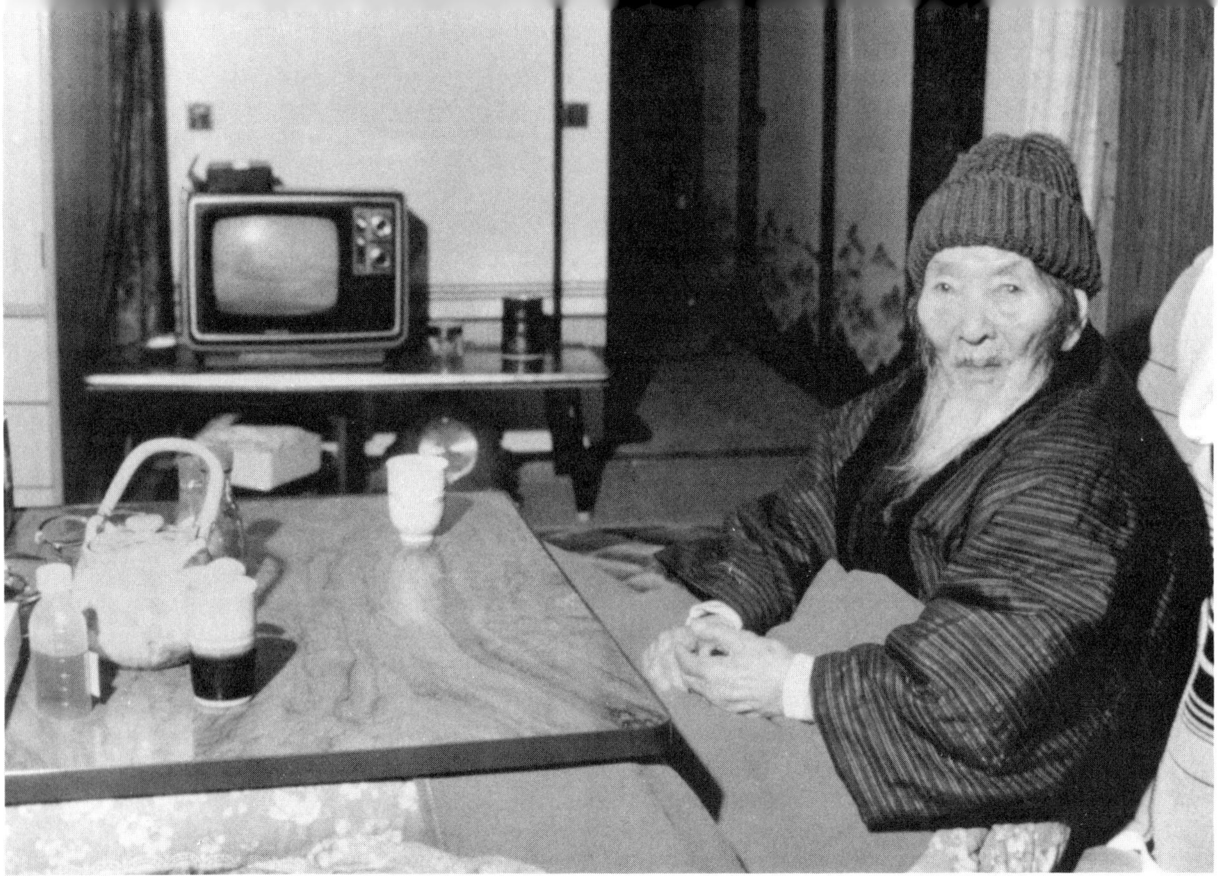

Shigechiyo Izumi of Japan was said to be the world's oldest living human when he reportedly celebrated his 120th birthday in 1985. He died months later, in early 1986.

maximum life span. Another argument for genetic determination is the finding that in humans, at least up to age 60, the difference in ages at death for identical twins (who share exactly the same genes) is less than for fraternal twins (who are not genetically identical).

According to the genetic approach known as the program theory, aging and longevity are determined by the genetic instructions contained in DNA, just as our growth and development are. Evidence in support of this theory is provided by a notable series of experiments carried out by Leonard Hayflick and Paul Sidney Moorhead at the Wistar Institute in Philadelphia in the 1960's. They showed that certain normal human cells, at least when grown in the laboratory, can reproduce themselves only a limited number of times. This is known as the Hayflick phenomenon, and it has been found in some but not all human cells.

Another approach, the somatic mutation theory, maintains that aging is not programmed ino our heredity but stems from cumulative damage to DNA (from radiation, for example), resulting in ever-increasing errors in the body's production of the proteins essential to life. Death comes when an "error catastrophe" occurs—that is, when an error (or errors) overwhelms the body's ability to function. But there is almost no concrete evidence for this theory. In fact, the instructions coded into DNA include much redundancy, and only a small proportion is active at any given time. Moreover, the body has a considerable ability to repair damaged DNA. Consequently, the longevity of an individual (or a species) may be determined by the extent of redundancy and by the capacity for repairing DNA.

Finally, some scientists think that the genetically determined development of substances called chalones—proteins that prevent cells from proliferating and ultimately cause cell death—may limit longevity at the level of the cell and, in turn, in the organism as a whole.

Free-Radical Theory

A number of researchers seek to understand the secret of aging by looking at the biochemical level, that is, the level of the chemical reactions that sustain life. One theory suggests that aging reflects cumulative damage to cells and tissues caused by oxidation reactions (oxidation is familiar to us as burning and the rusting of iron) triggered by free radicals—unstable molecules bearing a "free," or unpaired, electron. These reactions (involving, for example, polyunsaturated fat) may in turn account for such changes associated with aging as the accumulation within cells of a substance called lipofuscin ("age pigment"), decreased elasticity of connective tissues, and damage to membranes and DNA. Powerful antioxidants like vitamin E and an enzyme called superoxide dismutase have been claimed to prolong survival in mice and other animals.

Although the free-radical theory enjoys considerable popularity and remains under active investigation, there exists no evidence as yet that the basic process of aging is altered by antioxidants. It is possible that inhibiting the formation of free radicals may simply allow a greater proportion of animals to achieve their genetically determined life span.

Scientific research can help extend the average life span.

Worn-Out Systems

Physiological theories of aging focus on regulatory systems, particularly the immune system, which protects us from disease, and the neuroendocrine system—the complex interactions between the nervous system and hormone-producing glands. These theories suggest that the deterioration of such systems over time increases the effects of age on the body's functioning and, ultimately, survival.

Those who stress the role of the immune system note that with increasing age the system's response to factors that cause disease appears to decline progressively, while autoimmune responses, in which the immune system attacks the body's own cells, increase. As a result, the elderly are more vulnerable to certain diseases because of the immune system's diminished ability to tell self from nonself; these diseases include cancer, autoimmune diseases, and infections. The thymus, a gland that is central in the formation of disease-fighting white blood cells, peaks in size at adolescence and declines progressively thereafter. Furthermore, the ability of certain types of the white blood cells called T cells to replicate themselves declines with age.

Like other theories of aging, however, deterioration of the immune system cannot by itself explain all the phenomena involved. Certain primitive species that show signs of aging lack an identifiable immune system. Also, nutrition and the functioning of the neuroendocrine system have a major influence on the immune system.

The neuroendocrine system is equally plausible as the pacemaker of aging. It plays a central role in maintaining equilibrium within the body, and age-related changes are known to occur in such organs of the system as the brain. The total number of brain cells progressively declines with age. If this loss were random, the average individual's survival would not be jeopardized for perhaps several hundred years. However, the loss of neurons is selective, taking place at an accelerated pace in certain critical regions of the brain. This appears to be a prime cause of several common phenomena of old age (such as altered sleep patterns) and illnesses like Alzheimer's disease. Other phenomena related to the loss of neurons may include: changes in regulation of the hormone-producing glands by the body's "master gland," the hypothalamus; diminished regulation of thirst and appetite; and decreased regulation of the autonomic nervous system, which controls heartbeat and other internal body functions.

Combating the Aging Process

It is highly risky to draw conclusions, from basic research at its present stage, about how people age over time—and how this process might be retarded. Radically changing one's life-style or diet, or using vitamins or drugs in a frantic attempt to increase longevity, reflects fantasy and wishful thinking more than rational action, particularly if such efforts are begun at an advanced age or after serious disease has developed.

Programs for extending life that have attracted popular attention range from the unproven low-calorie and exercise approach espoused by Dr. Roy Walford of the University of California at Los Angeles to injections of animal tissue that amount to outright quackery. Walford draws on consistent findings concerning laboratory rodents. When given adequate nutrients but only about two-thirds of the calories they would consume if given all they wanted, the animals live considerably longer than their peers allowed to feed at will. The reasons for the effectiveness of such "undernutrition" are unknown, and there is no evidence that it would be successful in humans, but Walford aims to demonstrate that it would — with himself as a guinea pig.

Other programs do not have even the possibly inapplicable evidence to support them that Walford's does. For example, a book called *Life Extension: A Practical Scientific Approach*, which has sold more than a million copies since publication in 1982, advocates high doses of a grab bag of vitamins, nutrients, and drugs. The book's authors, Durk Pearson and Sandy Shaw, have virtually no scientific credentials, and their claims are dismissed by most doctors. Some of the other strategies that have been promoted for extending life include taking megadoses of the antioxidants vitamin E and superoxide dismutase to counteract the effects of free radicals, and, primarily in Romania, the administration of procaine (normally used as a local anesthetic) in a form known as Gerovital H3.

There is no reason to think that such approaches can lengthen life, although some people using them may derive psychological benefits from a belief in their effectiveness. A more rational way to seek increased longevity is through rigorous scientific research. This is less likely to result in extension of the maximum life span than in further increases in average longevity through reduction of premature death.

Efforts are being made to translate information already gained from basic research into widespread changes in people's behavior. Such measures include avoidance of smoking and alcohol and drug abuse, reduction of animal fat consumption, and appropriate exercise for all ages. Measures such as these, along with the prevention and treatment of hypertension and the prevention of accidents and violent deaths, are most likely to enhance human longevity in the industrialized world. □

Extending Your Life

You can try well-publicized schemes of no proven value, or you can take some medically sound hints that really are likely to help you live longer:

- Don't smoke and don't abuse alcohol.
- Do exercise regularly.
- Avoid overweight but eat a varied and balanced diet.
- Practice safety at home, at work, and in driving.
- Have blood pressure checked annually.

The

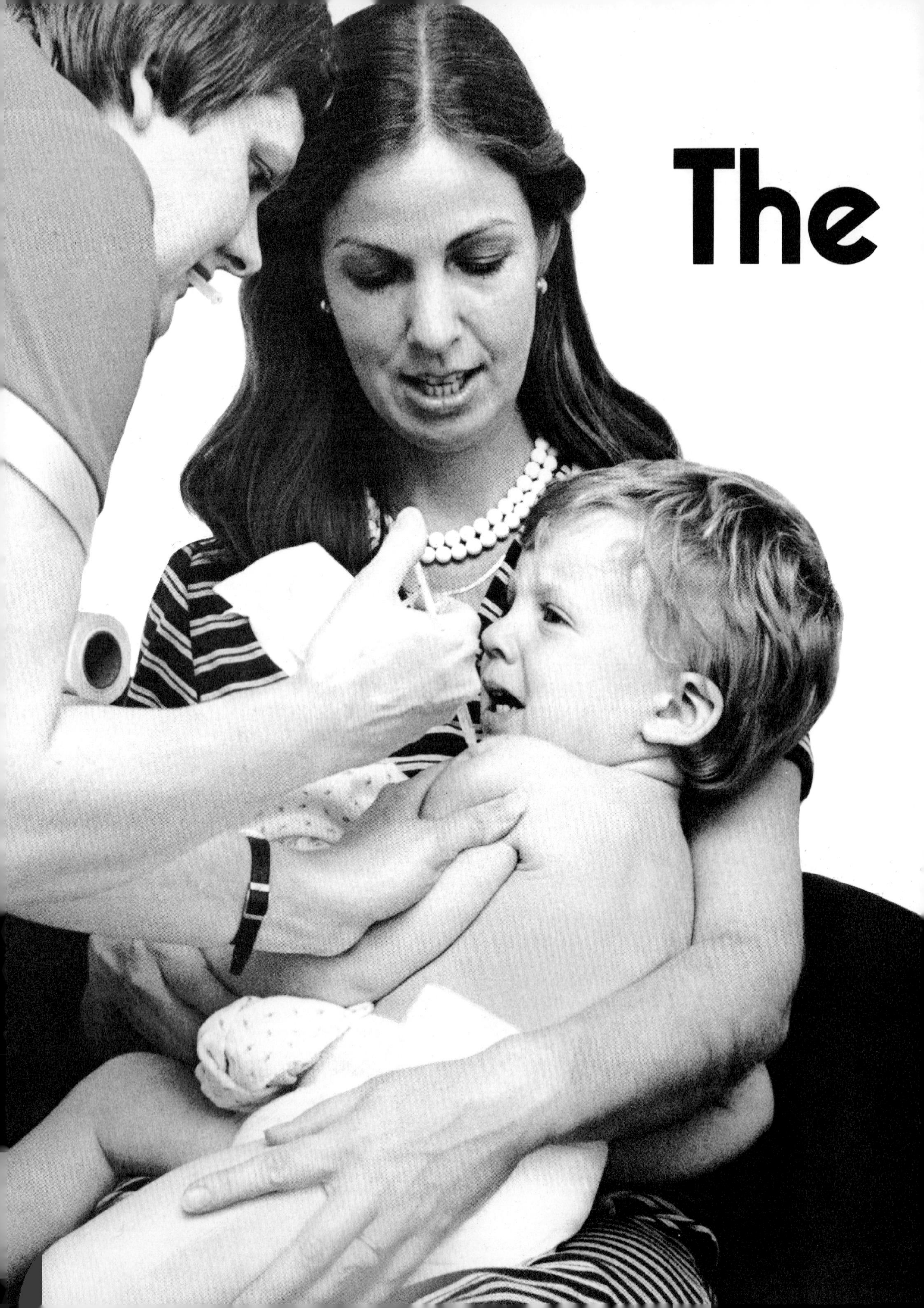

New Vaccines

Thomas H. Maugh II, Ph.D.

On a hot day in August 1952, 16-year-old Bill Kirkpatrick, the son of a Pittsburgh corporate executive, was looking forward to starting school and trying out for the football team. He was on his way home from his grandmother's when his neck became stiff and his throat began to hurt. By nightfall he could barely breathe or move. He was rushed to Pittsburgh's Municipal Hospital into an isolation area on the third floor, his illness diagnosed as poliomyelitis.

Bill was one of 57,900 individuals in the United States, most of them children, who contracted polio in 1952, the peak year in an epidemic that was the most serious U.S. public health problem of the decade. Children were forbidden by their fearful parents from visiting swimming pools, movie theaters, and other public places where the disease was thought to fester.

At the Pittsburgh hospital, two floors below Bill Kirkpatrick, Dr. Jonas Salk and his colleagues were working feverishly to develop a vaccine against polio. Since other researchers had recently isolated the three viruses known to cause polio, Salk and his group were seeking to use killed viruses to produce immunity, or protection against the disease, in individuals who had not yet been exposed to polioviruses.

Large-scale tests of Salk's vaccine were begun in 1954 under the direction of Dr. Thomas Francis, Jr., of the University of Michigan. By April 12 of the next year—just over three decades ago—Francis was able to announce that the vaccine was "safe, potent, and effective." The same day, the U.S. Public Health Service licensed the vaccine for manufacture. Throughout the country church bells rang and fire whistles blew in celebration. The following year the number of new polio cases fell to 15,100. By the late 1960's the United States was averaging about 50 cases a year. In 1985 the number was a mere handful, and most children had never heard of the disease.

A Wealth of Weapons Against Disease

Vaccines have made a monumental contribution to health throughout the world, although they have rarely been met with such unabashed enthusiasm as was the case for polio. Smallpox, once a deadly plague of the young, has been completely eliminated from the face of the earth by universal vaccination, and diphtheria and typhus are virtually extinct.

The most commonly used vaccines in the United States today are those that protect against influenza and the infectious childhood diseases polio, measles, mumps, rubella, diphtheria, tetanus, and whooping cough. In spring 1985 the U.S. Food and Drug Administration approved for use a vaccine against a bacterium that is the most common cause of serious childhood meningitis.

Other vaccines available are primarily for people at high risk of contracting a particular disease because of, say, their jobs or travel to foreign countries. These include vaccines for pneumococcal pneumonia, tuberculosis, rabies, Rocky Mountain spotted fever, yellow fever, typhoid, plague, typhus, and cholera.

More vaccines are on the way, some developed through such radically new approaches as genetic engineering. Vaccines against chicken pox and gonorrhea are now being tested in humans. Scientists are also working on vaccines against such disorders as herpes, acquired immune deficiency syndrome (AIDS), and even cancer.

Side effects or adverse reactions from a vaccine, if they occur, are ordinarily no more serious than a temporary fever or a swelling or redness at the site of a shot. More severe reactions are rare with current vaccines, and research promises even safer vaccines to come.

The First Vaccines

Today's vaccines are a far cry from the first efforts at vaccination, conducted more than 300 years ago. In 1713 the Italian physician Emanuel Timoni described for Britain's Royal Society the practice of inoculation for smallpox that had been carried out in Turkey for more than 40 years. Small amounts of fresh pus from pustules of young smallpox patients were injected by Turkish physicians into several little wounds in the arms and legs of healthy individuals. According to Timoni's report, the procedure almost invariably gave rise to a mild form of the disease that left no scars or pits on the face but conferred lasting immunity. The procedure was subsequently used to a limited extent in England.

At the end of the 18th century the English physician Edward Jenner took note of a local belief that dairy workers who contracted a certain relatively harmless animal disease called cowpox were protected from smallpox. This animal disorder is related to human smallpox. Beginning in 1796, Jenner injected several volunteers with pus from a victim of the animal disease and then, some time later, with pus from a smallpox victim; none of the volunteers contracted smallpox. Jenner did not know he was working with viruses, and he did not know anything about immunity. His careful observations, however, showed him how to provide protection against one particular disease and laid the groundwork for subsequent studies. His pioneering experiments led to the development of an effective smallpox vaccine based on the virus doctors now call vaccinia, from the Latin word for cow, *vacca*. Jenner's work is reflected in our terms "vaccine" and "vaccination."

Nearly a century elapsed before the next step in the development of vaccines occurred. The French biologist Louis Pasteur began experiments on chicken cholera, a disease caused by bacteria, in the spring of 1879 but left his cultures—the cholera bacteria he was growing—untended during the summer. When he returned to them in September, the cultures failed to produce cholera when injected into chickens. Pasteur obtained fresh bacteria and used them to inoculate both new animals and those that had been injected with the old bacteria. He observed that the new animals quickly contracted the disease while the previously injected animals showed no sign of cholera and remained healthy.

Pasteur was familiar with Jenner's work and was quick to see the connection. He formulated the general principle that a weakened or dead microorganism could provide protection against a disease even though the microorganism itself did not produce symptoms of the disease. Pasteur's principle has been the basis of all subsequent work on vaccines.

The Body's Defenses Against Infection

Vaccination brings into play the third of the body's three lines of defense against infection. The first line is the outer wrapping of skin and mucous membranes. These provide a physical barrier against infection.

If a disease-causing microorganism breaches that first line, it encounters a variety of agents carried in the bloodstream and lymphatic system. If the skin is cut, for example, the injured cells release histamine and other chemicals that cause nearby blood vessels to swell. Circulating white blood cells flow through the distended blood vessel walls, crowding into the site of the injury. The white blood cells called neutrophils engulf foreign invaders and destroy them. Blood clots begin to form, walling off the injured area. Pus—which is made up of white blood cells, both dead and alive, and tissue debris—accumulates. The temperature in the immediate area rises, creating an unfavorable environment for some infectious agents and assisting the work of the white blood cells.

If this inflammatory response, as it is called, is insufficient, the third line of defense comes into play—an immune system response that differs from the body's other defenses in that it is highly specific, tailoring its attack against the particular invader.

First it recognizes the invader. This is possible because the outer surface of all microorganisms—in fact, of all living cells—contains characteristic proteins called antigens. (Some fats and sugars can also act as antigens.) Each antigen has a unique shape. The immune system produces materials that are fitted to that unique shape. These materials include the white blood cells called lymphocytes, as well as antibodies, which are actually protein molecules produced by lymphocytes. Antibodies directly combat the invading

---

Thomas H. Maugh II is a science writer for the Los Angeles Times; *he is coauthor of* Seeds of Destruction: The Science Report on Cancer Research.

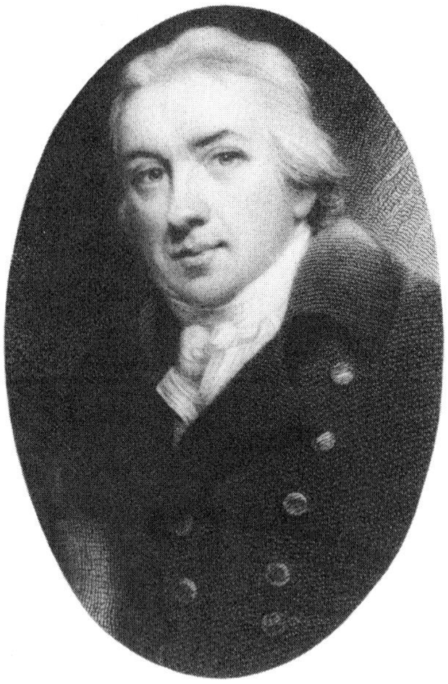

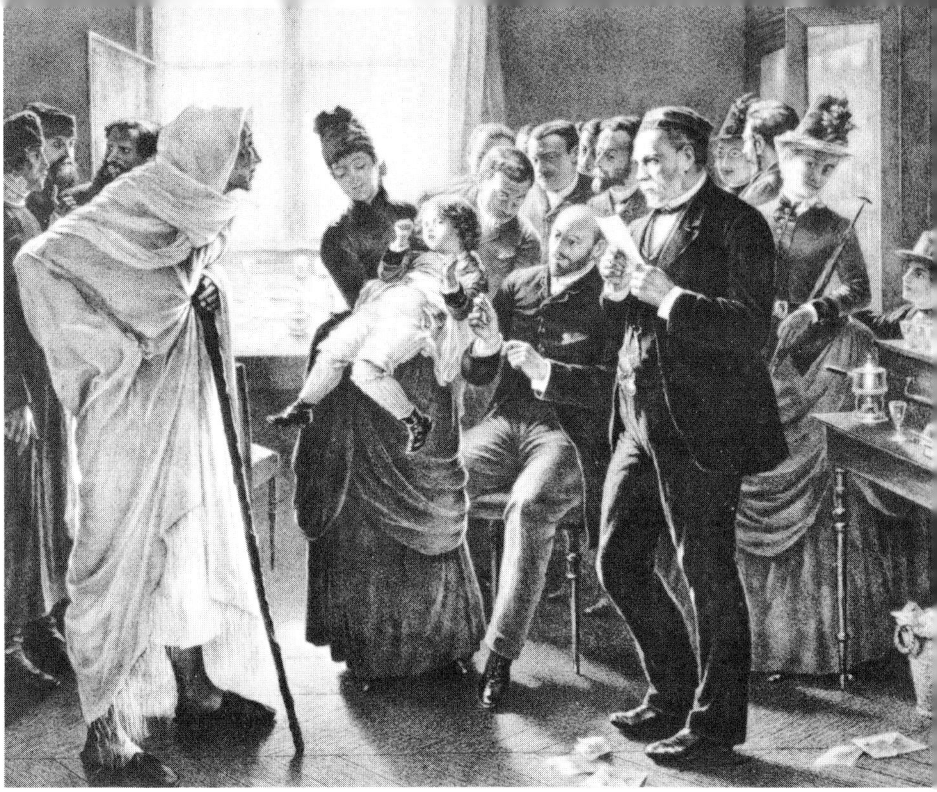

Pioneers in Vaccines

One of the early experimenters with inoculations was Edward Jenner (above left), who at the end of the 18th century developed a vaccine against smallpox. As a result of his work with cholera bacteria, Louis Pasteur (shown in the 1887 lithograph above right) formulated the principle behind vaccination. In the 1950's, Dr. Jonas Salk (at right) made the vaccine breakthrough of the century when he developed a killed-virus vaccine against polio.

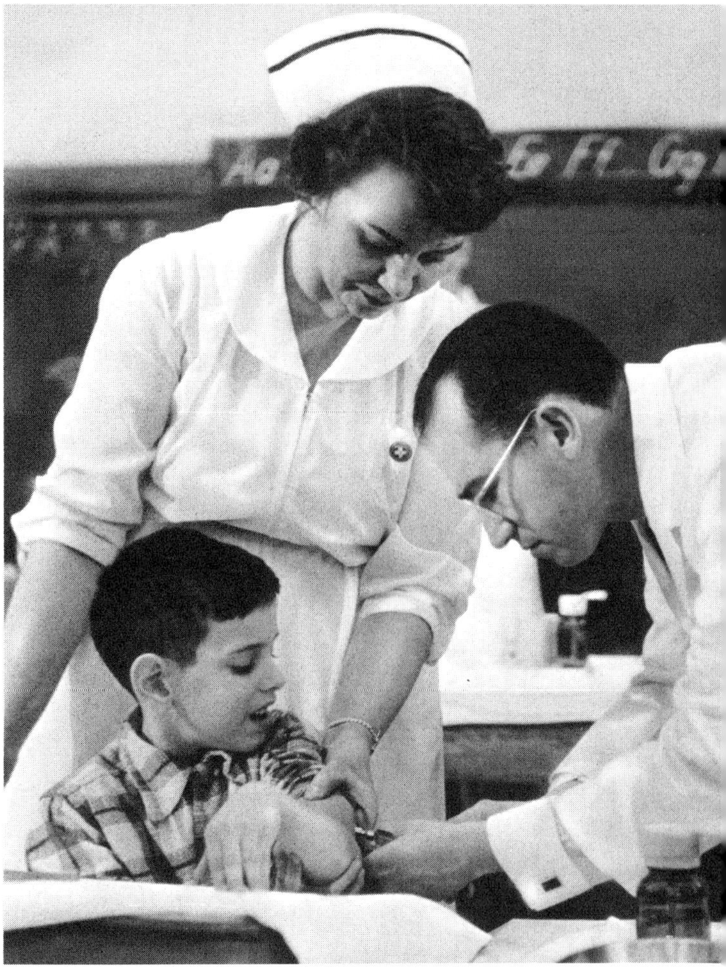

microorganisms against which they are targeted in three different ways. They bind to the intruders and mark them for destruction by neutrophils and other cells. They may also combine with the invaders in such a way as to block their activity; they might, for example, cover the site where a virus binds to a cell. And finally, they may themselves, in combination with other blood components, break open and destroy the foreign microorganisms.

Antibody production is initiated by the interaction of an antigen with the kind of lymphocyte called a B cell. This interaction converts the B cell into a plasma cell, which can make large quantities of antibodies that recognize and bind to the antigen. The interaction also causes the B cell to divide, thereby greatly increasing antibody production. It takes a B cell about ten hours to divide, and so the process is repeated approximately nine times in four days. If the invading microorganism does not proliferate rapidly, enough antibodies can be produced during the four days to halt the infection. If the organism does proliferate rapidly, the victim falls ill. If the disease is caused by a bacterium, it may be controllable with antibiotics. If it is caused by a virus, against which antibiotics are ineffective, little can be done.

After the first bout of infection the antibodies circulating in the body disappear, but memory cells sensitized to the antigen or antigens on the surface of the microorganism persist indefinitely. The memory cells provide long-term immunity because they are primed to begin immediate production of antibodies when the particular antigen appears. Creating these sensitized memory cells is the goal of vaccination.

Two Traditional Types of Vaccines

Until recently, most vaccines were made by one of two methods: the viruses or bacteria that cause a disease were grown in a laboratory and then killed for use in a vaccine, or a weakened form of the microorganism was isolated that could produce immunity without causing disease. (Vaccines against certain bacteria, such as diphtheria and tetanus vaccines, are made in a third way—from "toxoids," which are bacteria-produced toxic substances that have been rendered nonpoisonous.) Polio is unusual in that both of the principal approaches have been used successfully to make vaccines.

Salk's vaccine used polioviruses killed with chemicals. The antigens on the surface of the dead viruses provoke the body to produce large numbers of antibodies, thereby protecting the central nervous system against subsequent invasion by naturally occurring polioviruses. To be effective, the killed viruses have to be injected directly into the body.

In the late 1950's, Dr. Albert B. Sabin developed a polio vaccine that used attenuated, or weakened, polioviruses. Attenuated viruses can occasionally be found naturally—as with the vaccinia virus—but more often they are produced by cultivating the virus under conditions unfavorable to it. Genetic changes may occur that render the virus no longer able to produce disease although it still grows.

Attenuated viruses or bacteria proliferate in the body to stimulate immunity (typically longer lasting than for killed vaccines). They may give rise to a mild reaction, such as fever, but do not cause full-blown disease. Because they are alive, they can even be absorbed in a sugar cube and taken by mouth, which makes large-scale immunization much easier. The fact that the attenuated virus or bacterium is alive also means it can transfer from vaccinated children to unvaccinated people they come into contact with. This kind of "second-hand vaccination" can often induce immunity, further protecting the community. Theoretically, however, the attenuated microorganism can revert to a form closely resembling the naturally occurring one. This reversion has in fact occasionally been observed in attenuated polioviruses; it produces a very small number of cases of polio each year.

The Problem of Hepatitis

Several diseases—most notably herpes and the liver disorder hepatitis—have proved resistant to attempts to prepare a vaccine in the conventional manner, and scientists have had to adopt other approaches. One method began to take shape in 1964 when Dr. Baruch S. Blumberg of the Institute for Cancer Research in Philadelphia observed some unusual particles in the blood of Australian aborigines, a group with a high incidence of hepatitis. Blumberg and other researchers subseqently showed the particles to be pieces of the protein coat of the virus that causes hepatitis B. This is a severe form of the disease that is normally transmitted from person to person via body fluids, particularly blood.

In the early 1980's there were about 200,000 cases of hepatitis B in the United States each year; 10,000 patients required hospital treatment, and 250 died. About 10 percent of those contracting the disease become chronic carriers, able to infect others for the rest of their lives.

Studies by several groups of researchers showed that the particles isolated from the blood of aborigines are also present in chronic carriers and individuals with active hepatitis B. It was also found that the particles could by themselves produce immunity—could stimulate the immune system's defenses against hepatitis B. A vaccine prepared from the particles, which are now called hepatitis B surface antigen, went on the market in 1982.

Such vaccines that can produce immunity by using only a component of the disease-causing microorganism are called subunit vaccines. The new vaccine against childhood meningitis belongs to this group. It is made from the polysaccharide (an exceedingly large sugar molecule) in the bacterium's outer coating.

To make hepatitis B vaccine, surface antigen is collected from the blood of chronic carriers and then concentrated, purified, and treated so that any whole viruses present are killed. Nevertheless, some people have been reluctant to be immunized with the vaccine because of fears it might be contaminated with live hepatitis virus or possibly even the deadly AIDS virus (which can be transmitted through blood). These fears, however, have proved groundless. Unfortunately, the vaccine is too expensive—the required series of three injections costs $100 or more—for widespread use in the United States and for any significant use in developing countries. A possible way out of this difficulty was suggested by a preliminary study reported in late 1985. The researchers found that injecting the vaccine between skin layers, instead of into muscle as is usually done, seemed to provide nearly equal protection while requiring much smaller—and thus less expensive—doses.

Genetic Engineering to the Rescue

Genetic engineering techniques offer a different way of overcoming such problems. A key breakthrough was reported in 1981, when a biochemist at the University of California at San Francisco isolated the gene that "codes" for the hepatitis B surface antigen—that is, provides the blueprint for the virus's production of the antigen—and spliced the gene into the basic genetic material of a yeast cell. When the yeast was grown in a laboratory dish, it produced substantial quantities of the antigen. In 1983 researchers reported that a vaccine made from the surface antigen grown in yeast protected chimpanzees against hepatitis B. Initial promising results of tests of such a vaccine in humans were reported the following year.

The chief advantages of this genetic engineering approach are that the yeast-produced antigen can be purified more easily and more completely than the antigen derived from blood, there is no risk that the resulting vaccine will be contaminated by viruses, and the final cost of the vaccine should be lower. The same approach is being used to develop surface protein vaccines against other forms of hepatitis, foot-and-mouth disease (in animals), and rabies. The rabies vaccine should be a major improvement over the existing vaccine because it would be free of the contaminants that arise when the rabies virus used for the vaccine is grown in the laboratory; these contaminants produce the painful side effects that now accompany vaccination.

The development of a surface protein vaccine that protects against herpes infections in guinea pigs was reported in March 1985. The vaccine is now being tested in other animals.

Malaria

Perhaps the best example of the advantages of using genetic engineering to produce surface protein vaccines is represented by efforts to prepare a vaccine against malaria. Malaria has been very difficult to combat because of the complicated life cycle of the single-celled parasite, called a plasmodium, that causes the disease.

The two most important stages of the plasmodium life cycle are the sporozoite and merozoite. Sporozoites are the form in which the parasites are injected into the bloodstream of the victim by infected mosquitoes. They quickly invade the liver, where they are converted into merozoites. Merozoites invade red blood cells and reproduce, eventually rupturing the cells and producing malaria's characteristic symptoms of chills and fever.

Ronald C. Kennedy at the Southwest Foundation has been conducting research on anti-idiotypes—antibodies produced in reaction to other antibodies—for possible use in vaccines.

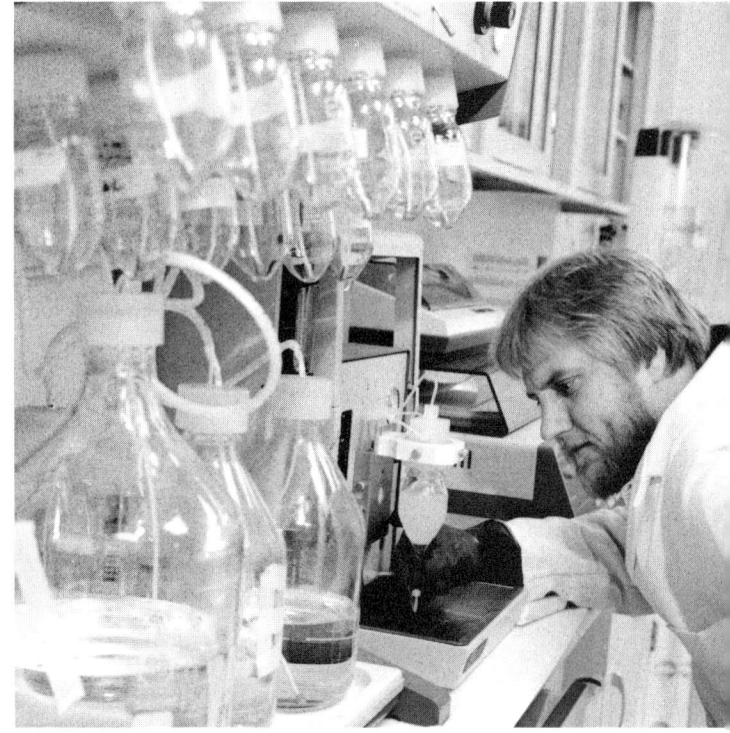

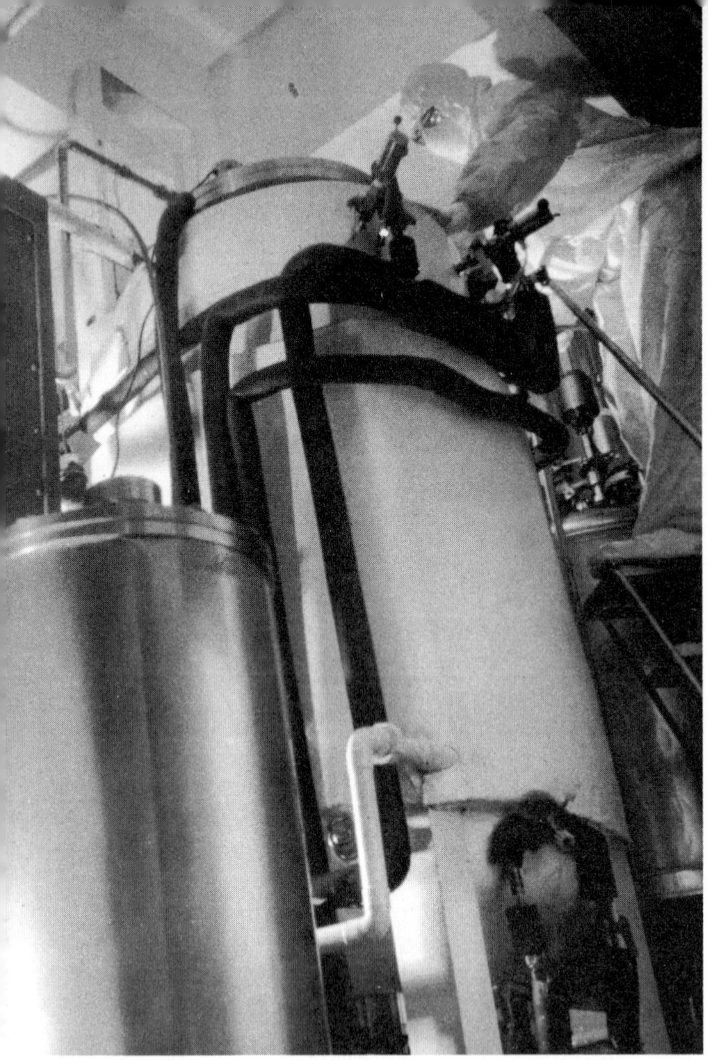

In giant fermentation tanks genetically altered yeast produces a protein for an improved hepatitis B vaccine, the first genetically engineered vaccine to be tested on humans.

Scientists have had great difficulty in growing sufficient quantities of either merozoites or sporozoites in the laboratory to produce experimental vaccines. But such efforts may no longer be necessary. A team of researchers from five institutions reported in May 1985 that they had inserted into bacteria the gene for a sporozoite surface protein of the major variety of plasmodia. When proteins subsequently produced by the bacteria were injected into mice, they stimulated the production of antibodies that blocked infection by sporozoites.

The antibodies produced by such a vaccine would have to be 100 percent effective in destroying sporozoites. If even one sporozoite were to escape the antibodies and reach the liver, it would be converted to merozoites, which would not be susceptible to attack by the immune system. Other researchers are, however, seeking to use the same approach to develop a vaccine based on merozoite surface proteins.

Vaccines From Pieces of Protein

Eventually, it may be possible to make a vaccine without even using microorganisms. Surface protein antigens are made up of building blocks called amino acids. These acids are connected in long chains that are folded upon themselves to form a globular structure. Since most of the amino acid chain is thus shielded from an antibody, some researchers have suggested that only the segments of the protein on the surface are important in stimulating an immune reaction.

Preliminary experiments have shown that a segment consisting of a string of as few as 10 amino acids—compared to the 150 or more amino acids in a whole protein—can trigger an immune response. In effect, the short string of amino acids tricks the immune system into thinking that an entire virus is present. Such short strings can be synthesized chemically, so there is no possibility that the resulting vaccine will be contaminated by cellular materials.

Experimenters at the U.S. National Institutes of Health in Bethesda, Md., have protected chimpanzees from hepatitis B with a synthetic vaccine involving a string of 27 amino acids that mimics part of the hepatitis B surface antigen. Another scientist has produced a similar synthetic vaccine that protects against foot-and-mouth disease. In June 1985 it was reported that a malaria vaccine effective in animals had been developed by synthesizing fragments of the sporozoite proteins.

There is one major drawback to using short strings of amino acids: by themselves, the strings are too small to produce much of an immune system response in humans. The response can be improved by linking the strings to a larger protein, but even that is not completely effective. What is required is a way of markedly enhancing the immune response. This can be done with materials called adjuvants. The most powerful adjuvants available today, however, are too corrosive for use in humans, causing sores and abscesses to develop where the vaccine is injected. The need to find better adjuvants means that it may be a while before synthetic vaccines made from amino acid strings come into common use.

Vaccines With Antibodies

Some scientists in recent years have been exploring the possibility of making a vaccine neither from antigen nor from pieces of antigen but from something that just appears (to the immune system) to be an antigen. Their starting point is the particular area of the antibody that recognizes the antigen. This site, called the idiotype of the antibody, is typically a string of 8 to 20 amino acids. It has a shape complementary to that of the antigen. Researchers have found that the immune system produces a set of antibodies, called anti-idiotype antibodies, that bind to this idiotype. (These antibodies are thought to have the function of eliminating superfluous antibodies from the body after an infection has run its course.) The part of the anti-idiotype antibody that binds to the idiotype has to have the same shape as the original antigen—it mimics the antigen; otherwise, it could not bind to the idiotype.

Because of this structural similarity, theoretically the anti-idiotype antibody can be used to make a vaccine causing the body to produce antibodies against the antigen. In a key study at the Southwest Foundation for Biomedical Research in San Antonio, Texas, rabbits were injected with an antibody to the hepatitis B surface antigen. The rabbits produced new antibodies directed against the idiotype of the injected antibodies. When these anti-idiotype antibodies were subsequently collected and injected into rabbits, mice, and chimpanzees, the animals produced antibodies that were specific for the hepatitis B surface antigen.

This approach has certain advantages over the use of strings of amino acids. For one thing, in synthesizing a string it is necessary to know the sequence in which the amino acids must be put together. Also, new techniques make it possible to produce large quantities of identical antibodies—called monoclonal antibodies—so that, in some cases, it may be easier for scientists to make antibodies than amino acid strings. Perhaps most important, the anti-idiotype antibodies are larger than the strings of amino acids and so may result in a greater response from the immune system. No one has yet shown, however, that a vaccine made in this manner will actually protect humans against disease.

New Uses for Old Viruses

The immune system responds more strongly to vaccination with a live virus than to vaccination with dead viruses, virus proteins, or protein fragments (unless an effective adjuvant is used). This means that live-virus vaccines provide greater protection against disease. Why not, therefore, modify familiar untroublesome live viruses to produce on their surface the proteins—antigens—of disease-causing microorganisms? A number of researchers have taken precisely this tack.

A major step forward was taken in 1983 when scientists at the U.S. National Institutes of Health reported that they had inserted the gene that codes for the hepatitis B surface antigen into the vaccinia virus (the one used for smallpox vaccine), which is very safe and easily grown. The hybrid vaccinia virus produced the hepatitis B surface antigen as well as its own surface proteins. When the new virus was injected into rabbits and chimpanzees, it stimulated the production of significant amounts of antibodies against hepatitis B in addition to antibodies against smallpox. Researchers subsequently used similar techniques to successfully insert into vaccinia viruses genes for surface proteins of the viruses that cause herpes and influenza, the virus that causes rabies, and the parasite that causes malaria.

Potentially, a single virus could be retooled in this way to produce immunity to several diseases at once. A team of New York State Department of Health researchers reported in 1984 that they had introduced into one vaccinia virus genes coding for proteins from the hepatitis B, herpes simplex, and influenza viruses; when tested in animals, the modified vaccinia produced antibodies against all the viruses.

Such multipurpose, or "polyvalent" vaccines could provide an easy and relatively inexpensive way to immunize large populations against several diseases at once. Inexpensive polyvalent vaccines would be especially useful in developing countries. Since it is relatively large, the vaccinia virus can accommodate considerable amounts of foreign DNA, so this approach appears to be viable.

Prospects

Scientists are hoping that one or more of the new techniques now in the experimental stage will yield vaccines against some of the severe illnesses that have not yet been conquered. With the variety of techniques now available, researchers frequently disagree about which of the new vaccine approaches is best for any particular disease. Sometimes several approaches seem to be equally effective. Virtually all scientists agree, however, that research on vaccines has never been more fruitful and that the prospects for controlling the diseases that still plague humanity have never looked better. □

UNDERSTANDING MEMORY

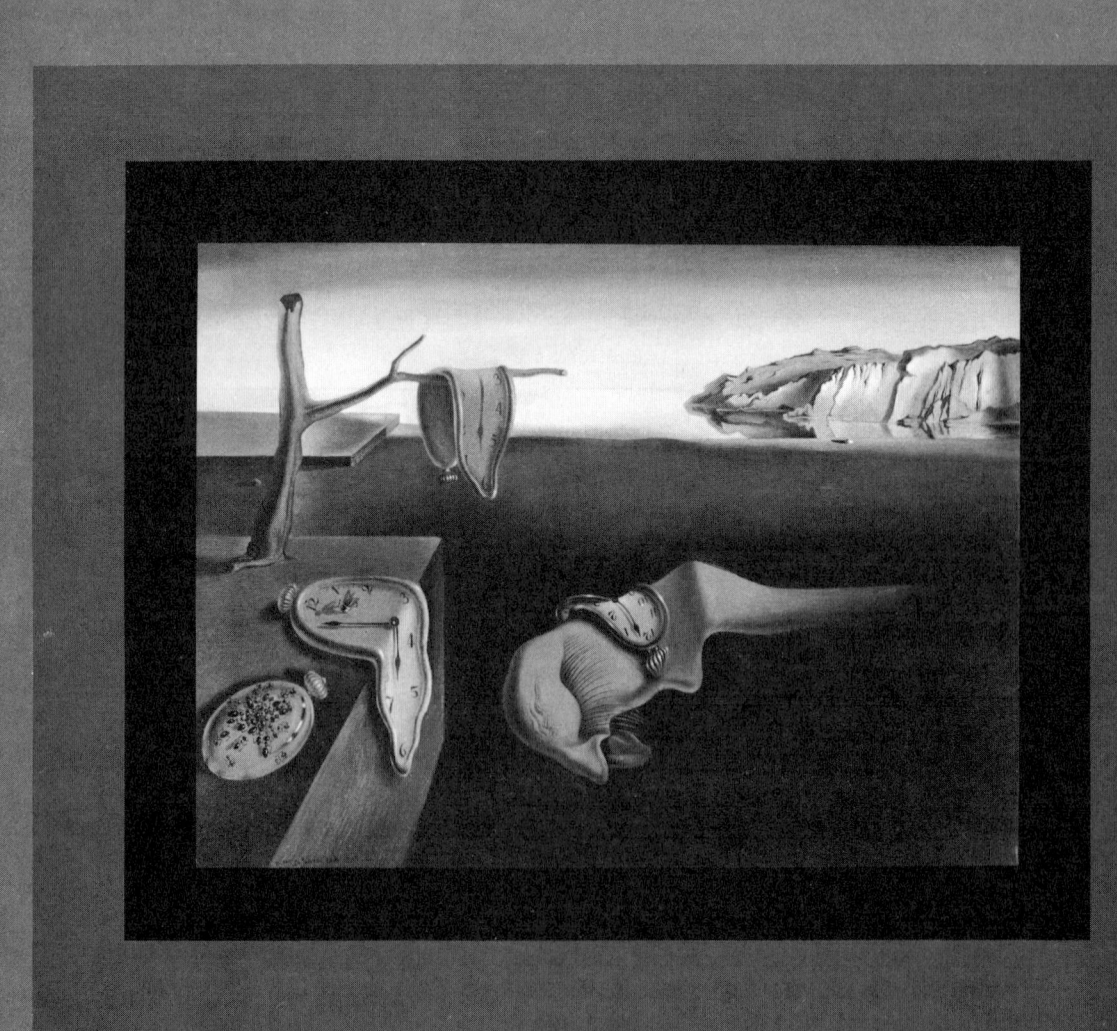

Mark Deitch

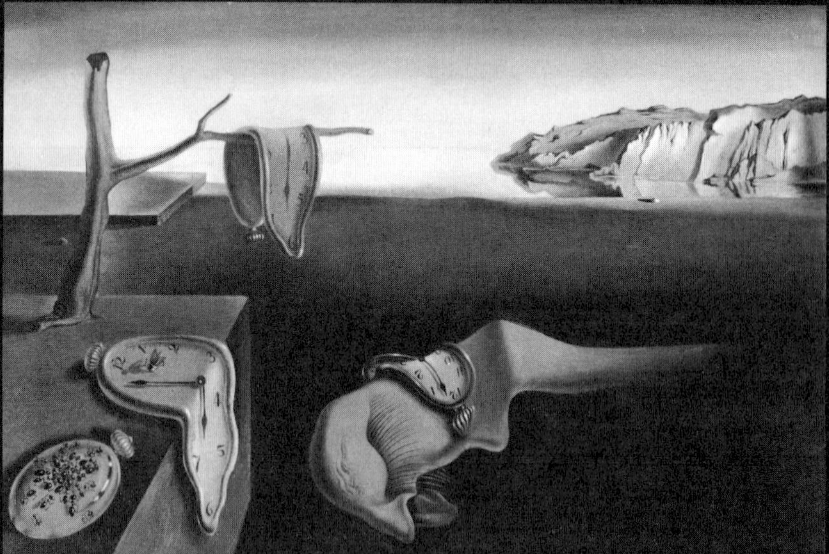

Memory is perhaps our most distinctive feature. The ability to retain, recall, and apply vast stores of information—everything from batting averages to love poetry to the best way to build a bridge—sets us apart from other species. Our memories also distinguish us from one another and provide each of us with a record of experiences that defines our individuality.

Memory has long been the province of poets and philosophers (and self-improvement salespeople), but it is only recently that scientific researchers have developed the tools and terminology to mount a systematic study of this central function. Although their work has produced some fascinating insights, nothing close to a comprehensive picture of how we remember has yet emerged. Instead, we have many different memory models, sketches of what memory might look like when the modest array of available facts are linked up by lines of speculation.

Basically, there are two ways in which contemporary researchers examine memory: from within and from without. The inside approach is taken by neurobiologists, who study the organic processes of the brain and try to determine, among other things, the physical properties of memory and the biochemical changes that are involved. The outside view focuses on the mechanisms of memory as they are used and demonstrated in human behavior, and this work is largely carried out by researchers in the relatively new field of cognitive psychology.

For the most part, neurobiologists and cognitive psychologists follow separate and only occasionally intersecting paths. One of the few areas of near-consensus, however, is that memory is not a unified function. We have different kinds and perhaps wholly different systems of memory in constant and simultaneous operation.

Types of Memory: The Short and Long of It

The most common classification of memory is by duration: short-term or long-term. This distinction has often been observed in people who have received electroconvulsive therapy (ECT) for depression or other mental disorders. Typically, people who have had ECT exhibit a limited and temporary retrograde amnesia—that is, they can't remember the event that immediately preceded their shock treatment, but their memory of more distant events remains intact. The same kind of limited memory loss often occurs in people who have been knocked unconscious by a blow to the head.

Salvador Dali's *The Persistence of Memory* (1931)

The exact boundaries of short-term memory—whether it should be measured in seconds, minutes, or hours—are not clear. Nor do memory theorists agree on whether short-term and long-term memory are part of the same continuum or should be considered as separate mental operations. Nevertheless, from a practical standpoint, the differences between temporary and lasting memories are obvious. When we look up an unfamiliar number in the telephone book, we can usually remember it (perhaps with the aid of a few repetitions) long enough to make the call. But unless we use that number regularly thereafter, it is unlikely that we will recall it more than an hour or so later, let alone after an interval of years. Yet there are some memories that last a lifetime, and without any apparent choice or effort on our part. A good example of effortless long-term recall for Americans in their late 20's or older is where they were and what they were doing when they heard the news of President John F. Kennedy's assassination.

It also seems clear that both types of memory are necessary for just about anything we do. To read these lines, for example, requires both temporary retention of the words as they are scanned and recourse to stored knowledge that will help make sense of the information. Every time we solve a problem or make a decision, we use short-term memory to maintain a picture of the details and options at hand, while calling on long-term memory to supply past experiences for comparison and analysis.

Knowledge or Know-how

Memory may also be categorized in ways that have nothing to do with length of retention. Recent research indicates that our brains, and indeed the brains of all primates, make a basic distinction between *declarative* memory and *procedural* memory, which translates roughly to the difference between knowledge and skill. Declarative memory encompasses facts, concepts, language, and meaning; procedural memory refers to learned behavior, such as how to ride a bicycle or how to swim. But the difference between them is not so simple as intellectual ability versus motor skills. Psychologists have studied individuals who, through injury or disease, have sustained brain damage that left them incapable of storing new factual knowledge. Just minutes after an interview, these patients will have forgotten the interviewer's name and face, the conversation, even the meeting itself. Yet with training and repetition they can learn to master new behavioral tasks, including mental challenges such as solving puzzles and reading words that are reversed in a mirror.

Researchers believe that declarative memory entails a process of learning by association, that is, the placing of new facts in familiar contexts. Our brains normally carry out this process almost automatically. Procedural memory, on the other hand, requires effort and conditioning and is more akin to building habits. Again, most human activities call upon both types of memory, a combination of "knowing that" and "knowing how." It seems likely, however, that the two systems develop separately and are controlled by different areas of the brain. Richard F. Thompson of Stanford University has tracked basic procedural memory activity in rabbits to the cerebellum of their brains; the brain's cerebral cortex is generally considered to be the seat of higher-order mental functions, which would include declarative memory.

This physical separation of memory functions would help to explain the common phenomenon of childhood amnesia, or the absence of memories extending back to our earliest two or three years. Freud theorized that early childhood memories are so emotionally charged that the mind represses them in self-defense. A simpler but less compelling explanation may be that while the procedural memory centers of infants are comparatively well-developed at birth—hence their capacity to learn and remember behavior—the declarative centers require more time to form the complex network of nerve cell connections necessary to sustain memories of the world around them. Interestingly, this neural maturation process seems to be at least partly responsive to the environment. Animal studies have shown that early development of the cerebral cortex proceeds more rapidly in "enriched," stimulating surroundings, less rapidly when the subject is in a sensorially barren environment.

The Geography of Memory

Although researchers have a general idea of which areas of the brain are involved in memory, the specific processes by which memories are established and how and where they are stored are only sketchily

---

Mark Deitch is executive editor of Rx Being Well, *the waiting room magazine.*

understood. The precise location of memory, in particular, is something like the neurobiologist's Holy Grail. The difficulty of this quest is illustrated by the work of Karl S. Lashley, a physiological psychologist who devoted the better part of his career to the search for an "engram," or the physical trace of a given memory. In 1926, Lashley initiated a series of experiments with the following rationale: He would train laboratory rats to run a maze, then surgically remove slices of their cerebral cortex until he had isolated the segment where the maze-running memory was stored. At the point when the rats no longer remembered how to run the course, the experiment would be complete. To his surprise and dismay, Lashley found that no matter what part of the brain he excised, the rats still managed to limp, stagger, or creep their way through the maze. Lashley was nothing if not persistent, however, and continued the experiments for 25 years, until in his final paper he concluded that the precise localization of memory is not possible at all.

Researchers following Lashley accepted his findings but looked for ways around his gloomy conclusion. For most of the 1950's and 1960's, it was widely believed that memories had no specific geographic location in the brain, but were somehow distributed equally throughout the cerebral cortex. Some adherents of this distributive theory compared the brain's functioning to holography, a laser-produced three-dimensional form of photography in which any segment of the film can reproduce the entire image. The distributive theory of memory has lost most of its support, however. Neurobiologists now take the view that memory involves the interplay of several different parts of the brain, each performing separate and specialized roles.

To start, there is the cerebral cortex, the thick outer layer of brain cells whose superior development in humans is our greatest evolutionary endowment. A marvel of compact complexity, the human cortex consists of some 10 billion nerve cells, or neurons, each equipped with branching fibers and receptors capable of communicating with up to 10,000 of its fellows. It has been estimated that this neural network is capable of holding 100 trillion bits of information, which is about 100,000 times the capacity of the most powerful contemporary computer. Scientists have identified sections of the cortex that are responsible for sensory perception and for the control of speech and motor activities. Surrounding these centers are regions of largely unknown function

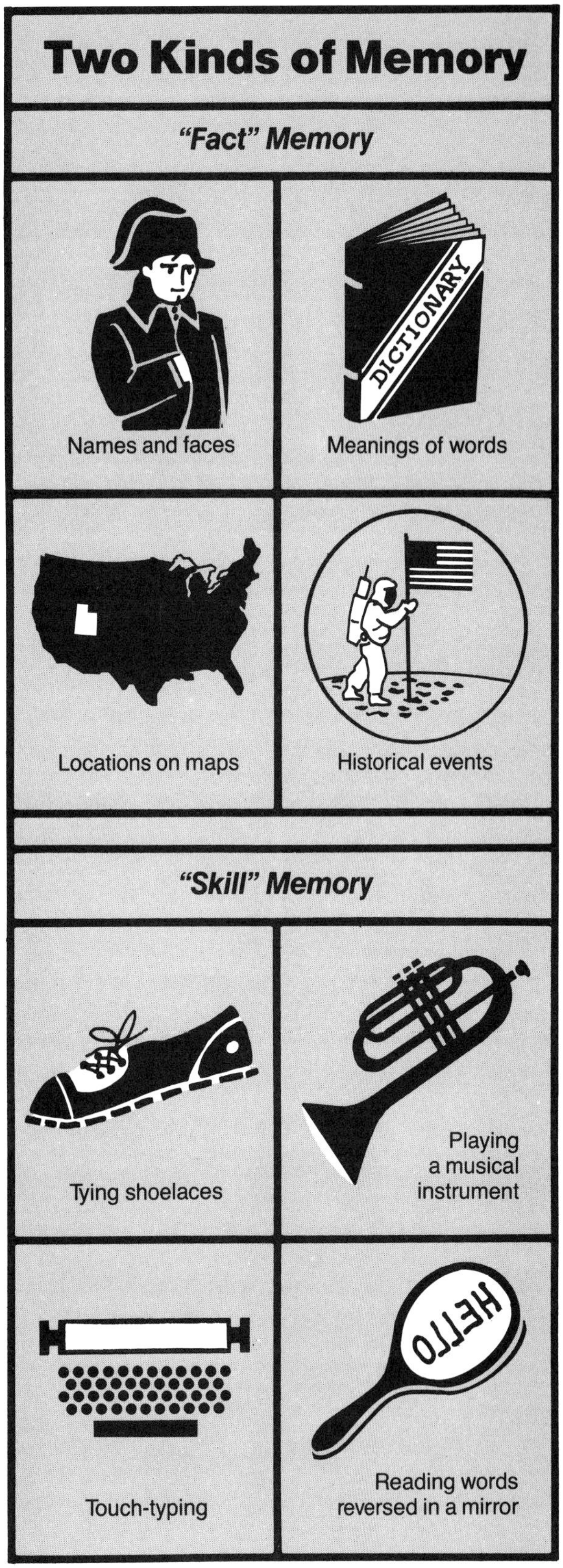

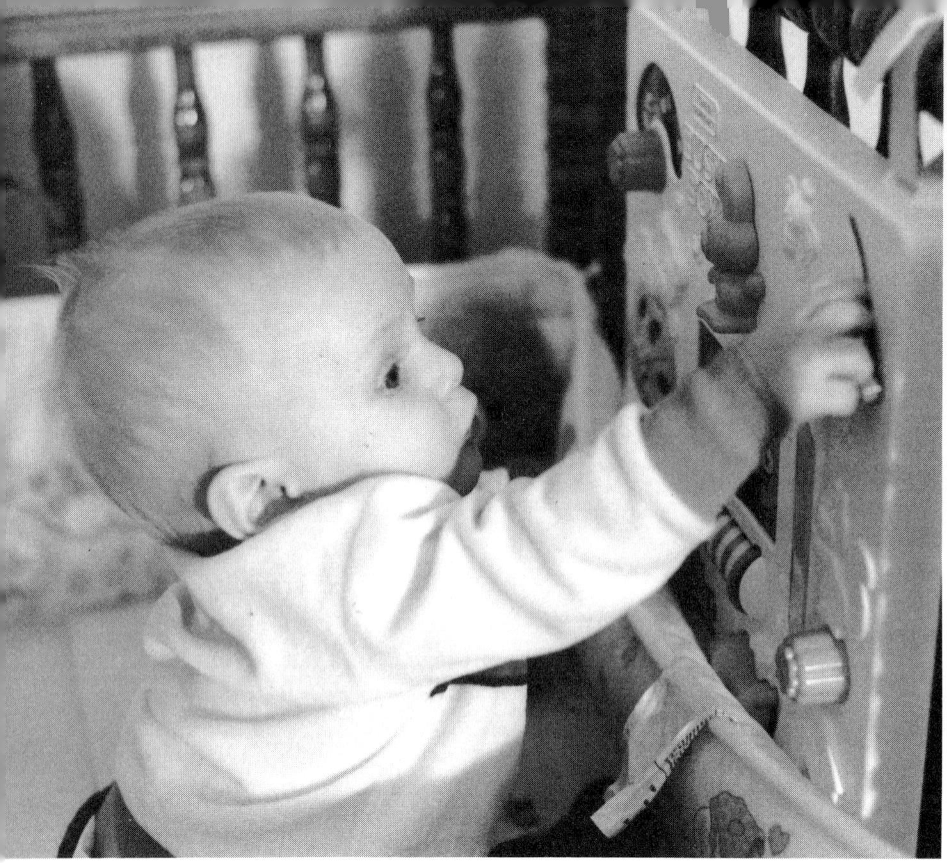

A Lifetime of Remembering

The accumulation of memories begins early (left), with the development of "procedural memories": knowing how to do things. Skills and knowledge are acquired and retained throughout life; even in old age people continue to learn and remember new things (right).

called the association cortices. In humans, these "silent" areas (so called because of their uncharted activity) occupy the largest proportion of the cortical surface, and it is there that long-term memories are believed to be stored.

Beneath the cortex of the temporal lobes (located roughly behind the temples) is a second layer of nerve cells comprising several smaller structures, including a horseshoe-shaped unit known as the hippocampus. The hippocampus has captured the fancy of memory researchers for several reasons. One is that certain of its cells have rather unusual properties. Some can "count," for example, while others are relentless novelty seekers. When stimulated in a certain way, the "counting" cells fire off a specific number of responses, then remember this pattern and continue to fire in numbered bursts for some time afterward. The "novelty" cells respond only to new stimuli and refuse to transmit familiar messages. The fact that no other brain cells seem to have this exclusive relationship with new stimuli suggests that the hippocampus plays a key role in new memory formation. And indeed, individuals who have suffered extensive hippocampal damage demonstrate a severe form of memory loss known as anterograde amnesia, in which they are unable to add new information to their long-term memory stores. The hippocampus is also the primary site of brain damage caused by Alzheimer's disease, an irreversible nervous system disorder, most prevalent in older people, whose symptoms include memory loss and general mental deterioration.

The hippocampus, researchers speculate, serves as a kind of halfway house for new memories. It takes in novel sensory perceptions, alerts the proper authorities, and shelters the perceptions during the consolidation process, a period of months or years in which recent memories are modified until they settle into place in the networks of long-term storage. The hippocampus also maintains a direct line to the thalamus, a ball-shaped structure situated almost exactly in the center of the brain. The thalamus's role in memory formation seems to be similar to that of the record button on a tape recorder. At the hippocampus's signal, the thalamus triggers chemical changes that establish new lasting pathways in the circuitry of the brain.

Tracing the Routes of Memories

A very tentative model of memory formation may go something like this: New sensory information—say, the image of an unfamiliar face—arrives via the retina of the eye and optic nerve at the visual perception center in the cortex. From there it is relayed through the association areas of the cortex to the hippocampus. The hippocampus then notifies the thalamus, which "prints" the circuit. Where, as

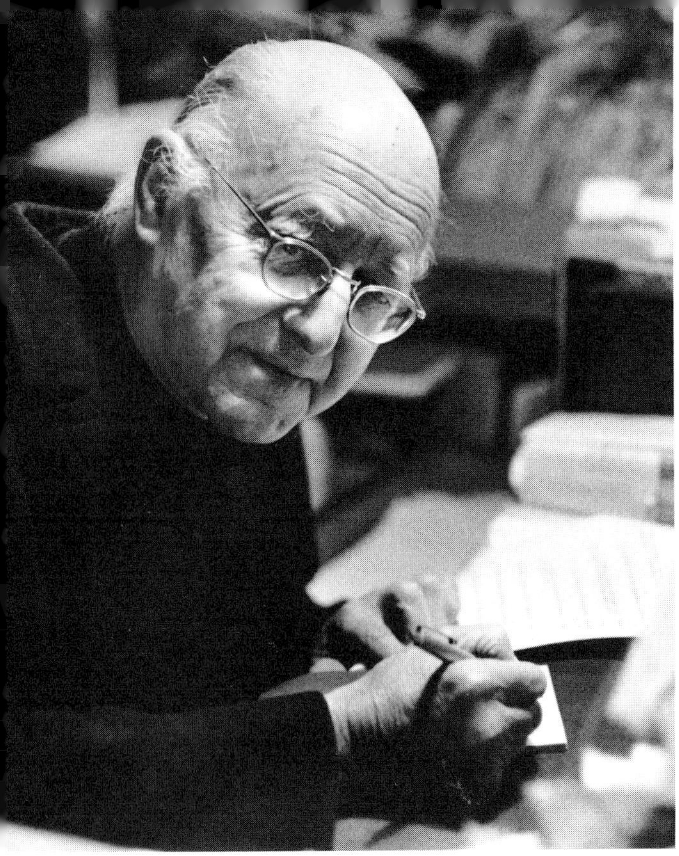

Lashley might have asked, is the engram—the physical trace—of this memory located? The best guess would be somewhere along, or throughout, the new pathway of nerve cell connections between the association cortices and the hippocampus.

More specifically, memory seems to occur at the synapses, which are the minute gaps across which neurons communicate with one another. Information travels through the nervous system in the form of electrical impulses; when an impulse reaches the end of one nerve cell, it must either leap the synaptic gap to another cell or die. In successful communications, a bridge is provided by chemicals called neurotransmitters, which are released at the nerve endings of the first (presynaptic) cell and stimulate tiny receptors on the extremities of the second (postsynaptic) cell. For memory to take place, neurobiologists believe, something must happen on one or both sides of the synapse to facilitate future communications.

Eric Kandel of Columbia University has found that the presynaptic cells of marine snails release increased amounts of neurotransmitter during simple memory functions, such as learning to withdraw their gills from a mild electric shock. Working with animals a bit closer to the human level, Gary Lynch and Michel Baudry of the University of California at Irvine discovered that immediately following intense stimulation, the postsynaptic terminals in rat hippocampi become rounder and more densely populated with receptors. These minute but lasting structural changes may be the closest scientists have yet come to isolating the physical stuff of memory.

Returning to Lashley's dilemma, it is important to note that the entirety of a given memory is rarely, if ever, entrusted to a single series of neural connections. Instead, aspects of the memory are stored in different circuits, which may take varying routes through the brain. National Institute of Mental Health investigator Mortimer Mishkin has demonstrated that in monkeys the cortex-hippocampus-thalamus circuit is used primarily in visual and spatial memory, or remembering the new image in terms of where in the environment it may be found. He concluded that the emotional quality of the memory—whether a remembered face is hostile or nonthreatening—is stored separately in a circuit that detours through the monkey's amygdala, one of the hippocampus's neighboring structures. It is quite possible, Mishkin suggests, that several other memory facets, such as color, sound, and verbal cues, may each have its own separate circuitry. In computer terminology, this kind of multiple storage of the same information is called redundancy. In higher animals, it appears to be a self-defense mechanism, a means of preserving information in case of localized brain damage, such as that produced by Lashley's scalpel in his long search for the precise site of memory.

The Cognitive Approach

Neurobiologists have made impressive advances in their study of the physical properties of memory, but the shortcomings of this approach are also substantial. The leading obstacle is the sheer complexity of the brain, with its billions of neurons and trillions of synaptic connections that make the charting of memory virtually impossible. Furthermore, neurobiological studies are largely restricted to animal experiments and observation of human subjects who have suffered specific memory impairments. The physical study of normal memory function in healthy human brains is, for obvious reasons, highly dangerous and all but nonexistent.

Discovering how human memory actually works in the world is one of the aims of the emerging field of cognitive studies. While neurobiologists study memory on a molecular and cellular level, cognitive psychologists look at memory as a mental activity and try to answer such questions as why we remember some things and not others, what circumstances are most favorable to learning and recall, and why memories tend to change over time.

One of the dominant approaches in cognitive studies is viewing the brain as a sophisticated information processing system, in which new knowledge undergoes a series of transformations along the way from external event to stored memory. In the information processing model, memory formation begins with the sensory register. This is the brain's capacity to hold a sensory impression—an image flashed on a screen, for example, or a word overheard in conversation—for a very brief period after the actual physical stimulus has passed. We are constantly bombarded with such vast amounts of sensory information that we cannot pay attention to all of it; the sensory register allows us a little time (less than a second with visual information) to recognize and tune in on items that interest us.

From the sensory register, selected information passes into short-term, or "working," memory, which cognitive psychologists define as the amount of new and unmemorized information we can keep in mind at any given time. Studies have shown that the capacity of short-term memory is surprisingly limited; on average, it can hold no more than 7 separate items, or chunks of information. Information may be retained indefinitely in short-term memory by "rehearsal," or repeating it over and over to ourselves. But rehearsal, by itself, does not seem to improve our chances of recalling the information some time later, after the repetition has stopped. For information to go from working memory to long-term storage, additional processing, or "elaboration," is usually required. Morton Hunt's book *The Universe Within* provides an excellent account of the elaboration.

> The elaborative processes . . . may, in some cases, consist largely of repetition—not the kind we do in rehearsal, but repetition in which we look for patterns, chunks, clusters of sounds, or associations that enable us to commit to memory a series of items with little meaning. It's what children do when they learn the alphabet by making a singsong jingle of it, using chunking, rhythm, and rhyme ("Ab-cd-ef-g; hi-jk-lmno-p," and so on). . . .
>
> But by far the greatest part of elaborative processing consists of quite a different kind of activity: the extraction of deeper meanings from words, sentences, images, and the like; classification of those meanings; and the linking of this new information to some part of our organized mass of long-term memories. All this can take place with remarkable speed. It's what has happened when, in a matter of seconds, you have forgotten the words of a sentence but registered its content.

Elaboration may be quite rapid, but the processing of new information continues for some time afterward. It may take years for a new memory to be fully consolidated, or shaped and slotted into a lasting niche in the long-term stores. The actual structure of long-term memory is obscure, but studies of the way and the rate at which people recall different items have provided some useful clues. Long-term memory seems to consist of overlapping networks of associations, in which a variety of diverse facts and propositions are arrayed around central and interconnected concepts. When we search our minds for a piece of information, we activate a chain of associations that starts with the central conceptual "nodes" and works its way down to the more peripheral data. Information that is closely linked with the central nodes is quickly and effortlessly recalled; more distant associations may take some time and effort to remember. As a rough example, remembering that an elephant is an animal will be far easier than recalling whether African or Asian elephants have larger ears (the answer is African).

Broad associative networks are sometimes referred to as cognitive structures, conceptual maps, or schemata; they are, in effect, organized bodies of knowledge. A well-developed cognitive structure can more efficiently store and retrieve information than can a poorly developed one. A mathematician, for example, may be able to rattle off complicated equations in the lecture hall but struggle to recall his checking account number at the bank. In the former case, he has built up a rich field of associations that give the equations meaning and context and facilitate recall; in the latter, he is faced with a random string of numbers without a supporting structure of related knowledge.

Shaky Testimony

One implication of the information processing model is that memories are not pure representations of external events but are altered to conform with preexisting knowledge and to fit into the web of

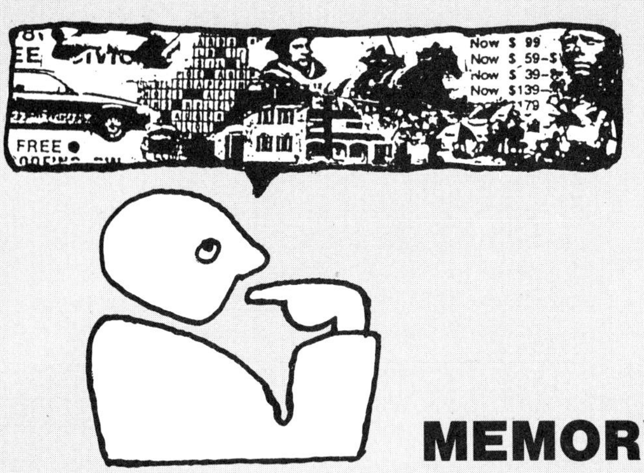

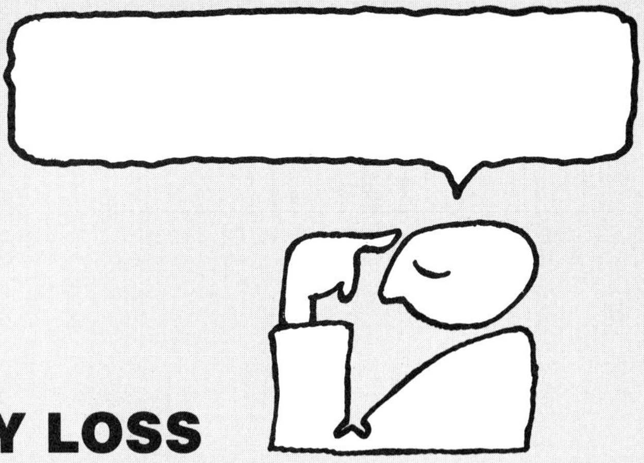

MEMORY LOSS

Amnesia, or memory loss, is one of the most puzzling disorders for health professionals and one of the most disturbing for the people who suffer from it. Depending on the circumstances, memory failures may be temporary and inconsequential or permanent and devastating, may involve past events or current experiences, and may be widespread or bizarrely selective. (One woman lost all conscious memory of her former acquaintances but continued to respond emotionally to those she had considered to be friends or enemies.) Some of the most important discoveries in memory research have come from the study of severe amnesiacs, yet medical cures for lasting memory loss are largely unknown. Following are some of the more common causes of memory failure.

Aging. For a variety of reasons, including arteriosclerosis ("hardening of the arteries"), people in their 50's or older often experience a gradual decline in their abilities to retain everyday details and to memorize or recall new information. Unless accompanied by disease or injury, these are *not* signs of serious mental deterioration and can be compensated for by making written lists or employing mnemonic devices.

Alcohol. Drinking to excess slows the brain and adversely affects memory. It's not unusual for heavy drinkers to have little or no memory of an alcoholic binge. Nutritional deficiencies associated with chronic alcoholism may bring about a more lasting and severe form of memory loss called Korsakoff's syndrome, whose victims may have difficulty learning and retaining new information.

Alzheimer's disease. The foremost cause of incurable loss of mental function in the elderly, Alzheimer's, which may also occur in younger people, involves failure to produce an important brain chemical and progressive destruction of brain cells. Loss of recent memories is a typical early sign of the disease; eventually it may cause total memory failure.

Brain diseases. Permanent mental impairment and attendant memory loss may result from various other diseases of the brain, including severe encephalitis (an inflammation of the brain), particularly in infants and the elderly; brain tumors or other cancers that spread to the central nervous system; and certain rare viral illnesses, such as Creutzfeldt-Jakob disease.

Head injury. Concussion or unconsciousness caused by a blow to the head often produces temporary loss of recent memories (retrograde amnesia) and failure to remember the events immediately surrounding the injury. There may also be a period of post-traumatic amnesia, in which the injured person has difficulty retaining new information. The extent and permanence of memory loss from severe head injury is unpredictable and seems to depend on the type of blow, degree of damage, and part of the brain affected.

Hysterical amnesia. Unlike the other memory impairments listed here (except stress), hysterical amnesia is of strictly psychological origin. It may involve repression of memories of particularly distressing events or a similar inability to acknowledge or retain aspects of current experience. It is usually treated by psychoanalytic techniques and/or hypnosis.

Medication. Sedatives, sleeping pills, narcotics, anticonvulsants and other drugs that act on the central nervous system may cause mental confusion and temporary memory failures, especially in the elderly.

Severe illness. Occasionally, there may be inability to remember the events surrounding an episode of severe, feverish illness (such as pneumonia or meningitis) or of diabetic coma.

Stress. Prolonged psychological stress causes people to do more than their usual amount of misplacing items, mistaking facts, and forgetting appointments. One theory has it that stress causes a mental traffic jam, reducing memory flow to a fraction of its usual capacity. Memory lapses may also accompany "performance anxiety" or stage fright, such as the sudden inability to remember a well-rehearsed speech or business presentation.

Stroke. Generally precipitated by a blood clot or cerebral hemorrhage, a stroke cuts off the blood supply to a portion of the brain. The type and degree of resulting mental impairment and memory loss correspond to the site and severity of the blockage. Some stroke patients lose their memory of how to perform basic physical tasks; others suffer from aphasia, a general term used to describe failures of speech, reading, writing, or recognizing words. Stroke is a leading cause of permanent severe memory loss in the elderly.

Surgery. People who undergo major surgery requiring general anesthesia may have failure to recall the events immediately preceding and following their operation.

cognitive structures. Such a conclusion would have considerable legal significance, especially in cases involving eyewitness testimony. Elizabeth Loftus of the University of Washington has conducted several experiments demonstrating that eyewitness memories are not only influenced by preconceived notions but are also susceptible to new information and suggestions made after the event. In particular, she has shown that the way a question is framed can alter an eyewitness's "remembered" response. If eyewitness testimony is to be used at all, Loftus suggests, witnesses should be allowed to reconstruct the events in sequence at their own pace, without leading questions or interruptions from trial attorneys.

Hypnosis does not seem to improve the reliability of eyewitness memory, despite a few isolated and well-publicized cases to the contrary. Hypnosis often succeeds in relaxing the witness and removing inhibitions that might hinder recall, but careful studies show that it also reduces the ability to distinguish between fact and fantasy, calling up real events indiscriminately with those that were dreamed, imagined, or seen on television.

A fascinating study of eyewitness memory was carried out by Ulric Neisser, the father of the cognitive movement, who analyzed the transcript of testimony by White House Counsel John W. Dean III at the 1973 Senate hearings on the Watergate scandal. Dean provided lengthy accounts of conversations he had had with President Richard Nixon and his associates concerning the Watergate break-in and subsequent cover-up. For a while, Dean's testimony was the only available evidence that Nixon was personally involved in the cover-up. When the secret tapes of these and other presidential conversations surfaced, Neisser compared the transcript of Dean's testimony with the transcript of the tapes and found a host of inaccuracies, both minor and major, in Dean's account of the conversations. Yet the "gist" (Dean's word) of the testimony—that Nixon know of and took part in the cover-up—was upheld by the tapes. Neisser concluded that in this case at least, Dean was not a liar. His testimony, with its discrepancies, time compressions, and self-serving distortions, all surrounding a central core of "truth," is an example of how we actually remember conversations and events.

Forgetting

The way memories alter over time may also help explain how information is forgotten. We retain only a very small part of the information we register in a lifetime. This is probably all for the best, for as William James wrote, "If we remembered everything

Eyewitness memories can be influenced by later suggestion. A person who was shown a film of an auto accident (left) was then asked how fast the cars were going when they SMASHED. That word affected memory to the extent of conjuring up the more dramatic (and false) image at right.

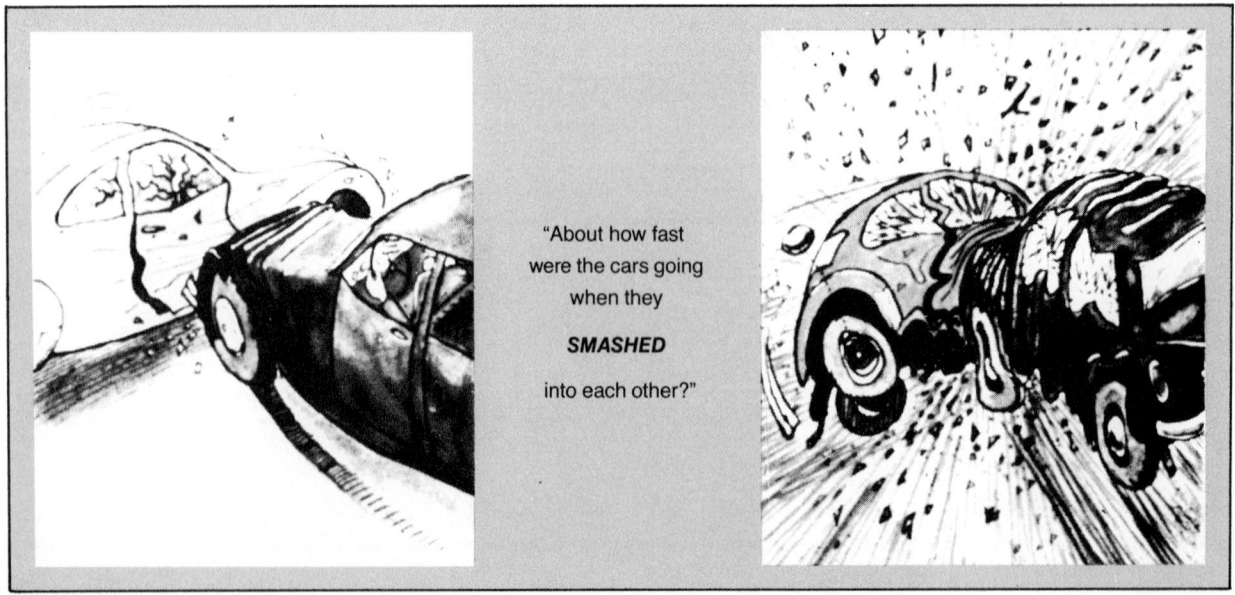

we should be as ill as if we remembered nothing." Perhaps the best-known case in the literature of memory studies is that of S., the Russian journalist chronicled by the psychologist Alexander Luria in *The Mind of a Mnemonist.* S. had an extraordinary capacity for making vivid and lasting mental associations, which rendered him virtually incapable of forgetting. The constant flood of memories that filled his mind interfered with his ability to concentrate and ultimately to hold a job. Eventually S. was reduced to an itinerant mnemonist, using his prodigious memory to earn his keep as a performer in sideshows and country fairs.

Unlike S., most of us seem to forget all too readily—not just passing details, but names, faces, facts, and events that we thought were securely stored away. Such memory lapses are often temporary frustrations caused by emotional stress or the "tip-of-the-tongue" syndrome, in which we know exactly the word we want but can't seem to locate the spot where it is hiding. Some "lost" memories reappear spontaneously in the unlikeliest of mental settings; others may be retrieved by concentrated effort or by trying different channels of word associations. But some are lost forever.

One theory of forgetting holds that memories are eroded by "interference" from other overlapping associations, the same way that using a word in a variety of contexts may obscure its original meaning. The interference theory has lost ground, however, and a more current view would be that some information simply isn't processed thoroughly enough to take a permanent place in long-term memory. The reason for this may be lack of use, lack of importance, lack of a cognitive structure capable of assimilating the information, or maybe even Freudian repression. A related explanation for certain kinds of forgetting may be that during the elaboration and consolidation processes, the external "packaging" of memories is stripped away so that the essential content can be got at more easily. Thus, as in John Dean's case, the precise details of a memory may be lost while the core concept is retained.

Stored information continues to be sifted and refined throughout our lifetime, in contradiction of the conventional wisdom that memory inevitably declines with age. It is true that older people lose some capacity to memorize new facts and remember details. But research indicates that the ability to store and recall *meaning* actually improves with age and experience. Our cognitive structures become better organized and more adept at extracting key concepts for as long as we stay healthy and intellectually active.

Masters of Memory

The role played by experience also calls into question the usual notions of what constitutes a good memory. Often, memory power is equated with the ability to memorize things like dates, lists, statistics, and quotations, quite apart from any other significance they may have. The mnemonist S. was clearly a giant in this domain. Some children, too, seem to have "total eidetic recall"—the capacity to conjure up a complete visual image of anything they have once seen. Curiously, this gift almost invariably fades by late adolescence.

Improving rote memorization is not difficult; anyone can learn to apply the basic techniques. All memory-building methods, including those used by stage performers capable of reciting pages from telephone books, boil down to variations on the elaborative processes of "chunking" and association. Psychologists at Carnegie-Mellon University have taught student volunteers with self-professed average memories to recall strings of numbers up to 80 digits long using these devices. One student, a runner, breaks the strings down to chunks of 3 or 4 digits, which he associates with times for different track events. The oldest mnemonic device on record is the "method of loci" used by ancient Roman orators. They would visualize a walking path whose features they knew by heart, then mentally link the main points of their speeches to the landmarks encountered along the familiar route. In ancient or modern guise, the rule of thumb for memorization is hanging new information on old pegs, using associations that are as vivid and unusual as possible.

Mnemonic devices, however, shed little light on a more fundamental function of human memory, which is the storing and arranging of our experience so that we can make use of it or just enjoy looking back on it. In some respects, Ulric Neisser writes, we are all minor masters of memory: "Everybody who is skilled at anything necessarily has a good memory for whatever information that activity demands. Physicists can remember what they need to know to do physics, and fishermen what they need for fishing; musicians remember music, art critics recall paintings, historians know history. Every person is a prodigy to his neighbors, remembering so much that other people do not know." □

REHABILITATION

Joseph Goodgold, M.D.

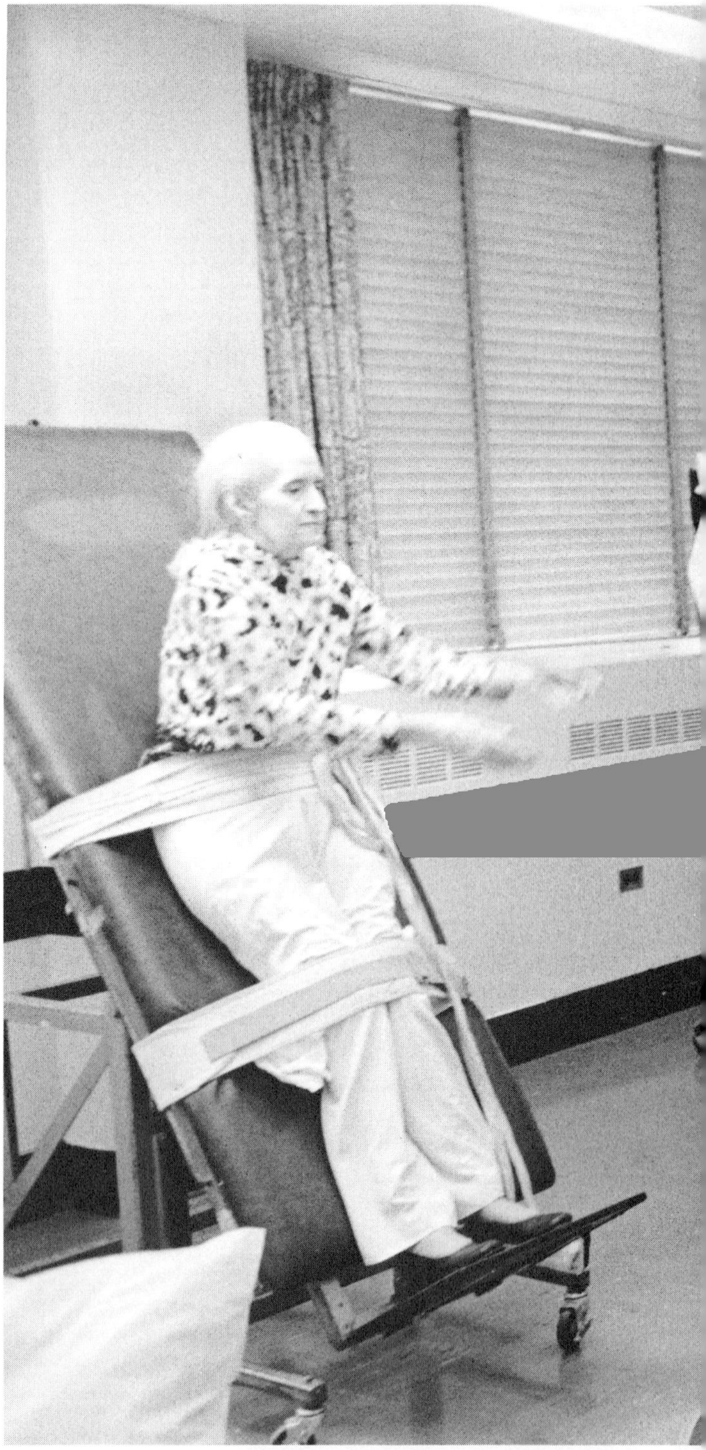

It was one of those ideal Sundays in July with a brilliant sun in a cloudless sky, a superb day to spend at the pool. From the house, John watched his younger brother Steve, age 17, dive off the side of the pool. But John felt ill at ease at how long Steve "swam" under water and how he then assumed a face-down, dead man's float.

Perhaps it was a premonition or an intuitive reaction that made John run outside to look at the boy. He immediately recognized that his brother was actually drowning in the "safe" end of the pool. Fortunately, John did not panic. He immediately removed Steve from the water and cleared an airway to restore his breathing. But all four limbs were immobile; they were paralyzed. The dive had been made into the shallow end of the pool, and the victim's head had struck the bottom with sufficient force to break his neck and injure the spinal cord. However, Steve *was* alive. His now uncertain future would ultimately reflect how badly he had been injured, the emergency care he received, to what degree his body was able to recover, and the availability of a good rehabilitation program.

Defining Rehabilitation

"Rehabilitation" is a word that has been applied across many areas, from the restoration of old buildings to the treatment of felons and drug addicts. The focus of this article is the rehabilitation of the disabled patient as it is carried out in a modern general rehabilitation center. In this context, rehabilitation may be defined in several ways. A narrow view might emphasize a purely physical approach, such as the use of light, heat, electricity, water, or exercise to treat disability. A broader, more

---

Tilt table basketball improves balance and dexterity, helping patients to regain eye and hand coordination.

CENTERS

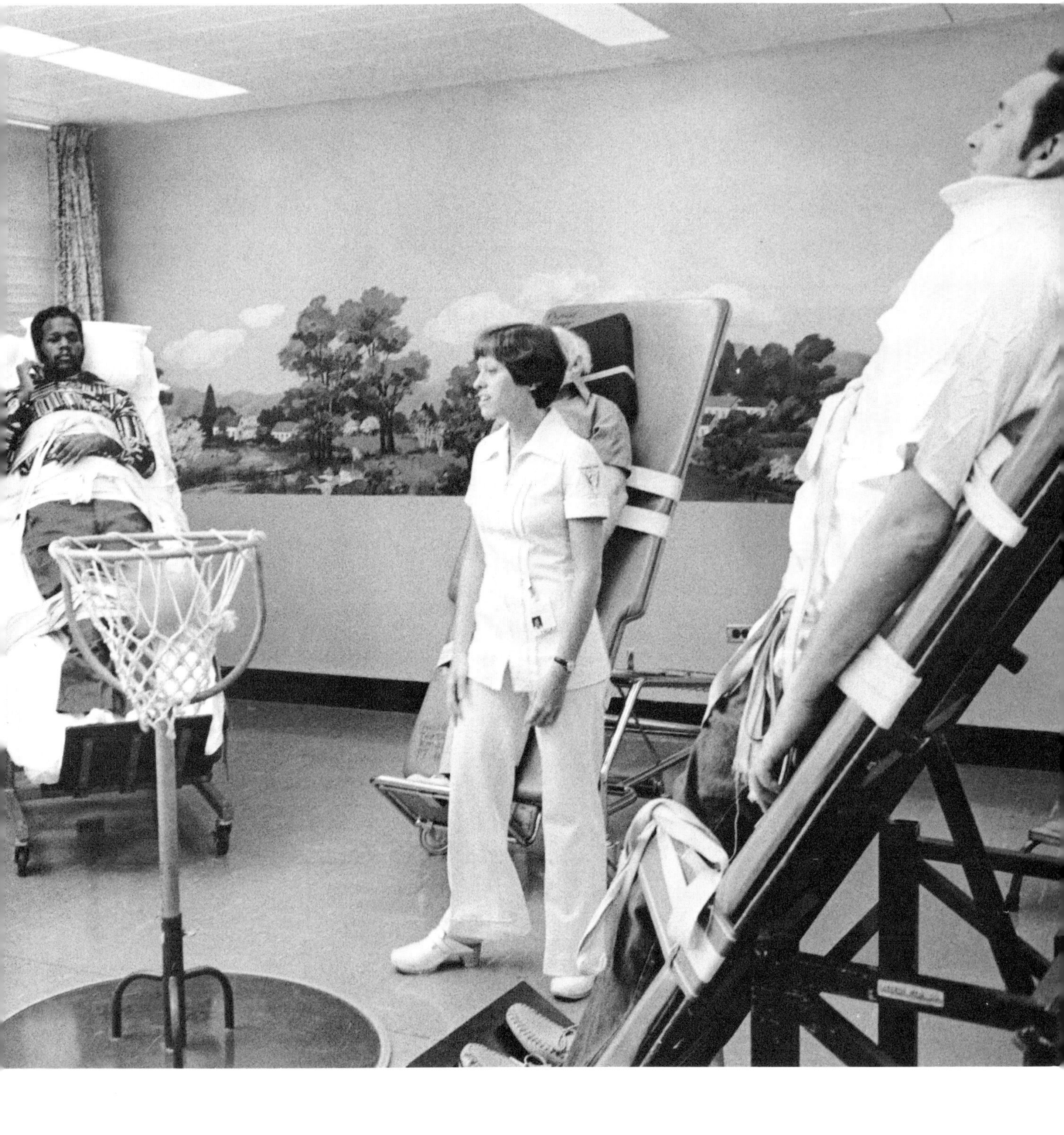

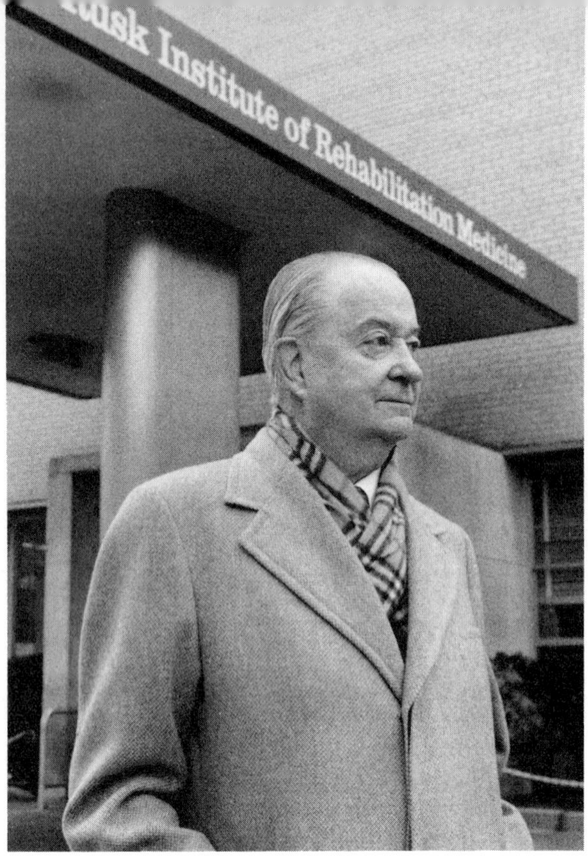

Dr. Howard Rusk, the "father of rehabilitation medicine," went beyond physical therapy to establish full reintegration into society as the final goal.

contemporary definition would encompass the sum of whatever treatment and training are required to help the patient attain the maximum possible restoration of a normal physical, psychological, social, and vocational life.

This broader concept is something of a departure in American medicine, which traditionally has seen the curing of disease as its overriding concern, while relegating the behavorial, social, educational, and vocational ramifications of sickness to a decidedly secondary, if not unimportant, status. Dr. Howard A. Rusk, the founder of New York University's Rusk Institute of Rehabilitation Medicine and often called the father of rehabilitation medicine, introduced the term "third phase of medicine" for the comprehensive, total care of a patient, the first two phases being preventive and curative care. Without this third phase—rehabilitation—especially in cases of disabling and chronic diseases, the process of restoring health is incomplete. A young amputee who has been excellently fitted with an artificial limb and then taught to use it may still remain outside the mainstream of society if his emotional reactions to an altered body image ensnare him in social and vocational isolation. Appropriate treatment of the whole person is the basis of rehabilitation medicine.

A Recent Specialty

Rehabilitation medicine is a relatively recent specialty in the United States, one that gained professional recognition only within the past 40 years. Physicians who specialize in this field are known as physiatrists (pronounced "fizz-ee-AT-rists"). From a handful of resident trainees in the late 1940's, physiatry has grown to the point where there are now 700 to 800 residency positions in about 80 accredited residency programs in the United States and Canada.

Rehabilitation medicine is carried out in a great variety of facilities. These include private offices, ambulatory clinics, acute-care hospitals, hospitals that specialize in treating chronic disease, some nursing facilities, and, finally, rehabilitation centers like the Rusk Institute. Ideally such centers are affiliated with academic medical centers, where clinical and consultation services are available and can be quickly mobilized. There is no precise count of the number of rehabilitation facilities in North America. Most moderate-sized hospitals provide some type of rehabilitation services, if only for orthopedic patients. There are probably about 80 major rehabilitation medicine centers in the United States.

The Patients

Who are the patients served in rehabilitation centers? Generally, they are victims of diseases or accidents that have resulted in severe physical disability and handicap. (An estimated 8–10 percent of the U.S. population falls into this category.) The most common disabling diseases are arthritis, nervous system disorders, and cardiovascular and respiratory ailments. Since the nervous system and the joints and muscles are often attacked by disabling diseases, the most visible handicaps among rehabilitation center patients are loss of arm and leg movement and an inability to stand and walk. Emotional problems resulting from these disabilities are common. Rehabilitation centers also deal with a number of disorders that particularly affect children; these

---

Joseph Goodgold is chairman of the Department of Rehabilitation Medicine at the New York University School of Medicine and director of the school's Rusk Institute of Rehabilitation Medicine. He is past president of the American Academy of Physical Medicine and Rehabilitation.

include cerebral palsy and other developmental defects, primary muscular diseases like some types of muscular dystrophy, and a host of congenital and acquired musculoskeletal problems.

Several categories of patients generally fill most of the 154 beds of the Rusk Institute, which can be considered a typical high-quality, comprehensive rehabilitation center:

- ***Stroke victims.*** Strokes are caused by a hemorrhage in the brain or by a clot or other blockage in a blood vessel nourishing the brain. The result is usually hemiplegia—full or partial paralysis of half of the body. For example, a stroke on the left side of the brain could result in paralysis of the right arm and leg.
- ***Paraplegics and quadriplegics.*** Paraplegia refers to paralysis of the lower half of the body, including both legs; quadriplegia is paralysis of all four limbs. Most paraplegic and quadriplegic patients are people in their late teens and early 20's who have been injured in auto or motorcycle accidents, diving accidents, and freak accidents, such as a hard spill during water skiing. A spinal fracture or a bone dislocation in the lower back that injures the spinal cord causes paraplegia, whereas quadriplegia is caused by similar trauma to the neck portion of the spine. The physical consequences of both conditions are often catastrophic; well before actual rehabilitation begins, correct emergency treatment and transportation, life-support measures, and hospital care are needed. If the patient does not receive the proper acute care, the spinal cord may be more severely injured or even severed. This results in loss of body function below the site involved, affecting muscle power, neurologic control of blood vessel expansion and contraction, bladder and bowel control, and sexual activity.
- ***Victims of brain damage.*** Aside from stroke, the most common cause of brain damage among rehabilitation center patients is motor vehicle accidents. Often the accident victim has been comatose for some period of time and was kept alive only by mechanical life-support systems. Use of the arms and legs may have been lost, and intellectual functioning and behavior may be affected as well. The patient may respond entirely inappropriately to everyday situations and may no longer be able to remember and think normally.
- ***Orthopedic patients.*** In a rehabilitation center orthopedic patients include accident victims who have lost arms or legs (multiple amputations are not uncommon), children born with limbs missing, and patients who have undergone surgery for scoliosis (severe curvature of the spinal column) or joint replacement. The replacement of an impaired hip or knee by an artificial joint is one of the truly remarkable advances in the care of patients with crippling arthritis or other conditions that damage the joints. Completely disabled patients are frequently

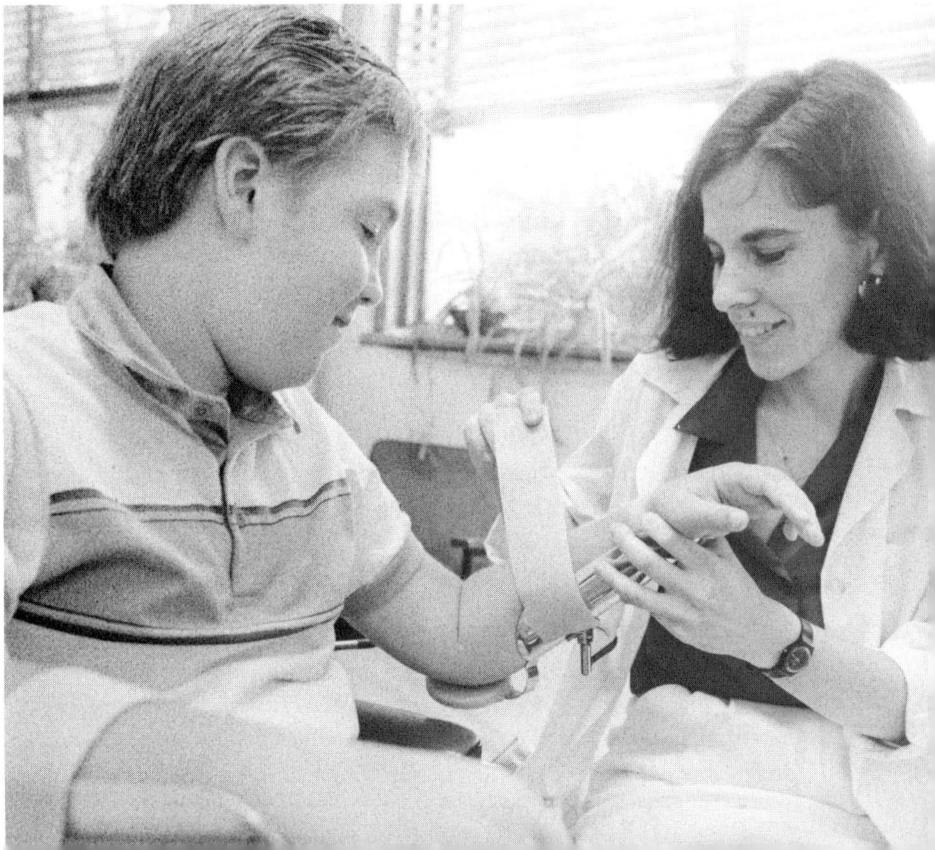

A young muscular dystrophy patient is fitted with a brace to help support the weakened muscles in his arm. Accident victims as well as those who suffer from debilitating diseases can benefit from therapy at rehabilitation centers.

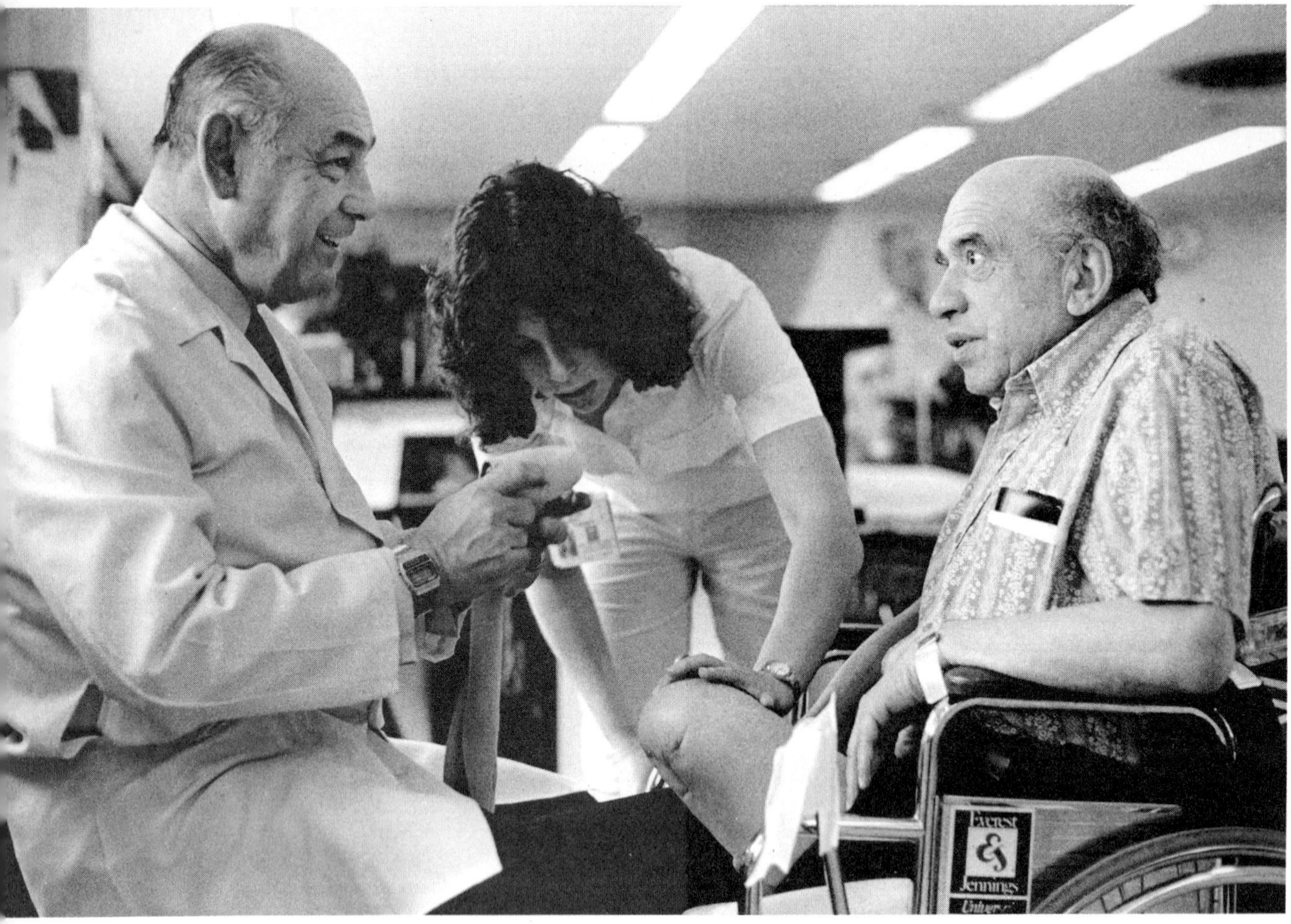

able to return to productive lives. However, surgery must be followed by a careful rehabilitation program to restore a full range of motion, muscle power, and joint stability.

• ***Cancer sufferers.*** At the Rusk Institute there is an active program of rehabilitation for patients with various types of cancer. Cases range from the young child with bone cancer of the leg, requiring amputation, to the patient with a severely invasive cancer of the lower abdominal cavity who requires radical surgery to remove body organs throughout the lower torso. There is also an active program for cancer patients who have had a breast removed; for these women, physical rehabilitation of the chest and arm must be accompanied by a program of psychiatric support.

Patients in the above categories represent a large portion of rehabilitation center cases, but a great many other diseases are represented as well. These include multiple sclerosis, Parkinson's disease, infectious polyneuropathy (Guillain-Barré syndrome), poliomyelitis, disease arising from deterioration of the spinal disks, arteriosclerosis with obstruction of blood vessels, muscular dystrophy, spinal atrophy, and congenital and developmental disorders in children.

Staff and Organization

An essential feature of rehabilitation medicine is its organization as a multidisciplinary team effort. In most specialized centers the director of the rehabilitation program is a physiatrist, although another specialist (an orthopedist or neurologist) sometimes holds this position. The staff of physician specialists in rehabilitation medicine is usually backed up by an extensive roster of consultants, since so many of the problems require input from other specialties. The most important of these are from neurosurgery, neurology, urology, orthopedics, internal medicine, pediatrics, and psychiatry.

Working with the medical staff are other important members of the rehabilitation team, a group

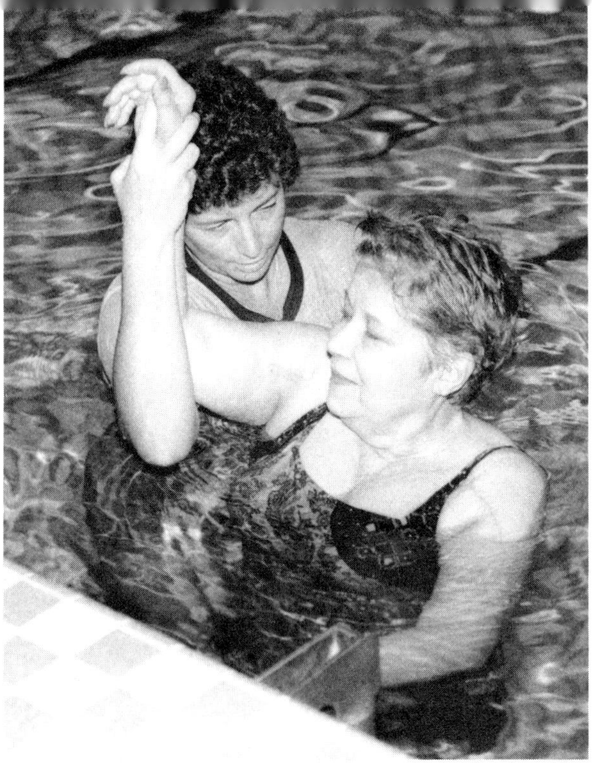

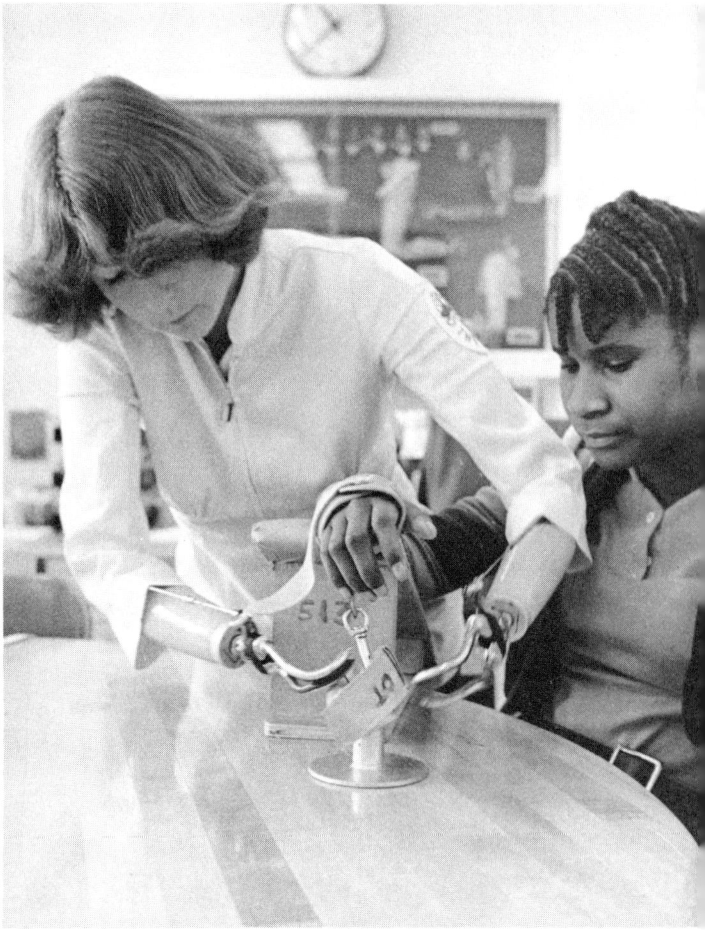

With Hearts as Well as Hands

Rehabilitated patients may become excellent teachers themselves; right, an occupational therapist, herself a user of prosthetic devices, provides emotional support as well as physical training for a patient. Above, the warmth of both therapist and water helps an arthritis sufferer move stiff joints. A doctor's reassurances (at left, Dr. Joseph Goodgold) are important in readying a patient about to receive an artificial leg.

frequently identified as allied health professionals. They include rehabilitation nurses, physical, recreational, and occupational therapists, speech pathologists, vocational counselors, social workers, psychologists, and specialists in orthotic and prosthetic devices (which improve limb function or replace body parts with artificial ones).

Most patients admitted to a rehabilitation center are referred by physicians and hospitals after having received emergency care and medical or surgical treatment. In some cases, however, especially those involving spinal cord injury, rapid transfer to a comprehensive rehabilitation unit is preferable since long-lasting complications may occur extremely early. For example, bedsores appear quickly and may penetrate tissue deeply (even down to the bone), requiring months of treatment and delaying the course of rehabilitation. Rehabilitation nurses have the awareness and know-how to prevent these sores.

Upon admission to the Rusk Institute, a patient's medical status is rapidly determined by the staff physicians. Each member of the rehabilitation team then carries out a detailed study of the patient for review at an initial evaluation conference, where a plan of treatment based on realistic and achievable goals for the patient is agreed upon. The complicated logistics involved in carrying out an individual's therapy program—which consumes most of the day other than mealtimes and requires that the patient be moved on schedule from one section of the center to another—is handled by a special scheduling group that accomplishes the difficult task for all 154 patients at the institute.

The patient's medical condition during therapy is monitored by daily physicians' rounds and by physician visits to the various treatment areas. Nursing services are delivered by specially trained rehabilitation nurses who are acutely aware of the particular needs of severely disabled people. Their skill is critical—for example, in recognizing complications affecting bladder and bowel functions and in immediately perceiving cardiovascular

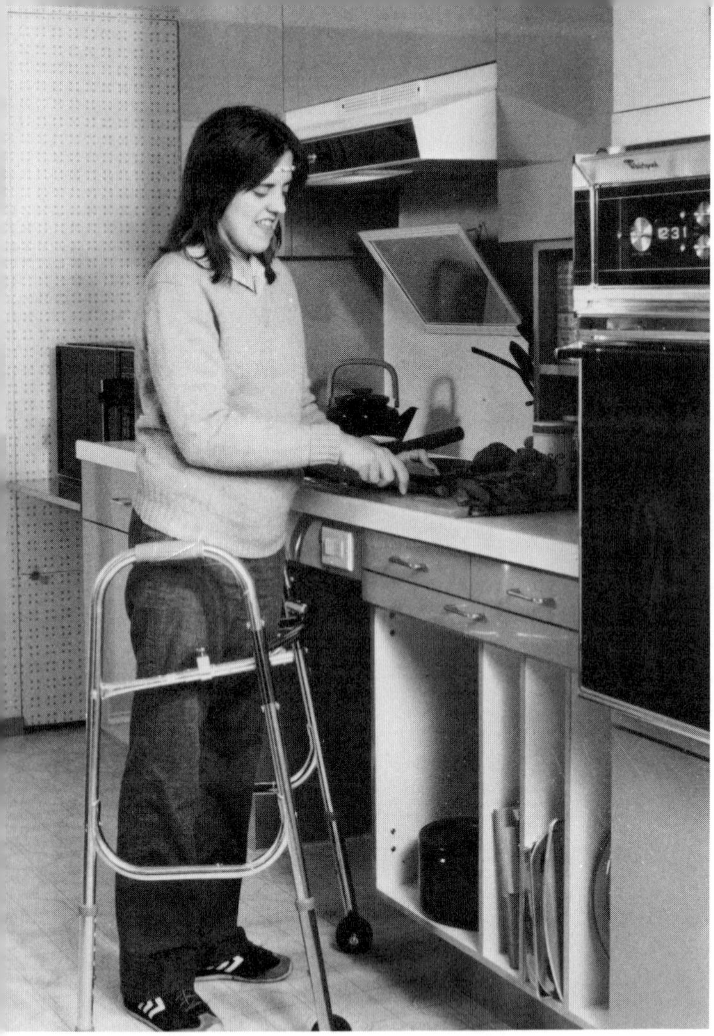

Many centers try to duplicate ordinary life situations to help patients adjust to the future. Above, a young patient cooks at a specially equipped kitchen at New York University's Horizon House; below, a wheelchair patient practices maneuvering herself into a car at Burke Rehabilitation Center.

problems, such as the sudden and potentially dangerous attacks of high blood pressure that occur with some spinal injuries. Nor are rehabilitation patients immune from general medical problems requiring skilled medical and nursing attention, especially since many patients are advanced in age. A stroke patient may have diabetes or heart disease.

Physical and Occupational Therapy

Physical therapy, an important component of rehabilitative care, may occur on a one-to-one basis, as when the therapist attempts to "reeducate" the muscles of the patient's hand, or in a group setting, like exercise classes for some stroke patients. The therapist may employ microwave diathermy (the therapeutic heating of body tissues using a microwave energy source), ultrasound, electrical stimulation, hydrotherapy, or carefully controlled exercise programs designed to improve endurance, strength, stability, and coordination. There is considerable emphasis on restoring the ability to move about (with or without mechanical aids) and restoring use of the arms. The stroke patient with a paralyzed leg may be fitted with a lightweight plastic brace, perhaps given a cane for additional balance, and then trained to walk without stumbling or falling and to negotiate level and inclined surfaces and stairs. The physical therapist's knowledge and skill are especially valuable in caring for children with neurologic and developmental disorders.

The goals of occupational and physical therapy often overlap. The occupational therapist's initial

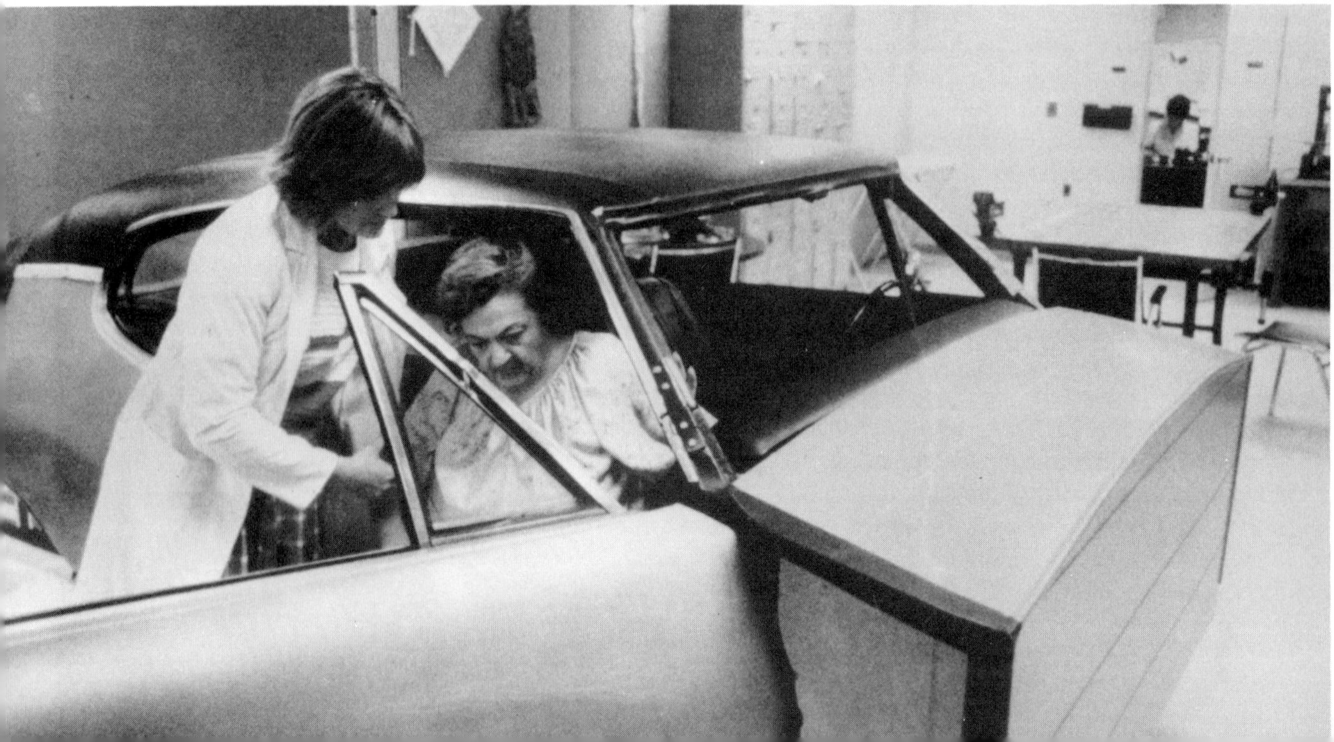

evaluation emphasizes the patient's ability to carry out specific functions, as well as the patient's capacity to respond to retraining. The therapist then plans activities that increase muscle power and coordination, restore the range of motion to impaired joints, and improve manual dexterity and eye-hand coordination. Occupational therapists also teach patients to use orthotic and prosthetic devices when these are needed. On occasion, therapists may even help design such devices.

Occupational therapy bears a great responsibility for teaching patients how to perform routine activities of daily living, in order to restore their capacity to function independently. These include getting dressed, getting in and out of a bed and a chair, and bathing. At the Rusk Institute an entire apartment has been set up, to retrain the handicapped homemaker before the patient's return home. In addition, the therapist visits the patient's home before the patient leaves the rehabilitation center to ensure that the patient will be able to maintain the independence attained at the center. Often, the therapist suggests that changes be made in the home to ease resumption of a productive and orderly life—installing ramps outside and stairway "lifts" inside for wheelchair-confined persons, or adapting appliance controls for the blind.

Therapy may also concentrate on the patient's vision. Many stroke victims and other brain-damaged patients lose half their perceived visual field; this loss, in both eyes, means the patient cannot see more than half of a written page, half a stairway, and, in driving, half the road—including oncoming vehicles! Until made aware of this deficiency, the patient may be completely oblivious to the problem. To compensate for the problem, patients learn head-turning techniques and thus avoid potentially dangerous consequences.

Although the psychological benefits of arts and crafts are still important, these activities are less prominent in therapy now than in earlier years. They have often been superseded by attention to communicative and computer skills.

Speech Pathology

Language has sometimes been defined in terms of expressive functions—speaking and writing—and receptive functions—understanding the spoken and written word. In a rehabilitation center the diagnosis and treatment of impaired language functions by a speech pathologist or therapist is an extremely common activity, especially with brain-damaged accident or stroke victims or the victims of some pediatric disorders.

About a third of stroke patients suffer from aphasia, a condition in which both expressive and receptive functions are impaired to varying extents. (In one type of aphasia, known as global aphasia, the loss of comprehension is extremely severe.) In some paralytic diseases that affect the muscles used in speaking, a condition called dysarthria results, in which abnormal articulation and stressing of syllables produces distorted speech. The successful treatment of speech-impaired patients requires a careful diagnostic workup that includes testing of the patient's hearing, since an undetected hearing loss would render speech therapy ineffective. The treatment of dysarthria focuses on improving articulation and often meets with some degree of success. Aphasia, often devastating to the patient, is far more difficult to treat. Some speech pathologists believe that the psychological counseling side of speech therapy is of prime importance in helping the aphasic patient learn to live with the limitations imposed by the disease.

Speech pathology programs may have an importance beyond their immediate clinical outcome. The normal processing of language, including the perception of sounds, integration of this "information" within the central nervous system, and the various responses to it can in some ways be seen as a microcosm of how the human brain functions. The thought has been advanced that if an understanding of this process were to be achieved, the knowledge gained could perhaps be applied to learning how to restore other functions affected by a variety of central nervous system diseases.

Social Services and Vocational Counseling

Social workers on the rehabilitation center staff help the patient accommodate to the unfamiliar world of the center, make contact with community and government support services, and prepare for eventual return to home and community. The immediate financial problems faced by the patient and family in paying for rehabilitation, nursing and attendant services, and devices such as wheelchairs and braces, as well as questions of supplementary income, are all within the province of the social worker. In many instances the social worker serves as the patient's advocate in dealing with government agencies and private insurance carriers, at least partly relieving the patient of often overwhelming concerns that can be a major distraction from the primary need to concentrate on treatment and retraining.

The social worker also organizes and participates in meetings of the patient, family members, and staff to promote mutual support and assistance. Yet another responsibility of the social worker is to take the lead in organizing a discharge plan almost as soon as the initial evaluation of the patient is completed, since a long lead time is required to arrange for follow-up services in the patient's home or in a nursing home. The relationship of the social worker to patient and family is often a sensitive one of confidant, friend, and advocate.

The management of patients' vocational problems is quite distinct from other social services. Vocational assistance extends so far beyond the stereotyped role of vocational testing and providing occupational information that the term "rehabilitation counselor" is more appropriate than "vocational counselor" for the provider of such aid. Successful counseling involves exploration by the counselor and patient of a wide range of issues that may include the patient's feelings of loss of adequacy, loss of dignity, and altered self-image. Counseling also takes into account the patient's degree of physical independence, social and economic status, educational and vocational background, and work interests. Vocational goals must focus on the patient's remaining abilities rather than on the person's disability.

Usually the counselor has a strong working relationship with state vocational agencies and private employment agencies. A successful placement can be difficult even under favorable economic conditions, and in an economic downturn there is a tendency for employers to give handicapped individuals the lowest priority in hiring. Yet the cost-effectiveness of returning handicapped persons to the work force has been conclusively demonstrated again and again. An investment in rehabilitation and subsequent vocational counseling and training often pays off if disabled workers can find jobs and achieve fiscal independence, earning taxable income rather than being welfare recipients.

Providing Emotional Support

Psychological problems are well recognized complications of many illnesses, but these problems are especially pronounced in severely handicapped or disabled patients and can profoundly affect the outcome of rehabilitation treatment. It is a rare patient who escapes such psychological reactions; most disabled individuals are at one time or another battered by some degree of depression, anxiety, anger, hostility, or withdrawal. The patient may become belligerent and uncooperative or, at the opposite pole, show an exaggerated, almost total dependence.

These problems warrant the earliest possible detection and treatment. The process begins when the physiatrist takes the patient's history and performs a physical examination. In general, the physiatrist is more alert to emotional and behavioral problems than are acute-care physicians. If the patient shows evidence of such problems, psychological or psychiatric examination and testing are scheduled, and if warranted, a treatment regimen is promptly begun.

Rehabilitation patients differ from patients with many other medical problems in that their disorder is essentially incurable: pneumonia and appendicitis can be treated and cured, but hemiplegia and paraplegia most frequently cannot. More so than patients with a chronic, progressive disability, those who experience the sudden onset of severe disability undergo a process of grieving and fear that often produces changes in personality. The treatment program must address these reactions and help the patient assimilate an altered self-concept, both physically and emotionally. In spite of difficulties that sometimes appear almost insurmountable, the majority of patients are able to accommodate to their situation and develop a life-style that takes maximum advantage of whatever ability remains to them, rejecting a life of mournful, lamenting surrender to disability.

A Complex Mission

The philosophy of medical practice has been enriched by rehabilitation medicine's concept of comprehensive and multidisciplinary patient care. The physiatrist functions as a responsible and responsive manager, working in tandem with other team members for the greatest benefit of the patient. At the same time that the rehabilitation center provides care for the patient, it also provides a milieu for training physiatrists during a four-year residency period and for conducting research in such fields as neurophysiology, bioengineering, and muscle physiology and pathology. □

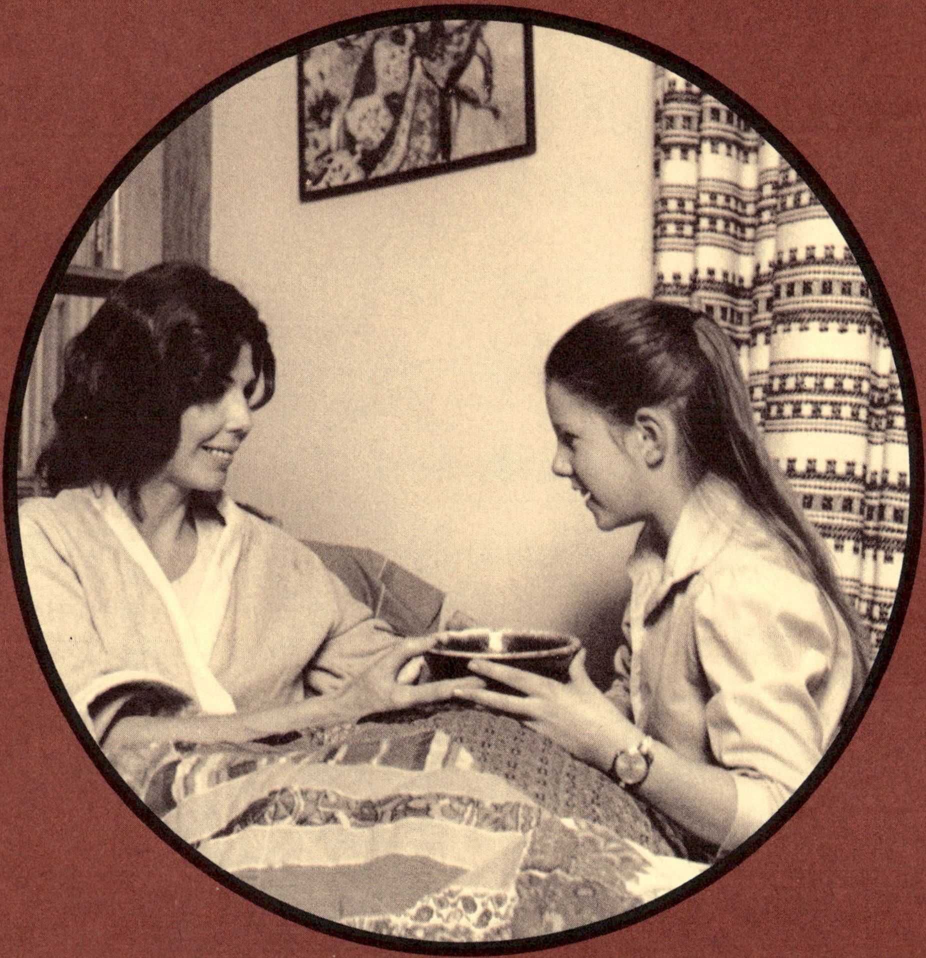

SPOTLIGHT ON HEALTH

Why You Need Eye Examinations

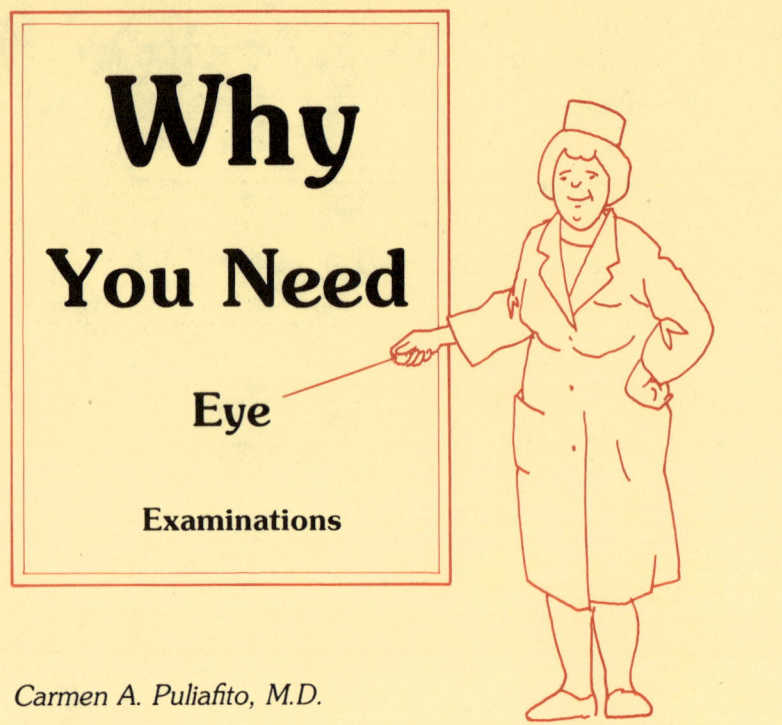

Carmen A. Puliafito, M.D.

Vision is a precious sense, and if we are to preserve it, we must protect and care for our eyes. Although the human eye is only an inch in length, it is a remarkably complex and delicate structure. No artificial device approaches its ability to sense the world around us, process the information it gathers, and make that information available to the brain.

Eye Examinations Are Crucial

How do we protect our eyes from diseases and injuries that can impair our sight? In the case of eye care, the timeworn adage "an ounce of prevention is worth a pound of cure" is particularly true. Because so many of the eye's structures are delicate, it may be difficult or impossible to restore vision to perfection if disease or injury occurs. (See the accompanying box for tips on preventing eye injuries.)

Eye examinations are crucial to protecting vision, because many eye diseases do not produce symptoms (and hence remain unrecognized by the patient) until vision has been irretrievably lost. Periodic eye examinations by an ophthalmologist are the key to both the detection and the treatment of eye diseases in their early stages.

Eye-Care Professionals

Ophthalmologists are medical doctors (M.D.'s) who have three to five years of additional training, after completing medical school, in eye diseases and surgery. It takes a great deal of training and experience to become skilled in examining the eyes and detecting the subtle, early signs of eye disease.

There is much more to a comprehensive eye examination than being fitted for a pair of glasses,. if necessary. An essential component is a test for glaucoma, a condition in which the pressure inside the eye is increased, with damage to the optic nerve that connects the eye and brain. The physician will also examine the retina (the light-sensitive tissue that lines the inside of the eye) after the pupil of the eye has been dilated with drops.

Because ophthalmologists are medical doctors, they have been trained to detect eye diseases. Other eye health practitioners are optometrists (doctors of optometry, not M.D.'s), who are trained to prescribe glasses, and opticians, who do not examine eyes or prescribe glasses but fill prescriptions for glasses.

Patients should routinely ask every healthcare provider about educational background, hospital affiliations, and participation in continuing education programs to keep skills up to date. Ask about the cost of services to be provided. You have the right to have answers to these questions, and any responsible healthcare professional will be happy to provide them.

When to Have Eyes Examined

All children should have medical eye examinations within the first three years of life. If there is a family history of childhood eye disease (for instance, strabismus, or "crossed eyes"), an eye examination should be performed within the first year of life. If a parent notes that a child is not

Children should have an eye examination before the age of three to diagnose and start treatment of common problems.

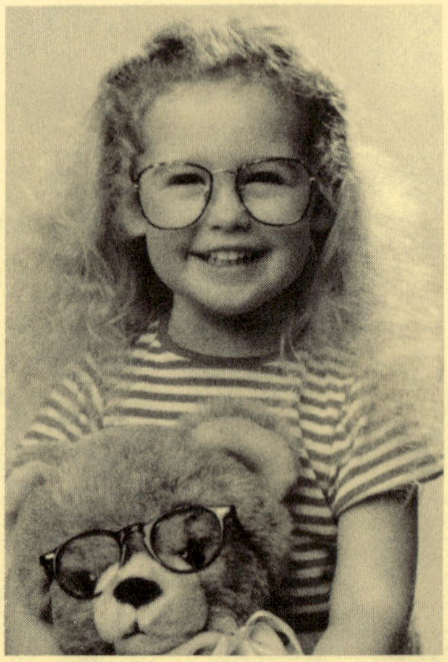

seeing well or that one eye is not straight, immediate consultation with an ophthalmologist is called for. Unless both eyes are straight, they cannot work in tandem, and one eye may be preferred. This condition is referred to as amblyopia, or "lazy eye," and can lead to poor vision in the eye that is not preferred. Unless the condition is recognized and treated before the age of seven, loss of vision in the affected eye can become permanent.

Throughout childhood and adolescence, periodic eye examinations (approximately once every two years) remain valuable. It is during the teenage years that nearsightedness, or myopia, is most often detected. This can usually be easily corrected with glasses or contact lenses.

Adults between the ages of 20 and 40 should have their eyes examined at least once every two to five years. Many ophthalmologists recommend annual eye examinations after the age of 40, since the risk of a number of treatable eye disorders increases with age. For instance, glaucoma occurs in about 2 percent of the population over age 40. Most often patients with early glaucoma have no symptoms. Periodic medical eye examinations are necessary if this disorder is to be recognized and treated early, before there is a loss of vision.

Special Cases

Any loss of vision, at any age, is an occasion for prompt consultation with an ophthalmologist. This is particularly true for individuals over the age of 60. Two of the most common eye diseases of older Americans are cataracts and a disorder called senile macular degeneration.

Cataracts are a clouding of the eye's natural lens. Cataract removal is one of the most commonly performed surgical procedures in North America today and one of the most successful as well. In most cases a plastic lens is implanted within the eye to replace the focusing power of the eye's lens.

Because cataracts are relatively common, many older people assume that any type of visual loss is caused by cataracts. This is not the case. For instance, macular degeneration is also a leading cause of severe vision problems in older people. In this condition, deterioration occurs in the central portion of the retina (the macula). This often leads to distortion in the center of the field of vision and a decreased ability to read or recognize faces. An ophthalmologist may be able to detect macular degeneration in its early stages.

Some forms of macular degeneration can be treated with lasers, which produce very bright light beams that can be precisely focused inside the eye, where they can destroy the abnormal blood vessels that cause these types of macular degeneration. If treatment is to be successful, however, early detection is essential. Older patients with any change in vision should have an examination very promptly. Waiting for the problem to disappear by itself has led many people to lose vision that might have been preserved had they sought medical help earlier.

Patients with certain medical disorders, like diabetes or high blood pressure, should be particularly careful to have frequent eye examinations. In general, patients with diabetes should be examined by an ophthalmologist every year since eye problems related to diabetes are a major cause of blindness. The disease may cause abnormal blood vessels to grow on the surface of the retina. These blood vessels are fragile and can break, producing bleeding inside the eye, with profound loss of vision. Laser treatment is highly effective in destroying the abnormal blood vessels, particularly in their early stages. Once again, it is clear that early detection of eye disease is the keystone of eye protection. □

PREVENTING EYE INJURY

Like disease, physical injury to the eye is a serious threat to vision, but most eye injuries can be prevented by proper precautions.

- Protective eyewear (goggles or safety glasses) should be worn whenever there is a threat of injury to the eyes. At work, such eyewear should always be used if it is provided or required by an employer. At home, such activities as hammering, sawing, and using power tools like drills or even lawn mowers call for protection. Sports like racquetball, squash, or hockey, in which a small, fast-moving ball or puck is used, should not be played without protective gear.
- Children and teenagers should not be allowed to play with fireworks or BB guns, which can produce exceptionally serious injuries that can lead to complete loss of vision in a damaged eye or even loss of the eye.
- The wrong kind of sunglasses can harm the eyes—glasses that let in relatively more ultraviolet radiation (UVR) than visible light. When there are low levels of visible light reaching the eye, the pupil dilates somewhat, allowing more UVR (which has been linked with cataract formation) to enter. Check to see that any sunglasses you buy screen out UVR.
- Good sunglasses are essential on the beach or in a sunny snowscape, where light intensity can be much greater than normal because of reflectance.
- Solar eclipses should never be directly viewed. Because the pupil dilates during the darkness of the eclipse, the eyes are especially vulnerable to the sun's rays when they return. The only safe way to see an eclipse is by projecting the sun's rays through a pinhole onto another surface.

New Ways to Take

Susan Carleton

When Mrs. Smith began taking nitroglycerin for occasional chest pains that had been diagnosed as angina, caused by an insufficient oxygen supply to the heart, she was afraid to go anywhere without a bottle of the little tablets. At the first sign of an attack, her doctor had told her, she was to pop a nitro pill under her tongue and try to relax until the pain subsided. The instructions were easy enough to follow, but Mrs. Smith, an 82-year-old widow who spent most of her day at home alone, was so anxious about losing the pills that her bouts of angina became more frequent.

Mrs. Smith's anxieties were eased a few years ago, when nitroglycerin became available in a new form—a patch that adheres to the skin, sold in the United States as Transderm-Nitro and Nitro-Dur. Now, by wearing a patch all the time, she doesn't have to worry about leaving her pills on her nightstand. As long as she remembers to change patches every night before going to sleep, her angina should remain under control. The patch, known as a transdermal drug delivery system, is designed to release nitroglycerin onto her skin at a steady rate for 24 hours; enough of the drug is absorbed through the skin and into the bloodstream to keep angina from occurring. The advantages are clear: transdermal delivery of nitroglycerin is designed to prevent rather than relieve the pain of angina and is also more convenient for patients like Mrs. Smith. (Some questions have arisen about the effectiveness of the patch, but it remains on the market while the manufacturers conduct additional tests at the request of the U.S. Food and Drug Administration.)

Pharmacology's New Frontier

This new way of taking nitroglycerin, a drug that has been used for most of this century in the treatment of angina, is part of a trend in pharmacology. Today's drug researchers are concentrating not only on the discovery of new compounds to treat diseases but also on the development of ways to make existing drugs available in more effective forms. By late 1985, besides nitroglycerin, one drug to fight motion sickness (scopolamine, sold in the United States as Transderm-Scōp and in Canada as Transderm-Z-V) and one high-blood-pressure medication (clonidine, sold as Catapres-TTS) were available in transdermal patches; a patch containing a synthetic form of estrogen for postmenopausal women was expected to be on the market shortly.

When delivery systems "target" drugs to specific sites in the body, lower doses can be used and dangerous side effects can be avoided.

Direct application of drugs to the skin is just one of the new routes for drug administration now in use or being tested. These nontraditional means of drug administration have become possible because of the development—in many cases, still experimental—of new devices that transport drugs to specific parts of the body. The devices, known as drug carriers, range from the deceptively simple transdermal patches to genetically engineered antibodies that deliver highly toxic drugs or radiation to specific sites in the body. Between those extremes are biodegradable membranes used to encase drugs and release them slowly and steadily after ingestion or implantation, as well as programmable electronic pumps that can be implanted beneath the skin, where, by means of a catheter, they infuse a drug to a specific site at a rate determined by the physician.

Advantages of New Methods

The traditional ways of taking drugs—orally, intravenously, or through injections into a muscle or beneath the skin—all have their problems, which vary from drug to drug. In general, the new technology overcomes these difficulties in three main ways.

- By targeting the drug, that is, getting the bulk of it to the place where it's needed without causing too many side effects. Most drugs in their present forms have a diffuse effect, working not only at the site of disease but in other parts of the body as well. In the case of some medications, such as anticancer drugs, this diffusion can cause serious side effects; with others, notably oral medications that must be processed by the liver, it simply means that a large dose is needed to get even a minimal effect. Delivery systems that target drugs to specific

Medicine

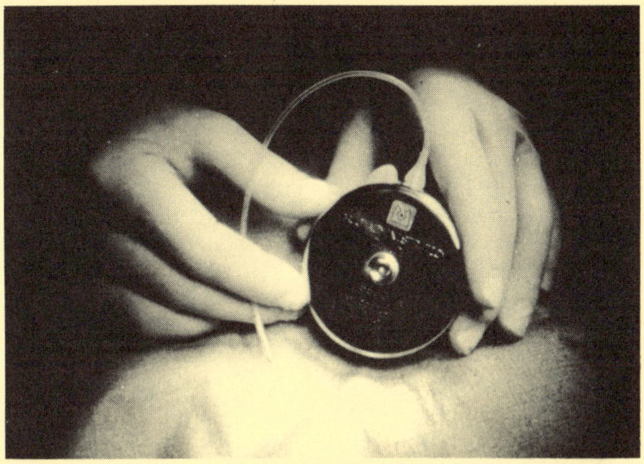

New drug delivery systems include (clockwise from right) a device implanted beneath the skin that pumps a supply of insulin, a disk worn in the eye like a contact lens that slowly releases a glaucoma medication, and a nitroglycerin patch for angina patients that adheres to the skin.

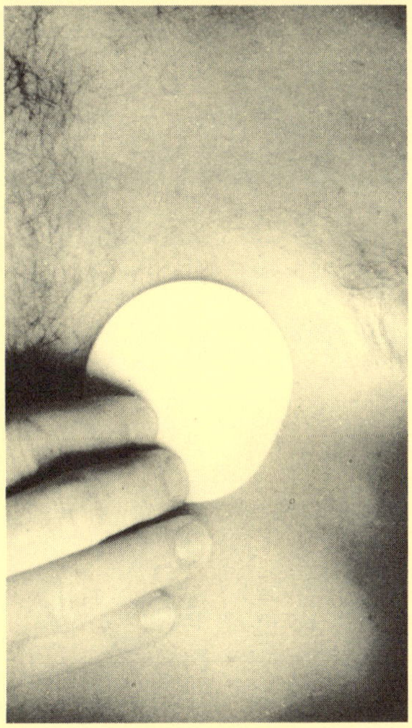

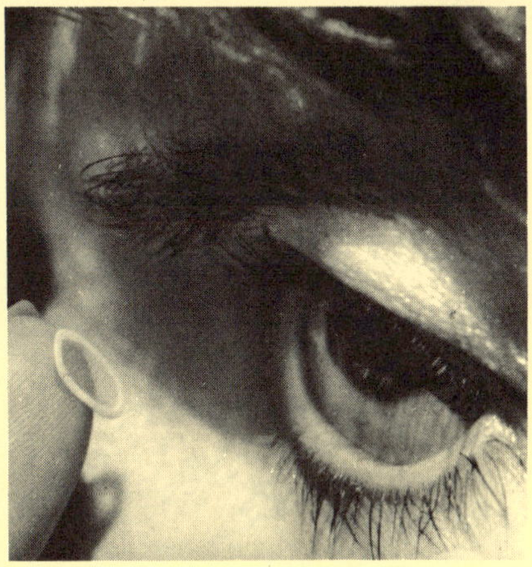

areas, however, permit larger doses of potentially toxic drugs to go directly to the area where their effects are desired. Drug targeting also permits medications to be given in smaller doses, since none of the drug's effect is lost as it passes through the digestive system.

- By controlling the rate of release, or delivering small amounts of the drug at a steady pace rather than large amounts periodically. The usual ways of taking drugs—pills and injections, in particular—make for a wide variation in the amount of medication in the bloodstream between doses. When the drug is at its low level, it may not be effective, whereas at its high level, it may cause side effects. Controlled release promises to even out these peaks and valleys and should also allow drug action to last indefinitely at its optimal level.
- By improving the odds that the drug will be used as intended. People are often lax about taking oral medications. Slow-release devices such as skin patches and permeable membrane coatings through which drugs can seep bit by bit sharply reduce the amount of attention a patient must pay to a medication schedule and thus minimize problems of patient compliance.

Making Adaptations

The process of adapting drugs to new delivery systems is slow because each drug has unique properties that must be taken into account. But rate-controlled devices are gradually being adapted to a wide range of drugs and uses, such as treating glaucoma: medication to decrease pressure in the eye is slowly released by a contact lens-type device worn for a week. In the area of contraceptives, a hormone-releasing intrauterine device sold as Progestasert is now commonly used in the United States and Canada. This IUD gets an enhanced contraceptive effect from the slow release of a synthetic form of progesterone, a hormone that makes the lining of the uterus inhospitable to fertilized eggs. Another contraceptive that uses synthetic progesterone is a beneath-the-skin implant developed by The Population Council. The device, called Norplant, consists of six separate rods of the hormone wrapped in a plastic-like material that allows the drug to seep out slowly. The rods, which are about 1½ inches long and a tenth of an inch in diameter, are implanted under the skin inside the upper arm. Within 24 hours, they begin providing contraceptive protection that can last up to five years. The drug usually prevents the monthly release of eggs by the ovaries. It also causes cervical and uterine changes that make it hard for sperm to fertilize any eggs that are released and for fertilized eggs to become implanted. Norplant has been approved for general use in several countries and has completed or is undergoing trials in 25 others, including the United States.

Several controlled-release oral medications have also made their way to the market. The concept of extending the time over which the drug in a pill is absorbed through the stomach is not a new one; slow-release forms of some medications in tablet or capsule form have been around since the 1950's. However, new controlled-released oral drug delivery systems employ a more sophisticated technology than the familiar "tiny time pills." One of the most interesting is called an oral osmotic pump, which consists of a core of drug and a semiporous plastic coating with a tiny, laser-punched hole in it. As water seeps through the coating, the drug is dissolved and released through the hole. By late 1985 a number of beta blockers (a type of heart medication) and an over-the-counter diet aid were already available in this form.

Implantable Pumps

One device that allows both rate control and targeting of medications is the implantable pump, several varieties of which have been developed. Although specific characteristics vary from one brand of pump to another, most of the pumps are round, measuring about 4½ inches in diameter and 1 inch thick. Within the pump is a drug reservoir with an opening for the catheter that delivers the drug, as well as some electronic circuitry and a power source, usually a battery. The physician implants the pump surgically, threading the catheter through an artery or vein to the area where the drug is to be delivered. Some of the devices beep when problems occur or when the drug level is low; when the drug runs out, the physician can refill the reservoir with a needle.

Patients are receiving several different drugs through implantable pumps. The pump system is ideal for anticancer drugs and is being used to deliver such compounds to tumors in the liver, breast, testicles, prostate, and lung. Physicians in several hospitals are also using pumps to deliver morphine to the spinal columns of cancer patients who need constant pain relief. Morphine administered this way has fewer side effects and provides a constant level of pain relief. Limited numbers of people with diabetes are receiving insulin through implantable pumps, and a few researchers are using pumps to deliver powerful antibiotics to treat severe infections. Other pump-delivered drugs include heparin, used to prevent or treat blood clotting; baclofen (Lioresal), an antispasmodic drug to control stiffness and spastic seizures; and dobutamine (Dobutrex), a drug for the treatment of congestive heart failure.

Slow-release oral medications now being developed are much more sophisticated than the familiar "tiny time pills."

More to Come

In the future, even more precise targeting of drugs should be possible with tiny molecular drug carriers called liposomes, which were first developed 20 years ago. The spherical liposomes, into which drugs can be placed, have an affinity for certain tissues, notably those of the liver and spleen. Researchers are investigating the use of liposomes to carry drugs to those areas.

Other investigators are looking at the possibility of combining drugs with laboratory-grown antibodies that can recognize and latch onto certain types of cells, such as tumor cells. Already, these antibodies are being used experimentally to carry radiation to tumors, and trials to determine how well they carry antitumor drugs are also under way. □

Six small rods of synthetic progesterone implanted in a woman's upper arm provide years of contraceptive protection.

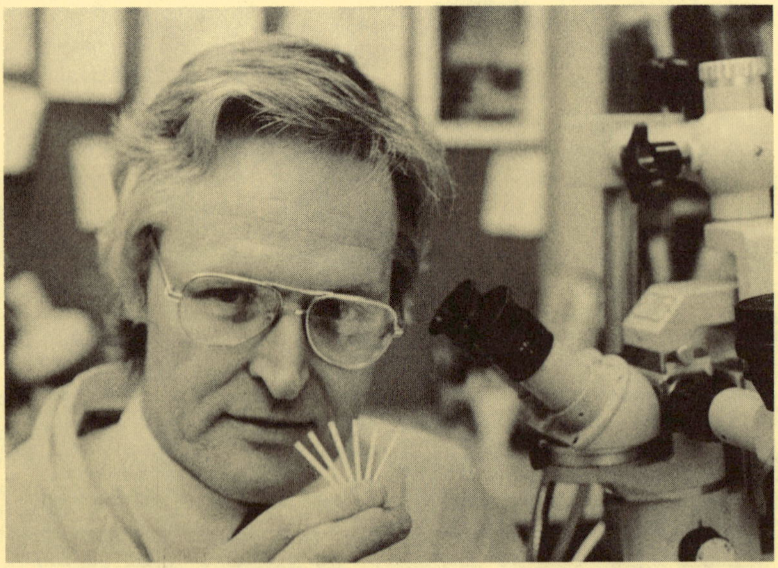

IUD's

Richard Hantula

Of all methods of contraception, the intrauterine device, or IUD, has been among the most controversial in recent years. No one doubts that it is highly effective. IUD's are used by millions of women around the world—as many as 60 million in China. In the United States, where they were introduced in the 1960's, IUD's were used by over 2 million women in 1982, the most recent year for which an authoritative estimate is available. But questions have been raised about their safety. Faced with a barrage of lawsuits alleging serious side effects from some IUD's, most manufacturers have withdrawn from the U.S. market.

The Device

The idea of preventing conception by putting an object in the uterus is centuries old. Development of the modern IUD began in the late 1950's with research on silver, stainless steel, and molded plastic devices of various sizes and shapes.

The modern IUD usually consists of a piece of plastic, around which, in newer versions, copper wire may be wound. Instead of copper, IUD's may also be "medicated" with silver (in some European types) or with a hormone. The medicating agent—metal or hormone—is slowly released from the IUD, enhancing its effectiveness. Although just how the IUD prevents pregnancy is unknown, it does so with a reliability of 95 to 98 percent. It is inserted by a physician in a brief office procedure. Manufacturers recommend that medicated IUD's be replaced every one to four years, depending on the device.

IUD's are almost as effective as sterilization and birth control pills and considerably more effective than condoms, diaphragms, foam, the sponge, or the rhythm method. Ideally, once the device is inserted, the woman can forget about it, aside from checking periodically to make sure it hasn't been expelled from the uterus.

Side Effects

Occasional side effects have always been associated with IUD's. Some women, particularly in the period after insertion, may experience bleeding or cramping, and there have been cases of the IUD puncturing the uterus, although this rarely happens when it is properly inserted.

Questions have been raised about the safety of IUD's.

The current controversy stems from other problems. IUD's bring an increased risk of infection—pelvic inflammatory disease (for most devices, largely in the first four months after insertion). PID ordinarily can be effectively treated with antibiotics but in some cases may lead to sterility and even death. A particularly high and long-lasting risk was found for the Dalkon Shield. This nonmedicated IUD, intended especially for women who had never had children, was sold from 1970 to 1974, when it was taken off the U.S. market by the manufacturer. Two studies published in 1985 confirmed that Dalkon Shield women had a relatively high rate of infertility caused by damage to the fallopian tubes from pelvic inflammatory disease. Two other nonmedicated IUD's, the Saf-T-Coil and the Lippes Loop, were also associated with subsequent infertility (although to a lesser degree) in women who had not had children. Little or no infertility was linked with copper IUD's.

Off the Market

The IUD industry's problems did not end with the withdrawal of the Dalkon Shield. The manufacturer (the A. H. Robins Company) in 1980 urged physicians to remove the devices from women still using them and in 1984 said it would pay all the medical costs of such removal. By the end of 1985, Robins had paid out $520 million in more than 9,000 lawsuits related to serious side effects, and some 5,000 suits were still pending. In August of that year Robins sought protection under Chapter 11 of the federal Bankruptcy Code.

The Saf-T-Coil was taken off the market by its manufacturer in 1982, and the Lippes Loop in 1985. According to industry sources, IUD sales accounted for less than 2 percent of the $1 billion U.S. contraceptive market in 1985. The Copper-7, which had become by far the most popular IUD, and the Tatum-T, another copper-bearing device, were removed from the U.S. market in 1986. G. D. Searle & Company, the maker of the two copper devices, attributed the withdrawal to the costs of defending itself against what it felt were unwarranted lawsuits—some 800 had been filed by early 1986—and the fact that liability insurance had become "virtually unobtainable."

Searle's move meant that the only IUD remaining on the U.S. market was the Progestasert, a T-shaped hormone-releasing IUD that was more expensive and had to be replaced annually. It had been selling at a rate of only about 100,000 a year. □

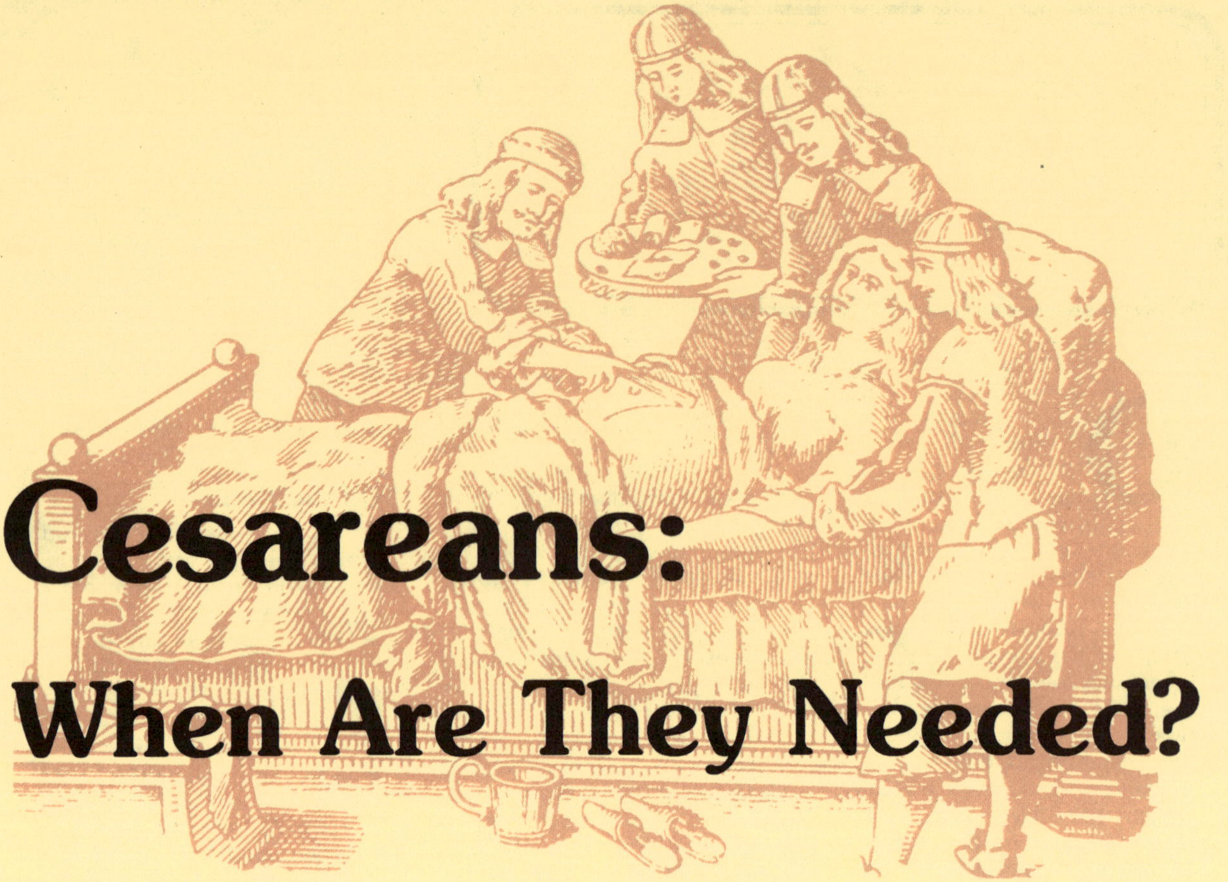

Cesareans: When Are They Needed?

Mortimer G. Rosen, M.D.

There are two methods by which an infant is born into the world: by natural birth through the vagina, or by cesarean, a major surgical procedure. During the past 20 years in the United States cesarean birth has, for many reasons, become increasingly common, growing from 4 to 6 percent of births in the mid-1960's to the current rate of more than 20 percent—one of the highest rates in the world. The trend has been similar in Canada, where cesareans accounted for nearly 18 percent of all births in 1983 (the latest figures available). The question of whether too many cesareans are being performed is now being widely debated.

What Is a Cesarean?

A cesarean is an abdominal operation performed under local or general anesthesia. The skin and the underlying fat and muscles are cut, and the abdominal cavity is entered. The uterus is then opened to remove the infant. There are two types of uterine incisions: the classical vertical incision, and the now far more common transverse (horizontal) incision in the lower uterus. The transverse incision is performed whenever possible, since it heals better and is less subject to rupture in a future attempt at labor and vaginal delivery.

Cesareans are relatively routine, but nevertheless, there are risks.

Surgical removal of a newborn through the abdomen is an ancient practice. Despite the popular belief that Julius Caesar was born by cesarean, this is not true. Roman law in the time of the Caesars, however, did mandate abdominal birth following the death of a mother in late pregnancy. In addition, the Latin *caedere,* "to cut," gives another possible origin for the word cesarean. The first successful cesarean, with survival of both mother and infant, was reputed to have been performed by a Swiss pig gelder about 1500, when his wife's midwife failed to deliver the baby because of an obstructed labor.

Maternal Risk and Infant Health

By the 1980's in the United States, cesarean delivery had evolved into a relatively routine operation, although a major one. Improved surgical techniques to maintain sterile conditions and control bleeding, greater safety in administering anesthesia and blood transfusions, and the availability of antibiotics for treating maternal infection have all combined to make cesarean childbirth a far safer option for mothers than ever before.

Nevertheless, there *is* risk. The incidence of maternal death in the United States is about 6 deaths per 100,000 live births after a normal delivery, while after an emergency cesarean delivery it is probably four times that. The maternal death rate after elective cesareans is twice that following vaginal birth.

Regarding the baby, if mortality rates from the 28th week of pregnancy to the 7th day of infant life over the past 50 years are reviewed, there is remarkable improvement. A great portion of that improvement is recent: in the United States the rate in 1983 was 11.2 deaths per 1,000 live births, compared with 23.2 in 1970; in Canada the 1983 rate was 9.5, compared with 21.8 in 1970. This improvement in what doctors call perinatal outcome has paralleled the rise in cesarean birth rates, and while direct proof is lacking, some of the improvement seems to be attributable to use of the cesarean procedure.

It must also be said, however, that a good deal more of the improvement in infant outcome is probably the result of advances in the medical care of pregnant women and, above all, the result of tremendous strides in caring for newborns. Fifty years ago a 5-pound baby was called premature and its life considered to be at risk. Today, the outcome for that child is as good as if it weighed 7 pounds. In fact, even a 1-pound baby has a good chance for survival today. Thus, only a small portion of the progress achieved can be ascribed directly to the increase in cesareans.

Reasons for Cesareans

The most common reason for a woman's first cesarean is difficult labor, known as dystocia and encompassing such problems as a birth canal that is too small, a fetus that is too large, or contractions of the uterus that are too weak to allow for a safe vaginal delivery.

The diagnosis of difficult labor is rather poorly defined and subject to wide variation in interpretation by the individual physician. The increased use of dystocia as a diagnosis is one of the major reasons cesarean birth rates have risen; it is thought to account for 30 percent of all cesareans.

Why Cesareans Are Done

Difficult labor: The birth canal is too small for the fetus, or contractions of the uterus are too weak.

Previous cesarean: The scar from an earlier cesarean could rupture during a vaginal delivery.

Fetal distress: The fetal monitor shows an abnormal fetal heartbeat, which could lead to oxygen deprivation and brain damage.

Breech birth: The baby's buttocks, rather than head, are closest to the vaginal opening.

Other reasons: Maternal illness, premature labor, low birth weight, rupture of the amniotic membranes, or blockage of the cervix by the placenta.

A prior cesarean is the second leading reason for a cesarean operation. Doctors have traditionally followed the practice of "once a cesarean, always a cesarean," primarily because of the fear that the uterine incision might rupture during labor. However, the low transverse incision that is in wide use today is much less susceptible to this risk. The 1980 consensus panel of the U.S. National Institutes of Health on cesarean births, as well as more recent investigators, have recommended that almost all women who have had a low transverse incision in a previous cesarean should be permitted to try labor and vaginal delivery, unless the circumstances that necessitated the first cesarean are expected to recur. A woman who experienced a breech presentation (a baby positioned backside first) in one pregnancy may not face the same circumstances with her next delivery. Similarly, dystocia that occurred in one pregnancy may not occur in the next (It should be noted as well that a previous cesarean adds risk, such as from premature labor or placental bleeding, to the fetus of the next pregnancy.)

Today, many more doctors are considering vaginal delivery for women who have had a previous cesarean, an approach supported by several lay groups formed around issues of cesarean birth. In most cases, allowing a mother a trial labor takes a willing doctor, an interested patient, and a hospital where a cesarean can be properly performed on short notice in case a previous uterine scar does rupture. A woman should discuss the options and risks with her obstetrician at the first office visit.

Fetal distress is another rather ill-defined diagnosis that often leads to a decision for a cesarean birth. If electronic monitoring devices used during labor indicate a possibly abnormal fetal heart rate, then the baby is considered to be at increased risk for various medical consequences. (Brain damage from an inadequate oxygen supply is one of the most serious of these consequences.) A cesarean may then be performed to avoid further risk to the baby. Most babies born by cesarean for fetal distress are healthy and grow up well. About 10 percent of all first cesareans are performed because fetal distress may be present.

Whether any baby in the breech position should be born vaginally is still an unsettled obstetrical issue. Today, 10 percent of all first cesareans in the United States are performed because of breech presentation, and about 60 percent of all babies in the breech position are born by cesarean (up from 12 percent in 1970). Explaining the risks and benefits of the two options to the mother often raises the fear, "What if the baby gets stuck by its head?" While this is certainly a risk, it is actually quite uncommon, as is brain damage from vaginal birth. However, when the baby is in the breech position, most physicians and patients choose cesarean delivery.

There are a host of other problems that may cause a doctor to choose the cesarean birth route, including maternal illness, premature labor with a low-birth-weight baby, and rupture of the amniotic membranes surrounding the fetus when labor has not started. It may sometimes be the method of choice in certain emergency situations, as, for example, in a condition known as placenta previa, when the placenta blocks the cervix, preventing normal birth. All such problems call for the doctor's best professional judgment, and choices other than cesarean may be available. When circumstances permit, the physician and family should discuss the specific problem ahead of time, to permit a decision that best suits the family's situation.

The Malpractice Issue

Surrounding the entire question of cesarean births—and probably influencing the number of cesareans—is the malpractice issue. A minimal risk of injury or death is the right of the fetus and the goal of the physician. To reach this goal—which in part reflects an increased societal emphasis on fetal health—physicians have resorted to cesareans more frequently than in the past.

It is also the case in the United States today that if anything has gone wrong during pregnancy, and especially during labor, the physician runs the risk of being sued for malpractice. In part this is the effect of confusion about the difference between malpractice, which involves negligence on the doctor's part, and a "poor outcome"—death or injury to the child or mother from any cause, including those that a physician might have little control over and that were once generally accepted as part of the normal risk

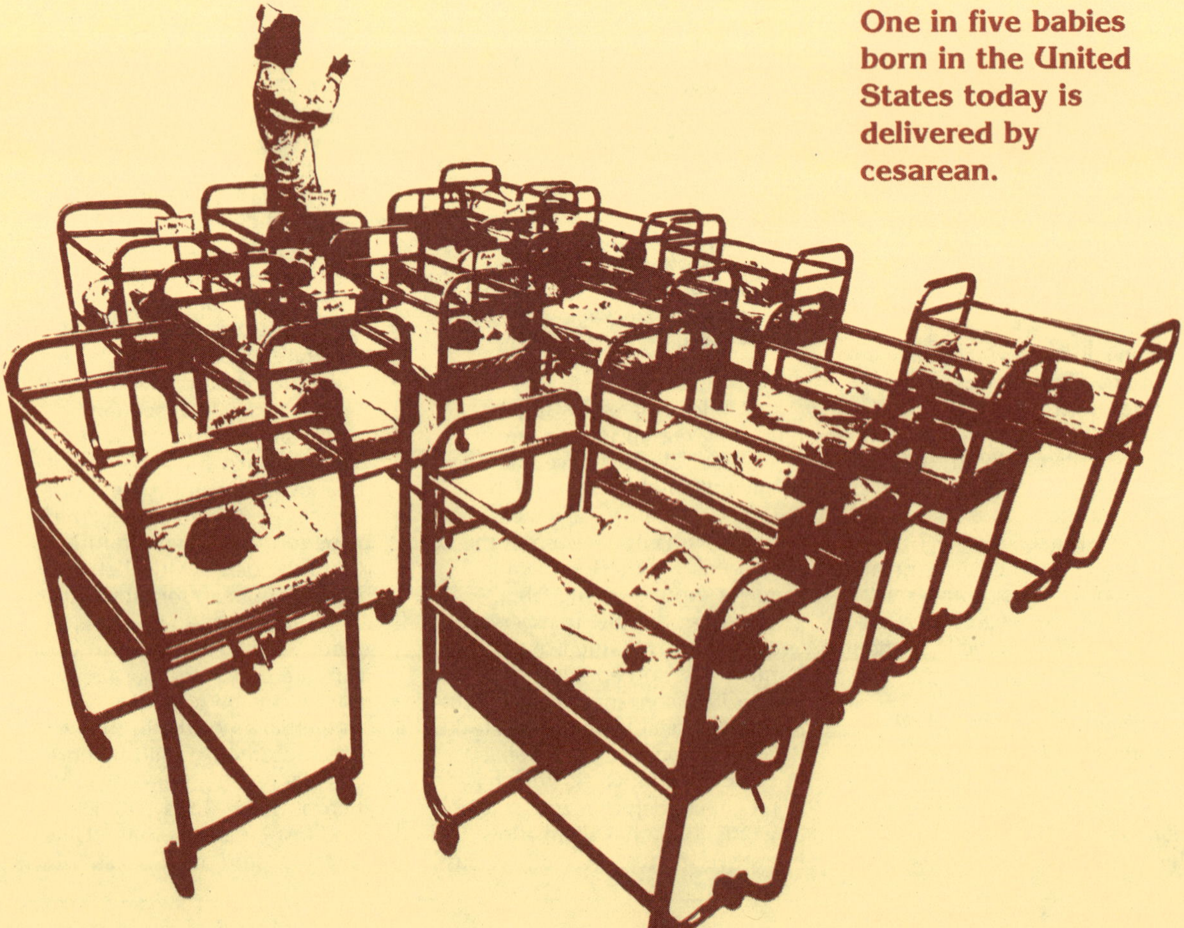

One in five babies born in the United States today is delivered by cesarean.

of having a baby. In the present legal environment it is quite likely that most instances of poor outcome will reach the litigation stage. Thus, fear of being sued influences how the birth is handled by the physician, who may feel more protected from a lawsuit if a cesarean has been performed. There is wide speculation that this nonmedical factor has altered obstetrical patient care and contributed importantly to the rising cesarean rates.

Recovering From a Cesarean

Convalescence following a cesarean is very different from that which follows a normal vaginal birth. After a vaginal birth, a mother often leaves the hospital in a day or two and resumes an almost normal level of activity. In contrast, after a cesarean, blood loss is at least twice that with a vaginal delivery, there is a higher incidence of infection, and, most important, the woman is unable to resume normal activity for perhaps two to three weeks or more. Hospitalization after delivery is two or three times longer, and there is a good deal of pain, which may persist for as long as a month. It may seem easier to have a baby by cesarean since delivery can often be scheduled and sometimes takes place before the onset of labor, but convalescence following surgery is slow and can be difficult.

Feelings After Delivery

The mother's emotional as well as physical reactions are different following a cesarean. The desire for a natural route of childbirth is very strong in most parents, and some mothers associate having a cesarean with failure in some sense. These women may experience prolonged depression in the postpartum period.

After a cesarean, future pregnancies often become an emotionally charged issue. A cesarean birth may lead to more limited family size, choice of a different physician, a search for different birthing environments, and—for a few families—the choice of home birth to avoid physician interference. Parents should seek information about what choices they have. However, choosing a home delivery in all cases places personal desires ahead of fetal rights. It does so by denying the fetus, in its sometimes risky passage through the vagina, the "safety net" of immediate emergency care that is available with a hospital delivery or with delivery in a birthing center affiliated with a full-service hospital.

Psychological studies of mother, father, and infant following a cesarean suggest that while the patterns of bonding (development of ties between parents and infant) that occur may differ from those following a vaginal delivery, they are not harmful. It appears that in the early postoperative period, although the mother may nurse and care for the child, the father gives more frequent and valuable care because the mother is under substantial and sometimes prolonged stress, pain, discomfort, and sedation. Once having entered the care-giving picture, the father remains there

Difficult labor is the most common reason for a first cesarean.

much longer, assuming more responsibilities during the entire first year than might otherwise be so. It must be stressed, however, that this possibly greater role for the father is not a reason for having a cesarean, even from the father's point of view.

A woman may wish to take the cesarean issue into consideration in choosing an obstetrician. She might inquire about the relative incidence of cesarean births at the doctor's hospital, whether previous cesarean mothers are offered an opportunity to deliver vaginally, what the physician's attitude is toward vaginal birth with breech presentations, and what the physician's rate is of cesarean deliveries. This kind of information should be available so that a woman may meet her personal needs in choosing a doctor.

Doctors today no longer automatically follow the traditional practice of "once a cesarean, always a cesarean."

An Ideal Cesarean Rate?

It is hard to believe that a 20 percent cesarean birth rate is medically required for American society. In some U.S. hospitals cesarean rates are higher than 35 percent; in contrast, other hospitals—even though they handle risky deliveries—have rates closer to 15 percent. Interestingly, it appears that the highest cesarean rates are in the healthiest segments of the population—those with the lowest incidence of risk.

Medical progress has brought a remarkable improvement in the safety of childbirth, both for the mother and for the newborn child. A parallel trend has been increased physician intervention in pregnancy and delivery, with one means of intervention being cesarean delivery. The cesarean has unquestionably contributed to the fact that so many more babies are now born alive and healthy. The question that remains unanswered is what is the "correct" cesarean birth rate in American society. The natural way of being born, and a more safe and appropriate way for the fetus as well as the mother, is still vaginal birth. □

How to Read Food Labels

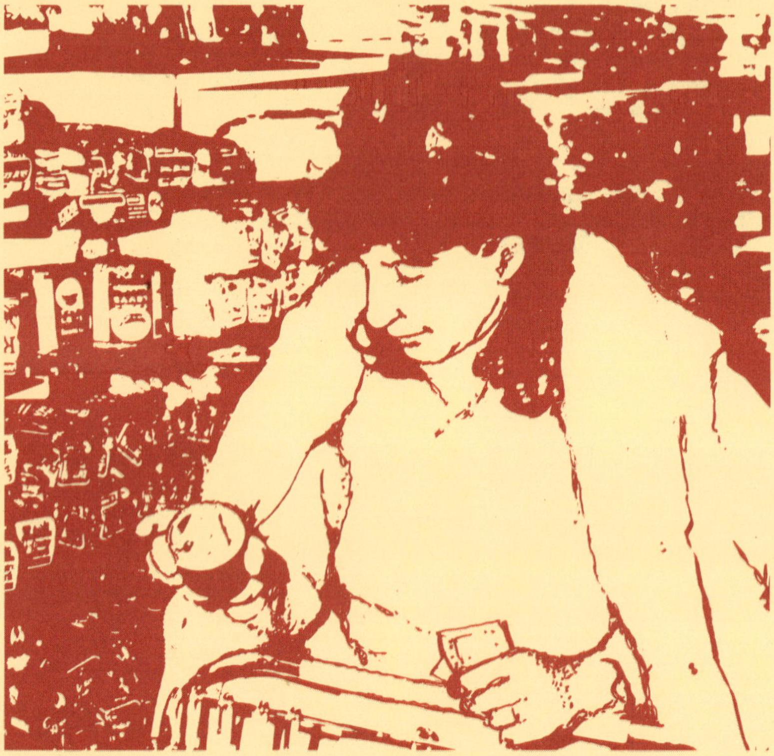

Robert Sorenson

In the not so distant past, it was a common practice to dilute milk with water or whiten bread with chalk—practices now outlawed by U.S. food regulations. However, a certain amount of knowledgeable caution can still be useful to consumers. The "light buttery taste" of pretzels may actually come from hydrogenated soybean and palm oils, and a cracker "made with whole wheat flour" may really have white flour as its most abundant ingredient. It is important for buyers both to read the fine print on food packages and to have some familiarity with the regulations that govern food labeling.

Label Information

The U.S. Food and Drug Administration (FDA) requires that all packaged foods display the name of the product, the net weight (for canned foods, this includes the liquid in which they are packed), and the name and address of the manufacturer, packer, or distributor. In addition, many foods must bear a list of ingredients, a nutrition label, or both. (Canadian regulations are basically similar to those in the United States but differ in many details.)

Many food processors have responded to the growing health-consciousness of consumers by lowering the fat, salt, or sugar content of their products. But sometimes only the label, not the product, seems healthier. While the use of many terms is regulated by the FDA, other terms are left to the discretion of a firm's advertising agency (see accompanying list).

Among the regulated phrases is "low-calorie" food, which can have no more than 40 calories per serving. According to regulations expected to go into effect in July 1986, "low sodium" will have to mean 140 milligrams or less per serving; "very low sodium," 35 milligrams or less; and "sodium free," less than 5 milligrams.

Food Standards

Most processed foods must carry a list of ingredients. However, products like ketchup and mayonnaise, which have had a "standard of identity" set for them by the FDA, are not required to do so. (Many manufacturers of these foods list ingredients on a voluntary basis.) About 300 such standards have been established, specifying mandatory and optional ingredients for products ranging from orange juice to blue cheese.

The standard for jam, for instance, stipulates that the product must be at least 45 percent fruit and no more than 55 percent sugar. Products that have too little fruit to meet the jam standard must be called by another name—like strawberry spread—or must include the word "imitation" on the label. A fruit beverage that is not 100 percent juice (aside from possible sweeteners) must be called a juice drink, or a fruit-flavored drink; the last need not contain any juice whatsoever. Items that are not manufactured according to the standards for various cheeses must be called cheese products or cheese foods—though some of these have standards of their own.

Any optional ingredients permitted by a food standard must be listed on the label if added by the processor.

The List of Ingredients

All processed foods except those that meet an FDA standard must list their ingredients on the package. The list must be in descending order (by weight), with the most abundant ingredient first and the least abundant, often a preservative or a dye, last. If you are attempting to cut down on your sodium intake, avoid foods with salt or other sodium compounds anywhere near the top of the list. People attempting to avoid some other types of foods—fats or sugar, for example—need to know more about what to look for.

Salad dressing, spaghetti sauce, and many snack crackers—to say nothing of breakfast cereals—are among the foods that often include a high proportion of sugar. But sugar is a substance with many aliases—including corn syrup, corn sweeteners, fructose, dextrose, sucrose, maple syrup, and honey—so a high sugar content may not be immediately obvious. If corn syrup, fructose, and dextrose all appear on an ingredients list, the total sugar content may be quite high even though each individual sweetener comes some way down the list.

Manufacturers may not add sugar to any product labeled "sugar-free" or "unsweetened," although these items may contain sugar that occurs naturally in some foods. The artificial sweetener saccharin requires a special label warning that it is associated with cancer in animals.

Cholesterol, a fatlike substance linked with heart disease, is found in meat, dairy products, and egg yolks; in addition, meat and dairy products can be high in saturated fats, which raise cholesterol levels in the blood. If you are concerned about cholesterol, you should look for any of these items on an ingredients list, as well as for various animal fats, like lard, suet, and tallow.

SLOGANS AND SUBSTANCE

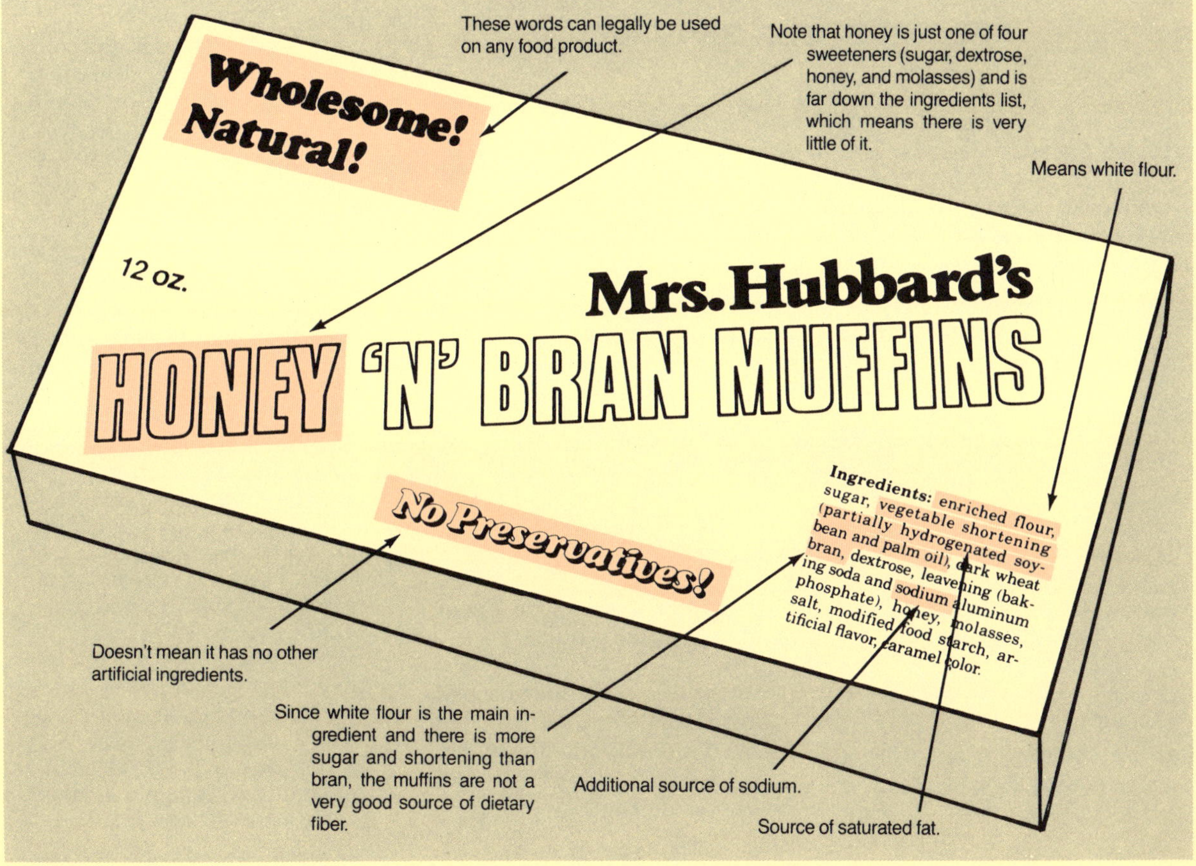

Coconut and palm oils are also high in saturated fats, as are any hydrogenated oils and shortening. Polyunsaturated and monounsaturated fats, for all the calories they can add to a diet, tend to lower blood cholesterol levels (monounsaturated fats may be preferable). Sunflower, corn, soybean, and safflower oils are highly polyunsaturated. Highly monounsaturated fats include peanut oil and olive oil.

Additives

Many ingredients lists conclude with chemical tongue twisters and exotic products home cooks never use, from propylene glycol alginate to guar gum. Additives like these are used to modify a food's texture, flavor, or color, improve keeping qualities, or increase nutritive value. Most additives have legitimate purposes and are safe, but a few can be cause for concern.

For example, about 100,000 people in the United States are allergic to the dye known as yellow No. 5, which must therefore be listed specifically if included in a product (other dyes may be listed as "artificial color"). Some people are allergic to and must watch for the preservatives sulfur dioxide and sodium bisulfite, and some consumers prefer to avoid other additives. The preservatives called BHA and BHT have raised concern because rats fed with them in a laboratory study developed enlarged livers. The nitrites that have been used for centuries in curing meats like bacon and ham contribute to the formation of cancer-causing chemicals called nitrosamines in our bodies, but they are important for preventing botulism, a deadly form of food poisoning. The FDA decided in 1980 that the benefits of nitrites outweighed the risk.

Only some terms that appear on packaged foods are regulated by the FDA.

Nutrition Labels

Any fortified food, and any food that claims to provide health benefits, must carry the following nutritional information: the number of servings in the package, the size of the portion, the number of calories each portion contains, and the weight in grams of protein, carbohydrates, and fat in each serving. The label must also show the percentage in each serving of the U.S. Recommended Daily Allowance (U.S. RDA) of protein, five vitamins, and two minerals. Regulations expected to take effect in July 1986 will require that nutrition labels also list the amount of sodium per serving. Manufacturers have the option of also giving the U.S. RDA percentage per serving of 12 other vitamins and minerals, as well as the amount of cholesterol and other types of fat.

Nutrition labels can help you ensure an adequate intake of nutrients and keep down your consumption of fats and salt. It should be understood, however, that the U.S. RDA's are based on average nutritional needs of people above the age of four; adolescents, pregnant women, and nursing mothers need more of several nutrients. On the other hand, the U.S. RDA's have been set at generous levels; many adults need only 75 percent of them. Nor is it necessary to take in the recommended amount of every nutrient every day; as long as your diet includes sufficient nutrients over a period of about a week, it should be adequate. □

LET THE BUYER BEWARE

Some words put on food labels have no legal meaning in the United States and may be used to describe any type of food:

Light (lite) does not necessarily mean the product has fewer calories than comparable items.

Natural does not necessarily mean the product contains no additives (although flavorings or colorings called natural must be derived from foods rather than synthesized).

Organic, health food can be used to describe foods grown with chemical fertilizers and pesticides.

Wholesome does not necessarily mean the product is better made or better for you than other food.

Some words don't mean exactly what they appear to:

Flavor, taste may be deceptive. "Cheese-flavored" does not necessarily mean real cheese was used, and there may be no butter in a product with a "buttery taste." (Check the ingredients list.) Also, a product with "100 percent natural flavor" may be otherwise 100 percent artificial.

Made with . . . means only that there is some of the ingredient named in the product; a muffin "made with honey" may be sweetened chiefly with sugar.

Sleepwalking

Anthony Kales, M.D.

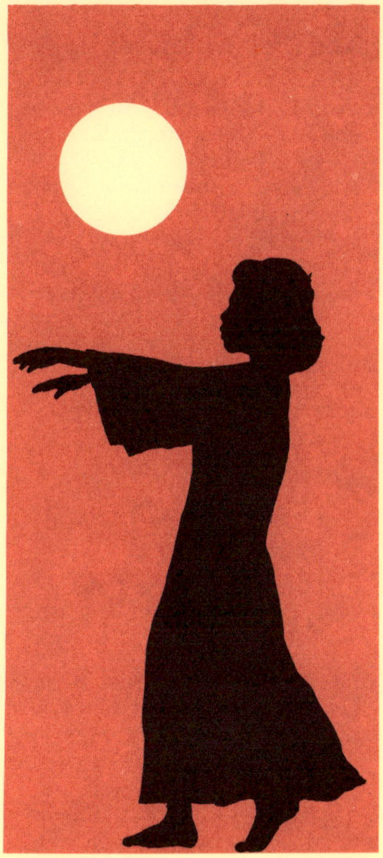

I have known many persons in sleep . . . some jumping up and fleeing out of doors, and deprived of their reason until they awaken, and afterward becoming well and rational as before, although they be pale and weak; and this will happen not once but frequently." This description of sleepers written by the Greek physician Hippocrates over 2,000 years ago reveals how long physicians have been concerned with the sleepwalking phenomenon. Examples of sleepwalkers (also called somnambulists) can be found in *Macbeth,* in which the sleepwalking Lady Macbeth relives the horrors of the night that murder was committed, and in Bellini's opera *La Sonnambula,* in which a woman's sleepwalking leads to comic entanglements.

Interest in sleepwalking has sometimes prompted extreme speculation about its causes. The influence of the moon was once thought to induce sleepwalking; somnambulists who walked when the moon was full were said to be "moon walking" or "moonstruck." Erroneous beliefs some people hold today are that sleepwalking represents the acting out of a dream or that the sleepwalker is capable of performing extraordinary physical and mental feats.

What Is Sleepwalking?

Sleepwalking is a disorder involving impaired arousal from sleep. During a sleepwalking episode, the person's motor functions and mental abilities are at very low levels. Basically, in sleepwalking the sleeping and waking states are combined.

The typical episode occurs within the first three hours of sleep. The sleepwalker sits up, gets out of bed, and moves about in a slow, poorly coordinated, automatic manner. Sometimes there is more complex activity, such as dressing, eating, or urinating, which takes place out of its usual context and reflects the sleepwalker's general lack of awareness.

During the episodes, which usually last for several minutes, the sleepwalker is exposed to potential injury because of the low level of coordination, thinking, and reactions to even strong stimuli. The somnambulist appears dazed, confused, and unresponsive and occasionally engages in repetitive and purposeless activity. Sometimes the sleepwalker's actions are agitated and—rarely—even violent. Although most sleepwalking events are confined to the home, in about 15 percent of the episodes the individual wanders outside.

Sleepwalking is a disorder involving impaired arousal from sleep: in essence, the sleeping and waking states are combined.

The sleepwalker is usually hard to awaken, and awareness returns only gradually; a sleepwalker who has just been awakened is often confused and disoriented. Unless sleepwalkers become fully aroused, they usually cannot remember the episode, although in some adult somnambulists there may be a partial recall of the event. There is rarely more than one episode per night.

Somnambulism generally—although not always—begins in childhood. About 5 to 15 percent of the population is estimated to have sleepwalked as children. In many cases the episodes are isolated and not likely to cause parents to become concerned.

Usually, in children who have more than isolated episodes, sleepwalking occurs frequently for several years, after which there is a gradual decline in frequency or an abrupt termination of sleepwalking. Sleepwalking that is outgrown almost always began before age ten. If sleepwalking continues into adulthood, as it does in about 20 percent of cases, the episodes usually occur less frequently.

The Risk of Injury

Although sleepwalkers do not often injure themselves during their episodes, when injuries do occur they can be extremely serious and even life-threatening. There have been incidents of sleepwalkers falling down stairs, off cliffs, and out of windows; burning themselves against a grill or oven; running through a screen door; and walking out the back of a moving camper. The risk of injury during sleepwalking poses special problems for adults, who may attempt to drive, and for those serving in the armed forces, especially in hazardous circumstances—on board ship, for example.

Children who sleepwalk generally do not have significant psychological problems and therefore need no treatment.

Causes

Although not a great deal is known about why sleepwalking occurs, a number of factors that contribute to its development have been determined. Hereditary, developmental, physical, and psychological factors all appear to play a role. The role of heredity is shown by the large number of families in which more than one person is or has been a sleepwalker. Physical factors are suggested by the occasional sleepwalking case that begins after a fever.

In children who stop sleepwalking by adolescence, an inherited predisposition and immaturity (that is, relatively slow development) of the central nervous system seem to be the primary factors. In people who begin sleepwalking in adolescence or especially in young adulthood, and in those who continue to sleepwalk as adults, psychological factors seem to be the predominant reason for the disorder. Regardless of the origin of the problem, psychological, physical, and environmental factors can affect the frequency and severity of episodes.

It is unusual for sleepwalking to begin in the middle aged or elderly; if it does, an underlying disorder, such as a brain tumor, may be the cause, and this possibility should be investigated by a doctor. A condition very similar to sleepwalking sometimes occurs in people taking the antimanic medication lithium carbonate and relatively high doses of so-called neuroleptic drugs.

Treatment and Protection

Because of the sleepwalker's minimal critical skills and relative unawareness of the surroundings, family members should take steps to reduce the risk of injury to the sleepwalker. Safety measures should include special latches for outside doors, sleeping accommodations on the ground floor, secure locks for bedroom windows, and the removal of potentially dangerous objects. Groups such as summer camps or boarding schools that are responsible for a child's safety away from home should be informed by parents if the child is a sleepwalker and instructed how to take appropriate safety precautions.

Safety precautions should be taken to reduce the risk of accidental injury to the sleepwalker.

Generally, sleepwalkers return to their own room; if not, they can usually be gently led back. Should a sleepwalker be awakened? Probably not: awakening somnambulists may frighten them, though more often it leaves them puzzled, confused, and at a loss to explain their behavior. Episodes should not be interrupted if previous interference has caused confusion or fright. Such attempts to intercede may actually increase the risk of injury.

In most cases sleepwalking begins and ends during childhood.

Since children who are sleepwalkers generally do not have significant psychological problems, and since they usually outgrow the disorder within a few years, psychiatric treatment is often unnecessary. It is important for the parents of a child who is a sleepwalker to be reassured of this and to avoid treating the problem as a psychological disturbance.

If, on the other hand, the episodes are frequent or persistent, or if there is evidence of disturbed behavior and sleepwalking seems to be triggered by stressful events, then parents should consult a family physician, pediatrician, or child psychiatrist.

Adult sleepwalkers are typically people who cope with frustrations by taking some action rather than struggling with problems within themselves. Psychotherapy to develop the sleepwalker's ability to react to stressful events constructively can be beneficial, and certain anxiety-reducing drugs may also help some adult somnambulists.

If adult sleepwalking is infrequent and has persisted from childhood or adolescence, generally no treatment is needed beyond safety precautions. However, if sleepwalking is more frequent or if it begins in adulthood, a physician should be consulted. □

What Is Hyperactivity?

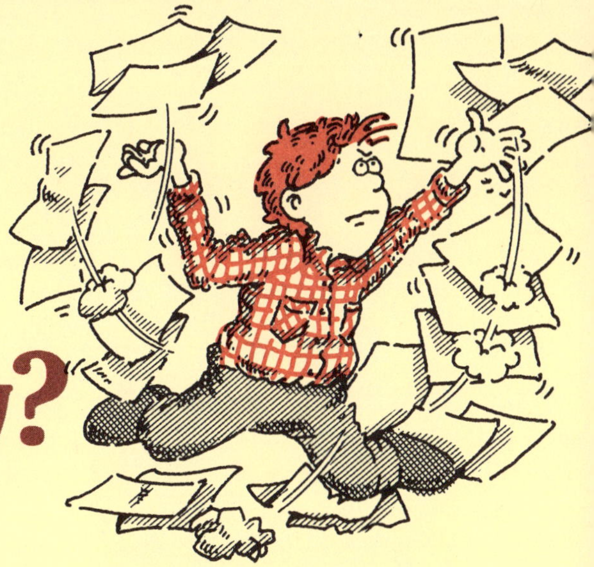

Daniel J. Kindlon, Ph.D., and
Michael Yogman, M.D.

Hyperactivity is one of the most common behavior problems that pediatricians, child psychologists, and child psychiatrists see among school-age children. The problem is technically known as attention deficit disorder with hyperactivity. The hyperactive child has a short attention span and is easily distracted, often acts without thinking, and seems to be constantly in motion. Short attention span and distractibility may also be present without the excessive motion of hyperactivity, in which case the problem is called simply attention deficit disorder.

Hyperactivity occurs in approximately 3 percent of preadolescent children and is ten times more common among boys than among girls. (The frequency of attention deficit disorder without hyperactivity is not known.) Parents will usually notice a problem by the time the child is three, but such children often don't get any professional help until they start school. Their behavior can vary, and they may appear quite normal at times, especially in structured situations, such as during a short examination in a doctor's office. The problem may or may not continue as the child grows older. All the symptoms may persist into adolescence and adult life, they may disappear completely at puberty, or the hyperactivity may cease at puberty while attention problems and impulsive behavior remain.

Poor Concentration

Children with attention problems have great difficulty concentrating and often fail to finish what they start—even tasks they enjoy or find interesting. Many are constantly distracted by other sights and sounds, as if it is impossible for them to filter out extraneous events. Thus, they cannot pay attention long enough to complete even simple tasks without adult supervision. A common complaint is that they cannot get dressed by themselves; they have to be told to put on each individual article of clothing.

With their tendency to act impulsively, children with attention problems may not be able to wait their turn in a game, may call out during class, or may not be able to stop themselves from using profanity. They often make careless mistakes in their schoolwork and find problems that require even a little reflection very difficult to solve.

Hyperactive children often have learning and emotional problems.

Always on the Go

True hyperactive children are always on the go, much more so than normal children—whose activity level, to begin with, is high by adult standards. Hyperactive children act as if they were driven by a motor. They have a hard time staying seated, and if they manage it, they often fidget or move about in their chairs. They may have trouble sleeping or move about excessively during sleep. Hyperactive children are usually accident-prone.

Because of their difficulties in paying attention and controlling their impulses, children with attention deficit disorder, whether or not they are hyperactive, often have academic and emotional problems. A classroom setting taxes their attention span severely, and they quickly fall behind—even though they may be of average or above-average intelligence. It is also not uncommon for these children to have other learning disabilities, such as problems with reading, spelling, or arithmetic, which make their academic progress that much more difficult.

Teachers and their fellow pupils often see them as bad, mean, or stubborn because of their difficulty in following rules. Other children tend to dislike them because they often seem immature and may be bossy and unable to control their tempers. Failure in school and poor relations with

What Parents Should Know

What is hyperactivity?

Hyperactivity, or more precisely, attention deficit disorder, is a condition whose main signs are an inability to pay attention, impulsive behavior, and seemingly constant motion. The attention problems may also occur without the excessive activity.

When is the child's problem detectable?

In most cases by the age of three.

How common is hyperactivity?

One in 35 children in the United States is hyperactive. The problem is ten times more common among boys than among girls.

What causes hyperactivity?

The exact cause is unclear, but many doctors believe problems within the nervous system are involved.

Can anything be done about it?

Yes. A range of treatments from behavior therapy to special educational services to psychotherapy can be beneficial. Certain drugs may be useful in some cases.

Is a special diet helpful?

Research has not established that a diet free of, say, food additives or sugar reduces hyperactivity.

peers can obviously lead to a poor self-image and emotional problems that may be manifested in various forms—including anxiety, depression, and antisocial or aggressive behavior.

The strengths these children have are often overshadowed by a constant focus on their attention problems. This is extremely counterproductive: focusing on and using such children's strong points is the way to improve their self-esteem and alleviate their emotional problems.

Causes

The precise cause of attention deficit disorder, with or without hyperactivity, is unknown. Many doctors believe that such behavior comes about because of problems within the central nervous system, and in the past attention deficit disorder was called minimal brain dysfunction. Children with attention disorders may show signs of poor coordination, which may reflect some nervous system immaturity. However, a specific neurological problem is diagnosed in only 5 percent of cases.

Recent research does suggest that chemical abnormalities in the nervous system may be responsible for the symptoms. Also, studies of families in which the problem is present and studies comparing its occurrence in identical twins (who have exactly the same genes) and fraternal twins (who have different genes) give evidence of some hereditary factor in the problem.

Making Sure of the Problem

One reason for the difficulty in determining the cause or causes of attention deficit disorder is that the condition has a wide range of symptoms, some of which can stem from other problems. A group of children to be studied may be selected on the basis of similar symptoms—for example, an excessive level of activity and impulsive behavior—with the researchers assuming that the children all have the same disorder. However, on closer examination, it may become apparent that the children's behavior can have different explanations. A child from a problem home, who has little opportunity to learn appropriate behavior and may have emotional problems as well, may be overactive, impulsive, and aggressive. Yet the child's problems may well be brought about by a poor environment, while those of other overly active children are believed to originate in the nervous system, even if precisely how is unknown.

It should be emphasized that a great many children who are hard to control and show some of the symptoms of hyperactivity have problems that are basically emotional; these children should not be treated in the same way as those with neurological problems.

Treatment

Effective treatment of attention deficit disorder is best achieved through a multidisciplinary approach, possibly including a number of different means of treatment.

- ***Behavior therapy.*** Providing a supportive, structured environment is a key ingredient in treating children with attention disorders. Parents should set clear and consistent rewards and punishments for specific desirable and undesirable actions, which helps children learn to control their own behavior. For example, parents can reward each step of the dressing sequence (pants, shirt, socks, and so on) with a token that can later be redeemed for something the child wants, such as time watching television. Such a system of rewards and punishments is usually established with the help of school personnel and a psychologist.
- ***Family counseling.*** Parents may need professional guidance in how to provide an appropri-

ately structured home environment. Children with attention problems often strain family relations, and counseling or family therapy can be beneficial for dealing with such strains. For example, counseling may help parents realize that they are angry with their child or that they are blaming each other for the problem.

- ***Special education services.*** Children with attention deficit disorder benefit from structured academic settings and strategies designed to help them learn organizational skills. Small classes or individualized instruction helps focus their attention, and learning simple, step-by-step procedures for completing assignments helps them develop their organizing abilities. In severe cases, the child may be best served by a residential treatment facility.
- ***Psychotherapy.*** Children who also have emotional problems often benefit from treatment by a psychologist, clinical social worker, or psychiatrist to help them recognize and cope more effectively with their difficulties.
- ***Drug treatment.*** Many children diagnosed as having attention deficit disorder are treated with drugs that reduce their activity level and impulsive behavior. Common medications are dextroamphetamine (sold as Dexedrine), methylphenidate (Ritalin), and pemoline (Cylert). Possible side effects of these drugs include suppression of appetite, mild slowing of growth, insomnia, and high blood pressure. There is evidence to indicate that some children become sad or less sociable as a result of treatment; on the other hand, peer relations may improve because the child becomes more well-liked with an improvement in behavior. Drug therapy should always be accompanied by treatments designed to improve the child's functioning in the home and school environments. As drug treatment makes the child more attentive, the psychological and academic measures taken to help the child should also become more effective.

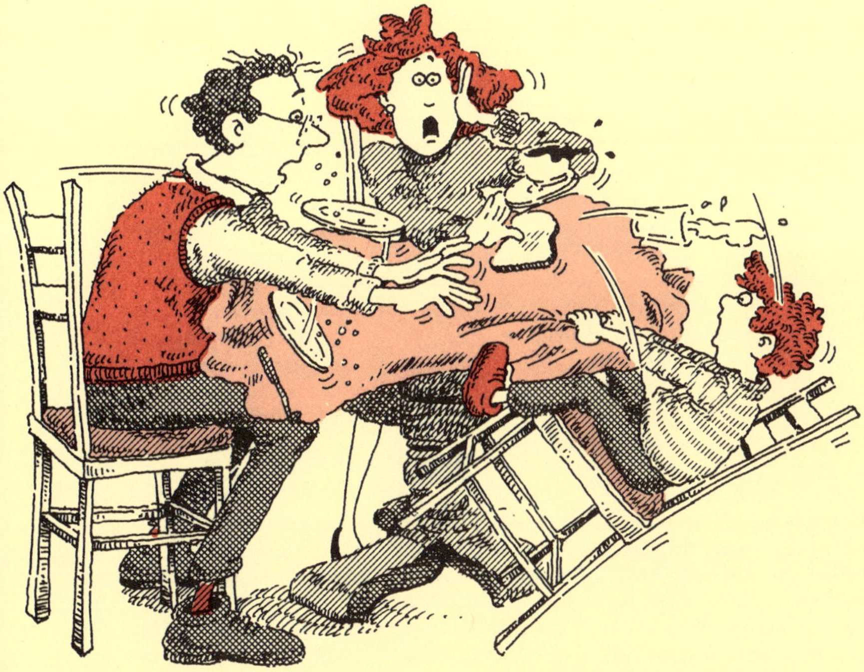

Parents may need family counseling to cope with the strain caused by a hyperactive child.

Diet and Behavior

Some doctors have suggested that diet—in particular, foods with artificial colors and flavors—may contribute to hyperactivity and that special diets eliminating such foods should be used as a treatment for hyperactivity (the best known is called the Feingold diet). A conference held on the subject by the U.S. National Institutes of Health found that no definite conclusions about the relation between diet and hyperactivity could be drawn at present, but the conference members did not rule out the possibility that some children could benefit from a special diet. The conference emphasized that traditional treatments should be carefully considered before any diet therapy program. Some doctors have suggested that the benefit children seem to get from a change in diet may actually arise from the increased attention they receive when their parents carefully select what they eat.

Although some doctors have suggested that eating sugar influences a child's activity level, there is no conclusive evidence for this. (In general, though, a high-sugar diet is not recommended for children unless there is a specific medical reason.) □

Suggestions for Further Reading

RENSHAW, DOMEENA C. *The Hyperactive Child.* Chicago, Nelson-Hall, 1974. Paperback: Boston, Little, Brown, 1975.

STEWART, MARK A., and SALLY W. OLDS. *Raising a Hyperactive Child.* New York, Harper & Row, 1973.

Prostate Problems

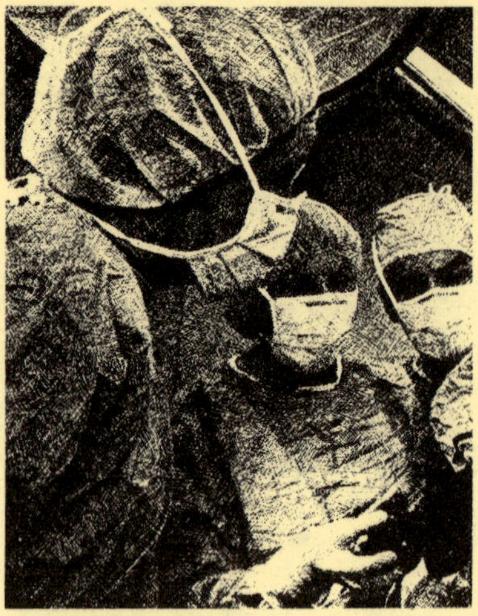

Leonard David Gaum, M.D.

The prostate gland is a male sexual organ whose sole function is to manufacture and store fluid that helps convey sperm during ejaculation. The prostate surrounds the urethra (the tube that carries urine from the bladder) at the point where it leaves the bladder. In size and shape the normal adult prostate gland resembles a horse chestnut; it is about an inch and a half in diameter and weighs less than an ounce.

For an organ with such a limited function, the prostate can cause a great deal of trouble, particularly in older men. Enlargement or inflammation of the prostate gland is increasingly common after the age of 40, and two out of three men over 70 have prostate problems of some kind. Cancer of the prostate is the third leading cause of cancer deaths, and the chances of developing it increase dramatically with age.

Benign Enlargement

Benign enlargement of the prostate (in medical terms, benign prostatic hypertrophy) is the most common cause of bladder obstruction in men. It is called benign to distinguish it from prostate cancer, but the effects can be quite serious. If the gland becomes large enough and presses on the urethra, the flow of urine can be impeded. Patients may have to urinate more frequently and may have difficulty beginning and ceasing urination, with dribbling afterward. (Sometimes these difficulties develop so slowly that they are hardly noticed.) The pool of residual urine that can result from failure to empty the bladder promotes infection and may ultimately lead to kidney failure.

The prostate gland manufactures and stores the fluid that carries the sperm during ejaculation.

Since the prostate is next to the rectum, rectal examination allows a physician to determine the size, shape, and consistency of the gland. Urine can be tested for infection, and X rays can supply information on how much urine is retained in the bladder. Other tests may be done as well. In a procedure called cystourethroscopy a fiber-optic tube is inserted into the urethra; this allows direct visual determination of the degree of bladder obstruction.

An enlarged prostate does not require treatment in every case. But if retention of urine in the bladder or incontinence is a serious problem, if kidney function is impaired, if there has been recurrent infection, or if there has been bleeding from dilated blood vessels near the prostate, surgery is generally called for. Various medications have been tried as an alternative, but the results have been too inconsistent and the side effects too troublesome to make drugs an acceptable treatment.

If an operation to remove excess prostate tissue is needed, two major approaches are available. Surgery may be done through the urethra (known as a closed approach) or through an external incision (open approach). The type of surgery performed depends on such factors as the size and shape of the prostate, the state of the urethra, and the presence or absence of other conditions, like bladder stones or obesity. In most cases, surgery for an enlarged prostate does not make the patient impotent.

Inflammation

Prostatitis, or inflammation of the prostate, has long been a problem, and despite recent advances, many doctors remain perplexed about how to diagnose and treat this condition. The cause of prostatitis is unclear, but it is probably most often precipitated by infectious organisms that ascend the urethra and are drawn into the prostate with infected urine.

Most inflammations of the prostate fall into one of four categories: acute and chronic bacterial prostatitis, nonbacterial prostatitis and a condition called prostatodynia. Diagnosis is based on examination of the prostate and analysis of the fluid it secretes. In bacterial prostatitis, the fluid generally yields bacteria that can be cultured in the laboratory and thus identified.

Treatments vary for different types of prostatitis, or inflammation of the prostate.

Patients with acute bacterial prostatitis tend to have chills and fever, pain in the lower back and in the region of the prostate, irritation on urinating, and varying degrees of urinary obstruction. The prostate gland itself will be tender and enlarged. Acute inflammation may require hospitalization. Aside from measures to control symptoms, the basic therapy is intravenous or oral antibiotics for at least 30 days to prevent the development of chronic bacterial prostatitis.

Although the symptoms of chronic bacterial prostatitis are variable, they are similar to those of acute inflammation. While symptoms may be controlled by antibiotics, they often reappear when medication is discontinued. Long-term therapy (12 weeks) with a combination of two antibiotics, trimethoprim and sulfamethoxazole, has proved more successful than short-term therapy. Some patients may benefit from continuous low doses of other antibiotics. If drug treatment is not successful, surgery to remove the infected portion of the prostate may be necessary.

Nonbacterial prostatitis is the most common form of prostate inflammation. In such cases, microscopic examination of the prostate fluid reveals a high count of white blood cells or other signs of inflammation. But, though the symptoms are about the same as in bacterial prostatitis, laboratory tests show no evidence of bacterial infection. Researchers have tried to identify nonbacterial organisms causing the condition, but the findings have been inconclusive.

Since the cause of nonbacterial prostatitis is unknown, therapy is difficult. Antibiotics may be tried if an infectious agent is suspected, but if they do not produce a response within a short time, therapy is limited to sitz baths (hot-water tub baths), drugs to relax the bladder, and anti-inflammatory drugs such as aspirin. The condition is not a life-threatening one, and the patient is encouraged to maintain normal sexual activity and exercise. There are no dietary restrictions unless it is found that spicy foods or alcohol increase irritation on urinating.

The Prostate's Location

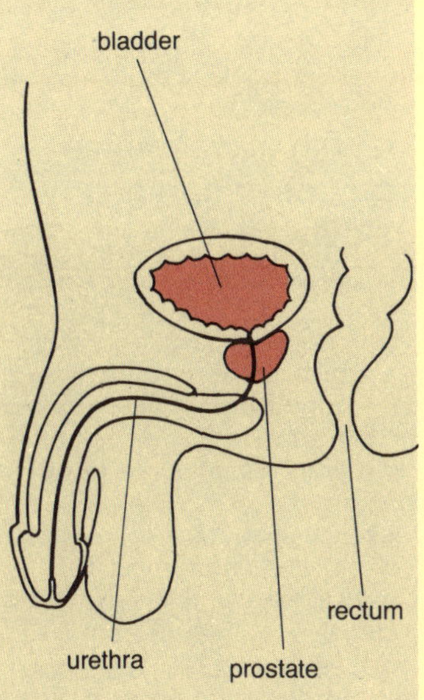

Since prostate cancer often shows no symptoms, it is important for men over 40 to get annual rectal examinations.

The patient with prostatodynia has symptoms of prostatitis, but with no microscopic evidence of inflammation and no sign of bacterial infection. In contrast to the other forms of prostatitis, this condition tends to affect young men, ages 20 to 40. Patients generally suffer from pelvic pain and pain on ejaculation, but complaints of impaired urinary function are less frequent. Many of these patients have personality problems, and studies indicate that emotional stress may be a major factor. Treatment is generally the same as for nonbacterial prostatitis. In some cases the patient shows signs of nerve impairment resulting in improper functioning of certain muscles near the bladder outlet. This problem can often be treated successfully with drugs.

Prostate Cancer

Prostate cancer is the most common type of cancer in the male genito-urinary system. An estimated 86,000 new cases were diagnosed in the United States in 1985, and there were an estimated 25,500 deaths from prostate cancer. Canada had an estimated 6,240 new cases and 2,230 deaths the same year. The frequency of prostate cancer increases with age, from 1 case per 100,000 men in their early 40's to 1,000 cases per 100,000 men in their early 80's.

Symptoms of Prostate Cancer

- **Painful urination**
- **More frequent urination**
- **Inability to empty the bladder completely**
- **Blood in the urine**
- **Constipation**
- **Pain in the rectum, bladder, prostate region, or bones**

Note: Because early prostate cancer often shows no symptoms, all men over 40 should have an annual rectal examination.

Symptoms of prostate cancer include pain on urinating, increased frequency of urination, urinary retention, dribbling, bloody urine, constipation, and pain in the bones, the rectum, the bladder, or the prostate region. In many cases, however, prostate cancer in its early stages shows no symptoms; this is one reason why men over the age of 40 should have annual rectal examinations as part of their regular medical care.

In patients with prostate cancer, rectal examination reveals a stony hard region of the prostate (the normal gland has a rubbery consistency). If there is a suspicion of cancer, the next step is a biopsy, or removal of some of the prostate tissue for testing. This can be done with a needle, under local anesthetic on an outpatient basis.

Blood tests may also be done, especially for levels of acid phosphatase, a substance produced by the normal prostate but often found in higher than normal amounts in the blood of patients with prostate cancer that has spread. X-ray examination is useful for determining how far the cancer has spread to other parts of the body.

Treatment depends on the extent of the cancer; doctors distinguish four stages: A, B, C, and D. Stage A cancers are not even detectable on rectal examination but are found in approximately 10 percent of all prostates operated on for benign enlargement. Stage B tumors are confined to the prostate and detected by rectal examination, while stage C tumors have spread through the capsule of the prostate gland (the fibrous case enclosing it) and into the tissues immediately surrounding it. Cancers that have spread well beyond the prostate—often into lymph nodes or bone—are called stage D cancers. The earlier the cancer is detected, the better the patient's chance of survival and a normal life. Unfortunately, nearly half of all prostate cancer patients have stage D disease by the time they are diagnosed, and for such people the median survival time is one to three years regardless of initial therapy.

A common symptom of prostate problems is urinary obstruction, which can develop very slowly.

Radical prostatectomy, or removal of the entire prostate gland together with the lymph nodes that drain fluid from the prostate is the mainstay of treatment for localized (stage A and B) prostate cancer. (If the cancer has spread, even into immediately surrounding tissues, prostatectomy is of little value.) Major complications of the procedure have included urinary incontinence and impotence; however, improvements in surgical technique now make it possible to preserve the nerves responsible for erections, so that most patients are not rendered impotent. (If potency is a problem, an artificial device can be implanted to restore erections.)

Radiation therapy has been used for prostate cancer in stages A, B, and C. This can be done with an external radiation source or the implantation of radioactive isotopes of gold, iodine, or iridium. Survival is around 70 percent—less than the chances for most patients who undergo surgery for stage A or B prostate disease.

If prostate cancer has advanced to stage D when first diagnosed, hormone therapy is the first choice for treatment. The prostate gland depends on the male hormone testosterone to function, and suppression of testosterone helps control the disease. The most direct approach to hormonal treatment is castration, or removal of the testes, which produce most of the body's testosterone, but this step is usually taken only when the patient has cardiovascular disease. In other cases, doses of the female hormone estrogen can be prescribed to lower testosterone levels. Side effects include fluid retention, breast enlargement, and blood clot formation (the reason that this therapy is not prescribed for patients with heart disease).

New drugs to suppress the body's production of testosterone without the side effects of estrogen are under investigation. One of them, leuprolide (sold as Lupron), was recently approved by the U.S. Food and Drug Administration and Canadian health authorities for use against prostate cancer. □

Music Medicine

Richard Amdur

Playing classical music for a living is not easy on the body. Instrumentalists commonly suffer from pain, cramps, spasms, numbness, or weakness in their fingers, hands or arms. Their vision may be damaged by poor lighting in orchestra pits. The high sound levels some musicians are exposed to can affect both hearing and blood pressure. And the psychological stress of performing—and competing for scarce jobs—also exacts a toll.

Orchestra conductors and some star performers, it is true, are blessed with unusual longevity. This may be partly because of the psychological benefits gained from being in a position of command. Conductors, moreover, derive strength and stamina from constantly exercising their upper bodies. But it is not uncommon for other musicians to give up their careers because of physical ailments. Fortunately, many health problems of musicians can be helped by medical treatment, if the musician seeks it.

Injuries

The physical injuries sustained by professional musicians are largely caused by overtaxing some part of the body. Sometimes the problem is bad playing habits. But even correct technique puts an extraordinary stress on particular nerves, muscles, or joints. In many cases, psychological stress compounds the risks: muscles that are tight because of anxiety are more susceptible to injury.

The variety of disorders that occur has given rise to a lengthy list of instrument-specific names for ailments: cymbal player's shoulder, pianist's cramp, tuba lips, horn player's palsy, fiddler's neck, violinist's jaw displacement, cellist's dermatitis, and so on. Horn players are prone to dental problems, and they may suffer cardiac arrhythmias and respiratory difficulties from the stress of producing high air pressure.

Sometimes the music itself is the problem. A number of Liszt and Rachmaninoff passages require pianists to perform long

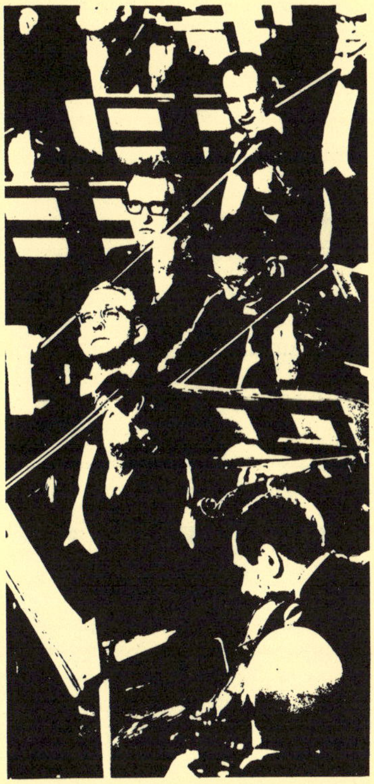

stretches that strain small hands. And large hands may be cramped by many Mozart passages. As one doctor says, "The Barber Piano Sonata ought to bear a warning from the surgeon general."

Treatment

While effective treatments are often available, many musicians do not seek help. Not wanting to admit that they have a potentially career-ending flaw, they hope the ailment will disappear.

If the musician seeks help, the treatment depends on the nature of the problem. In some cases, rest, followed by the adoption of less stressful playing habits, is all that is needed. In others, the treatment may include psychotherapy or such techniques as biofeedback, relaxation training, or readjustment of a player's bodily movements. Steroids or other anti-inflammatory drugs may sometimes be prescribed. Surgery is rarely necessary.

Self-treatment can create more problems than it solves. The drugs known as beta blockers, which have the ability to calm nerves while leaving motor functions undisturbed, have become so popular among musicians that a kind of black market has developed. Beta blockers, however, can be dangerous, especially for people with asthma or low blood pressure. The classic case of self-treatment is that of the 19th-century composer Robert Schumann. Schumann aspired to a career as a virtuoso pianist—until he crippled a finger while trying to strengthen his finger muscles with a mechanical device. He apparently never regained full use of his right hand.

A New Specialty

Medical science is now paying closer attention to musicians' needs than ever before. More studies are being performed. Symposiums are being held. Special treatment centers have opened in several cities, including Boston, New York, Cleveland, Los Angeles, and Victoria, Australia. These centers bring to bear the skills of such specialists as physical therapists, orthopedic surgeons, rheumatologists, neurophysiologists, and psychologists. A new field—music medicine—is establishing itself. □

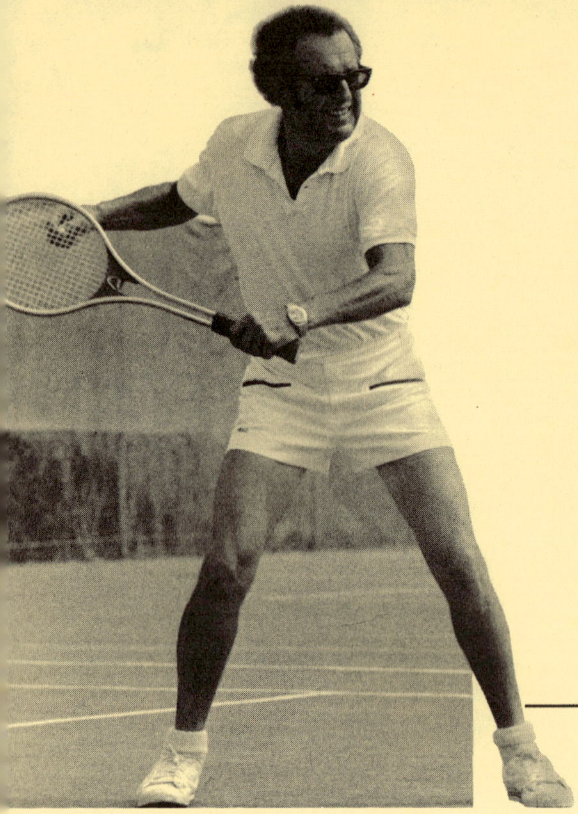

Racket Sports and Fitness

Marjorie Holt

You may want to get in shape but find the idea of monotonously running around a track or swimming lap after lap a bleak prospect. If so, the competition, excitement, and sociability offered by racket sports—tennis, squash, racquetball, badminton, platform tennis, and paddleball—may offer a more appealing way to start exercising and keep at it for a lifetime.

Racket sports generally do not provide the continuous prolonged exertion needed to significantly strengthen the heart and lungs—that is, to achieve aerobic fitness. But they do burn calories, especially fast singles tennis and the four-wall sports, racquetball and squash. Racket sports also develop aspects of general fitness—quick reflexes, eye-hand coordination, and fast thinking—that endurance sports like running and swimming usually don't require. In addition, the exhilaration of a good game may encourage novice players or those coming back to a racket sport after some sedentary years to follow a balanced fitness program that will give them the stamina to run down the shots at the end of a long match. This article will focus primarily on the way two very popular racket sports, tennis and racquetball, can be the basis of an all-around fitness program and can actually make exercise fun.

Shaping Up for the Game

To become proficient in the skills and strategy of a racket sport like tennis, and to become good enough to make playing it a test of stamina and agility, a player should try to play singles three times a week. Playing doubles can improve skills but involves less exertion and burns fewer calories than singles. Even in a singles game between skilled opponents, however, the vigorous activity of the game is interrupted by periods of waiting, which prevents it from being ideal aerobic exercise. Aerobic exercise requires continuous exertion and a constant high intake of oxygen and improves the body's ability to use this oxygen to produce energy, thus increasing the efficiency of the lungs and the cardiovascular system.

Tennis and racketball can make exercise fun and exciting.

Aerobic fitness will keep a player from "running out of steam" on the court. Players of racket sports should supplement their court time with 30-minute sessions of an aerobic activity like running, aerobic dance, stationary bicycling, or swimming. The aerobic activity, which should take place three times a week, doesn't have to be overly strenuous. A long walk at a brisk pace, perhaps to the court after work or school, is enough unless the player wants to train hard enough to shine in serious competition. If so, the more taxing endurance exercises are in order. To prevent strained muscles, pulled tendons, or nerve problems, the strenuous endurance exercises and time on the court should be preceded and followed by five to ten minutes of warm-up and cool-down exercises, such as easy stretches and light calisthenics.

Workouts for Tennis Skills

Tennis requires the most muscle power of the racket sports since the racket is heavier and the ball has to be hit and chased down over longer distances. To be in top shape, players, especially women, may want to work out with weights to increase upper-body strength. There is certainly no guarantee that weight training will make you a pro, but some of the world's top players, including Martina Navratilova and Chris Evert Lloyd, use weights as part of their training programs.

Weight training combined with a thorough stretching routine works the muscles on the non-hitting side of the body, which keeps the body in balance and helps prevent torn muscles or other injuries.

Weight training will improve hitting power, but it is also important to work specific muscles in the way that they will be used in a game. To strengthen the forearm, put the cover on your racket and swing for two minutes or until your arm tires, rest, then practice fast forehand and backhand swings for at least one minute. Squeezing a dead tennis ball 50 times will make your grip stronger, increasing control.

A powerful swing isn't good enough if you can't get to the ball in time to hit it back to your opponent. Aerobic fitness will provide the stamina to keep moving for shots, and running sprints (short, fast runs) will improve speed. Sprints can be part of a 30-minute conditioning run or can be done at home by running up and down stairs. It is also very helpful to practice running forward, backward, and from side to side on the court itself, preferably with racket in hand.

Hitting balls against a backboard can help develop consistent ground strokes, and taking over a court to serve a bucket of balls is great practice for the difficult skill of serving. In these practice sessions, a player can also work on getting as much of the body weight behind the stroke or serve as possible. To give the most velocity to the ball, it's best to get the back, shoulders, hips, and legs into the action instead of relying only on the strength of the arms and hands. This makes for a more fluid motion that can be performed with less strain. It also makes for a better workout.

Racket sports players should supplement their court time with an aerobic activity such as running or swimming.

Four-Wall Alternatives

Tennis may be more frustration than sport for some people, however. It usually takes many lessons and months of practice to become good enough to be able to challenge another player, or even to spend more time playing than chasing missed balls. In some areas, indoor tennis courts may not be easily available or may be too expensive for the average person to use three times a week all winter long. Racquetball is a challenging alternative, and because it has become so popular and court time is less expensive, racquetball may be more practical than tennis as a year-round sport. In addition, racquetball skills are much easier to learn than tennis fundamentals, giving near-beginners in racquetball a vigorous workout and the excitement of competitive play.

Since racquetball is played with a lively ball in an enclosed space the size of a handball court, 20 feet wide and 40 feet long, and since the ball can be hit against all four walls and the ceiling, the players can keep each rally going for a considerable time. The short-handled racquet also makes it easier for a player to hit the ball, avoiding the embarrassing complete misses common to novice tennis players, and easier to place the shot.

In racquetball, as in tennis, there are local tournaments for all age groups, and since racquetball gives a sense of mastery of the fundamentals more quickly than tennis, a racquetball player may be more willing to risk a competitive match. The thought of such a match coming up is likely to be an incentive to practice and get in top all-around condition. Although racquetball is a fast moving game, a player still generally stops and starts too often to get the 30 minutes of steady exertion necessary for real aerobic benefits. As with tennis, additional aerobic activity is needed for the player to be in the best condition. The arm strength, practice hitting, and sprint drills that help in tennis are likely to work wonders for racquetball too.

Playing Squash

Racquetball players looking for a somewhat different challenge, and people considering taking up a racket sport, might try the game of squash. This sport is losing its university club exclusivity with the opening of commercial squash facilities for the general public. Like racquetball, squash is played in an enclosed court, but it employs a lighter, longer-handled racket and a softer, less bouncy ball. This more controllable ball in part explains the major difference between racquetball and squash: squash requires more strategy, the use of a variety of shots and changes of pace to set up the "killer" shot that your opponent cannot return. The mental challenge may keep a player excited about the sport and eager to play regularly and master the subtleties of the game. □

New Surgery for Breast Cancer

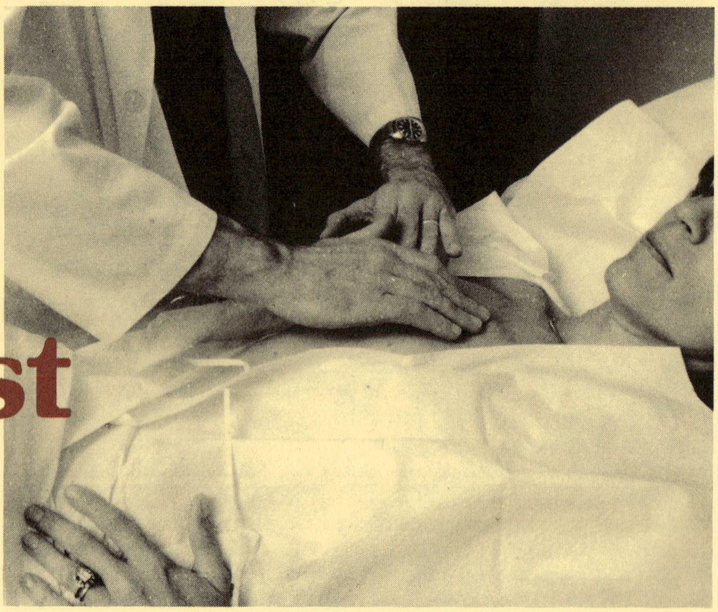

Katherine L. Griem, M.D., and Jay R. Harris, M.D.

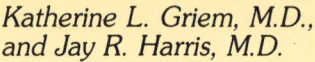

In the United States in 1985, 119,000 women were expected to be diagnosed as having breast cancer, and 38,400 were expected to die from the disease. In Canada, 9,450 new cases and 3,740 deaths were expected. One in 11 American women will develop breast cancer during her lifetime, and it is the disease women fear the most. The fact that breast cancer is potentially fatal is one reason for that fear—and the disfigurement that comes with a mastectomy is another.

Much work has been done on the early detection and treatment of breast cancer, and as a result, more and more women are surviving longer—and are even being considered cured. One of the treatment areas that has undergone the most change is surgery for early, or operable, breast cancer. More conservative surgical procedures have been developed that are beginning to be used today to treat patients for whom they are considered appropriate. These procedures appear to promise survival rates equal to the more extensive types of surgery and at the same time provide women with an alternative to losing a breast to cancer.

Radical Surgery

The breast is made up of 15 to 20 compartments that radiate out from the nipple. The compartments are separated from each other by fibrous tissue. Lymph fluid from the breast flows to lymph nodes located in the armpit (axilla) and under the breastbone; cancerous cells from a breast tumor can spread along these same lymph pathways to the lymph nodes—and from there, throughout the body.

In early breast cancer, the cancer occurs only in the breast or in the breast and lymph nodes, and has not apparently spread to other places in the body. Theoretically, all of the cancer can be removed by a single operation.

A new treatment for some patients is removal of the tumor and lymph nodes, followed by radiation therapy.

In the 18th and 19th centuries, breast cancer was treated by removal of only the tumor. The cancer often recurred, and few patients survived five years free of cancer. With better understanding of how cancer spreads, as well as improved surgical techniques and the mid-19th century discovery of anesthesia, came more extensive types of surgical procedures.

In 1894 a U.S. surgeon named William Halsted developed the radical mastectomy, often called the Halsted radical mastectomy. For many years—into the 1970's—it was the standard breast cancer operation in the United States. The operation involves the removal of a large area: the skin covering the breast, the nipple, and all the breast tissue, as well as the lymph nodes in the armpit (called the axillary lymph nodes) and two major muscles of the chest wall. (The lymph nodes under the breastbone are not removed; although they pose a cancer risk, they are very difficult to reach surgically.) Such extensive surgery is not without complications: women often suffer significant deformity, severe swelling of the arm, impaired shoulder movement and arm strength, and problems with wound healing. It was thought necessary, however, to remove so much tissue to reduce the chances of tumor recurrence and so increase the chances for cure.

As time progressed, though, it became apparent that even with such extensive surgery, many women, especially those whose cancer had spread to the lymph nodes at the time their disease was diagnosed, had a high risk of tumor recurrence, principally in distant sites such as the liver, lung, and bone. Despite the radical surgery, many of these women died. Some surgeons therefore began to wonder if less extensive and deforming surgery might be as good, especially if it were combined with radiation therapy to kill off whatever cancerous cells might remain.

In the 1940's an operation called the modified radical mastectomy was first performed. As it was originally done, the entire breast and the armpit lymph nodes were removed, but one of the major muscles of the chest wall was left intact; as the operation is done today, both of the muscles are usually preserved.

The modified radical mastectomy was virtually ignored by surgeons in the United States for many years, until studies began to show it to be as effective as the radical mastectomy in terms of cure rates for early breast cancer. It is clear as well that this less extensive surgery is better for the patient cosmetically and functionally. Wound complications are much less frequent than with radical mastectomy, the incidence of severe arm swelling is reduced to about 10 percent, and it is possible for reconstructive breast surgery to be done if the patient so chooses.

There has thus been a gradual change in the types of breast cancer operations performed. For instance, in 1969-1970 at Memorial Sloan-Kettering Cancer Center—one of the leading cancer centers in North America—77 percent of breast cancer patients were treated with radical mastectomies, only 14 percent with modified radical mastectomies. By 1978 the percentage of patients who underwent modified radical mastectomies had increased to 52 percent, compared with 41 percent treated with radical mastectomies. In 1982 modified radical mastectomies were performed in 83 percent of breast cancer cases at the center; radical mastectomies were done in only 15 percent. Two years later, radical mastectomies were performed in only 6 percent of cases, and modified radical mastectomies were done in 76 percent of cases; more limited operations were also performed.

Four Types of Surgery

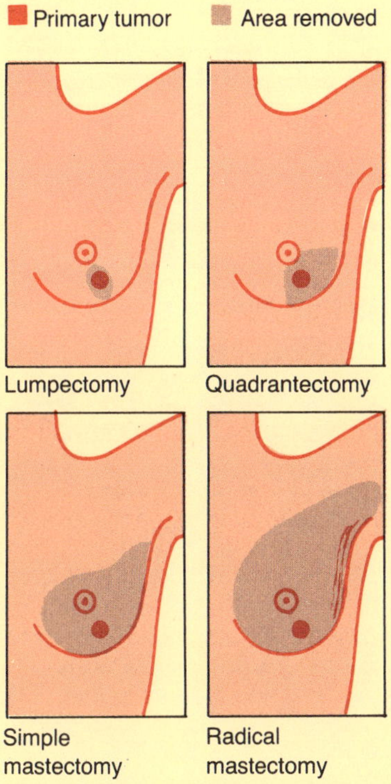

Lumpectomy
Quadrantectomy
Simple mastectomy
Radical mastectomy

Less Extensive Operations

An even less extensive procedure than the modified radical mastectomy is the simple mastectomy, also called a total mastectomy. This removes only the breast, leaving the lymph nodes and muscles intact. As early as 1948 a study in Scotland suggested that simple mastectomy followed by local radiation therapy was as effective as radical mastectomy.

Recent studies support this conclusion, including one by the National Surgical Adjuvant Breast Project, a cooperative group involving many U.S. and Canadian hospitals. In 1971 the NSABP began a study comparing radical mastectomy, simple mastectomy, and simple mastectomy followed by radiation therapy. Ten-year results published in March 1985 showed that women who had had simple mastectomies did as well as those who had had radical mastectomies.

In the NSABP study, women were divided into two groups: those whose lymph nodes showed evidence of cancer and those whose nodes did not. Women whose nodes showed evidence of cancer had either radical mastectomies or simple mastectomies followed by radiation therapy. The survival rate after ten years was 38 percent, regardless of which surgery was done. Women whose nodes did not show evidence of cancer had radical mastectomies, simple mastectomies, or simple mastectomies followed by radiation therapy. Their survival rate after ten years was 57 percent, regardless of which treatment they had had. Thus, whether the nodes are cancerous or not appears to be a more important determinant of survival at ten years than does the type of surgery performed.

Radiation Therapy

Shortly after the discovery of X rays in the 1890's, radiation therapy began to be used in the treatment of cancer. In the 1920's and 1930's, radiation ther-

How to Examine Your Breasts

step 1.

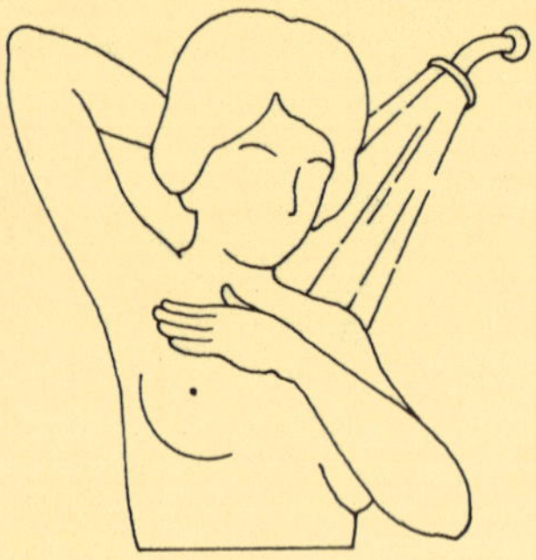

step 2.

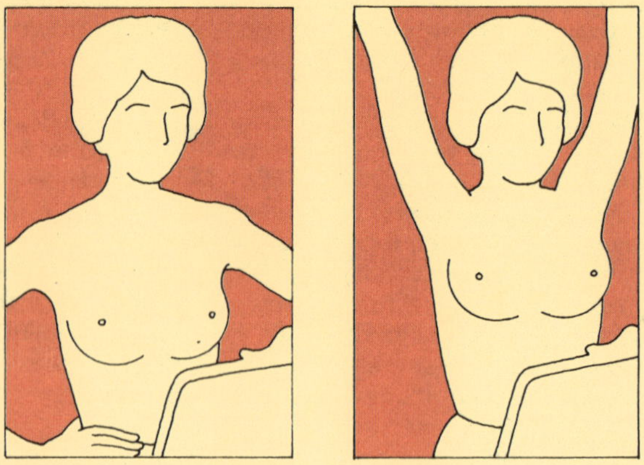

step 3.

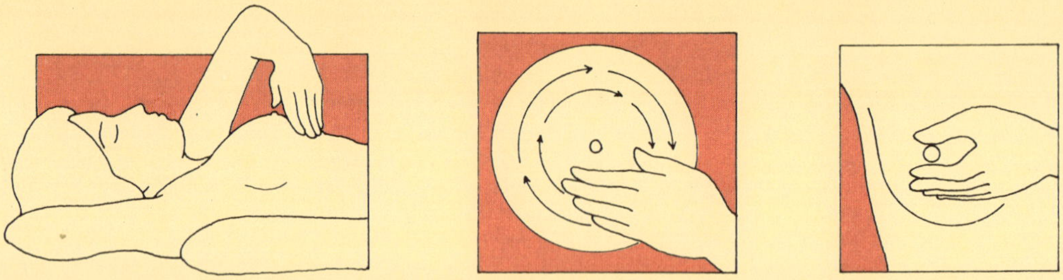

Every woman should examine her breasts once a month—ideally, right after her period. **(1)** Begin in the shower by feeling each breast for any lumps or thickening of tissue. **(2)** Stand in front of a mirror and look for any changes in the appearance of the breasts and nipples, such as a swelling or dimpling of skin. **(3)** Lie down with your right arm under your head and a pillow under your right breast. Use your left hand, fingers held flat, to examine the entire right breast, moving your hand in slow, clockwise circles. Do the same with your right hand and left breast. Then squeeze each nipple gently to see if there is a discharge. See your doctor right away if you find anything unusual.

apy for breast cancer—instead of surgery—was pioneered in Europe and Canada. Patients received very high doses of radiation, and the entire breast was treated. The radiation controlled the tumor but often left the breast hard and fibrotic. Because of these poor results, radiation treatment for breast cancer fell into disfavor and was used only infrequently (for instance, if the patient was not medically suitable for an operation).

However, in the 1970's it became possible to focus radiation on a specific part of the breast, with better cosmetic results. Recently, doctors have turned their attention to the use, in certain cancer patients, of lower doses of radiation as an adjunct to very limited surgery—so minimal that much of the breast is spared.

Breast-Sparing Treatment

The new, conservative treatment for breast cancer involving surgery and radiation is a three-step process. First, the tumor must be completely removed. This can be done in a number of ways, including local excision (lumpectomy) and quadrantectomy. Lumpectomy means the removal of the tumor along with a margin (usually about half an inch) of normal, healthy breast tissue. This excision is usually done through a small incision without removal of the overlying skin, and the breast to a large extent retains its normal appearance. If a quadrantectomy is done, the tumor is removed along with the entire quadrant (quarter) of the breast in which the tumor is located. This does involve removal of skin and the cosmetic result may not be quite as good, especially when the breast is small.

In addition to taking out the tumor, surgeons usually remove the underarm lymph nodes to determine if they contain cancer cells. Even lymph nodes that look normal should be removed since the physical examination alone may not detect nodal cancer. Removal of the nodes will not necessarily prevent the spread of breast cancer, but examining them is important because they act as a warning sign: patients with malignant lymph nodes (technically referred to as positive, or involved, nodes) are at a higher risk of developing cancer in distant parts of the body. Many physicians recommend that patients with involved nodes have chemotherapy in addition to local treatment of the breast.

If the doctor and patient decide on primary radiation therapy, no further surgery is involved if the tumor was fully removed when the lumpectomy or quadrantectomy was done. Shortly after that surgery, the patient begins her radiation therapy—the second stage of the treatment process. The standard treatment regimen at many American cancer centers consists of approximately 25 daily treatments lasting a few minutes each. The radiation is directed at the entire breast and sometimes the regional lymph node areas as well. The side effects are minor—only a slight reddening of the skin of the breast and perhaps some peeling; there is no nausea, vomiting, or hair loss. Patients can live at home and be treated on an outpatient basis, and the radiation therapy does not interfere with their usual daily activities.

In the third stage of treatment, a "booster" dose of radiation is given to the area where the tumor was located. The booster is given either by a machine that delivers a series of electron-beam treatments or by a radioactive implant. The implant requires a hospital stay and sometimes general anesthesia. After several days, the implant is removed; there is no residual radiation at the implant site.

One permanent effect of the radiation treatments is that the breast becomes firmer and loses its glandular structure, so that it can no longer produce milk. Since women who develop breast cancer are usually beyond childbearing age, this is not a major concern. The physical appearance following treatment is usually quite good. At the Joint Center for Radiation Therapy in Boston, for example, the cosmetic results were judged by physicians as good to excellent in 81 percent of patients treated, and the patients themselves tended to react even more favorably.

Promising Results

The results of conservative surgery with radiation therapy are quite promising: the treatment seems to produce local control of the breast cancer and survival rates equal to those achieved with mastectomy. In March 1985 the NSABP published the initial results of another of its studies, comparing three types of treatment—simple mastectomy, lumpectomy, and lumpectomy followed by radiation therapy—in over 1,800 women whose tumors measured about 1½ inches in diameter or less. The five-year survival rates were not significantly different in the three groups, but women who had had lumpectomies followed by radiation treatment did the best of all the groups in terms of overall survival and survival without recurrence of cancer. The follow-up period in the study is somewhat short. (In most types of cancer, patients who survive free of disease for five years following diagnosis are considered cured. However, breast tumors sometimes recur after more than five years.) Doctors are eager to see what will happen to the women in the NSABP study in the future; the recent five-year results are quite promising.

Regular breast self-examinations are critical.

Another study, done in Italy, showed similar results, and the patients were followed for a longer period of time—a median of 8½ years after treatment. There was no difference in survival rates between those who received a mastectomy and those treated with quadrantectomy and radiation.

These promising results notwithstanding, until further research has been done, some doctors prefer to perform traditional mastectomies.

Candidates for Conservative Surgery

Who can be treated with lumpectomy and radiation? Not all women with operable breast cancer are good candidates for conservative surgery. Women with a number of breast tumors, for instance, may be better treated with some type of mastectomy. This is also true of women with very large breasts, who are difficult to treat with radiation for technical reasons. In addition, not all hospitals have the facilities to treat breast cancer with radiation. The treatment requires a radiation therapist familiar with the technique, as well as high energy X-ray machines and the staff to run such equipment. The number of centers able to treat early breast cancer patients with radiation is growing, however.

Conservative surgery followed by radiation—the latest development in a field that has seen many changes in the last century—offers an acceptable alternative in selected women with early breast cancer. While the treatment does require a time commitment, it offers superior cosmetic and possibly psychological results. If women understand that many early cases of breast cancer can be treated effectively without leaving them disfigured, many may be more willing to perform monthly breast self-examinations. Catching more cancers early means more lives will be saved. Obviously, choosing conservative surgery involves a personal decision for the woman—but there clearly is a choice today. □

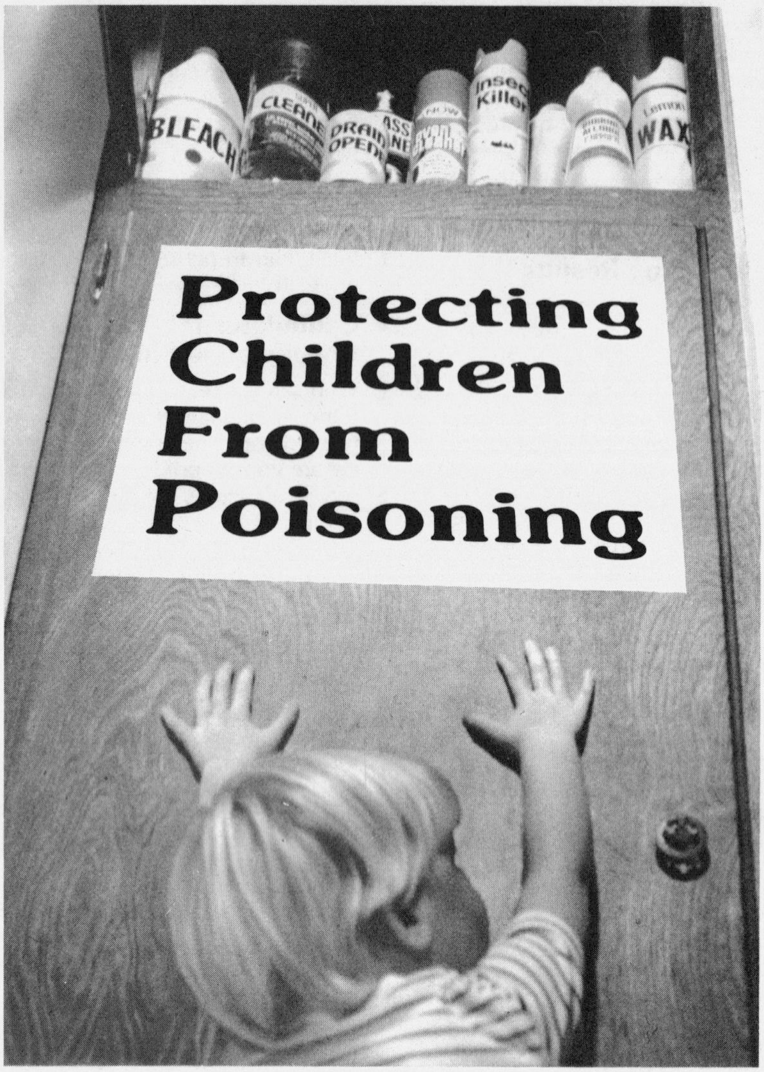

Protecting Children From Poisoning

Robert Sorenson

After having spent eight years with the U.S. Food and Drug Administration educating the public on how to protect children from accidental poisoning, Pauline Coker was sure she had made her own home a safe place for her two-year-old daughter, Kristen. But when Kristen's grandfather came for a visit, the little girl found some blood pressure medication in his suitcase and decided to give it a try. A dose of syrup of ipecac was immediately administered, and a crisis was averted. But the incident was a dramatic example of how even careful and informed parents may overlook a source of danger to their children.

The very young are especially at risk; in fact, the second year of life is the most dangerous for accidental poisoning. The problem is not only that small children, by nature extraordinarily curious, can't read warning labels and don't know what poison is, but also that they tend to be more sensitive to the possible toxic effects of substances. Sometimes an amount too small to harm an adult may be enough to hurt or even kill a young child.

What Can Be Poisonous

"All substances are poisons," wrote the 16th-century physician Paracelsus. "The right dose differentiates a poison and a remedy." Although this may sound extreme, it is a fact that in the United States common causes of hospitalization for poisoning among children under five are drugs for colds or pain and vitamins.

Besides adult medication, products that should be kept out of children's sight and reach include cleaning and laundry items and chemicals used around the house or in the garage, garden, and workshop. Particularly dangerous substances include rat poison and insect pastes, petroleum distillates (gasoline, kerosene, and paint thinner), weed killers, windshield-washer fluid, and antifreeze. Most such products have warning labels, and many have child-resistant caps. But some do not. Alcohol, particularly spirits, can be deadly to a small child; tobacco is also toxic.

Plants and Paints

A number of common houseplants, including caladium, dieffenbachia, philodendron, and the castor-oil plant, can make a child who eats them quite sick. Other poisonous plants occur in the garden or in the wild: members of the narcissus family, irises, hyacinth, foxglove, lily of the valley, henbane, certain mushrooms, and many other plants can be toxic if ingested. Before a child starts roaming the house and garden, find out exactly what plants you have and whether they are dangerous. A local nursery, library, or gardening club should be able to help.

Each year, thousands of children are harmed by lead poisoning, mostly from eating chips of lead-based paint flaking off walls or ceilings. Even household dust can contain tiny particles of paint. Lead poisoning can cause loss of appetite, personality changes, headaches, and even brain damage. U.S. government standards call for paint accessible to children to be no more than 0.06 percent lead. (Canadian standards allow a lead content of 0.5 percent.) Older homes, however, may have had many coats of paint applied before such standards went into effect. The best way to be sure of preventing lead poisoning is to keep painted surfaces in good condition, so that chips of old paint do not flake off. Frequent wet-mopping will help to keep dust levels at a minimum.

Breathing and Touching

Not all poisons need to be swallowed to cause harm: fumes from petroleum products, carbon monoxide from improperly vented fires or internal-combustion engines, and natural gas are all deadly if inhaled in sufficient quantity. This is why charcoal grills, for example, should be used only outdoors. Many aerosol products can also be dangerous if inhaled, particularly pesticides and oven cleaners.

Toddlers are especially at risk for accidental poisoning because of their curiosity and sensitivity to toxins.

Some poisons are powerful enough to be dangerous just through contact with the skin—these include many pesticides and naphthalene, which is found in mothballs and air fresheners. These and other chemicals can produce effects ranging from minor irritation to convulsions and death. The eyes are particularly sensitive to caustic substances. Aerosol cans are a special danger, since children playing with them can easily spray the contents into their eyes.

Baby's-Eye View

The first and most fundamental rule for preventing poisoning is to keep all toxic substances away from children. Before a baby starts to crawl, parents should survey their home from a baby's-eye view. Floor-level cabinets should be fitted with child-resistant safety catches (available in a hardware store or where children's products are sold). Even with safety latches installed, it would be wise to put the more dangerous household chemicals—bleach, drain cleaner, window cleaner, and so on—well out of reach, in case a child manages to open the catch.

Lower shelves in the bathroom should be cleared of shampoos, aftershave lotions, and hair-setting solutions, and drugs that are no longer being used should be flushed down the toilet. All medicine bottles should be equipped with child-resistant caps—which should always be replaced correctly after use.

It's a good idea to install a padlock on a cabinet in the garage, basement, or storage room so that especially dangerous substances can be locked up.

Paying Attention

All the precautions in the world won't do much good if the cabinet door is left open or the cap is left off a bottle of pills. Moreover, a great many poisonings occur while a toxic product is in use, which is not surprising, considering that a product being used is one that will attract a child's attention. If you have to answer the door or the telephone while adding bleach to the laundry or taking a medication, it is a

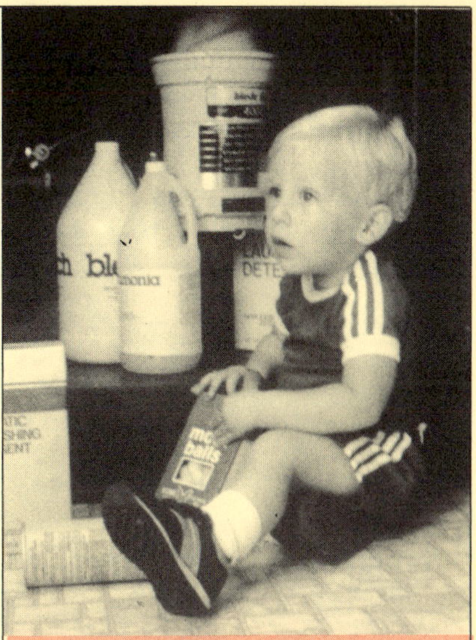

Guarding Against Poisoning

- Keep the phone number of your area's poison control center handy.
- Keep drugs, beauty products, and household chemicals out of children's reach.
- Install safety latches on cabinets.
- Buy products that come in safety containers.
- Rinse containers before throwing them away.
- Keep syrup of ipecac on hand.
- Never say medicine is candy.
- Put only food in food containers.
- Throw away old medicines.
- Never leave medicine or other dangerous products uncapped.
- Remember: a coat pocket or handbag can be a source of danger.
- Be alert when visiting homes not as child proof as your own.
- Teach your child about the dangers of accidental poisoning.

Poison, Poison Everywhere

Here are some examples of things often found around the home that can be poisonous.

- Aerosol sprays
- Aftershave lotion
- Ammonia
- Bleach
- Bubble bath
- Cigarettes
- Cologne and perfume
- Dishwashing liquid
- Drain cleaner
- Epoxy glue
- Furniture polish
- Hair dye
- Insect killer
- Iodine
- Kerosene
- Laundry detergent
- Liquor
- Makeup
- Medications and drugs
- Nail polish
- Nail polish remover
- Oven cleaner
- Paint
- Paint thinner
- Permanent wave solution
- Plants
- Rat poison
- Scouring pads
- Toilet cleaner
- Weed killer
- Window washing liquid

wise, sensible precaution to take either the child or the product along with you.

Poison Control Center

All parents should keep handy the telephone number of their local poison control center. (It can usually be found on the inside front cover or front page of the phone book.) Every area in the United States and Canada is served by such a center, which can provide information on preventing poisonings as well as give instruction in the event of an emergency. The poison control center is equipped to deal with a wide range of poisoning incidents, including bee stings, snakebites, and the like; in addition, each center has files on thousands of potentially toxic substances.

If you suspect your child has been poisoned, it is important to call the poison control center or a physician at once. Report the age of the child, what you think caused the poisoning, how much time has passed, and what symptoms, if any, have appeared. In cases where the child has eaten a poisonous substance, it will help if you can say how much was swallowed. You will be told what first aid steps to take and whether the child should be brought in for observation and treatment.

First Aid

Everyone should be familiar with the basic measures to take for poisoning. If the poison has been inhaled, get the child immediately into fresh air. The best treatment for contact poisons is usually to wash the affected area with large amounts of fresh water.

If the child swallows something poisonous, it may be necessary to induce vomiting. (This should be done only after consulting a doctor or poison control center.) Most doctors recommend that every home have a bottle of syrup of ipecac on hand for this purpose; it is safer and more effective than, say, the back of a spoon. (Using the old remedy of salt water can be downright dangerous.) The syrup can be bought without a prescription and will keep for two or more years.

To make your house safe, survey it from a baby's-eye view and put all potential poisons out of reach.

Vomiting should not be induced when a child has swallowed a petroleum product or a corrosive substance (such as acids, like toilet bowl cleaner or iodine, or alkalis, like bleach or ammonia), or if the victim feels pain or burning in the mouth or throat. Corrosives can injure the victim further on the way back up, while vomiting petroleum products may cause them to be drawn into the lungs, possibly leading to chemical pneumonia. In such cases water or milk is usually given to dilute the toxic material. No liquid should be given, nor vomiting induced, when a child is unconscious or in convulsions.

Do not induce vomiting if the child has swallowed a petroleum product or corrosive substance.

If the doctor or poison control center tells you to induce vomiting, make sure the child's mouth is cleared of all remaining toxic material (this should be done in any case), and administer a tablespoon of syrup of ipecac, followed by at least one glass of water. Keep the child facing forward with face down—a child lying face upward, or a drowsy child, can choke on regurgitated material. If the ipecac does not cause vomiting in 20 minutes, a second dose may be given, again with water.

If the child has to be brought to the doctor or the hospital, the container the poison came in should be taken along, as should a sample of any vomited material. This will make it easier to identify accurately what has been swallowed. Since a container's label sometimes has the key information needed to establish the cause of poisoning, potentially toxic substances should always be kept in their original containers. □

What to Do for a Hangover

Jacqueline Laks Gorman

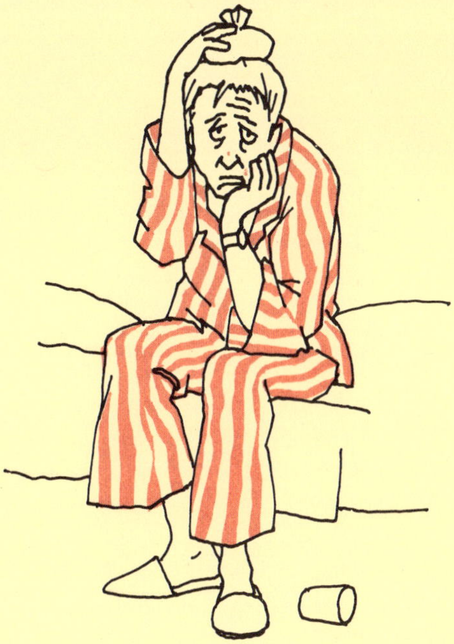

A dark brown taste, a burning thirst,
A head that's ready to split and burst. . . .
No time for mirth, no time for laughter—
The cold gray dawn of the morning after.

For even the most casual social drinker, there may be a rare night of alcoholic overindulgence followed by a wretched morning after, with the pounding headache, queasy stomach, and overall misery so aptly described by the American writer George Ade some 80 years ago.

Alcohol can, of course, have more alarming effects. A dangerous substance capable of causing addiction, serious diseases, and death, it is not something to be trifled with. Luckily, most Americans do not have serious drinking problems; when alcohol does affect them adversely, it is usually because they may have engaged in occasional overindulgence at a holiday gathering or other social celebration. (If such overindulgence occurs more often, or if you find yourself increasingly dependent on alcohol, you may have a more serious problem than you think and perhaps should consider seeking professional help.)

For sufferers of occasional hangovers, there is some good news and some bad news. The bad news is that there is no cure for a hangover, except time and rest. The good news is that there are ways to help prevent a hangover from occurring or to at least ease some of the symptoms.

Alcohol in the Body

Like any other food or drink, alcohol must be broken down in the body. However, alcohol is not digested in the slow, complicated way that most other foods and drinks are—which helps explain why you feel its effects so quickly. Just minutes after you take a drink, a small amount of the alcohol has already been absorbed into the bloodstream through the stomach walls. The rest passes to the small intestine, where it is absorbed into the blood only a bit more slowly. The blood carries and distributes the alcohol throughout the body, where its main effects are those of an anesthetic: at moderate levels, alcohol dulls parts of the brain. This can affect your ability to think clearly and make judgments, and it can also make you feel light-headed and carefree.

While there is no cure for a hangover, there are steps your can take to ease your misery: eat bland foods, drink fluids, take an aspirin . . . and relax.

Perspiration, respiration, and urination rid the body of a small amount of alcohol, but some 90 percent must be disposed of by the liver, the only organ in the body that metabolizes (in essence, burns up) alcohol. The liver metabolizes the alcohol in a typical drink (usually defined as a 12-ounce bottle of beer, a medium glass of wine, or a jigger of hard liquor) in roughly 60 to 90 minutes. This means that if you have more than one drink in that space of time, the liver will be bombarded with more alcohol when it hasn't yet burned up the first dose. The alcohol will stay in your bloodstream longer—and you will probably suffer all the more for it later.

The effects of all this will be worse for small people in general and for women in particular, because they have less water in their bodies to keep down the concentration of alcohol in their blood.

The strength of your drink apparently also has an effect. For instance, the alcohol in an ounce of 90-proof whiskey, which is 45 percent alcohol, will be absorbed somewhat more quickly into the blood than the alcohol in wine, which is roughly 12 percent alcohol, or in beer, which is only about 5 percent alcohol.

The Morning After

A hangover doesn't hit you until virtually all of the alcohol has left your system, so if you've had a hard night of drinking, you'll probably wake up to a painfully difficult morning. In fact, it may take several hours till you feel like yourself again. Of course, alcohol affects everyone differently, and consequently, hangover symptoms vary.

In general, though, your body feels miserable, and that is a direct result of what the alcohol has done to it. One classic symptom is the hangover headache—a throbbing pain that worsens when you tilt your head or make a sudden movement. The headache probably occurs because alcohol widens the blood vessels of the scalp and brain, which in turn stretches the nerves.

Nausea and stomach upset beset you because alcohol irritates the lining of the stomach and small intestine and causes an increased flow of acid juices. You'll probably be thirsty and have a "furry" tongue because alcohol interferes with a particular hormone in the body, causing a diuretic effect and upsetting the body's fluid balance. As for fatigue, chances are you were busy socializing and didn't get to sleep until late; since alcohol dulls reactions of the brain, you may well have stayed up a good deal later than common sense dictates in more sober situations.

Substances called congeners may also play a role in hangovers. These are chemicals, present in tiny amounts in alcoholic beverages, that add flavor, taste, and color. Some drinks—especially bourbon and brandy—are very rich in congeners and are thus said to produce more severe hangovers than, say, gin and vodka, which are low in congeners. Some people react more strongly to congeners than others.

What to Do

Humorist Robert Benchley once said that the only cure for a hangover was death. That's not exactly true, but despite all the folklore, there is no other surefire way to instantly end a hangover. The many weird remedies that at least some people swear by—rolling in the snow, rubbing a cut lemon in the armpits, or downing exotic concoctions containing oysters, raw eggs, and Worcestershire sauce—are not only ineffective but downright distasteful.

PREVENTING HANGOVERS

- **Don't drink to excess.**
- **Before drinking, eat a meal or substantial snack high in fat and protein.**
- **Eat while you drink.**
- **Space your drinks.**
- **Dilute your drinks with ice or mixers (but not carbonated mixers).**
- **Avoid liquors like brandy or bourbon that are rich in congeners.**

Only time and rest will end a hangover, but there are steps you can take to relieve the worst of it. If your stomach isn't too upset, aspirin or an aspirin substitute will help your headache. (However, exercise caution in taking these analgesics: there is some evidence that they cause internal bleeding in heavier drinkers.) You may also be able to help your headache by applying an ice pack or drinking coffee, since both ice and caffeine constrict the blood vessels involved in headaches. Contrary to popular belief, though, coffee will not sober you up right after you have been drinking, since it does nothing to get the alcohol out of your blood.

Bland, easily digested foods like soft-boiled eggs, broth, or toast can settle a churning stomach, and drinking (nonalcoholic) fluids will relieve your thirst. If nothing seems to work, simply rest and try to relax until you feel better.

One thing not to try is the proverbial "hair of the dog that bit you." An alcoholic drink in the morning may make you feel better at first, but you'll just be putting off the pain—and if you persist in the habit, you might well wind up with a serious drinking problem.

Prevention

You can avoid a hangover and save yourself a lot of discomfort by taking a few simple precautions. The first, of course, is don't drink to excess. Beyond that, don't drink on an empty stomach. Shortly before you start drinking, eat a meal or a substantial snack high in protein and fat—foods like cheese, milk, or meat. Fat and protein will coat your stomach and prevent gastric upset. It's also a good idea to snack while you drink, but not on salty chips and pretzels, which will make you thirsty.

Space your drinks, and dilute them with ice or mixers to lower the concentration of alcohol. But it might be best to avoid carbonated mixers; some investigators think the gas in such mixers will speed up alcohol absorption. It may be wise to avoid liquors rich in congeners if you know you'll be drinking a lot.

Be aware of where you are and of how you feel, because people are apt to drink more in tense social situations. Don't drink if you're upset—some doctors think that if you do, you'll be more likely to suffer a hangover or to have a severe one. □

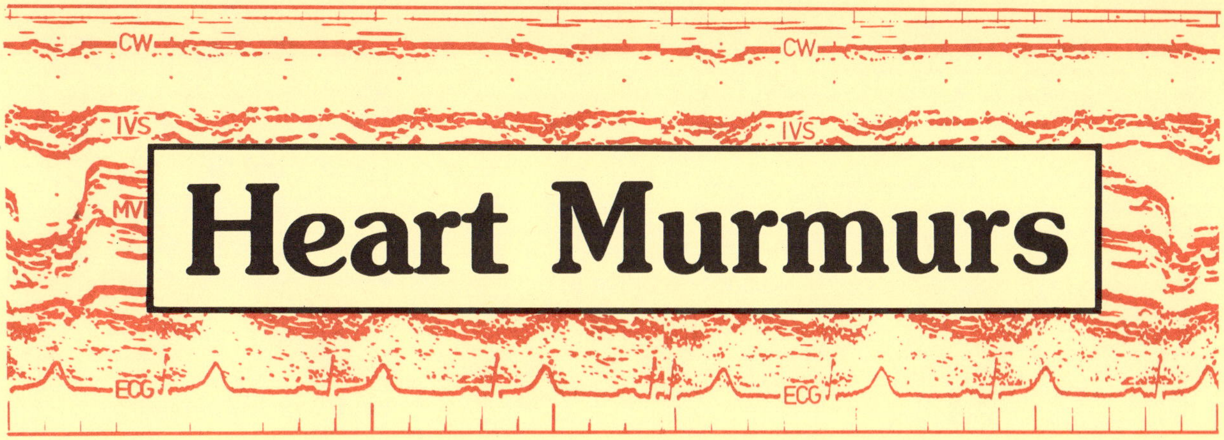

Heart Murmurs

Robert A. Kloner, M.D., Ph.D.

Heart murmurs are vibrations produced by turbulent blood flow within the heart or the place where a major blood vessel joins the heart. In general, murmurs are detected when a doctor listens to the heart with a stethoscope and hears a sound much like the noise made when one forcibly exhales with the mouth open. Some heart murmurs are described as functional, or innocent—there is usually no underlying heart disease. Other murmurs, however, provide important clues to the presence of various types of heart disease, including heart valve abnormalities.

Some heart murmurs are innocent; others indicate the presence of heart disease.

It is important to realize that a heart murmur itself is not a disease or even a diagnosis. It is a physical finding that must be explained. To determine whether a patient's murmur is innocent or potentially more serious, the physician must figure out why the murmur occurs—which parts of the heart or blood vessels are responsible for the sound.

Blood Flow

Understanding heart murmurs requires some basic knowledge of how the heart works and how blood flows through it. Key structures in this process are the heart valves, which are essentially flaps of tissue that open to allow blood to flow past them and then close to prevent the blood from flowing backward in the wrong direction.

Normally, unoxygenated blood carrying the waste product carbon dioxide from body cells flows into the right atrium (upper chamber) of the heart. From there, the blood flows through the tricuspid valve into the right ventricle, or lower heart chamber. This phase when a ventricle is filling with blood is called ventricular diastole.

The right ventricle pumps the blood through the pulmonary valve into the pulmonary artery (the phase in which a ventricle ejects blood is called ventricular systole). The pulmonary artery leads to the lungs, where the blood gets rid of the carbon dioxide and picks up oxygen.

The oxygenated blood is delivered to the heart's left atrium via the pulmonary veins. It then passes through the mitral valve into the left ventricle, which pumps the oxygenated blood through the aortic valve and into the aorta, the main artery from which oxygenated blood is delivered to the body's vital organs. (The left ventricle's diastole and systole phases occur at the same times that the right ventricle is filling and emptying.)

Heart Sounds

A doctor listening to the heart with a stethoscope does not normally hear the flow of blood. However, when the heart valves close, distinctive sounds are produced. Frequently, these sounds are described as "lub-dub." The first sound occurs when the tricuspid and mitral valves snap shut after the ventricles fill, the second when the pulmonary and aortic valves close after the ventricles empty. The time between the lub and the dub of one heartbeat is approximately that of ventricular systole. The time between the dub of one heartbeat and the lub of the next heartbeat is that of ventricular diastole.

Diagnosing Murmurs

A doctor detecting a murmur tries to determine various features of the abnormal sound. These include the loudness, "quality," and location of the murmur and the timing of the murmur in the heart cycle. The duration of the murmur and the direction in which it radiates are noted.

The loudness of the murmur depends on the speed and volume of the blood and also on the distance between the sound-producing area and the stethoscope. In a person who is very obese, an otherwise loud murmur might sound softer because of the amount of fatty tissue through which the sound must travel.

The quality of murmurs—described in terms like high-pitched, low-pitched, harsh, blowing, and musical—may provide clues to the nature of underlying heart problems. A high-pitched murmur of a particular type heard in the aortic area of the chest wall may indicate that the aortic valve leaks, or allows blood to flow backward—a condition called regurgitation. A harsh murmur heard in the same place may mean that the aortic valve opening is too narrow to let blood flow through easily; this is called stenosis. The location of the murmur in the chest also influences the diagnosis.

The sound quality of the heart murmur, such as its pitch or harshness, is important for the diagnosis of serious heart valve problems.

The timing of the murmur in the "lub-dub" heart cycle is crucial in figuring out whether there is valvular damage, and if so, what kind. If the patient has aortic stenosis, the murmur occurs during systole (between the lub and dub) because it is during this ejection phase of the left ventricle that the forward flow of blood meets the narrowed valve opening, producing turbulence. But if there is aortic regurgitation, the murmur is heard during diastole (between dub of one beat and lub of the next beat). It is during diastole that blood leaks backward from the aorta into the ventricle, causing the murmur sound.

Detection Techniques

The sound waves produced by murmurs can be recorded on an instrument called a phonocardiograph and printed out. Recording may be useful in difficult cases where the timing of the murmur in relation to other heart sounds is uncertain.

In the last several years a new noninvasive ultrasound technique has helped doctors determine the significance of murmurs detected during physical examinations. This technique, called Doppler echocardiography, uses transmitted and reflected sound waves to determine the speed and direction of blood flow. Doppler echocardiograms are used to confirm the presence of turbulent blood flow in narrowed valves and backward blood flow in leaky valves.

Drugs or surgery is needed when the murmur is a sign of faulty blood flow in the heart; otherwise, it can be left alone.

Underlying Causes

Defective valves are a common cause of heart murmurs. Some valve abnormalities are congenital; others, especially abnormalities of the mitral and aortic valves, may be caused by various conditions, including rheumatic fever, aging, and infection. Stenosis may occur if rheumatic fever causes thickening and fibrosis (an increase of fibrous tissue) of a valve, so that the valve does not open properly and the opening is narrowed. Regurgitation may occur if scar tissue, infection, or valve degeneration interferes with the closing of a valve.

Not all murmurs are caused by defective valves. Innocent, or flow, murmurs, those not associated with heart disease, are thought to occur when there is increased blood flow across a normal aortic valve. They are particularly common during the increased blood flow that occurs with exercise, pregnancy, or anemia. The murmurs tend to diminish or pass when blood flow returns to normal.

AORTIC VALVES: Normal and Abnormal

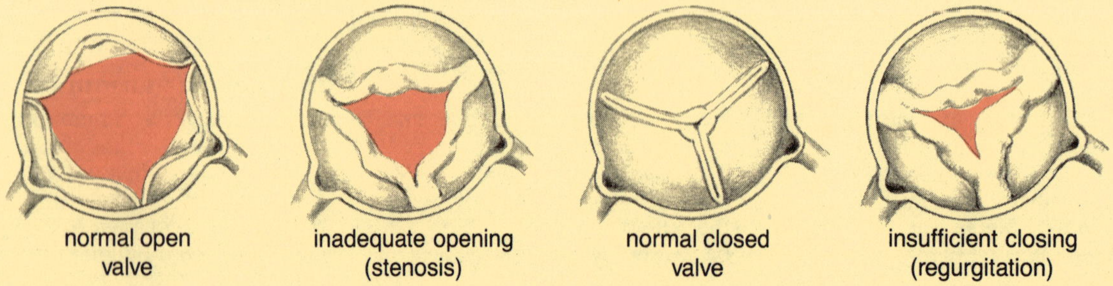

THE STRUCTURE OF THE HEART

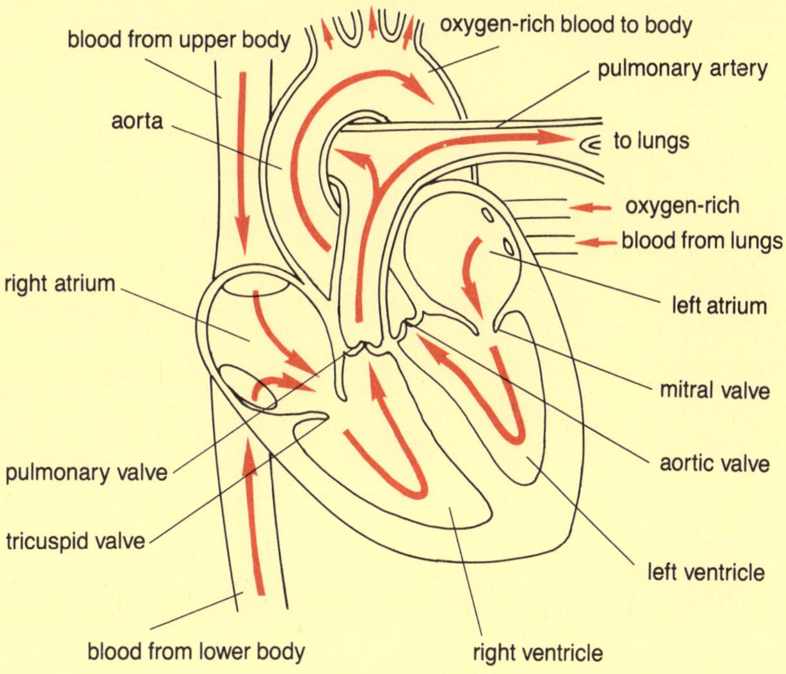

Another type of murmur is caused by a condition known as hypertrophic obstructive cardiomyopathy, in which there is a thickening of the muscle (the ventricular septum) that separates the left and right ventricles. This thickening acts as an obstruction to blood flow. A murmur may also be heard in cases where there is a hole in the ventricular septum (the hole may be congenital or develop after a heart attack) or as a result of several other types of congenital heart abnormalities.

How Does It Feel?

Sometimes patients are surprised when told that they have a heart murmur: they felt nothing wrong. People with innocent murmurs are likely to have no symptoms, and those with murmurs of other types arising from mild conditions may also feel perfectly well.

On the other hand, if the condition causing the murmur is severe, there are definite symptoms. Both severe aortic stenosis and hypertrophic obstructive cardiomyopathy can cause shortness of breath, chest pain, and blackouts. People with severe mitral stenosis or regurgitation may experience shortness of breath, fatigue, and palpitations. All of these conditions can cause a general feeling of weakness and seriously limit patients' daily activities.

Treatment

The treatment for a heart murmur depends on the cause of the murmur. People with innocent murmurs require no treatment at all, but in the case of other types of murmurs, medication and sometimes surgery is called for.

A valvular problem on the left side of the heart can eventually lead to heart failure. When there is aortic or mitral narrowing, pressure builds up in the chamber that is trying to pump the blood out. When there is aortic or mitral leaking, there is an overload of blood in the chamber to which the blood regurgitates. In all of these cases the heart cannot cope with the increased work load. Depending on the exact nature and severity of their condition, patients take different types of medication: digitalis to increase the heart's pumping force and to control irregular heart rhythm, diuretics to rid the body of excess fluid that accumulates when the heart cannot pump enough blood, and vasodilators to widen the blood vessels and thus lower the resistance against which the heart has to pump.

These drugs can help save lives and prevent serious complications. Sudden death may occur because of abnormal heart rhythms, especially in patients with aortic stenosis and hypertrophic obstructive cardiomyopathy. Blood clots can form when blood pools up in the left atrium because of mitral stenosis. If the clots travel and block arteries, they can do serious damage, as when a blocked artery to the brain causes a stroke.

If the valvular condition is especially severe or if drugs cannot control a patient's symptoms, surgery often will be needed to repair or even replace the damaged valve. Both artificial valves and chemically treated pig valves are used.

Preventing Infection

A potentially fatal complication for some patients—including those with various types of valvular abnormalities, artificial valves, and the common but rarely serious type of mitral regurgitation called mitral valve prolapse—is endocarditis, an inflammation of the heart that can result from bacteria in the body. To prevent endocarditis, patients with these valvular abnormalities should take antibiotics before and after undergoing any medical procedures that release bacteria into the bloodstream. These procedures include dental cleanings and tooth extractions, childbirth, and various kinds of surgery. □

Hay Fever

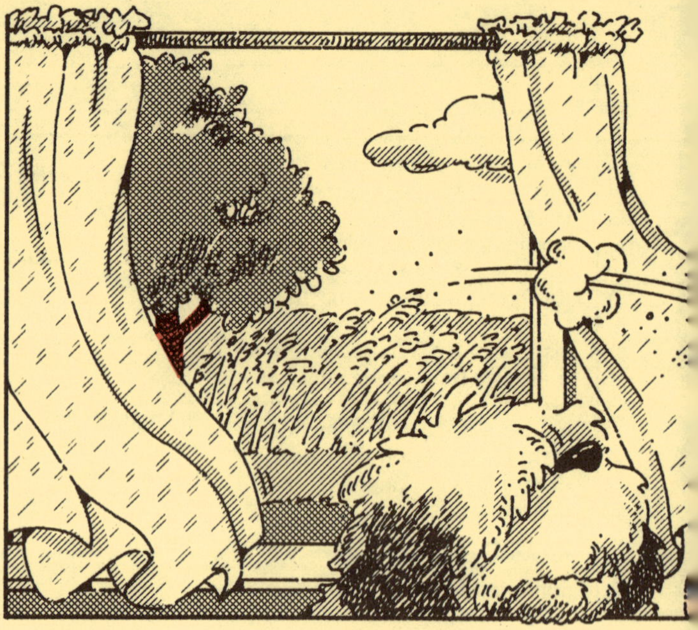

It's not just a seasonal sensitivity to pollen. Hay fever can be an allergic reaction to many other substances and can even occur year-round.

Theodore H. Sher, M.D., and Howard J. Schwartz, M.D.

Sneezing, a runny or stuffy nose, itchy eyes—this is the kind of misery hay fever works on its victims. According to one estimate, they number over 15 million Americans. Left untreated, the allergy can have an enormously disruptive effect on a person's daily life, sometimes making it impossible to go to work or to school for extended periods. Fortunately, a variety of treatments are available.

What Is Hay Fever?

Hay fever is a disease affecting the mucous membrane that lines the nose. It ordinarily is not caused by hay and does not directly produce a fever. Its medical name, "allergic rhinitis," is thus less misleading. Some victims have symptoms only at certain times of the year. (The term "hay fever" is in fact often used for just this seasonal allergic rhinitis.) Others suffer year-round. Most cases develop before the age of 30.

Like other allergies, allergic rhinitis is a hypersensitivity to (or intolerance of) some substance—called an allergen—that most people find harmless. When an individual sensitive to a particular allergen comes into contact with it, the body identifies the allergen as "foreign" and seeks to remove it. In the process, chemicals known as mediators—histamine is the best known—are released from certain cells of the body ("mast cells"), causing the allergy symptoms.

A person may become sensitized to an allergen at any age, even before birth. In the case of hay fever, what happens is that exposure to the allergen for some reason causes the body to make a type of antibody known as immunoglobulin E, or IgE. In contrast to the protective antibodies that form, for example, when an infection occurs, these special antibodies can trigger an allergic reaction when the individual again encounters the allergen.

Parents should not ignore a child's allergy; children tend to "grow into" their allergies, not out of them.

Although specific allergies are not inherited, the tendency to develop an allergy is much greater in families where allergy already exists. It is a mistake for parents to ignore a child's allergy in the belief that it will be "outgrown." Many children actually "grow into" their allergies, and so early identification and adequate treatment are important to avoid unnecessary discomfort.

Some Causes of Attacks

An attack is typically brought on by breathing in allergen particles floating in the air. A major offender is pollen—microscopic granules produced in enormous numbers by many plants. Pollen from trees, grasses, and weeds, including ragweed, is released into the air at specific times during the year, depending on local conditions and the geographic region. In the northeastern United States, tree and grass pollens are released during the spring and early summer, weed pollen during late summer and fall until the first frost.

Airborne allergens such as dust (and the microscopic mites that live in house dust), feathers, mold spores, and wool fibers may be responsible for symptoms that occur year-round, but they are especially likely to be troublesome during the winter months in cold areas, when the house is

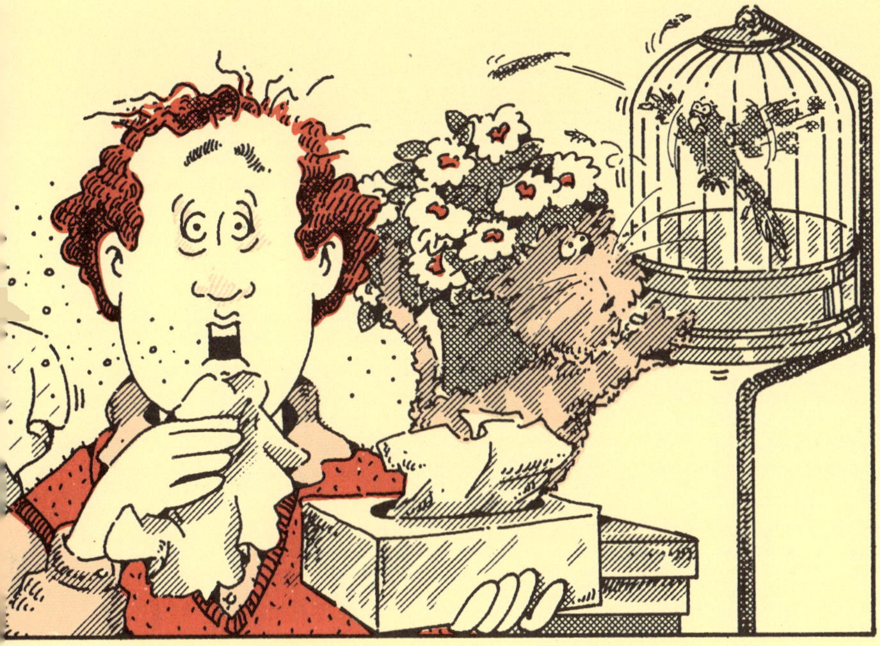

with a tiny sample of a suspected allergen, is generally the most sensitive. In some situations a properly used blood test (such as the one commonly known as RAST) may be of help, in addition to skin testing, in verifying an allergy. For suspected food sensitivity, an elimination diet may be used: the suspected food is first removed from the diet for a period of time and then added back as a "challenge test" to see if the allergic reaction recurs.

Several other conditions can produce symptoms similar to allergic rhinitis, including the common cold. But while a cold may cause congestion, the mucus is typically thick and yellow, not thin and clear as in allergic rhinitis, which also tends to be distinguished by itching and nonstop sneezing.

In making a diagnosis, the doctor will also consider the possibility of a sinus infection, especially if headache is a prominent symptom. Fever is not present in allergic rhinitis unless an infection has for some reason developed. Children who place objects in the nose may cause an obstruction producing symptoms that initially mimic allergic rhinitis. Occasionally, a person has allergy-like symptoms, but no specific allergen or infection can be found. The problem may be vasomotor rhinitis, a nonallergic condition sometimes brought on by temperature changes, strong odors, fatigue, anger, or anxiety.

relatively sealed. Other causes of year-round symptoms include animal dander (minute scaly skin material), hair, and lint.

For some people, eating certain foods can bring on an attack.

Symptoms and Complications

Among the many symptoms of allergic rhinitis are stuffed-up nose; postnasal drip (a persistent trickling of mucus from the back of the nasal cavity onto the surface of the throat); recurrent repetitive sneezing (as many as 20 sneezes in a row); red, itchy, and watery eyes; swollen eyelids; and itching of the mouth, throat, ears, and face. The itching may be quite severe at times, and infection can result from too vigorous scratching of the eyes and nose. Temporary partial loss of hearing, smell, and taste may occur, along with buzzing in the ears. A postnasal drip that doesn't go away can cause repeated throat clearing, hoarseness, a sore throat, and a dry cough.

Hay fever is not easy to diagnose since other conditions have similar symptoms.

Complications of allergic rhinitis are a risk if the condition is not treated. Infection can develop in the throat, ears, and sinuses. Tonsils and adenoids may become enlarged, and growths called polyps may develop in the nose. Also, fluid can build up in the middle ear, a condition called serous otitis media; if not detected and corrected, it can cause hearing loss in young children.

The allergy may cause a person to persistently breathe through the mouth, which can lead to gum disease. Poorly aligned teeth requiring orthodontic correction are another not uncommon result.

Making a Diagnosis

It's not always immediately obvious whether a person with hay fever-like symptoms has an allergy or some other condition. If the problem is an allergy, the offending allergens may not be easy to identify.

Laboratory tests can be a great help in making a diagnosis, particularly in determining the nature of the allergens. The skin test, in which the skin is scratched, pricked, or injected

Treatment Options

Medicine has made considerable progress in controlling the symptoms of allergic rhinitis. Three basic treatment approaches are used: avoidance of the allergen, medication, and allergy shots. In some cases only one approach may be required; in others all three may be necessary. It is important to remember that self-medication should be avoided; only those drugs recommended by a physician should be taken. All in all, today's treatment options promise a normal life-style, with minimal limitations, for virtually all hay fever sufferers.

Avoiding the Allergen

The ideal treatment for allergic rhinitis, because no drugs or injections are needed and results are guaranteed, is to avoid exposure to the allergen. Completely avoiding exposure is sometimes not easy, but it is often possible to at least minimize exposure.

People allergic to pollen, for example, should avoid long drives in the country or camping and hiking during hay fever season and should keep the windows closed at home. Those who live in an area of high pollen counts and can time their vacations to coincide with the pollen season will obtain relief by traveling to a place free of the allergens to which they are sensitive. Indoors, an air conditioner can be a big help, since by filtering the air it removes the pollen.

People sensitive to mold should stay away from barns and hay and avoid raking leaves and mowing grass. Dehumidifiers will help control mold growth in damp indoor areas.

Those allergic to dust should aim to make the bedroom a haven from heavy dust exposure. This can be done by such measures as using dustproof covers on pillows, mattresses, and box springs, among the commonest sites of house-dust mite infestation; covering hot air registers with dust-filtering materials; and using washable floor coverings. Some people may need to avoid such common household objects as stuffed animals, feather pillows, and toys made of fur or animal hair. Obviously, if a person has a significant animal-related allergy, it would be wise to remove the offending animal from the household, or at least from the bedroom.

Helpful Drugs

Many different types of medication are currently available to help control allergic rhinitis. Antihistamines, the mainstay of treatment over the years, block the effects of the body's histamine. Several kinds of antihistamine are on the market, and it may be necessary to change drugs if one stops working; this frequently occurs after prolonged usage.

Antihistamines are usually taken by mouth and therefore affect the body generally, sometimes causing drowsiness, a side effect that has limited their usefulness. This effect may lessen or disappear after a few days of continued use. Recently, several effective long-acting antihistamines have been developed that cause little or no drowsiness; terfenadine (Seldane), for example, has been approved in both the United States and Canada. Antihistamines can be used either preventively, before exposure to a known allergen, or as needed to control symptoms.

Oral steroid drugs are occasionally prescribed to alleviate incapacitating symptoms. They are extremely effective but have serious potential side effects when used at high doses for prolonged periods.

People with allergies should try to minimize exposure to the allergen; medication is available to help prevent and control allergic reactions.

Medication—in the form of nasal sprays—can also be administered locally, that is, to nasal tissue only. Several nasal sprays that have been introduced over the last few years can prevent symptoms from occurring. These preventive sprays are not decongestants and therefore do not cause "rebound congestion," the major problem with older decongestant nasal sprays. (Decongestants reduce swelling by shrinking the size of blood vessels in the nose; however, the spray irritates the nose lining, causing further congestion, the "rebound" reaction.)

The newer sprays must be used, under a doctor's supervision, on a daily basis in order to prevent symptoms from occurring, rather than on an "as needed" basis. With a seasonal allergy they are used during the season, and with year-round, or perennial, allergic rhinitis throughout the year. They are available in two major classes of drugs, cromolyn (sold in the United States as Nasalcrom and in Canada as Rynacrom) and steroids, for example, the drug beclomethasone. In many instances cromolyn may be used on a perennial basis, with steroids being reserved for seasonal symptoms, which are typically more severe.

Allergy Shots

When an allergen cannot be avoided, or when symptoms are severe, allergy shots may be given to lessen sensitivity, an approach known as hyposensitization. These are a series of injections containing small amounts (called an extract) of the material to which the person is sensitive. When injected, the extract causes the body to form protective antibodies that block the allergic reaction.

Injections are most successful in pollen allergies; they can also be given for such other allergens as dust, mites, and molds if necessary but are not helpful for food sensitivities. Up to one year of shots may be needed to produce results; if successful, the injections are continued, typically for a five-year period. Mild reactions such as swelling or itching at the site of the injection are quite common, but more serious reactions to the shots are fairly rare. □

Preventing Osteoporosis

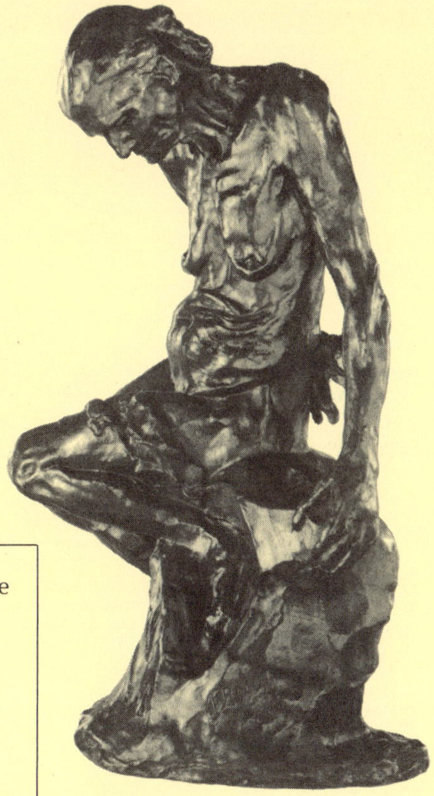

Auguste Rodin's She Who Was the Helmet-Maker's Beautiful Wife (The Old Courtesan), *1885.*

Jack Tohmé, M.D., and Robert Lindsay, Ph.D.

Osteoporosis, or thinning of the bones, is the most common bone disease in the United States. Affecting primarily older people, especially women, it makes bones more likely to break under minor stress. Osteoporosis often leads to fractures of the hip or wrist or to compression fractures of the vertebrae that can cause "dowager's hump" and make many women lose height as they age.

As many as 15 to 20 million Americans may have osteoporosis. The disease is responsible for more than a million fractures every year, including most of the approximately 300,000 hip fractures recorded annually; these are particularly serious because 10 to 15 percent of those who suffer a hip fracture die within a year as a direct complication of the fracture. The female-to-male ratio for fractures varies from more than ten to one for vertebral fractures to about two to one for hip fractures. The total U.S. health-care bill for osteoporosis is currently estimated at $3.8 billion a year.

The most common bone disease in the United States, osteoporosis affects primarily older women.

There is no general cure for the disease. But if those at risk of developing it take appropriate preventive steps, they can often slow its advance and minimize their chances of suffering a fracture.

Bone Remodeling

The skeleton is a complex system, made up of tissue undergoing a continuous repair process called remodeling. In this process calcium and other minerals are both removed from bone tissue and added back in. Until the ages of 20 to 35 the formation of new bone exceeds or equals the removal, or "resorption," of old bone, with men typically building up a higher skeletal mass than women. In time, however, bone formation lags behind resorption, and a steady decline in bone density occurs.

Types of Osteoporosis

Many doctors distinguish two major types of osteoporosis. Loss of the kind of bone that predominates in the vertebrae—called trabecular bone—appears to be closely related to hormonal changes in women after menopause. Loss of the kind of bone found, for example, in the hip—called cortical bone—together with loss of trabecular bone, occurs in both sexes with increasing age. It may be associated with a reduced ability of the digestive system to absorb calcium. This second type is superimposed on the first in the case of women. Together, the two types account for the vast majority of osteoporosis cases.

Occasionally, other factors may speed bone resorption or slow bone formation, thereby leading to a reduction in bone mass and so-called secondary osteoporosis. These factors include various gland disorders, the rare bone marrow cancer called multiple myeloma, vitamin D deficiency, and long-term use of cortisone drugs in the treatment of certain diseases. When such a secondary cause is present, dealing with it may help alleviate osteoporosis.

People at Risk

Women are particularly likely to develop osteoporosis because women have less bone mass when bone growth is complete, and because their bone mass decreases faster in association with the hormonal changes of menopause. In addition, a large body build seems to protect against osteoporosis, and thin women with slim builds run a notably higher risk of developing the disease.

Race also makes a difference. Osteoporosis is most common among whites and Asians, perhaps because blacks have greater bone mass. The disease tends to run in families. It is uncertain whether this is due to heredity or to "environmental" factors (like diet) that may affect all members of a family.

Soon it may be possible to routinely screen women for osteoporosis by measuring bone mass.

Among women, those who have an early menopause, whether occurring naturally or after surgical removal of both ovaries, are especially prone to develop osteoporosis. The body suffers a deficiency of the sex hormone estrogen after menopause, resulting in a loss of trabecular bone that may reach as high as 5 to 10 percent a year temporarily and in a loss of cortical bone as high as 2 percent a year. The rate of bone loss is greatest directly following menopause and tends to decline after four to eight years. It appears that the longer a woman retains her fertility, the less the risk of osteoporosis.

A diet low in calcium is another factor that raises the likelihood of osteoporosis. Most Americans do not get enough of this mineral; the average American woman consumes only about 500 milligrams of calcium a day. Many scientists believe that women may need 1,000 to 1,500 milligrams a day before menopause, and even more after. (Although the Recommended Daily Dietary Allowance set by the Food and Nutrition Board of the U.S. National Academy of Sciences is 800 milligrams, a revision is being considered.)

There is evidence that people with a sedentary life-style—a low level of physical activity—may experience accelerated bone loss. Also, alcohol abuse and cigarette smoking have been associated with osteoporosis, and research suggests that high intake of caffeine, protein, or phosphorus may also be contributing factors.

Measuring Bone Mass

At menopause about two-thirds of women have one or more of the various osteoporosis risk factors—body build, race, family history, early menopause, diet, life-style, and so on. Yet probably fewer than 25 percent of postmenopausal women will ever suffer significant fractures. If those who do develop osteoporosis could be identified at an early stage, preventive therapy could be started. Until recently, however, there was no way of making an early diagnosis; diagnoses took place when a fracture actually occurred or when thinning of the bones could be detected by a routine X ray, by which time 30 to 40 percent of the bone density was lost.

Over the past 15 or 20 years there has been an explosion of techniques for measuring bone mineral. In the fairly near future it may become possible to routinely screen women for osteoporosis with a measurement of bone mass at the time of menopause. Much improved measurements can already be made by using a combination of two techniques known as dual-beam and single-beam photon absorptiometry or by the sophisticated X-ray technique called computerized axial tomography (CT scanning). Dual-beam absorptiometry, however, is not yet universally available—though it may be soon—and CT scanning has the disadvantage (for use as a routine screening tool) of delivering a relatively high X-ray dose.

Prevention

Whatever technique is used, if a person's bone mass is found to be lower than normal, or if repeated measurements show the rate of bone loss to be greater than normal, the physician may want to start preventive therapy. Even without a bone mass measurement, special steps may be prescribed if any one of three major risk factors is present: poor diet (particularly calcium deficiency), sedentary life-style, and early menopause.

A key preventive measure is extra calcium in the diet. A total of 1,500 milligrams a day for most women is often suggested, especially after menopause. This can

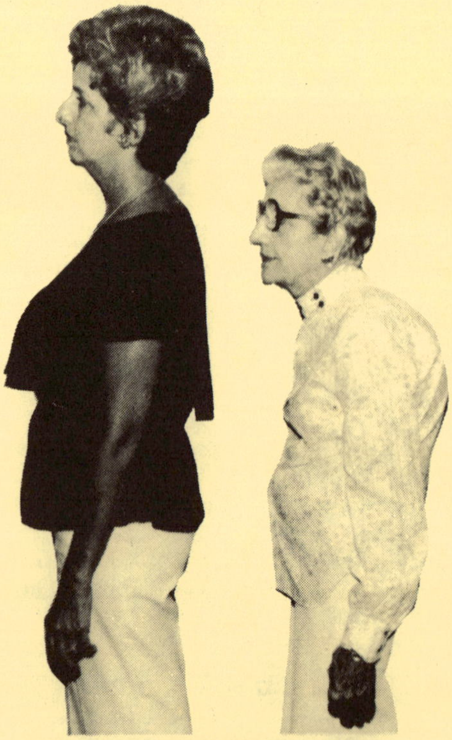

Bone loss resulting from osteoporosis caused the woman on the right (once only a half inch shorter than her daughter) to lose 5½ inches of her adult height.

be obtained by consuming more milk and dairy products—a glass of milk has about 300 milligrams of calcium—or by taking calcium tablets. (People with a history of kidney stones should take calcium supplements only under a doctor's supervision.) A normal

Getting enough calcium, exercising, and cutting back on alcohol and cigarettes are some preventive measures against osteoporosis.

intake of vitamin D is necessary for proper calcium absorption. Most people should get enough vitamin D from their skin, which makes the vitamin when exposed to sunlight. If sunlight exposure is limited, milk should supply it, since milk is enriched with vitamin D in the United States and Canada. For people concerned about their fat intake, low-fat milk can be used.

A second important preventive step is increased physical activity, if the individual's overall health allows it. Repetitive exercises in which muscles work against the pull of gravity, such as walking, jogging, and various forms of aerobics, may increase bone mass, especially in the central skeleton. Other helpful changes in life-style include reducing alcohol and cigarette consumption.

Estrogen may be prescribed for women after menopause, particularly if the menopause was early (when very many years have elapsed since menopause, however, estrogen is less effective, since estrogen can only slow the loss of bone, not rebuild it) or if there is evidence of continued bone loss after calcium and exercise therapy. Estrogen is the only treatment that has consistently been shown to be effective in reducing the occurrence of fractures. Estrogen will generally be given for at least five years. Careful follow-up by a gynecologist is important, because the estrogen may increase the risk of uterine cancer. Adding another hormone, progesterone, appears to reduce the risk, but the long-term results of the combination have not been fully evaluated.

Advanced Bone Loss

For people who have already suffered an osteoporosis-related fracture, meaning that the process of bone loss is already far advanced, treatment is also directed toward reducing pain and preventing further fractures.

Acute back pain is the most common symptom from vertebral fractures, requiring bed rest and painkillers. Hot packs and electrical nerve stimulation through the skin to control pain are often helpful; the aim is to minimize the period of bed rest and get the patient moving within a few days of the fracture. A back support may be temporarily needed to alleviate painful spasms of muscles near the spine. Fractures of the hip require surgery, but here, too, it is important for patients to move again as soon as possible.

A prime goal of researchers is an effective drug for strengthening bone. Calcitonin (sold as Calcimar) is a hormone that reduces bone resorption and has been approved in the United States for treating osteoporosis. But calcitonin merely retards further loss of bone. Patients with fractures would benefit most from therapy that stimulates the production of new bone and increased bone mass.

Researchers are trying to find a drug that will promote the formation of new bone.

Who Is at Risk?

Your chances of developing osteoporosis are higher if you:

- ☞ **Are a white or Asian woman**
- ☞ **Have a small build**
- ☞ **Have an early menopause**
- ☞ **Don't consume enough calcium**
- ☞ **Lead a sedentary life**
- ☞ **Abuse alcohol**
- ☞ **Smoke cigarettes**

Currently, there is no established drug treatment for achieving bone formation, although several approaches are under study. Fluoride in high doses has been found to induce bone formation, but doubts remain about the quality of the new bone. Also, fluoride can have undesirable side effects, such as stomach irritation, ulcers, and joint pain.

Vitamin D, which promotes the body's absorption of calcium, has been prescribed by some doctors, but in large doses it may increase bone resorption. In the body vitamin D is transformed into the hormone calcitriol. This substance (a synthetic form is marketed under the name Rocaltrol) may come to play a role in drug therapy in the future. □

The Importance of Iron

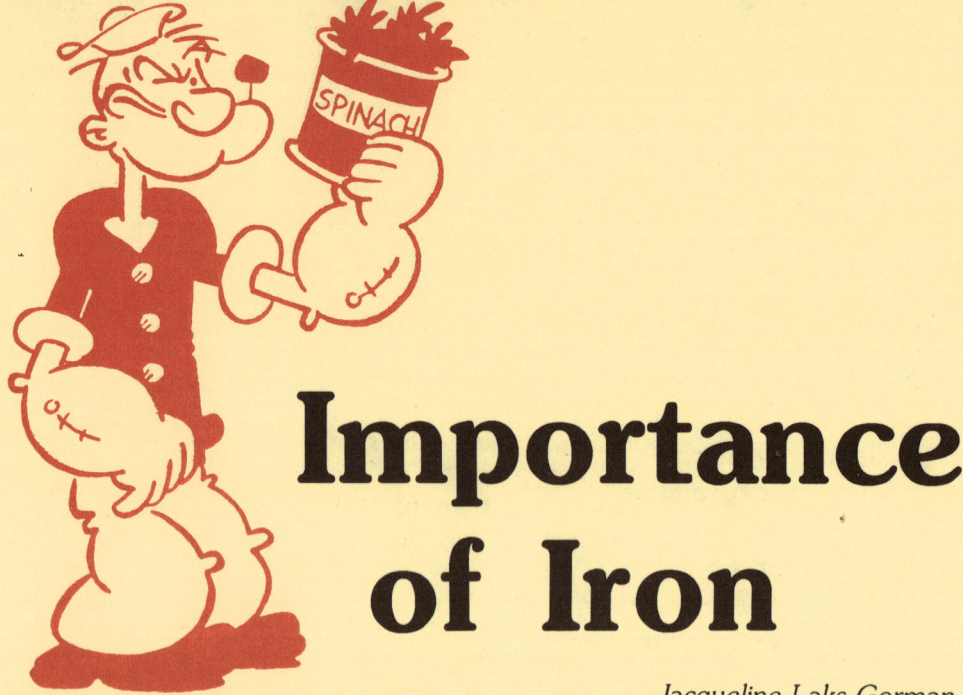

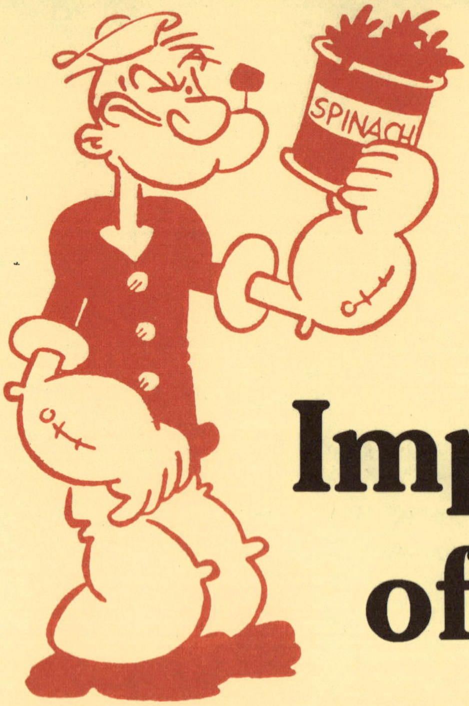

Jacqueline Laks Gorman

Popeye was wrong when he devoured a can of spinach, hoping the iron would give him an energy boost. Not only is spinach a relatively poor source of iron, but chances are the crusty old sailor didn't have an iron deficiency anyway. In adults, iron deficiency is far more common in women. Popeye should have shared his snack—imperfect source of iron though it was—with Olive Oyl.

Everyone needs iron in the diet, but adult men, like Popeye, need smaller amounts than infants and toddlers, teenagers, and menstruating women. Although most people should be able to get all the iron they need by eating the right foods, iron deficiency is the most common nutritional deficiency in both the United States and Canada.

Essential Element

Iron is a trace element, or trace mineral—one of a group of minerals (zinc and iodine are others) that the body requires in tiny amounts to perform important functions. Iron plays a critical role in supplying body cells with the oxygen they need to function and survive.

Most of the iron in the body occurs in hemoglobin, a molecule found in red blood cells that is the basis of the body's oxygen transport system. Hemoglobin is made of an iron-containing pigment called heme and a protein called globin. There are close to 300 million hemoglobin molecules in each red blood cell, and it is hemoglobin that gives these cells their characteristic color.

Hemoglobin can combine loosely with various gases, including oxygen and carbon dioxide, a waste product of body cells. When blood flows through the tiny blood vessels in the lungs, oxygen that has been inhaled diffuses into the blood and combines with the hemoglobin in the red cells. Then, as the blood travels through the body, it deposits oxygen with the body cells and picks up carbon dioxide. As the blood circulates back to the lungs, the carbon dioxide is left there to be exhaled. When at the end of their life span (about four months) red blood cells are broken down, the iron in them is saved and used again.

Hamburger, chili, or blackeye peas are better sources of iron than Popeye's spinach. A diet high in iron-rich foods can provide enough for most people.

Iron is also needed as part of certain enzymes and to form myoglobin, a pigment similar to hemoglobin found in muscle cells.

The Body Stores Iron

Iron stores—readily available surplus supplies of iron—are built up by the body at times when dietary intake exceeds the body's requirements. These stores are kept in the liver, spleen, and bone marrow. Maintaining iron stores is important because they provide a reserve the body can draw upon if dietary intake of iron is inadequate to meet specific needs. The larger the iron stores, the longer a person can tolerate a diet too low in iron.

For instance, if a woman enters pregnancy—during which iron requirements increase greatly—without adequate stores, it is unlikely that her diet will provide enough iron to meet her needs and those of the developing fetus. Without body stores to fall back on, she runs a strong risk of developing a serious iron deficiency. To prevent this, doctors routinely prescribe iron supplements for pregnant women.

"Tired Blood"

Contrary to the popular phrase, if you are deficient in iron, your blood isn't really tired—but you may be, because your body's cells are not getting enough oxygen. The condition is called iron-deficiency anemia, and its symptoms may include fatigue, weakness, paleness, light-headedness, and shortness of breath. Iron-deficiency anemia can also lower your resistance to various ailments, and studies have shown that youngsters suffering from it have reduced attention spans and may do poorly in school.

There are actually many types of anemia, which is any abnormal decrease in the amount of hemoglobin or number of red blood cells. Some types, like sickle-cell anemia, are hereditary. Others result if something goes wrong with red blood cell production. But iron-deficiency anemia is the most common.

Often, people suffer from an iron deficiency because there is simply too little iron in the diet and they do not have sufficient stores to meet normal needs, which vary from one population group to another. Young children, for instance, need a great deal of iron because of their rapid growth, and menstruating women need large amounts to replace the iron lost each month when blood leaves the body. In men, however, iron-deficiency anemia frequently occurs because of an intestinal tract disorder, an ulcer, or a tumor that causes abnormal bleeding.

If you think you may be anemic, you should see a doctor, who may do a blood test to determine whether you have anemia and, if so, what kind. If iron-deficiency anemia is diagnosed, you may be given iron tablets or perhaps even iron injections. The pills can cause intestinal discomfort and constipation, but you can help minimize these problems by taking the pills right after eating and adding to your diet high-fiber foods, including dried fruits, which have the added benefit of being rich in iron. Do not simply start taking iron pills without a doctor's recommendation if you have some of the symptoms of anemia. The symptoms may improve, but a possibly serious underlying disorder may go untreated.

Getting Enough Iron

Most people should not need an iron supplement if they eat the right combination of foods. A good deal of iron must be consumed to keep the body well supplied, since the body is capable of absorbing very little of the iron in food—about 30 percent of the iron contained in meat and only 5 to 10 percent of that in leafy vegetables.

Actually, the amount of iron that is absorbed depends to a large extent on how much iron

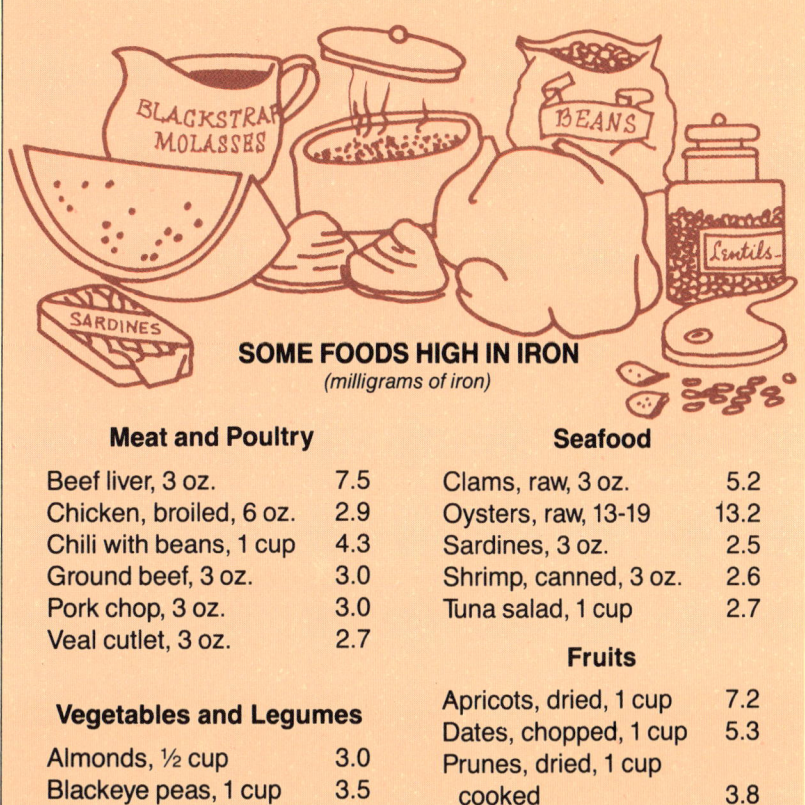

SOME FOODS HIGH IN IRON

(milligrams of iron)

Meat and Poultry

Beef liver, 3 oz.	7.5
Chicken, broiled, 6 oz.	2.9
Chili with beans, 1 cup	4.3
Ground beef, 3 oz.	3.0
Pork chop, 3 oz.	3.0
Veal cutlet, 3 oz.	2.7

Vegetables and Legumes

Almonds, ½ cup	3.0
Blackeye peas, 1 cup	3.5
Cashews, ½ cup	2.7
Kidney beans, ½ cup	2.3
Lentils, ½ cup	2.1
Lima beans, ½ cup	3.0
Navy beans, ½ cup	2.6
Sunflower seeds, ½ cup	5.2

Seafood

Clams, raw, 3 oz.	5.2
Oysters, raw, 13-19	13.2
Sardines, 3 oz.	2.5
Shrimp, canned, 3 oz.	2.6
Tuna salad, 1 cup	2.7

Fruits

Apricots, dried, 1 cup	7.2
Dates, chopped, 1 cup	5.3
Prunes, dried, 1 cup cooked	3.8
Raisins, 1 cup	5.1
Watermelon, 1 wedge	2.1

Sweeteners

Blackstrap molasses, 1 tablespoon	3.2
Sorghum, 1 tablespoon	2.6

Note: The amount of iron absorbed by the body varies with the type of food and other factors.

Source: Based on U.S. Department of Agriculture. *Nutritive Value of Foods*, 1981.

you need. If you are a menstruating woman and you have no iron stores, then your body will absorb as much iron as it can—perhaps twice as much as would be absorbed by a healthy man with sufficient stores. (The intestinal mechanism that controls absorption is not perfect, however. In the case of a relatively rare genetic disease, there is increased iron absorption that results in the buildup of excessive amounts of iron in and damage to the liver, heart, and pituitary gland. Healthy people can also suffer iron overload, especially if they take too many iron pills.)

The absorption of iron is also affected by other constituents of your diet. For instance, a substance called phytic acid, found in whole grains, combines with iron to form insoluble compounds that prevent iron from being absorbed. On the other hand, the presence of vitamin C favors iron absorption.

Since the absorption of iron depends on so many factors, generalizations about how much iron should be in people's diets are difficult to make. However, taking the variables into account, the Food and Nutrition Board of the U.S. National Academy of Sciences has drawn up Recommended Daily Dietary Allowances for different groups (see the accompanying table), indicating approximately the amount you must eat to absorb enough iron. If you eat little or no meat—the food from which iron is more readily absorbed—you may need to take in more iron than the amount recommended.

You can up your iron intake by eating more of such iron-rich foods as liver, red meat, and iron-enriched cereals, legumes, dried fruit, nuts, and leafy green vegetables. (See the accompanying chart for more detail on sources of iron.) Cooking acidic foods, like tomatoes, in iron pots can add iron to food. Alcohol, however, can interfere with iron absorption.

Greatest Needs

Infants, young children, adolescents, and women of childbearing age—not to mention women who are pregnant—need the most iron. As has been noted, women of childbearing age have a constant need for iron to replace that lost each month with menstruation. Most other cases involve the creation of new blood and body tissues.

Pregnant women need iron to supply the growing fetus and to support the development of the placenta—and also because their own blood supply is doubling. An iron deficiency can be especially serious during pregnancy; the mother will be more susceptible to infection and in increased danger if hemorrhaging occurs during delivery. Even if a deficiency does not develop, the mother runs the risk of exhausting her own iron stores in supplying the fetus. As a result, iron supplements are generally prescribed during pregnancy.

New mothers also need higher amounts of iron, and supplements are recommended—usually for two or three months. These make up for the iron the mother lost through bleeding at childbirth and add to her iron stores.

Babies and small children need relatively large amounts of iron because they are growing so rapidly. Until the age of four to six months, though, full-term infants get all the iron they need from the stores they are born with. After this time, to prevent iron deficiency, children must get iron from their diets or from supplements. (Premature infants have smaller stores and must be given iron supplements earlier in life.)

Although the iron in breast milk is well absorbed, the amount is too low to supply a baby with needed iron after four to six months of age. Infants who are bottle-fed may be given iron-fortified formulas from birth, but the iron is not actually needed until the baby's own iron stores are almost gone. Most physicians recommend iron-fortified cereals as the first food source of iron added to the infant's milk diet (at four to six months); later, green vegetables, liver, and other meats should be introduced as sources of iron.

A nutritious diet should provide children and adolescents with adequate amounts of iron. However, parents should be aware of how good or bad their youngsters' eating habits are. Iron supplements may be needed if diet proves inadequate. □

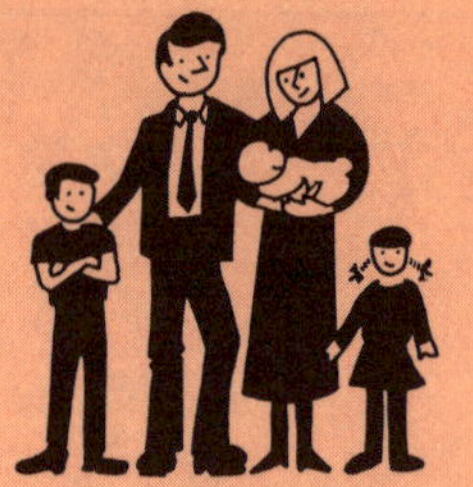

HOW MUCH IRON DO YOU NEED?

Recommended Daily Dietary Allowances

	Milligrams of Iron
Infants	
To 6 months	10
To 1 year	15
Children	
1–3 years	15
4–10 years	10
Males	
11–18 years	18
19 years and older	10
Females	
11–50 years	18
51 years and older	10
Pregnant	+30-60 mg supplement
Breast-feeding	+30-60 mg supplement

Source: Committee on Dietary Allowances, Food and Nutrition Board. *Recommended Dietary Allowances,* 9th ed. Washington, D.C., National Academy of Sciences, 1980.

Sex Abuse
What to Tell Your Child

Sally Cooper

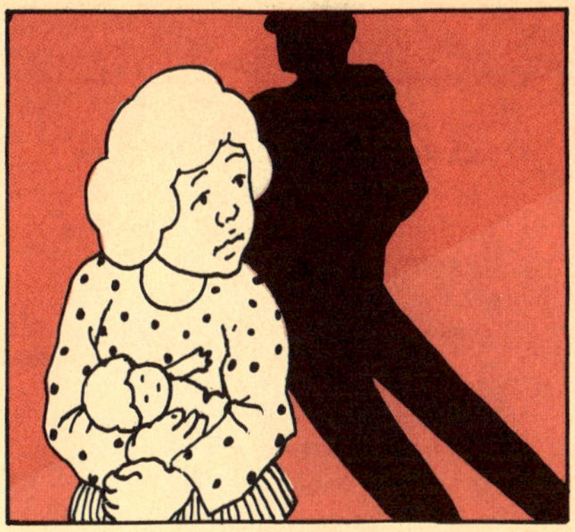

The sexual abuse of children is no longer an unmentionable subject. Revelations about sexual abuse in day-care centers, prime-time television shows about incest and child molestation, and a host of magazine articles have helped bring the subject out into the open.

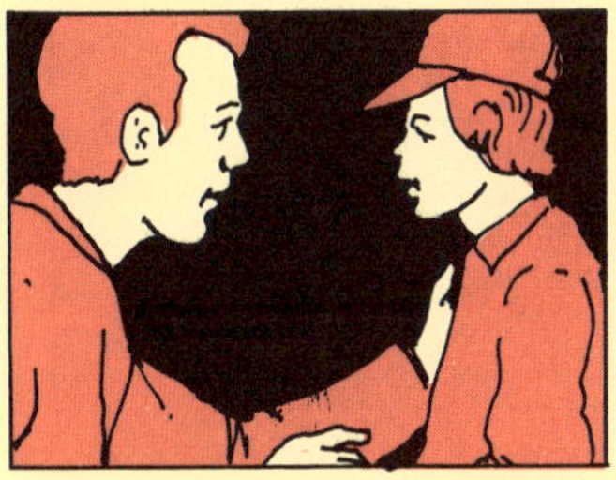

Many parents would like to talk to their children about preventing sexual abuse but don't know how. The topic is a difficult one. Parents are afraid they will say the wrong thing. Some feel a discussion of this topic could stir up excessive fears and anxieties.

Unfortunately, lack of knowledge about how to talk to a child leaves the child uninformed and consequently more vulnerable to assault. It is estimated that at least 100,000 and perhaps two to five times that many children in the United States are sexually abused each year. Recent studies indicate that approximately one out of every four girls and one out of every ten boys will be sexually assaulted before they reach 18 years of age. Victims come from every type of neighborhood and ethnic group and every economic class. No family is immune.

The warnings we were given as children—such as not to take candy from a stranger and not to get into a car with someone you don't know—are of little help when 80 percent of child victims are assaulted by someone they do know: a family member, neighbor, teacher, coach, baby-sitter, or leader of a church youth group. Children need to be prepared. Parents need to overcome their hesitations and speak directly to their children about ways to protect themselves from abuse.

Finding the Right Time

Parents don't have to call a big family meeting to talk about abuse prevention. Children as young as 2½ can be told that they shouldn't keep secrets from their parents. Television shows, a family trip, or a school program on child abuse can provide an opportunity for a parent to discuss the subject with the child in more detail. For instance, after the family watches a television show about a child who is assaulted by an adult, a parent could explain that sometimes children are hurt by people they know, even family members, and that keeping a secret that hurts prevents a child from getting help and support. Children who are afraid they won't be believed if they tell of such a thing should be reassured that they can trust their parents to accept what they say.

A Safety Issue

Parents teach children how to cross streets safely, what to do in case of a fire, and what to do and where to go if a storm or tornado threatens. Approaches used to teach these safety lessons can also be used to talk about assault prevention.

Focus on what your child can do. Sexual assault prevention information for women and children has traditionally focused on what *not* to do. This has meant that potential victims of assault often feel helpless in a dangerous situation. Children can follow all of the "don't" messages and still find themselves being threatened. Not knowing what to do may make them more frightened and leave them with feelings of guilt after an assault occurs.

Keeping the focus on what a child can do also prevents a parent from unnecessarily scaring a child. The discussion need not stray into graphic and horrible

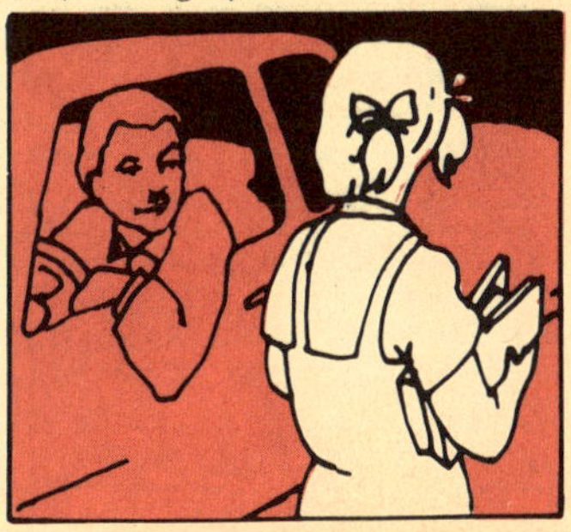

descriptions of what "some people" try to do to children. Instead, by learning real strategies for preventing assault, the child can come to feel capable and independent rather than defenseless.

Believe in your child's abilities. Self-confidence is 90 percent of prevention. When children believe they cannot prevent an assault, they probably won't even try. Parents should review prevention strategies regularly, always expressing their trust in a child's memory, ability, and quick thinking. Children have natural confidence that needs to be developed. Parents can reinforce that confidence by consistently giving the child "you can do it" messages.

Teach your child to say no. Parents should talk to children about their right not to be hurt or threatened. Using simple concepts and nonthreatening words, the parent can stress that a child has the right to say no even to an adult. (A child who can say no to eating green beans or going to bed may still be afraid to say no in an unfamiliar situation.) Parents may fear that children who are taught to say no will defy any adult authority, especially their parents. However, this is almost never true. Children need to understand, through clear and positive statements, that when they feel threatened they have parental permission *and encouragement* to stand up for themselves.

Children should be told that no one has the right to touch their bodies in ways that hurt, frighten, or confuse them. Direct information from parents about parts of the body can help them distinguish between "good touching" and "bad touching." Being tickled too long, having one's genitals touched, or being asked to undress without good reason are examples of adult behavior or demands that children can be told to reject. Adults who know the child they are assaulting often use bribes or threats to get the child to comply with their demands. Children must have confidence in their ability to say no even in these circumstances.

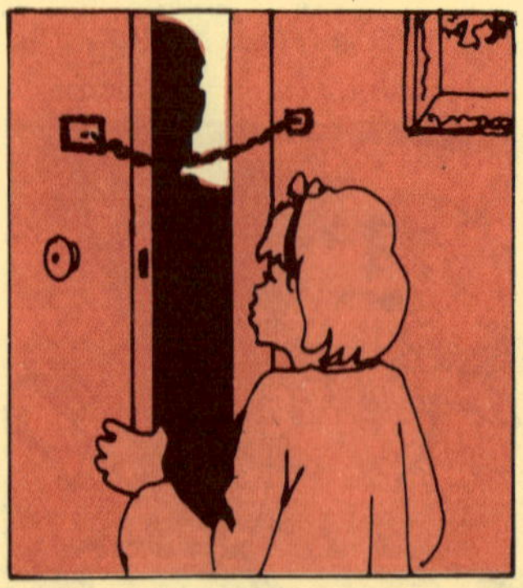

When It Does Happen

Even though parents should teach their children to prevent abuse, sometimes the worst may happen. When sexual abuse does occur, it is often difficult to detect. The child may be ashamed to reveal it or may have been told to keep the incident a secret. Children need to understand the difference between bad secrets and good secrets and to know that secrets about touching are bad secrets, which should not be kept. Children are often victimized repeatedly over a long period of time because of a belief that they had to keep a frightening secret.

Sometimes a child is afraid of not being believed. Perhaps the person responsible for the assault said, "I'll tell your mom you are lying, and she'll believe me." Children must feel confident that they can go to a parent with a painful secret and be believed. Experts agree that children rarely do lie about sexual abuse.

Signs of Abuse

When a child is too young or too frightened to tell anyone about abuse, it may still be possible to detect. Children who have been assaulted tend to share common characteristics:

- fear of going to a certain place or being with a certain person, or fear of adults in general
- unexplained bruises or bleeding
- self-destructive or self-mutilating behavior
- sleep disorders (bed-wetting, nightmares, sleeplessness)
- knowledge of sexual behavior at an inappropriate age
- sexually transmitted disease
- running away, promiscuity, stealing, drug use
- onset of school failure or discipline problems
- aggressive or withdrawn behavior

If you suspect a child is being abused, report it. Children rely on adults for intervention. In the United States, most state and county governments have a children's protective services office,

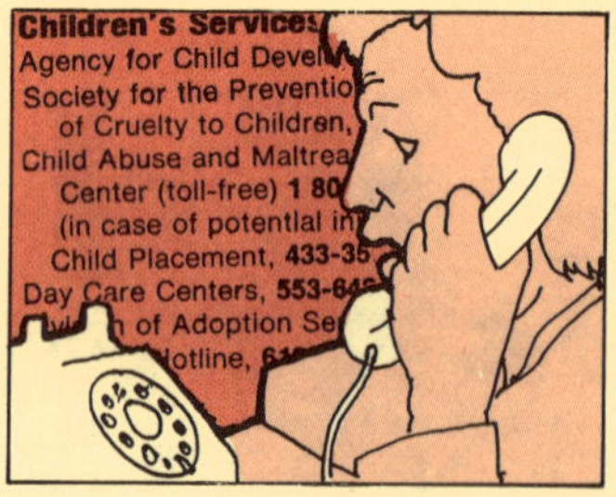

where suspected abuse can be reported. If you can't locate the number in your telephone book, call the governor's office or the state's child welfare department.

Residents of Canada can call an office of the Children's Aid Society.

Sexual abuse is a traumatic event in any child's life and can cause serious lifelong problems. Children are resilient, however, and if given love and support from family and friends can have happy lives after a frightening experience.

Certainly, all parents want their children to feel healthy and secure and to be free from the fears that abuse brings about. Parents who provide abuse prevention information for their children give them an important measure of protection. □

Why Teenagers Smoke

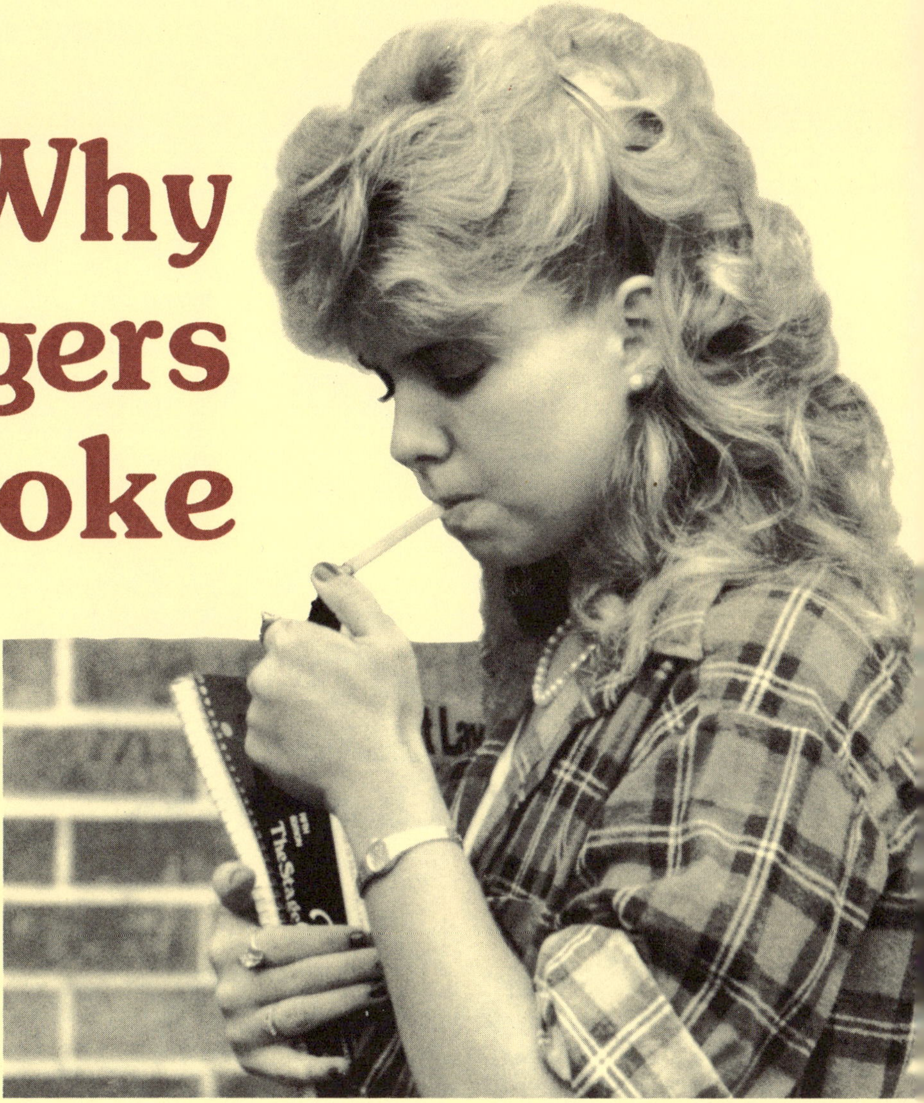

Richard I. Evans, Ph.D.

During the past several years there has been a substantial drop in cigarette smoking among adults: while approximately half of the adult U.S. population smoked in 1964, currently only about a third smoke. However, the news on the anti-smoking front isn't all good—the overall rate of smoking among teenagers is not dropping. There has been very little decrease in the proportion of teenage boys who smoke, and there has been an increase in smoking among teenage girls. Smoking by teenage girls is of particular concern because, presumably, these girls will continue to smoke when they get older. There has been a general increase in the proportion of adult women who smoke, and as a result, lung cancer has passed breast cancer as the most prevalent type of cancer among women. (It has long been the most common cancer among men.)

There is another potential tragedy in teenage smoking: teenagers who smoke may be more likely in the future to turn to drugs and alcohol.

In the University of Houston Social Psychology/Behavioral Medicine Research Group, several years of research have enabled us to determine some of the major reasons why, in the face of the obvious dangers connected with smoking, teenagers begin to smoke. These findings, which in general agree with those of other U.S. and British research groups, are based on information obtained from hundreds of interviews with teenagers, as well as on general knowledge of adolescent psychology. The findings have enabled us to devise strategies to help teenagers resist pressures to begin smoking.

Before we look at the reasons for teenage smoking, we should consider two interesting findings that have emerged from the research. First, virtually all teenagers now accept as fact that smoking cigarettes is dangerous to one's health. Indeed, younger children, between the ages of 4 and 11, are so concerned about the dangers of smoking that they actively try to get their parents who smoke to quit the habit. Second, most teenagers believe that more of their peers smoke than really do. In fact, most youths aged 13 and 14 smoke very little or not at all.

Peer Pressure and Role Models

Perhaps the reason most often given by teenagers for beginning to smoke is peer pressure. Teenagers who smoke place varying degrees of pressure on nonsmoking teenagers to begin smoking as one price for acceptance into the "in" group. Many teenagers seem unable to say no to these pressures.

Another reason teenagers begin to smoke is one they themselves only rarely recognize: the effect of "modeling"—for example, of seeing one's parents smoke. Studies by various research groups have found that if both parents smoke, the likelihood of a teenager smoking is much greater than if only one parent smokes or if neither parent does. And if both parents and an older brother or sister smoke, there is a four times greater likelihood that a teenager will begin smoking than if none of these family members smokes. Other models besides family members who exert a powerful influence on teenage smoking habits are the attractive, dynamic individuals who appear in cigarette ads and characters in television programs or films, who are shown smoking.

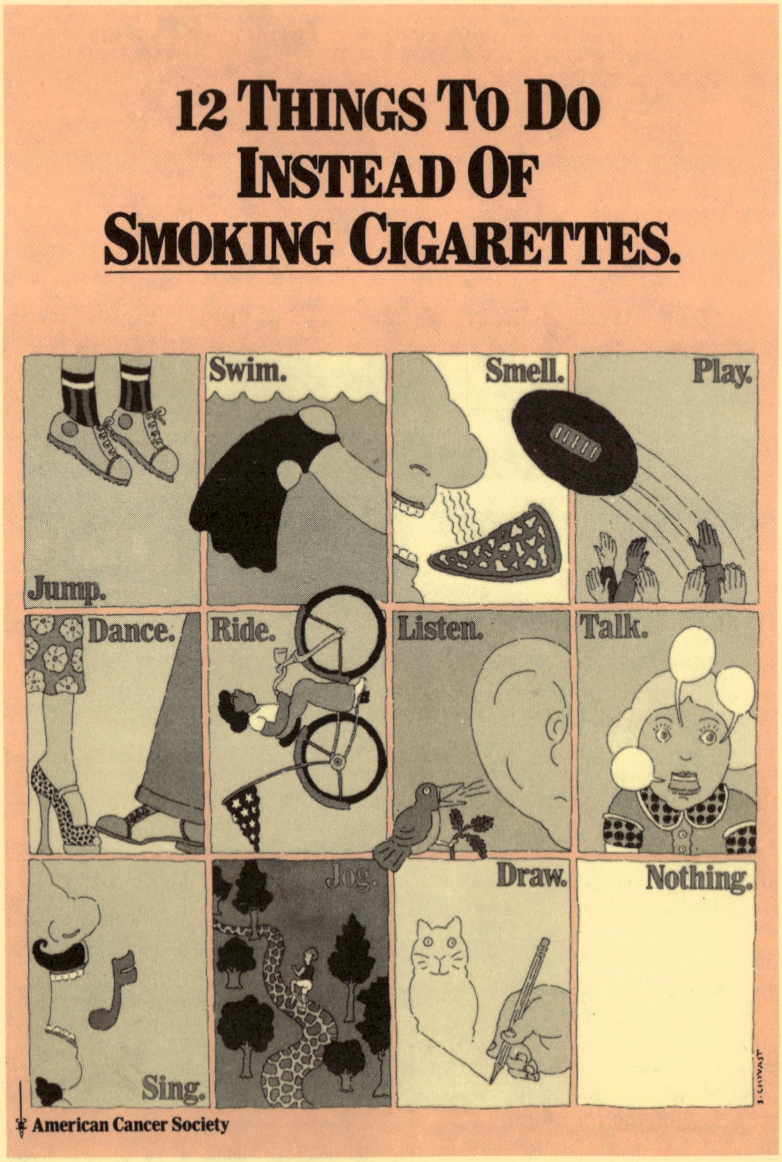

Taking Risks

One way in which teenagers attempt to assert their independence is by taking risks, particularly when this behavior does not meet with their parents' approval. Knowing the dangers of smoking, therefore, may be precisely the reason that some teenagers smoke, and in fact, much of the peer pressure to smoke is a challenge to engage in risky behavior. The relationship between risktaking and declaring one's independence from parental control may play a particularly strong role in the growing prevalence of smoking among teenage girls. Young women may feel a greater need to assert their independence by engaging in activities like smoking that were more likely to be considered male behavior in the past.

Scare Tactics

In order to help teenagers cope with both the obvious and the more subtle pressures to smoke, we in the Houston research group looked at previous approaches to preventing teenage smoking and developed new strategies; other researchers have proceeded along similar lines. It appears that too much of the health education to which teenagers have been exposed depends on arousing fear of the long-term consequences of smoking, namely, contracting serious illnesses like cancer or heart disease. But teenagers are more concerned with the present, and scare tactics are simply not enough to persuade many of them not to smoke.

As an alternative approach, we developed a series of films, around which are built sessions of discussion, skits, and role-playing activities. The aim is to raise teenagers' awareness of the pressures to which they are vulnerable, of some of the immedi-

A new tactic with teenagers is to stress immediate consequences of smoking, not long-term dangers.

ate risks of smoking, and of techniques for "fighting back."

Saying No

We learned from teenagers themselves the kinds of situations in which they were confronted with peer pressure (our discussion sessions use filmed simulations of these situations). We also asked a number of teenagers who did not smoke how they managed to resist the pressure to do so. From this information we were able to present teenagers with a "saying no" strategy in response to low, medium, and high peer pressure.

When faced with a relatively casual degree of pressure to smoke ("Hey, how about a cigarette?"), the teenager will usually find it sufficient to simply decline the offer assertively. Medium peer pressure, frequently phrased as a more direct challenge ("We're all doing it. What are you afraid of?") more often requires that a reason or excuse be given for refusing: "It'll ruin my track time" or "It's too messy." The nonsmoker may also exert counterpressure, placing the challenger on the defensive by asking, "How come you smoke?"

To resist a high level of peer pressure, which may occur as an organized effort (against girls as well as boys) in which the nonsmoking teenager is constantly taunted as being "gutless" and afraid, the nonsmoker must be prepared to resist actively by saying, "Why are you putting pressure on me?" or "Look at all the kids who *don't* smoke." At this level of pressure, self-esteem plays an important role in resistance, since by refusing to smoke a teenager is essentially refusing a kind of "social entrance ticket." The present climate of growing social conservatism in society at large and the growing militancy of adult nonsmokers against those who smoke in public places provides a valuable atmosphere of support for this kind of resistance.

This new "saying no" program—called the social inoculation approach—appears to be more successful than simply trying to use scare tactics in persuading teenagers not to begin smoking.

Also effective are films and a discussion program we designed to train teenagers to recognize how they are influenced by role models who smoke—whether parents, people in ads, or media celebrities. This increased awareness lessens the impact of such models.

Immediate Dangers

Finally, the Houston research group's approach stresses the immediate physical and social consequences of smoking rather than the long-term dangers. There are many drawbacks that make an impression on teenagers: eye and throat irritation, bad breath, tobacco stains on teeth and fingers, a smoke odor that permeates clothing, falloff in athletic performance, rejection by a nonsmoking girlfriend or boyfriend, effects on the unborn child should a teenage girl smoke during pregnancy, serious complications that may arise when smokers take birth control pills, and even economic consequences, since a growing number of employers are advertising for nonsmokers.

What about youths who have already begun to smoke? Since most teenagers who smoke are relatively light smokers, the same techniques used for prevention are often effective in deterring continued smoking as well. (The comparative few who have developed a full-fledged nicotine addiction may have the same withdrawal problems as addicted adult smokers who try to stop.)

Even without films and organized discussion groups, the new approaches to preventing teenage smoking can be applied by parents, physicians, and others. At the same time, many parents have been active in bringing the film and discussion programs into their local school systems, where health education programs provide a ready vehicle for the antismoking programs and where the students are in effect a captive audience.

For the Future

The Houston research group is currently involved in a large project to apply its antismoking techniques to discouraging teenagers from using drugs and alcohol as well. We also have found a new problem: the use of chewing tobacco and snuff by teenagers. This may be an increasing health threat because while teenagers believe that "smokeless tobacco" is safer than cigarettes, recent research indicates that it may be directly related to the development of various types of oral cancers (cancers of the lip, tongue, mouth, and pharynx), to tooth loss and gum disease, and even to heart disease.

Nonsmoking teenagers must learn how to resist pressure from their peers.

In the case of smoking, however, with our increasing knowledge of why teenagers begin to smoke and the development of the new social inoculation techniques for training teenagers to resist pressures to smoke, there is some basis for optimism that smoking among teenagers will decline significantly during the next few years. □

Is Fever Good?

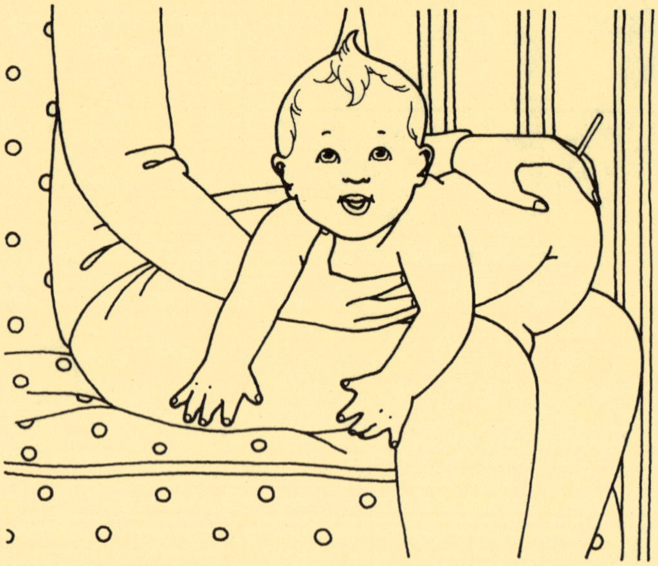

Matthew J. Kluger, Ph.D.

Fever is something we have all experienced at one time or another, and we are familiar with its unpleasant effects. In fact, not only humans but many other living things—lizards, fish, and birds, as well as all mammals—develop fevers. But despite fever's commonness, little has been known until recently about what it actually is and how it works. Research now shows that fever may not be the villain it's been cast as for so long.

Temperature Regulation

To fully understand the nature of fever requires some knowledge about how body temperature is regulated. Birds and mammals—the so-called warm-blooded animals—have the ability to maintain a relatively constant internal temperature despite temperature changes in their environment. When a person is out in the sun on a hot day, the body responds in various ways to help keep internal temperature down. Excess heat is carried to the skin by increased skin blood flow. This causes tiny blood vessels in the skin to dilate, thereby increasing the area over which heat can be dispelled. Also, large amounts of heat are lost from the skin surface through the evaporation of sweat, which is secreted by specialized glands.

In addition, the hot weather may trigger a number of behavioral responses: the person may seek out a cooler place, remove some clothing, and perhaps spray the body with water, which is cooling as it evaporates.

Fever sets in motion elements of the immune system that fight infectious bacteria and viruses.

When a person is exposed to the cold on a winter day, the body takes different steps to keep internal temperature up. The surface blood vessels contract to prevent heat loss. The muscles begin to quiver—that is, the person shivers—and the energy generated is converted to heat. Of course, one may also respond by putting on more or heavier clothes and by drinking hot liquids. It is through the body's heat-regulating (thermoregulatory) reflexes, plus behavioral responses, that humans are generally able to maintain a body temperature close to the normal 98.6°F.

The regulation of body temperature is controlled by the body's thermostat, which is located in the part of the brain known as the hypothalamus. The body's thermostat can be compared to the thermostat that runs a home heating system. The temperature the home thermostat is set for and that it maintains is called the set-point temperature; any significant deviations above or below this temperature will cause the thermostat to turn the furnace on or off.

The body's thermostat also has a set point, generally at a temperature of about 98.6°F. This set point varies by about a degree among individuals—and within a given person, depending on the time of day. Body temperature is generally lowest in the early morning and highest in the late afternoon or early evening. When the outside temperature differs from the internal set point, it is the hypothalamus that sets the body mechanisms going to produce or get rid of heat.

Resetting the Thermostat

Fever occurs when, because of the presence of certain substances in the body, the body thermostat is turned up to a higher set point. Many things can trigger a rise in set point, which can increase 7°F or more. These include physical injuries, adverse reactions to drugs, and, most commonly, infections.

The invasion of the body by viruses or bacteria sets off many defenses. Among them is the activation of various phagocytic white blood cells that engulf and destroy the infectious agents. When one such white cell, the macrophage, is stimulated, it begins to synthesize and release a protein once called endogenous pyrogen, or EP. (A pyrogen is defined as a substance that produces fever.) Recently, after it was found that dozens of other body responses to infection are also triggered by EP, the protein was renamed interleukin-1.

Interleukin-1 travels through the bloodstream to the brain, where it raises the hypothalamus's thermoregulatory set point—and thus causes fever—by stimulating the production of prostaglandins, a class of naturally occurring chemicals. Drugs that reduce fever, called antipyretic drugs, do so by preventing the production of prostaglandins.

The initial resetting of the set point makes the individual feel cold. This is because the body temperature has not yet risen to the higher set point. To raise body temperature, the hypothalamus sends out impulses that cause decreased blood flow to the skin (which prevents heat loss) and that cause shivering (which produces warmth). Moreover, behaviorally the person reacts in many ways to help raise body temperature, like putting on warm clothing. Soon the chills end, and the individual with fever feels hot, because the higher set point has been reached. The person may also feel uncomfortable, experiencing fatigue, headache, muscle aches, and loss of appetite. These discomforts are not caused by the fever itself but by the effect of interleukin-1 and prostaglandins on various parts of the body.

When the infection ends, the fever "breaks"—that is, it declines as the thermoregulatory set point returns to normal. Blood flow to the skin increases; the person may look flushed and sweat profusely; excess clothing is removed. All this helps body temperature go down to normal

Does Fever Have a Function?

From a purely practical standpoint, a fever is extremely useful—body temperature is easy to measure and provides a quick indication of health. (It should be noted, however, that fever is not the only thing that increases body temperature. Exercise or sitting in a sauna or hot tub also does, but this rise is actually a condition known as hyperthermia. During hyperthermia the set-point temperature is not elevated—only the body temperature. The body's physiological and the person's behavioral responses are all designed to return body temperature to the normal set point.)

Recent research has shown that

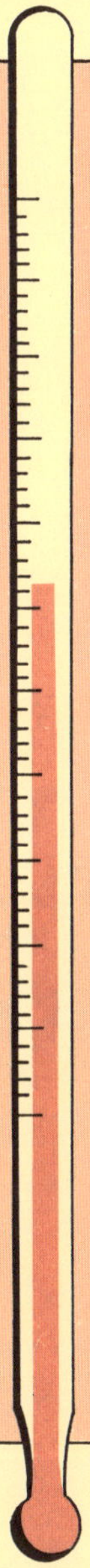

THE FEVERISH CHILD

Children tend to run higher fevers than do adults: in most cases a fever in a child is not considered high or dangerous until it reaches 105°F. On the other hand, parents should never ignore a fever. Some tips on when to call the doctor:

- **When a baby under six months of age runs any kind of fever.**
- **When a temperature of 100°F or 101°F persists for more than a day.**
- **When a fever of 104°F or higher lasts for more than four hours, even after the child is given a fever-reducing drug.**
- **When any fever—even a low one—lasts as long as four days.**
- **When any fever is accompanied by symptoms like lethargy, extreme drowsiness, breathing difficulty, or a rash, earache, or sore throat.**

If a temperature goes above 102°F and the child is uncomfortable, many doctors recommend fever-reducing drugs to ease the aches and pains associated with a fever. Use aspirin substitutes instead of aspirin if a child has chicken pox or the flu.

Taking a small child's temperature orally is difficult. Alternatives: putting the oral thermometer under the child's armpit, which will give a reading 1°F lower than the oral method, or using a rectal thermometer, which will give a reading 1°F higher than the oral.

fever is an integral component of the body's defense armament—its immune system—and that fever sets in motion processes that fight bacteria and viruses. The notion that fever is beneficial is not a new idea. In ancient times, fever was thought to help "cook" the poisons that caused infection. This belief was held by Hippocrates over 2,000 years ago and was taught by physicians until the mid-19th century, when antipyretic drugs like aspirin were first developed. At this point the belief that fever was beneficial began to wane, probably because of the fact that antipyretic drugs are also analgesics—that is, they reduce the aches and pains that often accompany a fever. Since the reduction of the fever coincided with less discomfort, it was concluded that fever itself is bad and causes pain. Medical research, however, does not support the claim that in general fever is harmful.

Stimulating the Immune System

There have been numerous studies in recent years demonstrating that small elevations in body temperature stimulate the body's immune system. When an infectious agent breaks through the skin or the mucous membranes that line the respiratory or digestive tract, the next line of defense is probably the activation of neutrophils. This class of white blood cells rapidly travels to the site of the infection and begins ingesting the infectious agents. There is also a burst of activity leading to the production of many antibacterial substances within the body. Studies have shown that when there is a fever, the neutrophils travel more rapidly to the site of the infection and ingest the foreign particles more readily. There is increased production of antibacterial chemicals as well.

Fever also stimulates the body's cells to start producing interferons, which are proteins that have potent antiviral, antitumor, and antibacterial effects. In addition, fever speeds up the production of T lymphocytes—a group of white blood cells that not only attack foreign agents themselves but also stimulate other cells to fight infection.

There have been studies of how fever affects the survival rate of various animals suffering from bacterial and viral infections. In general, these studies have shown that moderate fevers have a beneficial effect. Lizards, goldfish, and certain newborn mammals with infections have higher survival rates when they run fevers, while the suppression of fever in bacterially infected rabbits results in increased mortality.

Can Fever Be Harmful?

It is important to emphasize that although fever plays a role in the body's response to infection, not all fevers are beneficial. In individual cases, fever may be harmful. For people with heart conditions, fever might pose an unmanageable stress since it increases the heart rate. High fevers during pregnancy increase the risk of birth defects. But for most people it is likely that moderate fevers—up to about 102°F—rev up the body's defenses and speed recovery.

What to Do for Fever

What should you do the next time you have a fever? If it is low or moderate, getting plenty of rest and drinking sufficient liquids to replace the fluids lost through sweating may be all that is necessary; the fever can be allowed to run its course and help combat the infection. However, if you are extremely uncomfortable, an antipyretic drug like aspirin or acetaminophen may be taken. Since most infections are not life-threatening, the relief the drugs provide may be more important to you than the benefits of the fever. For children suffering from flu or chicken pox, it is advisable to avoid aspirin since it has been linked to the dangerous disease Reye's syndrome in such cases.

High or persistent fevers generally indicate the presence of a more severe infection. A physician should be consulted if a fever rises particularly high or lasts more than a few days. While a high fever should never be dismissed, parents should remember that children tend to run higher fevers than do adults. □

Fever sufferers of all ages should get plenty of rest and drink sufficient liquids to replace any fluids lost through sweating.

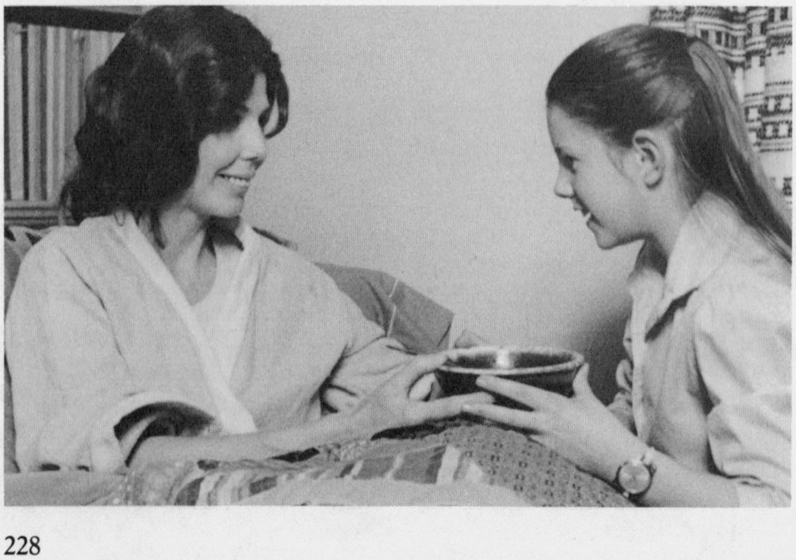

High-Tech Surgery

Sharon Begley

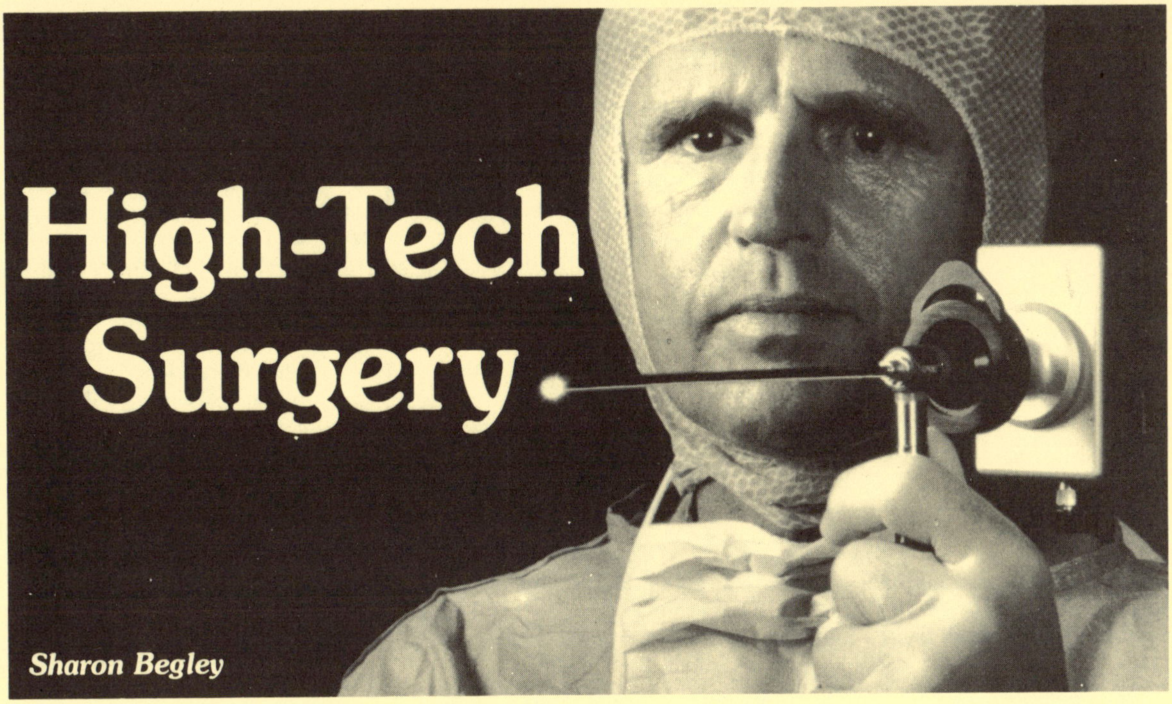

When the gold medals were being awarded at the 1984 summer Olympics in Los Angeles, two of the U.S. winners had more than their coaches to thank for helping them to the victory stand. They also owed a big debt to their orthopedic surgeons. Both Mary Lou Retton, winner of the women's all-around gymnastics competition, and Joan Benoit, who took the gold in the first women's Olympic marathon, had undergone arthroscopic knee surgery just a few months before. A decade ago their injuries would have required open-knee surgery and would have sidelined the athletes for perhaps 12 weeks. With the burgeoning use of arthroscopy, however, they were back in training within a few days.

Arthroscopic surgery is only one of the procedures classified under the catchall phrase "endoscopic surgery." There are endoscopes for the lower gastrointestinal tract (sigmoidoscopes and colonoscopes), for the genitourinary system (cystoscopes and nephroscopes), and for other parts of the body. The instruments have basic similarities: they are thin shafts, sometimes flexible and sometimes rigid, crammed full of light-carrying glass or plastic strands called fiber optics. When inserted through a tiny incision or natural opening in the body, the scopes allow the physician to see inside the colon, knee, or other body part. Most of the scopes have additional channels through which miniaturized operating tools can be passed; in this way a physician can cut out a potentially cancerous polyp in the lower bowel without subjecting the patient to open abdominal surgery.

Although primitive endoscopes have been used since the 19th century, the devices did not become widely popular until the development of fiber optics in the 1950's. Thinner than a human hair, the fibers carry a bright light into the joint or organ the doctor is examining. The image can be viewed directly through an eyepiece, or, in a high-tech variation, projected onto a television monitor for a magnified picture. Once used only for diagnosis, endoscopes are now also used in surgery; they are even being paired with lasers, which seal off the blood vessels, for essentially bloodless surgery, often on an outpatient basis.

Patients recover faster from an endoscopic procedure than from conventional surgery.

Like much of medicine lately, endoscopic diagnosis and surgery is driven not only by technology but also by the urgent need to hold down medical bills. Because some endoscopic surgery is now being performed on an outpatient basis in clinics or even in doctors' offices, and because even the operations done in hospitals require a much shorter stay, the technique appeals to budget-conscious healthcare providers. In 1985 there were an estimated 500,000 arthroscopic procedures, and 6,000 of the 14,000 orthopedic surgeons in the United States now perform such operations.

Surgery Inside the Knee

Some 90 percent of the knee operations in the United States are now performed with arthroscopes. Usually, these are operations to remove torn cartilage, the tough, rubbery tissue between the bones of the knee that acts as a shock absorber, or to remove bone chips lodged in the joint. The arthroscope has been used for diagnosis for about a decade and combined with microsurgery for about eight years.

In a typical procedure, the patient is placed under general anesthesia. The surgeon then makes three tiny incisions in the knee, each usually no bigger than a quarter-inch. A tube is inserted into the first incision, and a saline solution is injected to flush bits of tissue out of the knee, which in effect enlarges the joint for examination. The arthroscope, a steel cylinder some 10 inches long, is inserted into the second incision. Its fiber-optic system, connected to a tiny video camera, transmits movie-quality images of the joint to a television screen. The surgeon scrutinizes the picture to pinpoint the areas needing repair.

To make the repairs, the surgeon threads microsurgical tools through the third incision. The surgical instruments include hand-held scalpels and forceps, power-driven drills to which surgical blades are attached, and electrosurgical instruments that cut tissue and stop bleeding by means of a radio-frequency current. Using any of these tools, and guided by the picture on the TV screen, the surgeon can do a number of repairs.

It isn't hard to account for the popularity of arthroscopic surgery for knee injuries, which, in this fitness-conscious age, are no longer the bane only of football running backs. Each year, more than 200,000 Americans need to have damaged knee cartilage removed, and this has become the most common application of arthroscopic surgery. Damaged cartilage can injure other parts of the joint and allow the knee bones to rub against each other in a very painful way.

With scopes, growths and obstructions in the GI tract can be removed without full-scale surgery.

Fixing damaged knees used to require major surgery, in which the physician opened up the joint. The patient spent several hours in the operating room, a week in the hospital, and three to four months recovering at home. Arthroscopic surgery, in contrast, takes about an hour, can be performed on an outpatient basis, and in most cases keeps the patient on crutches for just three to five days. Some recoveries are even faster: Retton was back training the day after her operation, and Benoit had completed two one-hour runs just a week after her surgery. Another benefit is that arthroscopic diagnosis is often more accurate than X rays, which can be obscured by shadows in the knee and thus do not always pinpoint the extent and location of joint damage.

Arthroscopic surgery is used now in ankles, elbows, and shoulders, too. It can shape or soften cartilage that has been roughened or worn down by overexercise, to treat the arthritis-like condition called chondromalacia. Arthroscopic surgery is also being used to repair ligaments (which brace the joint and hold the bones together), removing torn ones, reattaching them, or even replacing them with synthetic or transplanted tissue.

The widespread enthusiasm for arthroscopic surgery can, however, conceal some of its drawbacks. Although many surgeons have learned the techniques of this type of surgery, operating on a delicate joint while watching a TV screen for guidance requires a dexterity and experience that not all possess. Also, arthroscopic diagnosis can miss problems originating outside the joint. Even the promise of quick recuperation can backfire; patients may be tempted to get back on the jogging path too soon, jeopardizing their recovery.

Scopes for Internal Organs

Other types of endoscopes offer similar advantages over conventional diagnosis and surgery, but for internal organs instead of joints. For the past decade these endoscopes have been used increasingly in conjunction with surgery. Today, sophisticated technology is making them even more useful.

Each endoscope, which costs around $10,000, has a diameter and length adapted to the organ it will be used for—the stomach, for example, or the colon. But the basic elements of each endoscope, such as the fiber-optic channel and operating-tool channel, are identical. One manufacturer recently introduced a scope with interchangeable shafts of different lengths and diameters so that, for the price of one scope and light source, the physician has the capability to examine both the colon and the upper gastrointestinal tract by simply using shafts of the appropriate size. One of the latest advances is an ultrasonic endoscope—an endoscope equipped with an ultrasonic probe, which uses sound waves to create an image of an organ, called a sonogram. When the probe is placed close to the target organ, it produces a better image than many through-the-skin sonograms and can detect minute tumors within organs such as the liver and the pancreas. An endoscope alone can detect only abnormalities visible on the surfaces of organs.

Into the GI Tract

One major application of endoscopes is in the gastrointestinal (GI) tract. To perform an examination of the upper GI tract, which includes the esophagus, stomach, and duodenum (the first portion of the small intestine), the physician has the patient swallow a long, flexible endoscope, called an upper endoscope, which is then maneuvered into place. (The patient is usually given a sedative or an anesthetic spray on the back of the throat to numb the gag reflex.) The scope reveals inflammation, ulcers, tumors, or polyps so well that some physicians use it as the first line of attack against gastric complaints. It is more accurate than X rays in detecting gastric and duodenal ulcers, and it may reveal cancers too small to show up on X rays.

If small polyps or tumors are found, the physician can thread a wire snare down the operating channel of the scope and remove the suspicious-looking growth, or the doctor can take a snip of the growth with a biopsy forceps, for laboratory examination of the tissue. Alternatively, if there is an unhealthy-looking mass of cells, a small brush can be passed through the endoscope to wipe cells from the spot for later laboratory testing—in essence, a GI Pap smear-type test to detect cancer.

In another application, an upper endoscope can be used to detect and alleviate a troublesome condition in which a gallstone becomes stuck in the common bile duct, obstructing the flow of bile from the liver and causing liver damage, jaundice, or a dangerous bacterial infection. Dye is injected directly into the bile duct, through a catheter passed through the endoscope's operating channel, making the stone (or stones) visible on an X ray. The physician can then remove the obstruction by passing through the scope's operating channel an instrument that resembles a wire basket, which opens and snares a stone. The

Doctors performing delicate arthroscopic surgery on the knee watch the video monitor for a view inside the joint, transmitted by the scope's fiber-optic system.

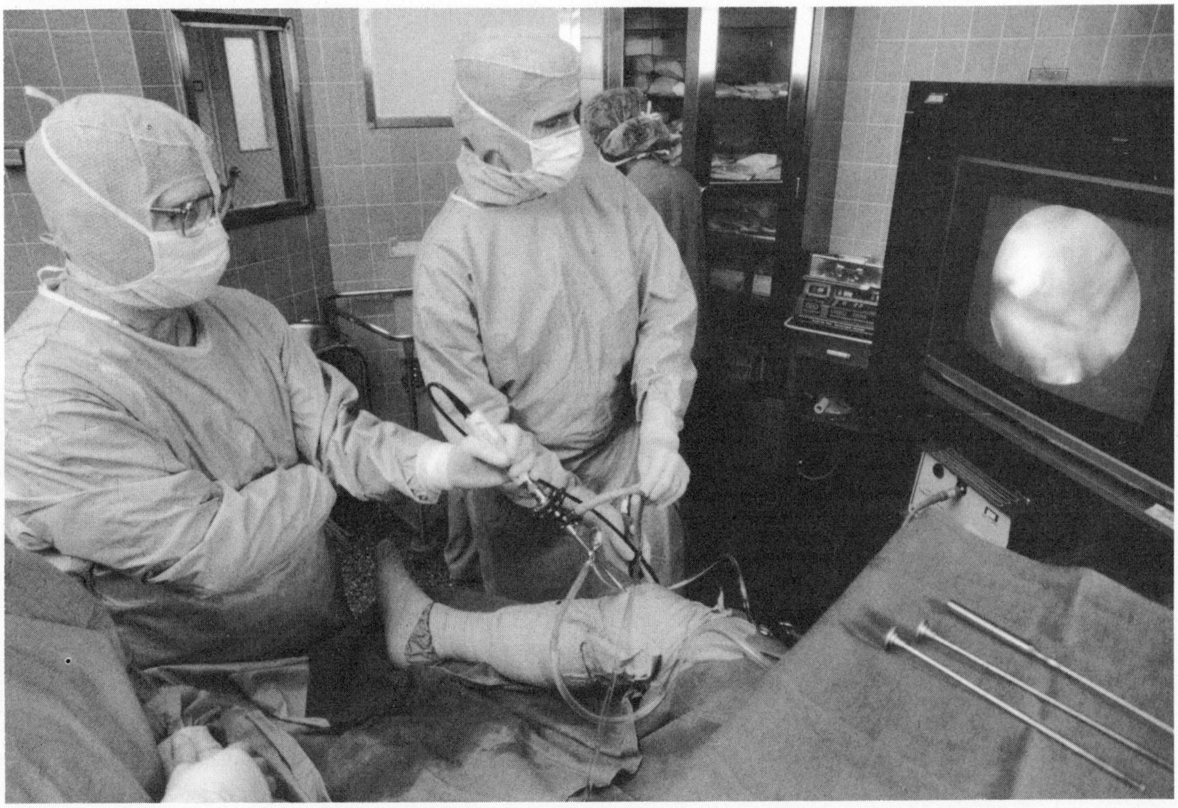

physician also can use other microsurgical instruments in the operating channel to enlarge the duct opening, letting the stone pass through. Although this is one of the most technically difficult areas of endoscopy, its use has been growing in the last few years.

In another important advance in the treatment of GI problems, some endoscopes are now being fitted with a laser light source: the fiber-optic bundles carry the laser beam to the stomach, where it can stop bleeding, or to the esophagus, where it can burn away some tumors.

Colon and Rectum

In the lower GI tract, colonoscopes and sigmoidoscopes are used to examine and remove growths from the colon and rectum. Physicians are particularly alert for signs of cancer in these organs, since colorectal cancer has become very common in the United States and Canada. Despite advances in diagnosis and treatment, mortality from colorectal cancer remains high, largely because the disease is often not detected early enough. The sigmoidoscope, which is used to examine the lower part of the colon, can help detect cancer in early or precancerous stages; as a result, sigmoidoscopy has become part of the standard physical checkup, especially for people over age 50. The sigmoidoscope is inserted through the rectum, without the patient being anesthetized.

The colonoscope is more invasive—that is, it goes farther into the colon—requiring up to 90 minutes for a diagnosis, and the patient receives a mild sedative. It is therefore less desirable as an initial screening tool for abnormalities of the colon but quite useful to determine the cause of an already detected symptom, such as bleeding, or to study in detail abnormalities suspected from an X ray. Again, should the physician find a polyp, a wire snare can be laced down the scope to the polyp to sever the growth with a radio-frequency current carried through the wire. The current simultaneously coagulates the blood vessels. Alternatively, a small brush passed through the scope can collect cells for a Pap smear-type cancer test. A colonoscope can be used to detect larger tumors as well. This was the case with President Ronald Reagan, who in July 1985 underwent conventional surgery to have a malignant tumor removed from his colon after a colonoscopic examination had revealed its presence.

Endoscopes may be more accurate than X rays in detecting gastric and duodenal ulcers.

The flexible endoscope, equipped with its operating channel and augmented by radio-frequency current or laser light, offers obvious advantages over traditional gastrointestinal surgery. (However, the endoscopic form of treatment cannot be used in all cases.) Most obviously, it saves time and money, since endoscopic procedures can often be done on an outpatient basis. Also, it can save lives: before endoscopic diagnosis and surgery, many GI polyps went undetected until they became cancerous. The only choice in the event of bleeding or other symptoms of uncertain cause was to open up the patient for exploratory surgery. And before colonoscopy, major abdominal surgery was the only way to remove polyps. As the scopes become smaller, they are more comfortable for patients, and as their optics improve (the current models pack some 15,000 to 30,000 fibers in a bundle), they are giving physicians better views, thus making possible more accurate diagnoses.

Other Applications

In the urinary tract, many conditions that previously required open surgery can now be performed endoscopically. Bladder stones and cancers can be detected by cystoscopes. Moreover, cystoscopes can be paired with a source of sound waves that can literally blow up the stones. Urethroscopes that examine the entire length of the ureter from the kidney to the bladder are being used to detect tumors and stones; once found, the obstructions can be removed by forceps threaded through the urethroscope instead of by conventional surgery. Similarly, nephroscopes pushed through a catheter into the kidneys are finding kidney stones that can then be destroyed with sound waves.

In a recent application of endoscopic surgery, physicians at the Johns Hopkins Hospital treated patients suffering from sinusitis. Using forceps inserted alongside the illuminating endoscope, they removed the damaged sinus tissue, which seems to cause nagging inflammation, postnasal drip, and a stuffed nose. If further tests prove its usefulness, this outpatient procedure could replace conventional surgery in which the entire sinus lining is removed during an expensive hospital stay.

Like most new medical technologies, endoscopes do have their limitations. Most significant, they can tear the stomach or the intestine; if the tear allows intestinal fluids to leak out, surgical repair may be required. Although widely touted for their cost-effectiveness, endoscopes can also be overused—particularly for diagnosis—when a cheaper method such as X rays would perform just as well. But there is no doubt that as physicians and surgeons substitute scopes for full-scale surgery in more and more procedures, the outlook indeed seems to be for lower patient bills, earlier diagnoses, and faster recoveries. □

Pregnancy and Exercise

Mona M. Shangold, M.D.

Women today are more active than ever, running in marathons, swimming daily laps, and lifting weights. But what happens when a woman becomes pregnant? Is it all right—even good—for an expectant mother to continue her exercise program? And should a woman who has not previously exercised regularly take up a physical activity when she becomes pregnant?

In general, pregnancy is not a good time to begin a new training program or to intensify an old one. However, women who before pregnancy were accustomed to any type of aerobic exercise (activities like jogging, swimming, or stationary bicycling that raise the heart rate and keep it elevated continuously and that increase the body's intake and use of oxygen, thus conditioning the heart and lungs) can probably continue the sport throughout pregnancy. Various other sports can be continued as well. This assumes that a woman has no medical or obstetrical complication, like heart disease, a cervix that opens too easily, or a multiple pregnancy. Of course, any woman should check with her obstetrician before engaging in an exercise program during pregnancy.

Which Exercises to Do

Pregnant women should avoid any sport that involves a strong possibility of falling or of trauma to the abdomen. Beyond that, many sports can safely be continued during pregnancy by women who became accustomed to them beforehand, and a few activities may even be taken up during pregnancy.

As noted, pregnant women can continue any type of aerobic exercise, although they should probably exercise at a slower pace. If a woman was accustomed to running seven-minute

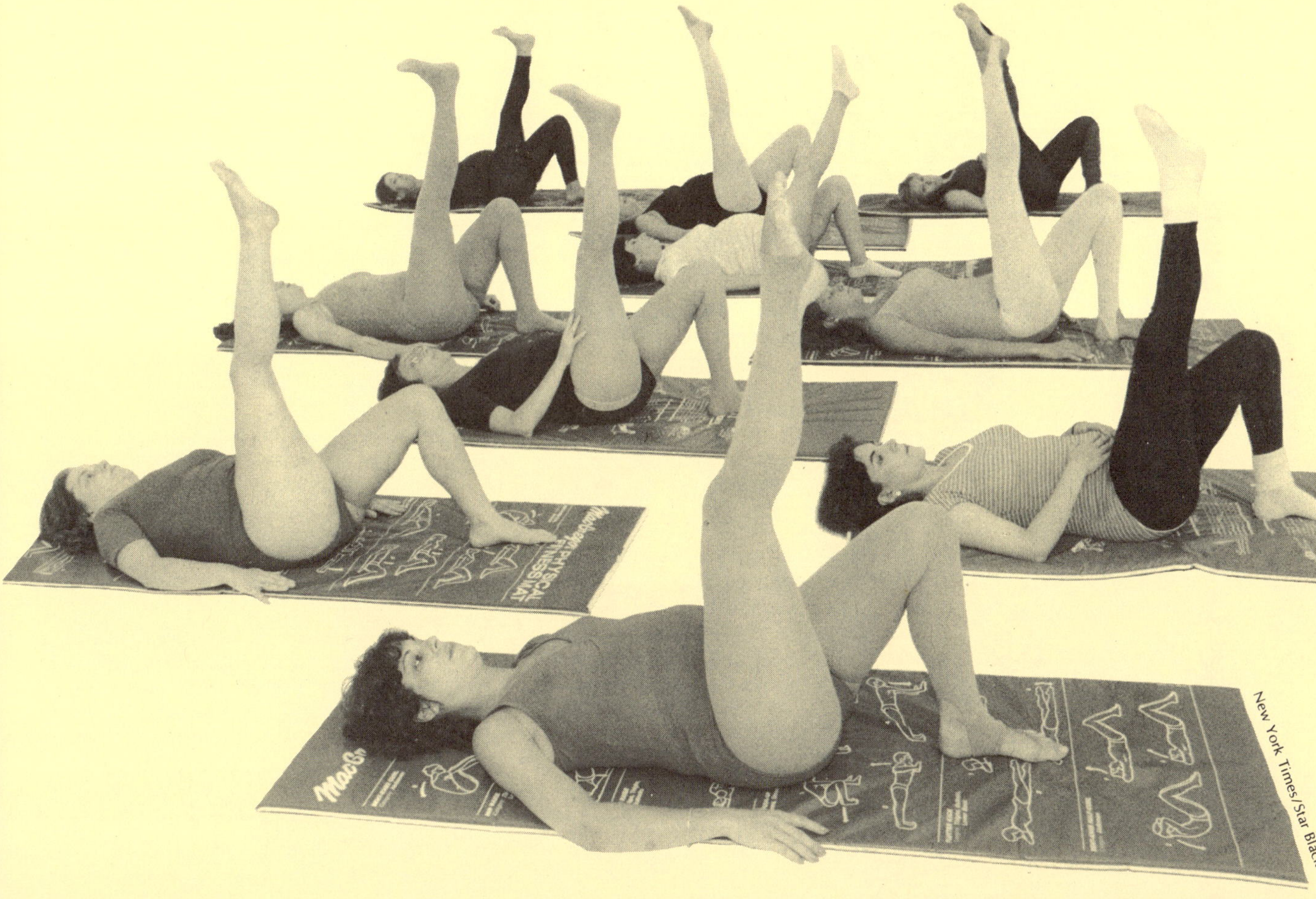

New York Times/Star Black

miles prior to pregnancy, she will probably have to slow down to a nine-minute-mile pace. Slowing down will be particularly necessary toward the end of pregnancy; the woman will be carrying considerably more weight by that time. Of course, if any aerobic sport, even one a woman is already accustomed to, causes discomfort, it should be discontinued.

Other sports that may safely be continued during pregnancy include golf, bowling, softball, basketball, and racket sports (tennis, racquetball, or squash). A pregnant woman can go ice-skating or roller-skating if she is good enough to avoid falling. Among competitive track and field sports, both javelin and discus are fine.

Among the sports that probably should be avoided during pregnancy are hang gliding, parachute jumping, and boxing. Nor should pregnant women go diving (either deep-sea or springboard), since changes in pressure can be dangerous. Also to be avoided are tackle football, fencing, hockey, soccer, and most competitive track and field sports.

Expectant mothers can participate safely in many different types of sports and activities.

Although pregnancy is not a good time to take up any aerobic sport more strenuous than walking, some other types of activities—calisthenics or weight training, for example—can be started by someone who was not an exerciser before pregnancy. Mild stretching exercises are quite safe. However, calisthenics are unlikely to promote fitness since they do not condition the heart and lungs and do not increase muscle strength. (After the fourth month, a woman should not do any calisthenics—or other exercises—that involve lying on her back, which could compress a major vein and interfere with the fetal blood supply.)

For women with no medical or obstetrical complications, weight training is an excellent way to strengthen the muscles of the arms, legs, chest, and back (although it also won't improve cardiovascular fitness if it is done with heavy enough weights to strengthen the muscles significantly). Stronger muscles will help a woman carry her added weight and cope with the altered center of gravity during pregnancy, and so she will be less likely to experience many of the aches and pains common among pregnant women, particularly low back pain. The muscle strength acquired during pregnancy will make it easier to carry the baby around after birth too.

Weight-training machines are safer and more comfortable and efficient than free weights for both pregnant and non-pregnant women, but either can be used to attain and maintain stronger muscles. Women who have never lifted weights before will find it helpful to have an instructor present during the first few sessions. After this, supervision is probably unnecessary for women using weight-training machines; women using free weights may benefit from always having an instructor present if they are lifting very heavy weights.

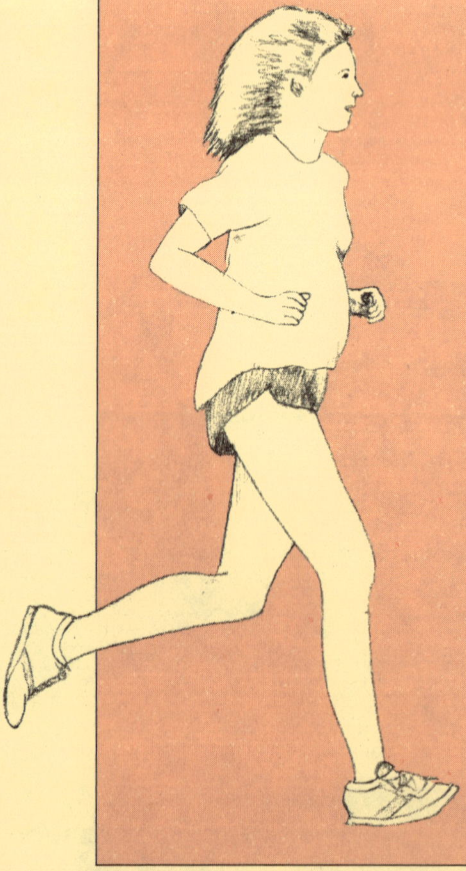

PRECAUTIONS DURING PREGNANCY

- **Don't do any type of exercise that causes discomfort.**
- **Avoid any sport that involves a strong possibility of falling or of trauma to the abdomen.**
- **Slow down if you are continuing an aerobic exercise you did before becoming pregnant.**
- **Limit aerobic exercise sessions to a maximum of 30 minutes.**
- **Don't let your temperature rise above 101°F.**
- **After the fourth month, don't do any exercises that involve lying on your back.**
- **Stop exercising and see your doctor immediately if you develop pain, bleeding, dizziness, shortness of breath, palpitations, or ruptured membranes or if you stop feeling the baby move for more than 12 hours.**

Playing It Safe

Pregnant women continuing a fitness program should avoid extremely vigorous or tiring exercise, because it is still not known exactly how much maternal exercise is safe for the baby. Two major concerns deal with possibly diminished blood flow to the uterus and with heat accumulation.

In any individual, blood flow is altered during exercise. While more blood goes to the exercising muscles and the skin, less blood flows to the liver and kidneys. Doctors do not know at what intensity or duration of exercise the blood flow to a pregnant woman's uterus also decreases. Since the blood going to the uterus supplies oxygen and nutrients to the developing baby, a decrease in this blood supply could have a harmful effect. In fact, some studies have shown that pregnant animals who exercise run a greater risk of premature labor (going into labor too soon, before the baby is fully matured) and that their offspring run increased risks of stunted fetal growth, stillbirths, and death shortly after birth. Although no detrimental effects from exercise have been shown in humans, the animal findings are worrisome.

Women who enter pregnancy in a good state of fitness are better able to meet the challenges of pregnancy, labor, and delivery.

Therefore, pregnant women must be cautious and sensible. Because speed work is most likely to divert blood toward the exercising muscles, these women should avoid sprinting or otherwise exercising very intensively for more than a minute or two.

During aerobic exercise, the exercising muscles get warmer and raise the temperature of the entire body. High body temperatures in the first two months of pregnancy can increase the chances of birth defects, and in the last five months, increased temperatures can promote premature labor. Therefore, it is important for pregnant women to avoid overheating—probably throughout the pregnancy. They should probably limit any aerobic exercise sessions to a maximum of about 30 minutes. Significant temperature elevations can occur shortly after 30 minutes of continuous exercise; however, they are unlikely to occur within that time.

Women exercising during pregnancy should check their temperature at the end of a customary workout. If it is greater than 101°F, internal temperature may be too high for the baby. In that case, the woman should take measures to keep cooler when exercising: working out at a cooler time of day and for a shorter period of time, wearing lighter clothing, and drinking more fluids.

The best way for an exercising pregnant woman to judge the intensity of her exercise is by her breathing effort. As long as she does not have to breathe so rapidly and heavily that it interferes with her ability to carry on a conversation during exercise, she is not exercising too intensively.

Weight Gain

Exercise during pregnancy should not burn up so many calories that it prevents the mother—and the baby—from gaining enough weight. A woman should gain approximately 20 to 30 pounds during pregnancy (including the weight of the fetus). The baby's growth can be measured by the growth of the uterus and, if necessary, by the use of the visualizing technique ultrasound, or sonography. If the mother is gaining weight too slowly and/or if the baby's growth is inadequate, the woman may need to alter her habits, eating more or exercising less.

Being Fit For Pregnancy

Some women become interested in fitness for the first time when they are pregnant. However, they would have been much wiser to strive for fitness before pregnancy, because pregnancy itself is hard work—more easily performed by someone who is already physically fit. Merely nourishing the fetus and carrying it around require a great deal of exertion on the body's part.

Extremely vigorous or tiring activities should be avoided, as should those that cause any discomfort.

Any activity that a woman performs while carrying the extra weight of pregnancy represents a much greater work load than it otherwise would, and women who enter pregnancy with weak muscles and poor cardiovascular fitness are ill equipped to meet the additional demands of pregnancy. Those who enter pregnancy at higher levels of fitness should be better able to meet this challenge. Fit women will also be better equipped to handle the exhausting experiences of labor and delivery.

Listening To One's Body

Whether a woman is starting or continuing an exercise program while pregnant, she should always listen to her body, which will tell her when she is overdoing it. She should stop exercising immediately and see her obstetrician promptly if she develops pain, bleeding, dizziness, shortness of breath, palpitations, or ruptured membranes or if she stops feeling the baby move for more than 12 hours. She should not resume exercising until her doctor tells her it is safe. □

Treating Epilepsy

John M. Pellock, M.D.

Once it was known as the falling sickness. People suffering from it were sometimes thought to be possessed by demons. Even today epilepsy is a disorder that may bring social stigma and discrimination because of wide public ignorance about the nature of the disease.

The fact is that epilepsy is a relatively common brain disorder—affecting 1 to 2 percent of the population—and its symptoms are often mild. It is not contagious. It is characterized by recurring attacks, called seizures, that may range in severity from brief staring spells to prolonged, violent convulsions. The seizures may occur at any age but most commonly begin in childhood.

Medical science has made great progress in improving the lives of epileptics. While a general "cure" is not yet in sight, for most people available treatments can result in complete control of seizures with minimal side effects.

Misfiring Neurons

Epileptic seizures can be considered as a symptom of a malfunction of nerve cells, or neurons, in the brain. Neurons communicate with each other by electrical signals; a seizure is the result of abnormal or excessive discharge of such signals by a group of neurons. Exactly why the neurons misfire remains unexplained. It is known, however, that a malfunction of the cell membranes is at least partly responsible, probably because of an interruption of the normal passage through the membrane of many chemicals—such as sodium, potassium, chlorides, and calcium. Research suggests that recurring seizures may damage surrounding normal brain cells.

An accidental injury to the brain or a brain disorder is sometimes involved in the neuron malfunction. Some cases of epilepsy appear to be associated with a brain tumor, an infection (such as meningitis, encephalitis, brain abscess, or tetanus), a chemical imbalance in the body, a very high fever, poisoning, or a congenital brain defect.

Types of Seizures

To treat epilepsy effectively, a determination needs to be made of the kind of seizures the patient has. Although some people experience two or three types of seizures, most have only one.

An important advance helping neurologists to diagnose seizures was the adoption in 1981 by the International League Against Epilepsy of a new, standardized classification system. In this system most attacks fall into two broad categories: partial seizures, which are the most common, and generalized seizures. Partial seizures start in an area within one side, or hemisphere, of the brain, while generalized seizures from the beginning involve both sides. In some cases a partial seizure develops into a generalized one; such attacks are said to be secondarily generalized.

In simple partial seizures (which used to be called focal seizures), there is no impairment of consciousness. An arm or a leg may jerk, or there may be a tingling or numbness in some area, or a hallucination may occur, such as an image or flashes of light. In one subtype (Jacksonian seizures), the seizure begins in one place—say, with the twitching of a finger—and then "marches" up the arm to the shoulder; it may spread to the leg and in some cases go on to affect the entire body.

In complex partial seizures (formerly called temporal lobe or psychomotor seizures), consciousness is typically impaired for only a few minutes. After losing touch with the surroundings, the individual may experience automatisms—coordinated, repetitive movements such as chewing, licking, or kicking—or may have hallucinations or a feeling of unreality or dreaminess.

With generalized seizures, the second broad category, consciousness is always impaired. This group includes the violent convulsions, once known as grand mal seizures, that many people associate with the word "epilepsy." Such attacks, now called tonic-clonic seizures, begin with an outcry and loss of consciousness. In the first, or tonic, phase, the body is rigid. This is followed by uncontrollable jerking—the clonic phase. The attack may last two to five minutes.

Also in the category of generalized seizures are absence seizures (formerly called petit mal attacks), which usually do not occur after age 20 and are characterized by a general cessation of activity or simply by staring for several seconds. Among other generalized seizures are atonic (drop) attacks, where the person suddenly falls down; myoclonic seizures, involving quick, jerking movements; and infantile muscle spasms, in which a baby's head and knees may come together like a jackknife.

Forming a separate category in the seizure classification system is a sometimes life-threatening condition known as status epilepticus, in which seizures come one after another, with no recovery between attacks, for a period of hours or even days.

Diagnosing Epilepsy

In the past, people suspected of having epilepsy were often quickly placed on medications and then kept on them for many years. Now neurologists analyze the origin and nature of the seizures before a drug is prescribed. The electroencephalogram, or EEG, an electrical recording of brain wave patterns (on paper or a screen), is a key tool for this purpose. Only patients whose EEG's indicate that their seizures originate in the brain are treated with antiepileptic drugs. This means that people with seizure-like symptoms caused by fainting, abnormal heart rhythms, or low blood sugar usually are not given antiepileptic medications, nor are those whose symptoms are caused by anxiety or other psy-

FIRST AID

If you see someone having an epileptic seizure, the first rule is to make sure the person is not in physical danger. With the convulsions of a tonic-clonic, or grand mal, seizure, you should:

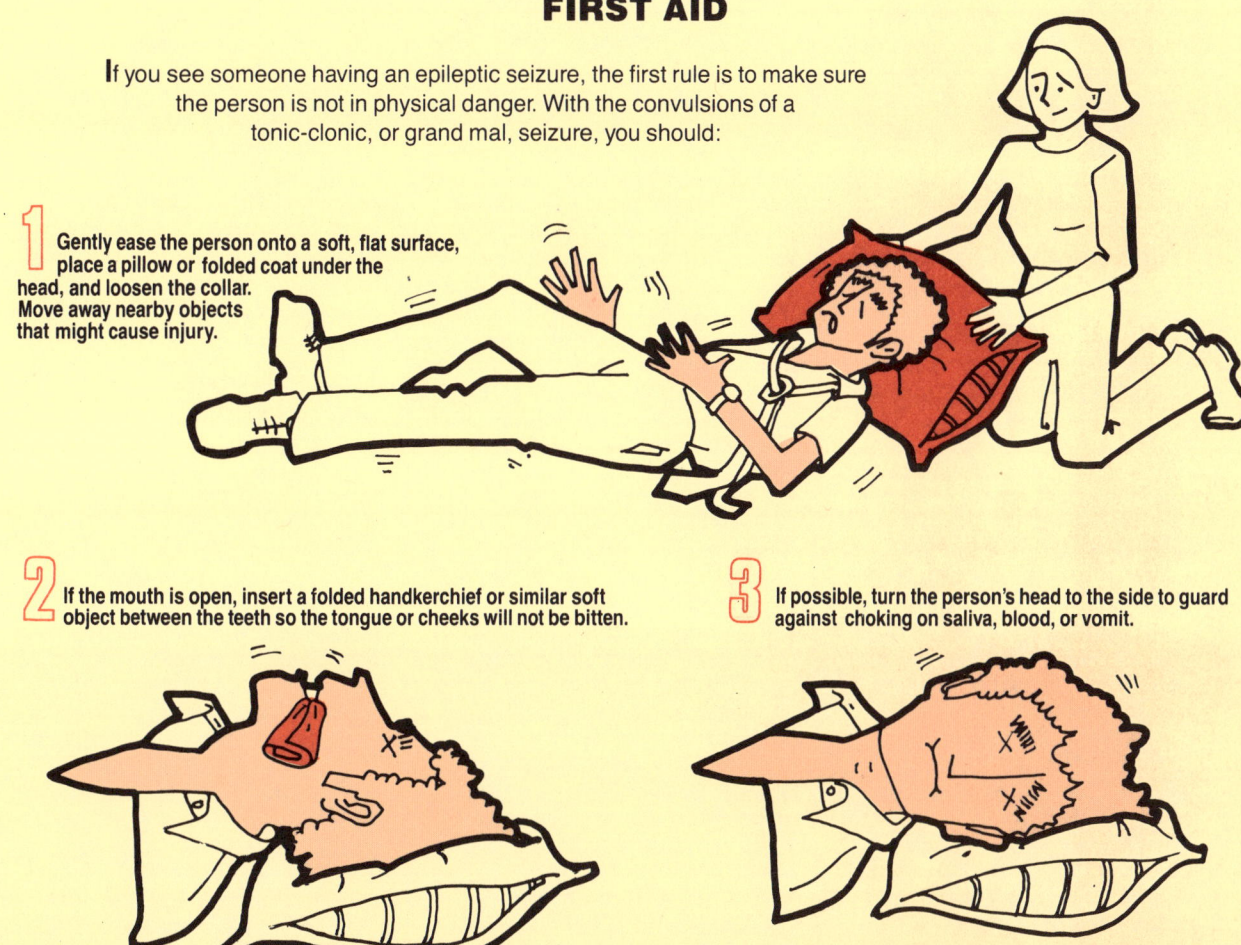

1 **Gently ease the person onto a soft, flat surface, place a pillow or folded coat under the head, and loosen the collar. Move away nearby objects that might cause injury.**

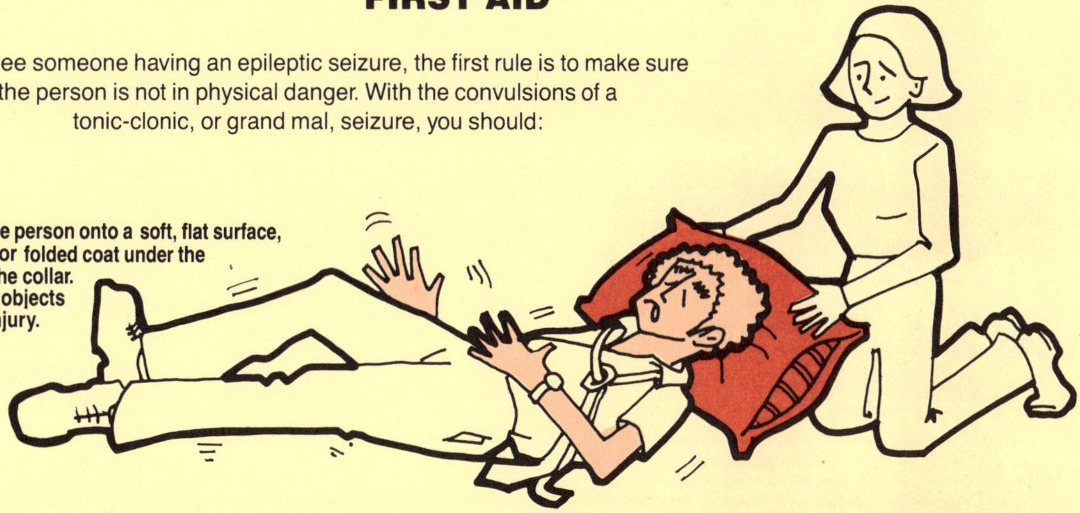

2 **If the mouth is open, insert a folded handkerchief or similar soft object between the teeth so the tongue or cheeks will not be bitten.**

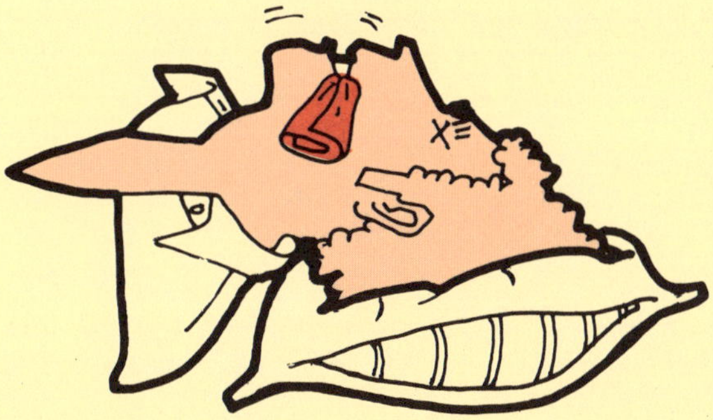

3 **If possible, turn the person's head to the side to guard against choking on saliva, blood, or vomit.**

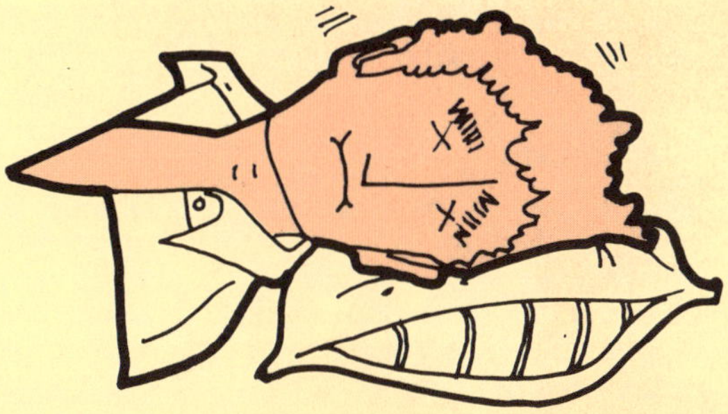

You should never try to restrain or hold down a person having a seizure, nor should you try to pry open the mouth if it is closed. If a seizure lasts for more than a few minutes or a new seizure begins, call for medical help immediately.

chological conditions that can mimic epilepsy.

Abnormalities in a routine EEG help to diagnose epilepsy in about 75 percent of patients with seizurelike symptoms. Recent variations on the traditional EEG, such as recordings made for 24 hours or longer, have proved valuable in many cases. Sometimes these are done with simultaneous videotaping, so that the EEG tracings and the actual seizures can be seen together. Portable EEG units have been developed that allow brain waves to be recorded for 12 to 24 hours on a cassette tape recorder worn on the belt, while the patient goes about normal daily activities.

An array of other techniques have also brought advances in diagnosing epilepsy, as well as in research on its causes. Computerized tomography (a CT, or CAT, scan) measures the density of various brain tissues by using X rays and then constructs images from this information that show "slices" of the brain. Magnetic resonance imaging (MRI) measures the differences of magnetic energy in body tissues to give similar pictures. Positron emission tomography (PET scanning) reveals how chemicals are used, or metabolized, in various areas of the brain, both during and between seizures. Sonography (ultrasound) can show parts of the brain in newborns and infants who still have an open soft spot at the top of the head (the fontanel). Together these techniques make it possible to identify very small areas from which seizures may develop.

Medication

Approximately 70 to 75 percent of all people with epilepsy can become completely seizure-free by taking one or more antiepileptic medications. Recent studies indicate that in certain cases where seizures have been completely controlled for two to four years, medication may be stopped with little chance of the seizures ever recurring. This is particularly true for children.

A new approach in treating epilepsy is to use a single drug rather than multiple drugs, thus reducing the number of potential side effects and adverse consequences from drug interaction. Whenever possible, the epileptic patient is now prescribed the one best medication to control the type or types of seizures experienced.

In most cases epileptic seizures can be completely controlled with few side effects.

Partial seizures are usually treated with drugs like carbamazepine (Tegretol), phenytoin (Dilantin), or primidone (Mysoline). Absence seizures can usually be controlled with ethosuximide (Zarontin) or valproic acid (Depakene or Depakote), but may not be improved or may even be made worse by such drugs as phenytoin. Patients with generalized tonic-clonic convulsions are commonly treated with phenytoin, phenobarbital, carbamazepine, primidone, or valproic acid.

Since individuals vary greatly in how their bodies "use" a drug, throughout the course of therapy blood samples from the patient are routinely analyzed to determine if the antiepileptic drug is at the proper concentration in the body, allowing maximum antiseizure action with a minimum of toxic side effects. The amount given may be raised or lowered accordingly. However, even with this blood level monitoring some people develop sufficiently serious side effects from an antiepileptic drug to require a change to another medication.

In the development of new antiepileptic drugs, increasing attention is being paid to side effects that were once considered unavoidable, especially changes in behavior and intellectual functions. Such relatively recent medications as carbamazepine and valproic acid seem to cause fewer side effects like drowsiness, depression, and learning disabilities than do some of the traditional antiepileptic drugs.

Other Therapy

In cases of severe seizures that cannot be controlled with existing drugs, surgical removal of the abnormal brain tissue may be considered, especially if the seizures all seem to arise from a small area of the brain. To help outline the location of the abnormal brain activity, special EEG electrodes may be surgically positioned inside the skull above the brain's surface and even inside the brain itself.

A so-called ketogenic diet, low in carbohydrates and high in fats, sometimes helps control certain kinds of seizures in children. Epileptic patients are usually advised to avoid any particular situation or activity that seems to lead to seizures.

Toward Greater Understanding

It is not widely enough appreciated that many people with epilepsy are completely normal and able to function as well as others in society. Educational campaigns to make the public aware of these facts are sponsored by the Epilepsy Foundation of America and similar organizations around the world. Legal steps have been taken to protect those with epilepsy from discrimination in employment and elsewhere.

Additional information on all aspects of epilepsy can be obtained in the United States from the Epilepsy Foundation of America, 4351 Garden City Drive, Landover, MD 20785; and in Canada from Epilepsy Canada, 2099 Alexandre de Seve, P. O. Box 1560, Station C, Montreal, Quebec H2L 4K8. □

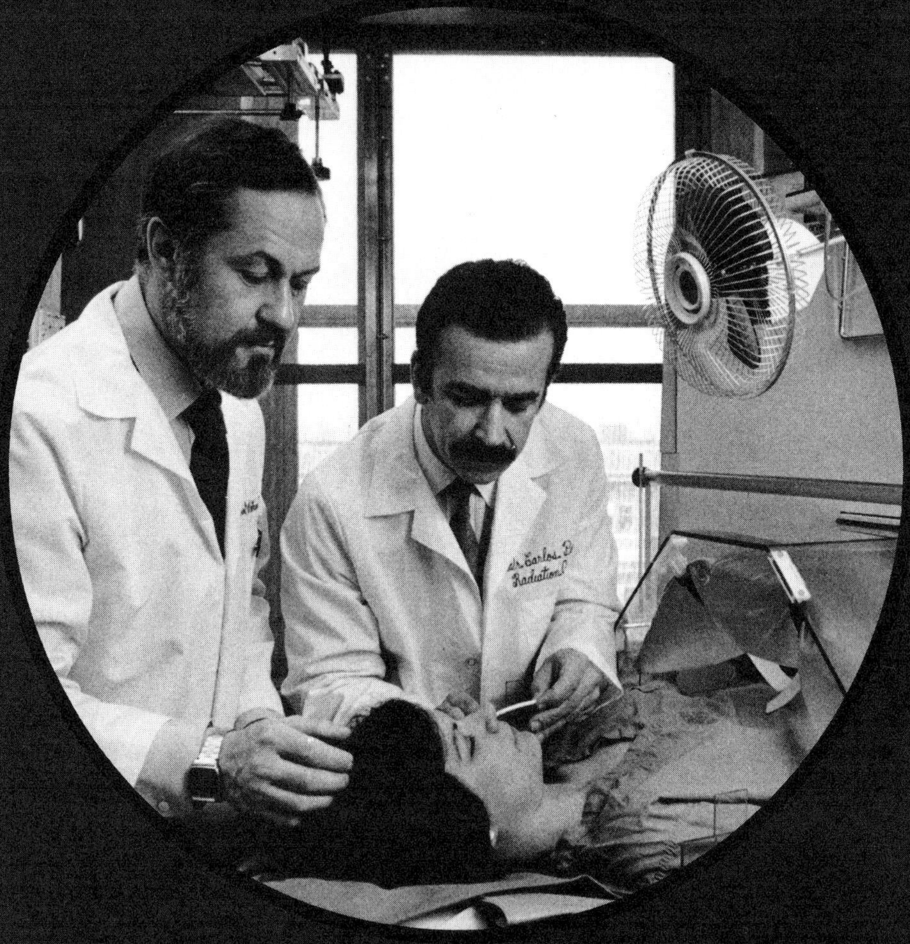

HEALTH AND MEDICAL NEWS

Alcoholism

Moderate Drinking Unlikely for Alcoholics • Weakened Bones in Alcohol Abusers • A Broad Front Against Drunk Driving • Alcohol on Campus

Can Alcoholics Drink Again?

It is highly unlikely that alcoholics will ever be able to control their drinking, limiting themselves to just a few drinks a day. This was the conclusion of a group of researchers at Washington University in St. Louis, who found that once an individual's use of alcohol has reached the point of requiring medical or psychiatric treatment, changing over to a moderate level of drinking is "strikingly rare." Various reports over the years have said that such "controlled drinking" by alcoholics might be possible, and the issue has been very controversial.

The St. Louis researchers looked at over 1,000 alcoholics five to seven years after they had received treatment at a medical or psychiatric facility. Fewer than 2 percent were able to return to long-term, stable, moderate drinking, generously defined in the study as consuming up to six drinks daily; nearly 79 percent still drank heavily. These findings suggest that people in alcoholism treatment programs should not be encouraged to believe that they someday may attain a controlled level of drinking. Alcoholics should aim instead for total abstinence.

Alcohol and Disease

A rise in blood pressure. Evidence that drinking can cause a rise in blood pressure is mounting. The relationship between alcohol use and hypertension has been difficult to determine because other factors may also affect blood pressure levels. However, Australian researchers who investigated this relationship designed their study to eliminate the influence of a number of risk factors, including obesity, age, and cigarette smoking. They found a greater prevalence of hypertension with increasing alcohol consumption. This confirms a larger, earlier U.S. study which showed that consumption of more than three drinks daily resulted in higher blood pressure levels.

Strokes in alcoholics. Swedish researchers in 1985 identified one possible reason for the increased incidence of strokes that has been reported in alcoholics: their blood clots more easily, at least at certain times. The researchers studied a group of alcoholic men who also were cigarette smokers, together with a group of nonalcoholics that included both smokers and nonsmokers. Neither the nonalcoholics nor the alcoholics, who were undergoing inpatient detoxification (treatment to stop drinking that entails an abrupt cessation of drinking), had had any alcohol for one week. Tests of blood clotting processes showed that the alcoholic group had an increase in the "clumping" together of blood platelets—structures that play an important role in blood coagulation—and a shortening of bleeding time, as well as an increase in thromboxane, a substance that causes blood vessels to narrow. These changes were not observed in any of the nonalcoholic subjects, and clotting functions were not influenced by cigarette smoking in the nonalcoholic group.

The most common types of strokes occur when a blood clot blocks a blood vessel supplying the brain, so an increase in blood clotting and vessel narrowing could make someone more susceptible to a stroke. Thus, it appears that for a brief period following the abrupt cessation of heavy drinking, when clotting-associated changes are known to occur, alcoholics may have an increased risk of problems like strokes (and heart attacks) that are sometimes related to clot formation.

Dangers for heart patients. The traditional "prescription" of small amounts of alcohol by many physicians for its supposed benefit to the heart may be a mistake for patients with heart disease, according to recent research. Investigators found that as little as 2 ounces of whiskey had a depressant effect on heart muscle function in patients recovering from a heart attack. This effect occurred in healthy subjects only after they had had 4 ounces of whiskey. The adverse effect in heart disease patients was most prominent at the site injured during the heart attack.

Bone disease. Several explanations, including calcium and vitamin D deficiencies, have been offered by scientists for the weakened bones (a condition called osteopenia) that make alcoholics vulnerable to fractures. A group of California researchers who studied eight alcoholic men have proposed another explanation. They suggest that alcohol directly inhibits the way bone remodels itself—that is, the processes by which old bony material is absorbed into body tissue while new bone is deposited. This inhibition is particularly prominent in the spinal region. Other factors, such as the influence of hormones and the effect of alcohol on the absorption of calcium, may also contribute to the reduced bone mass seen in alcoholics. The investigators note that regardless of the particular mechanisms involved, long-term abuse of alcohol has a detrimental effect on bone.

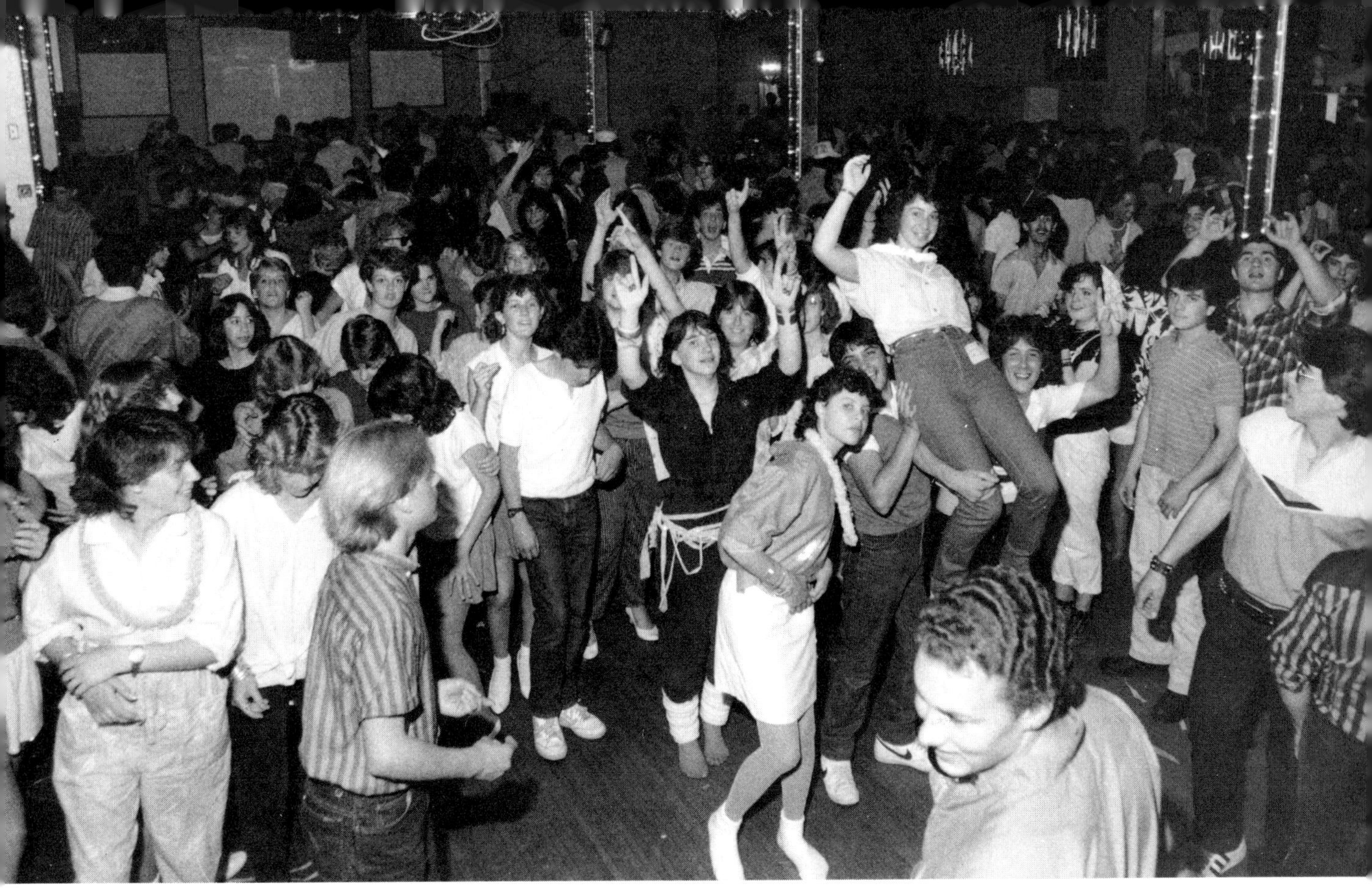

Teenagers have an uproarious time at a Fairfield, Conn., disco that serves no alcoholic drinks. Various programs to combat growing alcohol use among young people stress that little or no alcohol is needed to have fun.

Fetal Alcohol Syndrome

Physical and mental abnormalities suffered by a child whose mother drinks heavily during pregnancy appear to be long-lasting, according to a recent report. The complex of birth defects and medical problems—known as fetal alcohol syndrome—includes facial deformities, eye and ear problems, and severe underweight, as well as below-normal intelligence.

Fetal alcohol syndrome was first identified in 1973, in a group of 11 children born to chronic alcoholic women. In 1985 a ten-year follow-up of this original group was published. Two of the 11 were dead (one died of breathing difficulties five days after birth, the other in an accident when she was 3½), and one could not be found. The remaining eight children were small for their age and still had facial abnormalities (although the heart murmurs and other heart problems they had suffered from had disappeared). Intellectual development was below normal for all eight children: four were mildly handicapped and were attending a combination of regular and remedial classes, while the other four, more seriously affected, were attending classes for the retarded and needed constant supervision outside the home. While some of the children's mental abilities improved over the years, this was not the case with the most severely affected boys and girls—despite the adequate home environments of some of the children (often with adoptive or foster families).

Combating Drunk Driving

According to the U.S. National Highway Traffic Safety Administration, at least half of the 44,200 deaths in automobile accidents in 1984 (the latest figures available) were alcohol-related. There are signs of progress, however. While the number of drivers who died in all car accidents fell 11 percent from 1980 to 1984, the estimated number of fatally injured drivers who were drunk dropped by a higher rate—24 percent—during the same period, from more than 14,000 to 11,000. In 1980 half the drivers who died were drunk; in 1984 the figure was 43 percent.

Attempts to reduce drunken driving continue. Massachusetts became the first state to adopt a ban (dubbed the "happy hour regulation") on all bar and restaurant drink promotion gimmicks. Some bars have adopted a "designated driver" program: on a given night, the designated driver in a group consumes no alcohol and is responsible for getting the others home.

In other cases, intoxicated patrons are sent home in a cab. A miniature "breath analyzer" has been marketed, permitting motorists to measure their own alcohol level before they start their cars.

Other approaches are being tried as well. One is to promote consumption of nonalcoholic beverages such as the "beer" Moussy. A growing number of states—39 by March 1986—have adopted a minimum drinking age of 21 (some were influenced by a scheduled reduction in federal highway funds to states with an under-21 limit by October 1, 1986). In some states, driver education manuals include information on the effects of alcohol. An educational program called Starting Early, jointly sponsored by the American Automobile Association and the Canadian Automobile Association, has been introduced at many U.S. and Canadian schools. It includes a series of games, films, and puzzles for children through sixth grade, aimed at fostering an awareness of the dangers of drinking and driving.

Alcohol Use Among Youth

A 1985 Gallup poll indicates that 74 percent of those 18 to 29 years old in the United States and 90 percent of the same age group in Canada consume alcoholic beverages. In addition, according to the 1985 report of an annual survey of U.S. high school seniors, nearly 80 percent say they do not view one or two drinks daily as potentially hazardous, and the majority do not view five or more drinks at a party as hazardous. The number of students who say that they use alcohol as an escape has increased from 12 to 18 percent since 1975, and those who use it to deal with frustration and anger increased from 11 to 16 percent during the same time. A survey of deans of student affairs at 181 U.S. two-year and four-year colleges that was published in 1982 indicated that 16 percent of students at these schools were excessive drinkers, nearly 6 percent needed treatment for alcohol abuse, and 2.3 percent left college because of an alcohol problem.

A variety of campus alcohol-awareness programs are under way. One attempt to combat the problem is a Canadian project known as CAPE (Campus Alcohol Policies and Education), which employs posters, buttons, ads, and exhibits to stress the need for moderation in drinking. Many colleges have formulated specific policies about where and when alcohol may be served on campus. An important stimulus to much of this activity is the growing number of states raising their legal minimum drinking age to 21, making the majority of students underage. This has led to the planning of more campus social events that emphasize music and food rather than alcohol.

See also the Spotlight on Health article WHAT TO DO FOR A HANGOVER.

T. M. WORNER, M.D.

Bioethics

Life or Death Rules for Sick Newborns • Landmark Decision on the Right to Die • Dilemma of Children With AIDS • Profiting From the Human Body

Final Rule for Baby Doe

Almost three years after the first efforts by the federal government to intervene in decisions on whether or not to treat seriously ill newborns, the U.S. Department of Health and Human Services issued a regulation requiring doctors and hospitals to provide life-preserving treatment for these babies unless death seems inevitable. The government action that led up to this "final rule"—which went into effect in mid-1985—was first prompted by the so-called Baby Doe case. Baby Doe, an infant born in Bloomington, Ind., in 1982, had Down's syndrome and an abnormality of the throat and esophagus that prevented taking food or drink by mouth but was surgically correctable. At the urging of the child's physician, the parents refused the surgery. Baby Doe died at the age of six days, as legal appeals were being filed on his behalf.

The case started a series of political struggles as the administration of President Ronald Reagan became involved. These struggles culminated in Congress's passage of the Child Abuse Amendments of 1984, often called the Baby Doe Amendments, to the Child Abuse Prevention and Treatment Act. The amendments—hammered out between the administration, right-to-life groups, advocates for the disabled, doctors, and hospital representatives—in turn authorized the 1985 final rule.

Technically, all the rule does is create a new condition that state agencies must meet in order to qualify for federal grants directed at preventing child abuse. The new stipulation requires states' child protective agencies to set up mechanisms for receiving and investigating complaints of alleged cases of "medical neglect." It also requires the state agencies to have programs or procedures for obtaining, in accordance with state law, court-ordered treatment when the agencies decide that treatment is being wrongfully withheld.

A key element of the rule is the new category of medical neglect, which includes "withholding of medically indicated treatment." Essentially, the rule says that any medical treatment that "reasonable medical judgment" deems appropriate for a life-threatening condition must be given unless:

- the infant is chronically and irreversibly comatose,
- treatment would merely prolong dying and would not ease or correct all of the baby's life-threatening conditions, or
- treatment would be virtually futile in terms of the baby's survival and, under such circumstances, the treatment itself would be inhumane.

Withholding treatment under other circumstances would be considered medical neglect under the rule.

The political fight was chiefly over the definitions of key terms in the rule. Right-to-life advocates wanted to define phrases such as "medical neglect," "reasonable medical judgment," and "merely prolong dying" so strictly that virtually all parental and physician discretion would have been eliminated. Pressure from a number of sources, not the least of which was the coalition of U.S. senators who had sponsored the legislation, forced the Department of Health and Human Services to issue a final rule leaving much more room for discretion. While not everyone is satisfied with the rule, some of the heat has dissipated from the controversy—at least until the next Baby Doe captures attention.

Right to Die Cases

Not feeding the dying. In a major decision on the right to die, the New Jersey Supreme Court ruled in early 1985 that feeding tubes could be withdrawn from

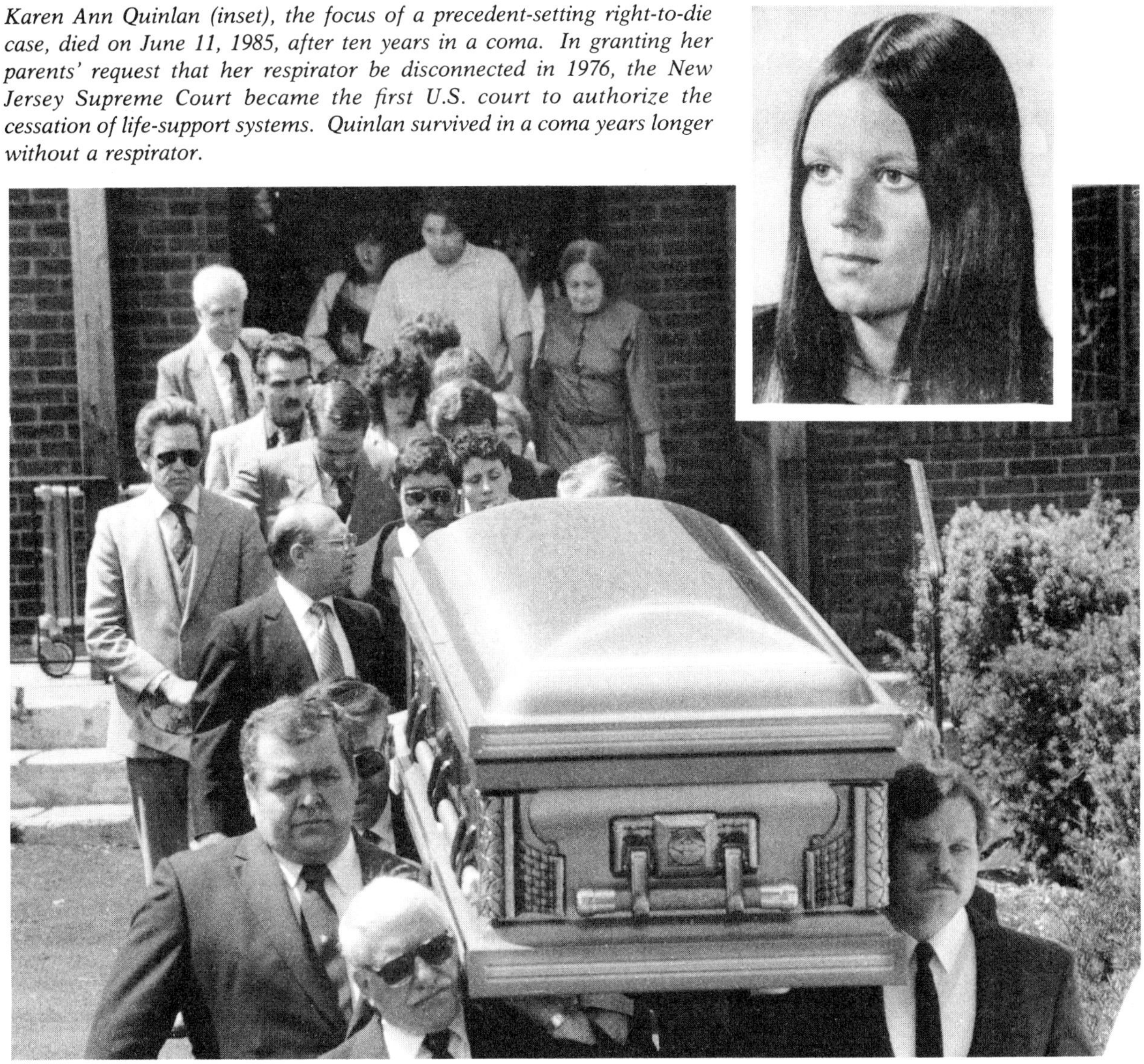

Karen Ann Quinlan (inset), the focus of a precedent-setting right-to-die case, died on June 11, 1985, after ten years in a coma. In granting her parents' request that her respirator be disconnected in 1976, the New Jersey Supreme Court became the first U.S. court to authorize the cessation of life-support systems. Quinlan survived in a coma years longer without a respirator.

an incurably ill nursing home patient. Most right-to-die cases—like the landmark one involving Karen Ann Quinlan, which also took place in New Jersey—have centered on removing patients from respirators or other life-support systems, not on something as basic as simply deciding to stop feeding these people.

The court case involved Claire Conroy, an 84-year-old nursing home patient who was irreversibly ill with a number of conditions, including diabetes, heart disease, gangrene, severe organic brain disorder, painful bedsores, and hypertension. She had been reduced to an immobile, uncommunicative state, weighed less than 50 pounds, and other than giving an occasional moan or smile, seemed unaware of her surroundings. She did not need complex technology to stay alive, but since she could not eat, she did require a feeding tube.

Conroy's nephew—her only living blood relative—had been her legal guardian since 1979 and had earlier opposed ending life support. But having become convinced that keeping her alive with tube feedings was no longer in his aunt's interest, he petitioned the court to permit the tube to be removed. Court records reveal that the nephew had no financial interest that would have influenced his judgment on the issue.

A New Jersey trial court heard the Conroy case and granted the nephew's petition, but the decision was reversed by an intermediate level appeals court in 1983. The state Supreme Court then took the case under review and in January 1985 ruled in favor of removing the tube. The court did set up a series of tests that would have to be met before feeding could be discontinued. These include an attempt to determine what the patient's wish would have been. If there is insufficient basis for determining this, the family, physicians, and a state-appointed "ombudsman" would decide whether the pain of the patient's life outweighed any benefits the patient derived from life. The ruling applied to severely ill, incompetent nursing home residents with a life expectancy of a year or less.

Uncertainties linger about the wisdom of the Conroy decision. The trial court judge had suggested that Claire Conroy's life had become "impossibly and permanently burdensome" to her, but the New Jersey Supreme Court explicitly rejected any "quality of life" criteria other than the patient's own pain and suffering. Yet critics of the ruling wonder how a society can ever make the judgment that some other person's life has become so burdensome that the person would prefer to be dead. Another concern is that in the name of compassion, but really in the interest of economizing, society will deny nutrition to people like Claire Conroy as "the only effective way to make certain that a large number of biologically tenacious patients actually die," as bioethicist Daniel Callahan has put it. Finally, there is a worry that feeding—even by a tube through the nose to the stomach—is much more than a "medical" intervention. From earliest infancy, and in many, perhaps all, cultures, feeding has a powerful symbolic value. It is the first way we demonstrate care for the infant, and it remains throughout life an important means of communicating care and concern for others. What does it mean for a society when it in effect permits people to starve to death?

One fact overlooked in the first criticism—that we can never be certain how burdensome someone else's life is—is that we do not have the option of *not* making a decision. To keep tube-feeding someone implies a judgment that the person is better off living under the circumstances, however painful and hopeless. It makes excellent sense to err in the direction of protecting and sustaining life when we are uncertain. But are we always deciding in the patient's interest if we refuse to consider removing feeding tubes from devastated people such as Claire Conroy?

In the ironic tradition of landmark legal cases in bioethics, Claire Conroy died of natural causes, tube still in place, before the final court ruling was issued. Another New Jersey nursing home patient, 65-year-old Hilda Peter, in a coma since a massive heart attack in late 1984, became the first test case of the procedures set forth in the Conroy decision when legal efforts were mounted in 1985 to have her feeding tube withdrawn. In March 1986 the state ombudsman rejected removing the tube, because state-appointed doctors had determined that Peter might live for years with it in place. An appeal to the courts remained a possibility.

In a separate development in March 1986, the American Medical Association put forth the opinion that it "is not unethical" for doctors to withhold "all means of life-prolonging medical treatment," including food and water, from patients in irreversible comas, as well as from those who are terminally ill.

Quinlan death. Karen Ann Quinlan, the young woman who in the 1970's became the focus of an impassioned debate on the right to die, died on June 11, 1985, at the age of 31. Ten years earlier, Quinlan had become irreversibly comatose from a combination of drugs and alcohol. In a landmark lawsuit her parents asked that the respirator she was on be disconnected to allow her to die "with grace and dignity," and in 1976 the New Jersey Supreme Court ruled in their favor. The respirator was disconnected but Quinlan (fed with a tube) survived years longer.

AIDS and Schoolchildren

Should children with AIDS be allowed to attend school? This is a difficult and emotional question.

One of the saddest aspects of the AIDS crisis is the children who have become afflicted with the disease.

By the beginning of 1986 there were over 300 reported cases of AIDS in the United States among those 19 years old or younger. Most were children born to mothers who had AIDS or were in one of the "at-risk" groups, particularly intravenous drug users or sexual partners of men with AIDS. Other children have acquired AIDS from transfusions of blood or, in the case of children with hemophilia, of the clotting factors derived from blood. The ethical and policy dilemma arises from the desire of some families of children with AIDS to send them to public school. Parents of unaffected children worry that the presence of a child with AIDS threatens the health of their own children.

Several factors exacerbate the conflict over whether children with AIDS ought to be permitted to attend school. Fearful parents stress the uncertainty in statements by medical scientists about whether the AIDS virus could be transmitted in the classroom. The virus has been found in tears and saliva as well as in blood (although evidence that it can be transmitted by tears or saliva is lacking—the vast majority of documented AIDS cases have been transmitted through blood, either directly or during sexual contact). At present there is no known means of preventing AIDS, or of curing or even arresting the progress of the disease.

All these things urge a policy of conservatively protecting against even the most remote possibility of infecting schoolmates. On the other hand, most scientists familiar with AIDS believe that the danger of infection is so remote, if not actually impossible, in school settings (unless a child with AIDS bites another youngster or has open wounds) that they are strongly in favor of permitting children with AIDS to attend school, on a case-by-case basis. A child is probably in much greater danger of dying from a school bus or auto accident or from football or diving than from AIDS.

One of the difficulties in crafting ethically and scientifically sound public health policies is that scientists are trained not to say that they are absolutely certain about something. It is intrinsic to the process of science to be open to new evidence. But parents terrified of the specter of this relentlessly fatal disease will settle for nothing less than a guarantee of absolute safety.

See also the feature article AIDS: TWO EPIDEMICS.

Profiting From the Human Body

A lawsuit filed in 1984 raises the issue of whether people "own" their bodies and can profit from them. In 1976 a man named John Moore had his grossly enlarged spleen removed as part of the treatment for hairy-cell leukemia, a rare form of blood cancer. Like many other patients, Moore signed a vague consent form permitting his spleen (which produces such white blood cells as lymphocytes) and blood cells to be used for medical research. Through genetic engineering, two scientists at UCLA managed to isolate and reproduce an apparently valuable line of cells derived from Moore's lymphocytes. They received a patent in 1984 on the cell line, which may prove useful in stimulating the immune system against cancer. Moore's attorney filed a complaint that the cells—which were given the name Mo cells—were, after all, Moore's, and that he should be entitled to a share of any profits from the cell line.

The Mo cell case raises significant ethical issues about our relationship to our bodies. Do we "own" them? Can we sell our body parts? How should we think about tissues that are taken from us: as commercial property? as surplus? or as a very special sort of gift? Our approach to organ donation suggests that we do not regard parts of the body as commodities fit for sale: we forbid the profit motive to taint our system for procuring organs for transplants, assuring that tissue removed from human bodies is treated respectfully and that no one gains undue profit from it.

The most likely view is that we regard our removed tissues as a gift to be given to the socially valued enterprises of medical education and research. The question, then, is whether someone given a gift of human tissue later found to be commercially profitable has any moral obligation to share those profits with the source of the gift.

THOMAS H. MURRAY, PH.D.

Blood and Lymphatic System

DNA Analysis Helps Hemophilia Families • Eliminating Hepatitis Virus From the Blood Supply • Progress in Treating Hodgkin's Disease

Identifying Hemophilia Carriers

Researchers have recently succeeded in finding specific gene abnormalities that govern the development of hemophilia in its classic form, hemophilia A. Their work is expected to permit identification of carriers of the disease, helping affected couples to plan their families with a better understanding of the potential risks.

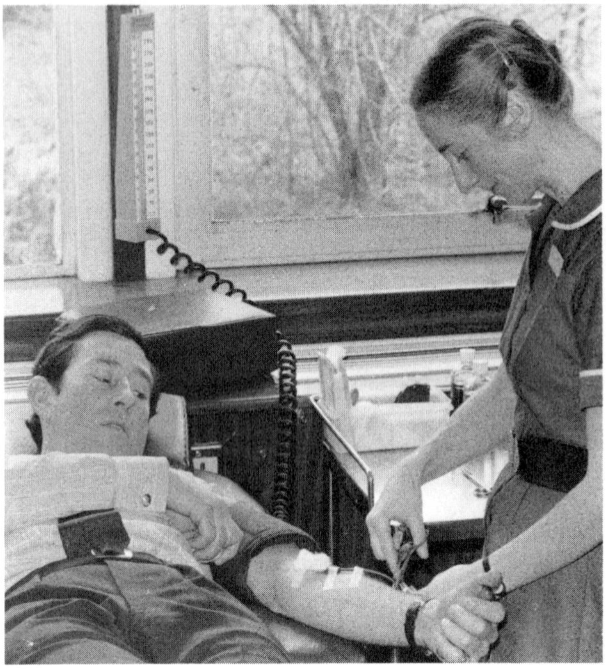

RED-BLOODED ROYALTY

British blood banks got a royal assist in their campaign to dispel the notion that blood donors run the risk of contracting AIDS. With blood donations declining throughout Great Britain because of groundless fears, Prince Charles stepped forth in March 1985 to donate a pint at the North London Transfusion Center—the first member of the royal family ever to give blood. Before the royal vein was punctured, the Prince of Wales answered, with aplomb, some indelicate questions about whether he belonged to a major risk group for AIDS.

Asked who would be the lucky recipient of the regal fluid, a doctor at the center said that the prince's blood "will not be specially labeled. It will be totally anonymous and will go to any patient in need." And was the royal blood blue? Said Charles in mock apology, "I'm afraid it's red like anyone else's."

Hemophilia A is caused by a deficiency or abnormality of a blood clotting protein, factor VIII. Hemophiliacs usually require regular transfusions of factor VIII concentrate to prevent excessive bleeding.

The development of hemophilia A is determined by the presence of abnormalities in a gene located on the X chromosome, one of the rodlike bodies within a cell that determine a baby's sex as well as other characteristics. In males, these abnormalities lead to low levels of factor VIII in the blood and consequent bleeding problems. Females with this genetic trait, on the other hand, rarely suffer from bleeding problems but can pass the trait on to their children; such women are called carriers.

Existing methods of detecting hemophilia carriers leave much to be desired. Since there is a wide variation in what is considered a normal level of factor VIII, it is difficult to determine whether a woman is a carrier on this basis alone. At present the best a doctor or genetic counselor can do is to estimate the probability that a woman is a carrier, making it difficult to advise couples about the likelihood of passing hemophilia on to their children.

In recent research, the exact gene area responsible for the production of factor VIII has been studied, characterized, and cloned (copied). Building on these studies, a team of investigators from several U.S. research centers reported in 1985 their use of recombinant DNA techniques to reveal specific abnormalities in the gene for hemophilia. (In recombinant DNA work, the substance of which a gene is made—DNA—is "taken apart," then reconstructed with DNA from another organism.) At the present level of sensitivity, if DNA analysis of blood from a woman yields a positive result, then she is a carrier; a negative result, however, does not rule out her being a carrier.

These techniques can also be applied to find out before a baby is born whether it has hemophilia or is a carrier, by using amniocentesis to analyze cells of the fetus for the presence of the abnormal gene. Until now hemophilia A could be diagnosed prenatally only by measuring factor VIII levels in the blood of the fetus; it was impossible to learn whether the fetus carried the gene. Measuring fetal factor VIII levels may be more accurate than DNA analysis for diagnosing hemophilia. But fetal blood sampling is a dangerous procedure; it is relatively easy to do amniocentesis.

Toward a Safer Blood Supply

The transfusion of blood products—including plasma, red blood cells, platelets, and coagulation factors—has been extremely useful in the treatment of bleeding patients and in cancer patients, whose ability to make blood components is temporarily impaired because of their disease or the treatment they receive. For patients who lack specific blood coagulation factors, transfusion of concentrated blood factors has been life saving. With these benefits, however, there have come a number of risks, including the transmission of blood-borne diseases, notably hepatitis. An estimated 5 to 9 percent of the 3 million people transfused with blood products in the United States each year contract hepatitis; a small but significant proportion go on to develop cirrhosis.

Screening blood for hepatitis. Routine testing of donated blood to determine whether a donor may be a carrier of the hepatitis virus is being instituted by a growing number of blood banks. Hepatitis is an inflammation of the liver that occurs in several forms. The great majority of cases transmitted by transfusion are non-A, non-B hepatitis, a form for which no specific test yet exists. Although individuals who contract non-A, non-B hepatitis rarely develop symptoms of the disease, over half would probably have abnormal results on liver function tests. Some of these patients—up to an estimated 10,000 to 40,000 Americans each year—may develop the severe liver disorder cirrhosis as a result of the hepatitis infection.

To reduce these risks, a number of blood banks are now adding another procedure to those already used to screen donated blood for various contaminants. The test measures the level of a liver enzyme called alanine aminotransferase (ALT) in the donor's blood. Although an elevated level of this enzyme does not necessarily mean that the donor has hepatitis (high ALT levels can also be caused by the use of alcohol, birth control pills, or other drugs), a strong correlation has been found between elevated levels of ALT in a donor's blood and an increased risk of hepatitis in the donor. Blood in which ALT levels are abnormally high is therefore discarded. Proponents of the procedure hope that it will reduce the incidence of post-transfusion hepatitis by at least 30 percent.

Viral inactivation process. In September 1985 researchers at the New York Blood Center patented a method of inactivating the viruses that commonly contaminate blood products used to treat clotting disorders. Patients with hemophilia, for example, who require frequent transfusions of clotting factors throughout their lifetime, are exposed to blood components from thousands of donors and consequently face an extremely high risk of contracting hepatitis. The new method is used during the preparation of blood products from plasma. It takes advantage of the fact that most blood-borne viruses, including those causing non-A, non-B hepatitis and hepatitis B, are sheathed in an "envelope" composed of lipids, fatty substances that occur in the body. The new method strips away the lipids, rendering the virus noninfectious without affecting the function of important blood coagulation proteins. The viral inactivation process is now being licensed to firms and blood centers in various countries that prepare blood products.

Lymphatic Cancers

New treatments for two lymphatic cancers, Hodgkin's disease and chronic lymphocytic leukemia, are helping patients who do not respond to more established drug therapies for these disorders.

Hodgkin's disease. Researchers from Johns Hopkins University reported in 1985 that a radioactively "tagged" antibody against the protein ferritin showed promise in hard-to-treat cases of Hodgkin's disease. This malignant disorder of the lymph nodes is often fatal if left untreated. Modern treatment with a combination of drugs cures more than half of patients in advanced stages of the disease; for those patients not cured with combination chemotherapy, however, there have been few effective alternatives available.

The new method of therapy involves antibodies (protective substances produced by the body) called isotopic immunoglobulins. The specific antibody employed acts against the protein ferritin, which is found in some normal body tissues but is made in greater quantity in the malignant cells of Hodgkin's disease patients. The researchers added radioactive iodine particles to the antiferritin antibody and injected their patients with the combination, thus specifically directing the radioactivity against the tumor cells. They found there was significant response, with few side effects, in almost half the patients who had not been cured with standard chemotherapy.

To date, there has been much enthusiasm about the use of antibodies to treat cancer. Unfortunately, until now few successful results have been seen when these methods were applied to patients. Although the results of isotopic immunoglobulin therapy in Hodgkin's disease are still preliminary, they do offer hope that immunological methods can be effective in treating lymphatic cancers.

Chronic lymphocytic leukemia. Low doses of a compound called deoxycoformycin (dCF) appear to be effective in combating chronic lymphocytic leukemia (CLL), a cancer of the lymphatic system that most often occurs in older people. In its earlier stages, CLL may not cause any symptoms or require any treatment, but patients with advanced cases often experience anemia and bleeding and an increased susceptibility to infections. When these problems arise, corticosteroids or combinations of standard anticancer drugs may be given. However, many older patients are too frail to tolerate such drugs, and for others the treatments may not be effective over extended periods.

High doses of dCF, a compound that inhibits an enzyme necessary for the metabolism of the malignant cells found in CLL, had previously been found useful in treating the disease, but patients could not tolerate the drug's side effects at these dosages. In the new approach to dCF use, low doses have brought improvement, without serious side effects, to CLL patients who were no longer responding to standard drug therapy. The use of dCF in therapy is still considered experimental, however.

Cause of "Bubble Boy's" Death

Autopsy results released in 1985 for David, the boy who had lived all 12 years of his life in a germ-free "bubble" at a Texas medical center, revealed that his death the previous year was from a B cell lymphoma, a cancer in which certain white blood cells multiply rapidly. The Epstein-Barr virus that was found to have caused the tumor is an extremely common virus; it had apparently entered David's system when he received a bone marrow transplant from his sister four months before his death. David was born with a condition called severe combined immunodeficiency, in which the body has almost no immune defenses. Doctors emphasized that almost any virus might have had the same effect.

WILLIAM L. STERNHEIM, M.D.

Bones, Muscles, and Joints

Better Ways to Replace Joints • Treating Bone Tumors Without Amputation • Restoring Blood Supply to the Hip

Progress in Joint Replacement

Substantial improvements have been made since the era of joint replacement began in the early 1960's, when an English surgeon, Sir John Charnley, developed the first artificial hip joint. The result has been better function and comfort for people whose joints have been damaged by injury or diseases like arthritis.

Hip replacement. Charnley's artificial hip used stainless steel and polyethylene plastic to replace the hip joint, which consists of a ball and socket: one bone forming the joint has a spherical end that fits into the cuplike socket of the other bone that is part of the hip. The lower part of Charnley's joint was a metal ball with a stem, which was inserted into the upper end of the thighbone (femur). The upper component, replacing the socket of the natural joint, was made of high-density polyethylene. Both portions were held in place with methyl methacrylate, a substance originally used as dental cement. It is not a true cement, but rather a grout that makes a fit between the synthetic joint components and the person's bone. Although today's hip replacement surgery does not substantially differ from when it was first performed, many refinements have been made.

The basic problem with hip replacements is their limited longevity. Unlike living bone, which repairs the wear and tear that happens every day, methyl methacrylate, metal, and plastic are unable to maintain themselves. Eventually they will undergo fatigue (the tendency of a material under repeated stress to break) and failure, resulting in recurrent hip pain.

Another basic problem is that the components can loosen. Advances in preventing loosening have included getting the cement further into the porous bone by using a thinner formula and increasing the pressure on the implant while it sets. Moreover, design changes have been made to decrease long-term stresses on the cement, including adding a metal backing to the plastic socket—which was originally just a simple shell—thus spreading forces over a larger surface area. Increasing the surface areas of the metal inserted into the femur by making the components with much broader surfaces and more rounded edges has a similar effect on the lower portion of the artificial joint.

Loosening of the implants in the femur may be caused by the way bone responds to the replacement. Occasional daily stress is important to stimulate bone to repair itself and remain strong, but since the metal implant is stiff, most of the stress it places on bone is in its lowest portion, and the top end of the femur may lose some of its strength. When this occurs, the implant may loosen. Although selecting a more flexible metal may increase stress on bone cement, which could itself cause loosening, some doctors believe that increasing the stress in the upper end of the femur by this means will be of long-term benefit by stimulating the bone and thus keeping it strong.

As better cementing techniques are expected to increase the longevity of hip replacements, designers are becoming more concerned about possible fracture of the metal component. Stainless steel, for example, is no longer used in the lower component because of its poor fatigue properties. But chrome-cobalt alloys shaped by special forging techniques show improved fatigue properties in laboratory tests.

Much recent research has focused on designs that require no cement at all. In the past, "press fit" implants have been designed. These were partial artificial hips that were simply pressed into the femur to replace the ball component of the hip. Because of the less-than-perfect fit, however, a number of patients had considerable thigh pain. Some improvement has come by making the fit as good as possible.

The method that may ultimately give long-term fixing of the new joint without cement is to place a coating on the component that allows bone to adhere to it. Options being explored include beads or wire mesh on the surface of the component. This allows bone to grow into the spaces between the beads or in the mesh. Another possibility is a ceramic made—like bone—of calcium and phosphate, which will allow natural bone to adhere to the coating and ultimately replace it. This last approach involves one old risk and one new one. The old risk is metal fatigue and fracture. This is actually quite rare, but if the metal-bone attachment becomes very strong, the weakest link in the artificial joint may turn out to be the metal just outside the bone. If it broke, removing the buried metal component would be so difficult that such a fracture would be a far more serious problem than it is today. A new problem that may occur with the porous-coated artificial joint is possible metal poisoning, since the greatly increased surface area of the new type of joint exposes more metal to body fluids.

New knees. Total replacement of the knee joint was at first unsuccessful because the designs lacked sufficient flexibility. Normally, much of the shock of walking is absorbed by ligaments and soft tissues around the knee. The first metal knee joints did not have this cushioning, and stress quickly wore down the cement, resulting in loosening and infection.

Patients' experience with a variety of newer, more flexible designs is encouraging; these joints provide pain relief and last significantly longer than earlier artificial knees. Some of the newer models have retained the basic flexibility but modified the design slightly to reduce shifting back and forth in the knee joint. Restraint is provided by either a plastic post inside the knee or by saving one of the knee ligaments. These designs seem to improve function—especially climbing stairs. Long-term follow-up is needed to determine how long the new designs will last.

Hands and fingers. A variety of hand components is available. The most commonly used are simple silicone rubber implants whose major function is to act as a flexible "spacer" between bones to allow movement. The body forms a new joint capsule, like the tissues around a natural joint, around this spacer so that even if it should break later, the finger joint can continue to function.

Another important component is an artificial tendon, which was at first used simply to allow the body to form a new sheath to house a tendon transplanted from another part of the body. Recent modifications have concentrated on the artificial tendon itself: it is hooked to muscle at one end and finger bone at the other, so that it can function as a normal tendon while the body is forming the sheath around it. If the artificial tendon breaks, it can then be replaced by a tendon taken from another part of the body.

Saving Limbs From Bone Tumors

It is becoming ever more possible to salvage a limb in which bone cancer has appeared, rather than resorting to amputation, which was the only real hope for a cure in the past. Better surgical techniques, as well as chemical and radiation therapy, have changed the treatment picture.

Ewing's tumor, a malignant bone tumor that usually affects children, is now being treated increasingly with a combination of surgery, chemotherapy, and radiation therapy. Radiation therapy was an important early advance in treatment for these patients, but it carries some risks for young children: it may interfere with further growth of the irradiated limb, and it may predispose some patients to developing other bone tumors in later years. While radiation therapy is still very important in treating Ewing's tumor, its exact use is being reevaluated.

For Ewing's tumor as well as other bone tumors, including osteosarcoma and chondrosarcoma, surgical techniques have advanced to the point that amputation, once a major part of treatment, is not necessarily done. Instead, limb salvage is taking a more important role. Limb salvage is the surgical removal of the tumor and a safety margin of normal tissue to make sure all of it has been taken out, combined with surgical reconstruction of the limb so that it functions well and appears as natural as possible.

The major problem with limb salvage in the past has been finding the best way to replace the bone lost in surgery. Good techniques are now available to use the patient's own bone from elsewhere in the body or donor bone (from cadavers), and artificial replacements are also becoming better and more widely used. The advantage of using the patient's bone or donor bone is that the longevity of the reconstructed segment of bone is excellent once it heals completely after several years. The major drawback is that frequently the function of at least one joint, commonly the knee, is lost, leaving the patient with a stiff knee.

Blood Supply in the Hip

Better treatments are being developed to restore lost blood supply to a portion of the hip. This disorder—

avascular necrosis of the hip, the loss of blood supply to the top of the femur—can be a complication of various conditions. People at risk include kidney dialysis and sickle-cell patients and people being treated with steroids, as well as anyone who drinks alcohol or is exposed to the bends (decompression sickness) from deep sea or high atmospheric pressure activities. After such a loss of circulation, the femoral head, which supports the body's weight within the hip joint, is no longer able to bear the necessary weight, and it collapses and disintegrates. This causes considerable pain for the patients, who tend to be relatively young people for whom artificial hips are not a suitable alternative: the artificial joint would not last long enough.

There are several surgical procedures for treating the problem. Core decompression, or drilling to remove a central core of the dead bone to allow an improved blood supply to the remaining bone, has had some success. Some surgeons also add a bone graft to try to support the weight-bearing area of the top of the femur while it heals. Others transplant bone still connected to its surrounding blood vessels. Such a bone graft will support the top of the hip, and, more important, bring in a new source of blood supply.

A recent innovation that shows promise in improving blood supply is the use of external electrical coils strapped to the hip, which induce an electrical current and a magnetic field within the bone. The major advantage of this form of treatment, if it is proved successful by further testing, is that it involves no surgical procedure and no patient discomfort.

See also the Spotlight on Health article PREVENTING OSTEOPOROSIS.

ERIC L. HUME, M.D.

Brain and Nervous System

First Effective Treatment for Guillain-Barré Syndrome • New Drug for Parkinson's Disease? • Stroke Surgery Questioned

Guillain-Barré Syndrome

A method of separating antibodies from blood, called plasmapheresis, has emerged in recent years as the first effective therapy for Guillain-Barré syndrome, a puzzling condition that is one of the most common disorders of the peripheral nerves. There are about 3,000 new cases of Guillain-Barré syndrome each year in the United States, and it is thought to be the single largest cause of paralysis in young people.

The peripheral nerves are those that extend from the brain and spinal cord to all parts of the body, carrying motor information to the muscles and returning sensory information from the skin, joints, and muscles back to the central nervous system. The peripheral nerves can be damaged by general medical conditions such as diabetes mellitus, by toxins such as alcohol, and by a number of neurological conditions, including Guillain-Barré syndrome. Although the cause of Guillain-Barré syndrome is unknown, it often follows a viral illness, such as influenza or gastroenteritis. It may also occur after an immunization or as part of AIDS (acquired immune deficiency syndrome), but many cases have no apparent provocation.

Typically, an affected individual feels a progressive weakness that begins in the legs and over a period of several days spreads to the arms and sometimes the face and eyes. The weakness may be preceded or accompanied by numbness or tingling in the fingers and toes. When weakness is severe, the muscles used in breathing and swallowing are affected; this occurs in about 20 percent of Guillain-Barré patients, who then require mechanical breathing support in an intensive care unit, often for weeks. The weakness may also progress to total paralysis. Fortunately, nearly all individuals recover within a period of months, most without drugs, surgery, or other specific therapy. However, since these individuals are gravely ill at the time of the most severe weakness or paralysis, serious or even fatal complications are possible.

Recent progress in managing neurological patients who require breathing assistance and intensive care has greatly improved the chances for eventual recovery for these patients. In addition, plasmapheresis, a "blood cleaning" technique in which a large amount of plasma (the liquid part of blood) is withdrawn and then returned to the body after antibodies are removed from it, has been found to hasten the recovery of muscle function, shortening the duration both of intensive care and the overall hospital stay. Plasmapheresis is the first treatment shown to be of unequivocal value in Guillain-Barré syndrome, and it is in increasingly wide use. Patients are usually referred to neurological centers for a series of plasmapheresis treatments, since specialized equipment and staff are required. Plasmapheresis has also been used in a number of other neurological disorders, including myasthenia gravis, multiple sclerosis, and other diseases affecting the peripheral nerves, although its value has been proven only for Guillain-Barré syndrome.

Parkinson's Disease Update

Researchers in 1986 are beginning U.S. clinical trials of a drug that some European neurologists have used for Parkinson's disease.

While many older people have difficulty with walking and balance and feel generally "shaky," in some these problems are actually symptoms of Parkinson's disease, a degenerative condition that most commonly affects people over 50 and that leads to generalized stiffness, a slowing of movement (bradykinesia), and an inability to move at will (akinesia). Many patients have a tremor as well. Although intellectual deterioration (dementia) was not historically recognized as part of Parkinson's disease, recent research has shown that 5 to 10 percent of patients suffer some loss of mental functioning in the early years of the condition, while as many as 50 percent experience the same effect as the disease progresses. Dementia is also the hallmark of Alzheimer's disease, another condition that affects primarily the elderly. It is well known that the destruction of certain nuclei—collections of brain cells—at the base of the brain leads to these two diseases. What is not known, however, is what causes such destruction.

In recent work with laboratory animals, using a variety of substances injurious to nerve cells (neurotoxins), scientists have begun to explore the vulnerability of these cells to chemicals that may be present in the environment, as well as possible ways to forestall cell damage. In carrying out this work, researchers have found that the Parkinson-like condition caused in humans and animals by MPTP, a neurotoxin found in some forms of synthetic heroin, can be prevented if the drug deprenyl is given at the same time that the animal is given MPTP. Deprenyl has been tried in Europe as a treatment for Parkinson's disease. It has not yet been proved by studies to be effective. The Food and Drug Administration in 1985 granted permission to conduct the first U.S. trials of the drug in humans.

Clinical trials using small numbers of patients are now under way in several countries to answer the question of whether deprenyl or similar drugs may forestall the progression of Parkinson's disease. Answering this question will require many years of analysis. It is widely expected that during that time animal research will shed new light on mechanisms of the disease and on possible remedies.

Progress in Treating Stroke

Stroke is the third most common cause of death in the United States, following only heart disease and cancer. According to recent studies, however, the incidence of stroke has declined about 10 percent over the past decade. (A declining trend has also been found for heart

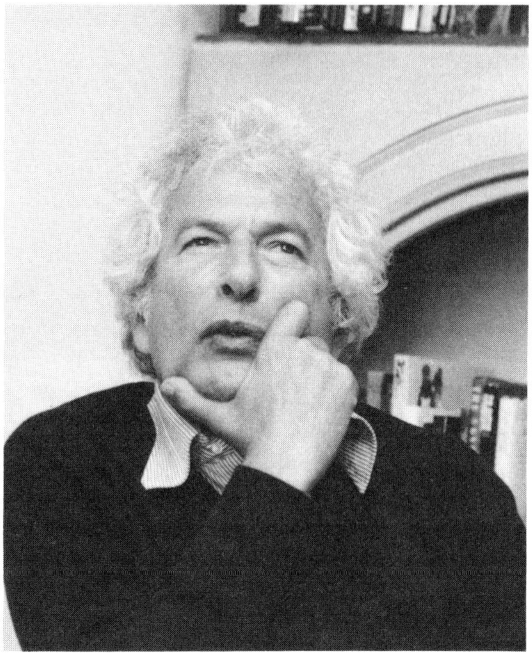

NO LAUGHING MATTER

Joseph Heller, the author of such best-selling comic novels as *Catch-22* and *God Knows,* suffered an ordeal that had to have tested his famed sense of humor. Heller was 58 and in excellent physical condition when Guillain-Barré syndrome suddenly struck a few years ago. This disorder attacks the body's peripheral nerves, those outside the brain and spinal column. One day Heller felt an extreme weakness in his limbs; the following day saw him in the intensive care unit of New York City's Mount Sinai Hospital. The disease quickly progressed to the point where he could do no more than slightly move his hands, feet, and head. He became so helpless that simply transferring him from his bed to an adjacent stretcher-chair mechanism was a six-person job. Yet inside of a year, after months of therapy at the Rusk Institute, Heller was back at his typewriter. He eventually made what is regarded as a complete recovery, although his muscles, as he says, "don't work as well as they did before." With his old friend Speed Vogel, who cared for him as he recovered, Heller wrote a book about his struggle with Guillain-Barré. The title: *No Laughing Matter.*

disease.) The incidence of both stroke and heart disease is clearly related to hypertension (high blood pressure), as well as to overweight, diabetes, cigarette smoking, an elevated cholesterol level in the blood, and a family history of these diseases. Blood pressure is the most important risk factor, however, and the decline in the rate of stroke has been attributed primarily to more effective treatment of hypertension and to changes in the American diet, especially a decline in consumption of saturated fats and an increase in the consumption of polyunsaturated fats.

Stroke is actually not a single condition; rather, the term is a general one that refers to several quite different mechanisms by which the blood supply to the brain is interrupted. One major kind of stroke occurs when an artery that supplies blood to the brain is blocked by a clot, either one that has traveled from the heart or another blood vessel (such a clot is called an embolism) or one that has formed in an artery inside the brain and attached itself to the artery's interior wall (a type of clot known as a thrombus). A second cause of strokes is rupture of an artery within or outside the brain, leading to a leakage of blood from the vessel. If an artery bursts inside the brain, the result is called an intracerebral hemorrhage. Rupture of an artery outside the brain causes a clot to form within the arachnoid, the fluid-filled covering that surrounds the brain; such a stroke is known as a subarachnoid hemorrhage. In all of these types of stroke, neurological injury results from a combination of insufficient blood flow to the brain, the presence of the waste products of brain metabolism that are normally removed, and swelling of the brain that leads to an increase of pressure within the skull; all of these factors lead to still further injury to the brain cells.

Both thrombotic and embolic strokes can be prevented by drugs that affect the clotting mechanism, once the patient has experienced certain warning signs of being vulnerable to a stroke. The substance most widely used for these patients, common aspirin, is also one of the most effective in decreasing the risk of stroke in men although—oddly—not in women (it also prevents certain kinds of heart attack and sudden death). Other drugs, such as sulfinpyrazone and dipyridamole, have also been used, but their value is not as well proven. Several collaborative studies in Britain, Australia, Canada, and the United States are under way to clarify the role of these drugs.

Surgery is also sometimes employed for thrombotic and embolic strokes. The value of one of these surgical procedures, in which the blocked vessel is bypassed by connecting an artery from the scalp to one on the surface of the brain (the operation is called an extracranial-intracranial arterial bypass), was called into serious question by the results, published in 1985, of a major international study. Stroke patients who had the operation suffered at least as many later strokes as those not operated on (all patients in the study received drug therapy), and the operation itself may have increased the patients' risk of stroke. However, a much more commonly performed operation called carotid endarterectomy, in which fatty deposits are removed from inside a hardened artery in the neck, remains an important treatment for preventing stroke in patients who have had prior warning signs of a blocked artery.

Subarachnoid hemorrhage, a common cause of stroke in all age groups but especially in young people, usually occurs without warning and with devastating effect. Although in many cases it is amenable to surgical therapy (a procedure in which the neurosurgeon applies a clip to the defective blood vessel), the effectiveness of this surgery in improving the patient's overall prospects has been limited because patients are often gravely ill at the time it is performed, having already suffered great injury to the brain. Progress in caring for critically ill neurological patients, especially in the computerized monitoring of blood pressure, respiratory function, brain activity, and general neurological status, is now allowing neurosurgeons to operate with a greater margin of safety and at the soonest possible time. Recent work has also focused on new drugs that stabilize blood vessels, thereby preventing vessel spasms that might lead to a second stroke. For example, nimodepine, a drug that is one of a class called calcium channel blockers that are commonly used to treat heart disease, has been shown to prevent secondary stroke after subarachnoid hemorrhage. At present it is undergoing clinical testing.

See also the Spotlight on Health article TREATING EPILEPSY.

HAMILTON MOSES III, M.D.

Cancer

The Promise of Interleukin-2 • Innovative Treatments for Bone, Liver Cancer • Studying Cancer Genes • Research Into Cancer Prevention

Stimulating the Immune System

Utilizing a substance called interleukin-2, scientists at the National Cancer Institute have been able to turn patients' white blood cells into "killer cells" that apparently can help shrink tumors in their bodies. This innovative—and still highly experimental—technique, developed by Dr. Steven Rosenberg and his colleagues, was the most publicized advance in cancer treatment in 1985.

Many cancer patients, like healthy people, have circulating white blood cells called lymphocytes that are capable of reacting with and destroying tumors. In an attempt to increase the numbers of such cells with "killer" activity, Rosenberg and his colleagues treated lymphocytes with small proteins called lymphokines that are capable of stimulating lymphatic cells. The lymphokine they used is called interleukin-2; it is present in the body naturally in only very small quantities, but relatively large amounts of it are now being produced by genetic engineering technology. When interleukin-2 is added to normal blood lymphocytes that have been removed from an animal or a person with a tumor, it causes normal lymphocytes to develop into so-called lymphokine-activated killer (LAK) cells. When transfused back into the animal or patient, the LAK cells sometimes result in reduction of tumor size. These LAK cells were shown to be different from killer cells produced naturally by the body: they were derived from a particular group of lymphatic cells normally present in the blood, lymph nodes, and bone marrow that are not the same as other types of killer cells. In animal experiments, LAK cells produced major reductions in cancer that had spread to the lung or liver from a wide variety of malignancies, and without damage to normal tissue.

Interleukin-2 had been tried alone to treat cancer patients, but it had not been effective. In the new approach, 25 patients with a variety of advanced, apparently incurable cancers that had resisted standard therapy had their blood lymphocytes removed, stimulated with interleukin-2 to produce LAK cells, and then transfused back. In addition, patients received extra doses of interleukin-2 by injection. Of the 25 patients, 11 had partial remission: their tumors shrunk by more than 50 percent. One had a complete remission: the cancer completely disappeared. Side effects, however, were substantial, with the most serious problem being severe fluid retention that could cause breathing failure. The treatment also remains extremely expensive, at tens of thousands of dollars per patient. In addition, the time for follow-up study of the patients has been short, and even patients with partial tumor remission are often helped only modestly by treatment.

Thus, although it is exciting news, the research results must be considered preliminary and should be viewed with caution. Interleukin-2 research will be expanded during the coming year. New data will be obtained that should make it possible to better evaluate the new treatment's effectiveness and safety.

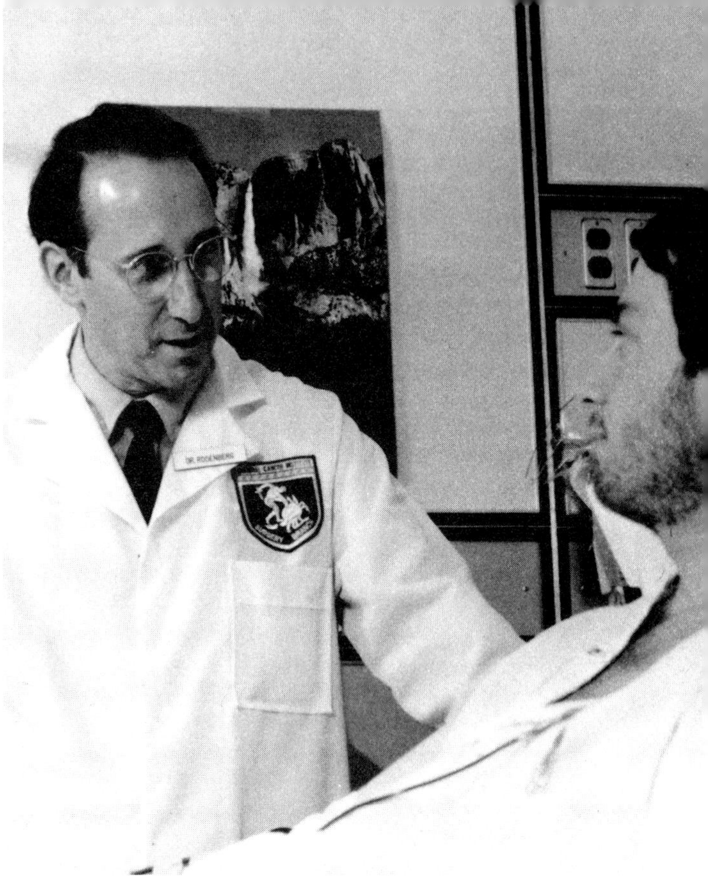

Dr. Steven Rosenberg of the National Cancer Institute has won national attention with his experimental work on a new kind of cancer therapy; the treatment uses the hormone interleukin-2 to stimulate the body's own immune system to attack the cancerous cells.

Other Progress in Treatment

Improving bone cancer survival. Chemotherapy following surgery can help improve the chances for curing osteosarcoma, a highly malignant form of bone cancer. Osteosarcoma is most commonly seen in adolescents. It usually begins in the growing portions of arm or leg bones. In the past, treatment generally required surgical amputation of the limb. In spite of such drastic measures, only 20 to 40 percent of patients could be expected to survive longer than five years. Recently, two important studies comparing surgery followed by chemotherapy with surgery alone demonstrated that postoperative chemotherapy can improve patient survival significantly. This important finding should help resolve many years of controversy about the value of chemotherapy for this cancer. All patients with this illness should now have postoperative chemotherapy unless other medical considerations prevent it. Another advance in the treatment of bone cancer is surgery that spares the affected limb. Newer procedures using bone grafts, prosthetic devices, and other means of preserving the long bones may eliminate the need for amputation.

See also BONES, MUSCLES, AND JOINTS.

Hyperthermia plus radiation. The use of hyperthermia (heat therapy) in combination with radiation therapy can lead to better treatment for a variety of malignancies. High temperature is capable of destroying cancer cells.

Localized areas of the body, such as the head and neck, chest wall, and cervix, can be heated externally using ultrasound (high-frequency sound waves), electromagnetic waves, or even microwaves. The entire body can be heated using warmed air breathed by the patient, special suits containing hot water, or heated blankets, or by heating the blood outside the body by means of a device similar to a kidney dialysis machine. Used alone, hyperthermia does little to destroy cancer cells, but it can increase the damage radiation does to cancer cells without increasing damage to normal tissue. So far the most impressive results of this combination have come in cancers of the head and neck and recurrent cancers of the breast. In advanced cases, such treatment has resulted in a rate of complete remission that is twice that gotten with radiation alone. Hyperthermia also enhances the effects of several cancer chemotherapy drugs; studies evaluating the effects of whole-body hyperthermia in combination with chemotherapy are under way.

New treatment for liver cancer. Genetic engineering has made a promising new approach to treating liver cancer possible. Cancer beginning in the liver (as opposed to cancers that spread to the liver) is usually rapidly fatal. Although rare in the United States and Canada, liver cancer, or hepatoma, occasionally occurs as a complication of cirrhosis, chronic hepatitis, and other liver diseases. Most patients with this illness get little benefit from standard radiation treatment or chemotherapy. But the development of antibodies that adhere to an iron-containing protein called ferritin, which is found in high concentration in both tumor cells and the surrounding normal tissue of the liver in hepatoma patients, has provided a new treatment tool for doctors at the Johns Hopkins University. (An antibody is a protein that reacts specifically with a substance called an antigen; scientists can produce antibodies that react with different substances—in this case, ferritin.)

The antiferritin antibodies are combined with radioactive iodine and given to patients with advanced and otherwise incurable liver cancers. Once injected, these antibodies travel to the liver, where they combine with the ferritin in the cancer cells while sparing the normal liver cells and the surrounding normal tissue. This allows for a dose of radiation that could not be given by other standard techniques to be delivered directly to the tumor. Of 66 patients evaluated, almost half had greater than 50 percent reduction in the size of their liver cancer, and 7 percent had complete remission. Unfortunately, the median survival of patients whose tumors shrank was only 11 months, though 15 percent did survive longer than two years. The results are nevertheless impressive, since earlier therapy had failed with all the patients. Future research will attempt to improve the treatment by combining the antibody with different sources of radioactivity, by developing more specific antibodies using genetic engineering techniques, and by combining the antibody treatment with chemotherapy.

Bone marrow transplants. Progress in bone marrow transplants promises to make this therapy useful for treating more patients with more types of cancer. Bone marrow is essential to the body's production of blood cells, and bone marrow transplants (BMT) have been a major advance in the treatment of many diseases that affect it, most notably aplastic anemia (a condition, usually of unknown cause, characterized by a decrease or absence of normal bone marrow cells). The procedure involves using a needle to draw marrow cells from within the bones of a donor and then injecting the cells into the bones of a recipient. At present, the main role of BMT in cancer therapy has been in treating leukemia patients who have gone into remission after chemotherapy. Another use for BMT is in treatment that uses very high doses of chemotherapy or radiation that—because of the extent to which they destroy bone marrow—would be lethal without its use. The use of BMT after high-dose chemotherapy or radiation could save patients from the lethal side effects. Such approaches are now being tried in a variety of human cancers.

A common problem with BMT is finding appropriate donors: too great a genetic difference between donor and recipient will result in rejection of the transplant as foreign tissue by the recipient's immune system, generally making it necessary to use identical twins or siblings whose tissues have been carefully matched for major immune-system factors. In general, the chance of finding a relative who is immunologically matched for four major genetic factors is only one in four. But in 1985 scientists at the University of Washington reported success in bone marrow transplants using siblings who were not this closely matched for these factors. The new research suggests that more of a patient's relatives may serve as potential bone marrow donors. Although there were more problems with transplants from less closely matched donors, the long-term survival of patients who received such transplants was just as good.

Instead of using bone marrow from a related donor after high-dose chemotherapy or radiation treatment, it is also possible to take the patient's own bone marrow in advance for retransplant. The patient's bone marrow is frozen, stored, and then later thawed and retransfused into the patient after high-dose therapy. Retransplantation is an attractive technique since it eliminates the possibility of rejection of the bone marrow as a foreign tissue. The fact that there may be cancer cells in a cancer patient's bone marrow represents the major drawback of such a transplant. This may in turn be overcome by new procedures that use chemotherapy or other methods to remove cancer cells from the marrow without altering the normal cells. These new transplant techniques are likely to lead to many new treatment programs using potentially curative but otherwise lethal doses of chemotherapy or radiation.

The Causes of Cancer

Although the causes of most cancers remain unknown, continued research into how certain genes trigger malignant cell growth continues at an explosive pace. Experiments with cell cultures and animal tumors have led to the recognition that certain genes called oncogenes ("onco" means tumor) are involved in the transformation of benign cells to malignant ones. Such genes have now been shown to be present in a variety of human cells, both benign and malignant. In normal cells these oncogenes appear to be prevented from functioning, but if changes that allow such genes to function occur, they cause the cells to produce proteins that lead to malignant growth. It has now been demonstrated that specific gene rearrangements commonly occur in several human cancers, including small cell lung cancer, lymphoma, neuroblastoma, and chronic granulocytic leukemia. Such rearrangements make for a relocation of oncogenes to chromosomes where they are able to function and transform a normal cell to its malignant counterpart.

Much research is now focused on how oncogenes become capable of triggering this cell transformation. In addition, the isolation and purification of the proteins produced when oncogenes become activated is progressing rapidly. Once such proteins are isolated, it should be possible to design therapy to block or modify their harmful effects. One strategy in this effort is the development of genetically engineered substances called monoclonal antibodies that are capable of blocking the proteins associated with oncogenes, but not normal cellular proteins. Such antibodies could prevent or stop malignant growth.

Genetic research has also led to the discovery of genes that are responsible for resistance to chemotherapy—that is, for preventing chemotherapy from destroying previously sensitive cancer cells. Such genes serve as blueprints for the production of enzymes and other proteins capable of interfering with anticancer drugs. Researchers are looking for methods of preventing the activation of these genes.

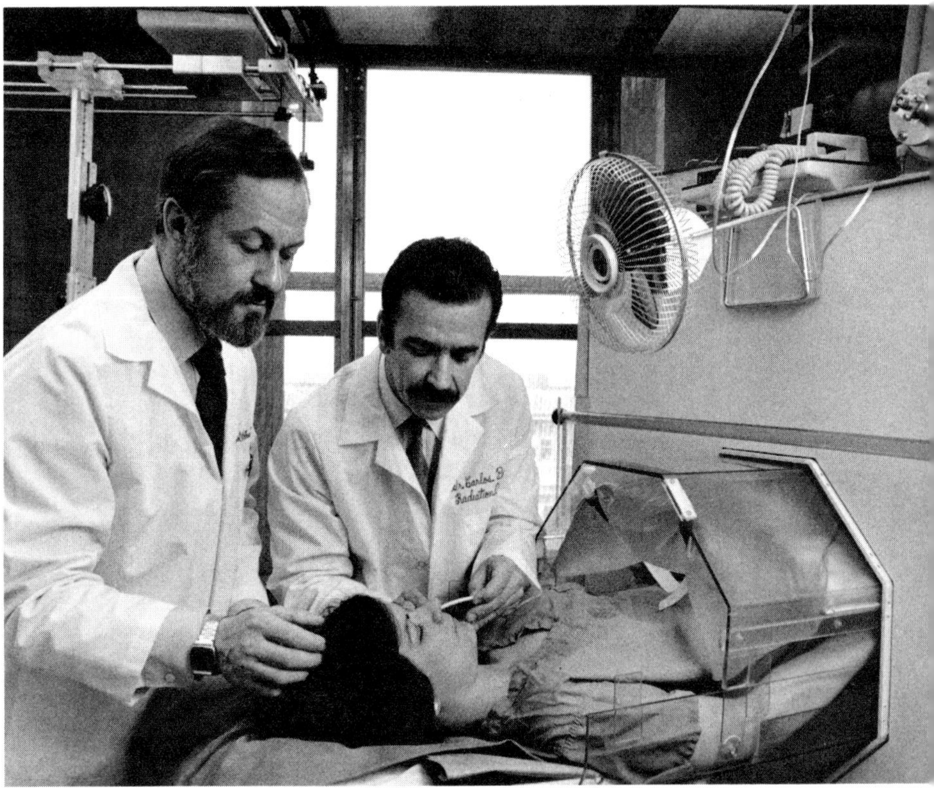

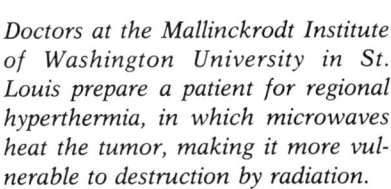

Doctors at the Mallinckrodt Institute of Washington University in St. Louis prepare a patient for regional hyperthermia, in which microwaves heat the tumor, making it more vulnerable to destruction by radiation.

Prevention and Early Detection

Diet and cancer. Vitamin A, beta-carotene (the substance from which the vitamin is formed), and synthetic derivatives of vitamin A called retinoids have been shown in several animal and human studies to decrease the frequency of cancer. Several long-term trials are currently exploring the role of the vitamin or its derivatives in preventing cancer of the lung, cervix, and skin. Other types of cancer targeted for study include breast, colon, bladder, and head and neck cancer.

Much evidence supports the idea that diet plays a role in the development of breast and colon cancer. A major study will compare the risk of breast cancer in women who consume a diet in which 20 percent of the calories are provided by fat compared with those who eat a standard North American diet, with 40 percent of calories provided by fat. Another trial will assess the benefits of a low-fat diet in preventing the recurrence of breast cancer in women who have already had breast cancer. The role of dietary fiber and colon cancer will also be studied.

Smokeless tobacco. The apparent decline in cigarette smoking may be offset by the growing use of snuff and chewing tobacco. Although such smokeless tobacco has not been as convincingly shown to be a cause of cancer as cigarette smoking, it appears to be clearly associated with an increased incidence of mouth and oral cavity cancer. Of great concern is the use of such products by teenagers. In one study, almost two thirds of teenage users had abnormalities that could be detected by oral examination.

It appears likely that smokeless tobacco will prove to be a major carcinogen (cancer-producing substance), and its use should be discouraged. Users of such products should be examined regularly to detect potentially malignant changes in the mouth. In January 1986 a panel convened by the U.S. National Institutes of Health warned that smokeless tobacco was a danger to health and posed an increased risk of mouth and throat cancer. Federal legislation enacted in February requires that smokeless tobacco products bear warning labels similar to those on cigarette packs.

Cancer of the testicles. The importance of self-examination and early detection for success in treating cancer has received widespread publicity in recent years, but one cancer has perhaps not received sufficient attention in this regard. Testicular cancer is the most common cancer in males between the ages of 15 and 35. Early detection depends on finding a mass attached to the testicle. Such masses are frequently painless and may not cause concern when detected, but new information has suggested that a delay in diagnosis lowers the probability of a cure and that men be made aware of the importance of any testicular mass. Self-examination of the testicles—something like female breast self-examination—should be performed by all males on a monthly basis. Any mass or lump should be brought to the attention of a physician.

See also the feature article COLON CANCER: PREVENTION AND TREATMENT *and the Spotlight on Health article* NEW SURGERY FOR BREAST CANCER.

HYMAN B. MUSS, M.D.

Dentistry

See TEETH AND GUMS.

Digestive System

New Ulcer Drug Shows Promise • Why Smoking Is Bad for Ulcers • Relief for Irritable Bowel Syndrome • Back Slaps Out, Heimlich In

Prostaglandin Drug for Ulcers

A potential new source of relief for ulcer victims is on the horizon: the drug misoprostol (Cytotec). It has shown good results in tests, and in 1984 Mexican health authorities approved it as safe and effective in the healing of ulcers in both the duodenum (the first part of the small intestine) and the stomach. In mid-1985 an advisory committee of the U.S. Food and Drug Administration recommended that the FDA approve misoprostol for marketing as a treatment for duodenal ulcers. The drug was approved in Canada in early 1986.

A gastric or duodenal ulcer is a kind of inflammatory sore in the lining of the stomach or duodenum, respectively. It may develop because an excess production of stomach acid overwhelms the lining's natural defenses or because the defenses are defective—and cannot cope with normal amounts of acid. Drugs used up to now to treat ulcers—antacids, cimetidine (Tagamet), and ranitidine (Zantac)—work by reducing or eliminating stomach acid. Misoprostol is the first medication designed both to inhibit stomach acid production and to bolster the lining's defenses.

Misoprostol is a synthetic drug belonging to the class of substances known as prostaglandins. First thought to come from the prostate gland, prostaglandins are now known to be made throughout the body from fatty acids. They affect nearly all the body's physiological functions, including the gastrointestinal system's secretion of acids. Moreover, high levels of prostaglandins are normally found in the lining of the stomach and intestines and appear to play a role in protecting the lining against damage by such substances as acids and alcohol. It is this kind of beneficial effect, called cytoprotection, that misoprostol is said to offer in addition to inhibiting acid secretion. Side effects of misoprostol include diarrhea and possibly, in some pregnant women, bleeding or even miscarriage.

Smoking and Ulcers

Cigarette smoking definitely has negative effects on ulcers, but how it produces these effects has remained a question. Recent findings from studies in the United States and in Japan, however, may shed light on the reasons why smokers' ulcers heal more slowly and why smokers have more ulcer recurrence.

HOW TO DO THE HEIMLICH MANEUVER

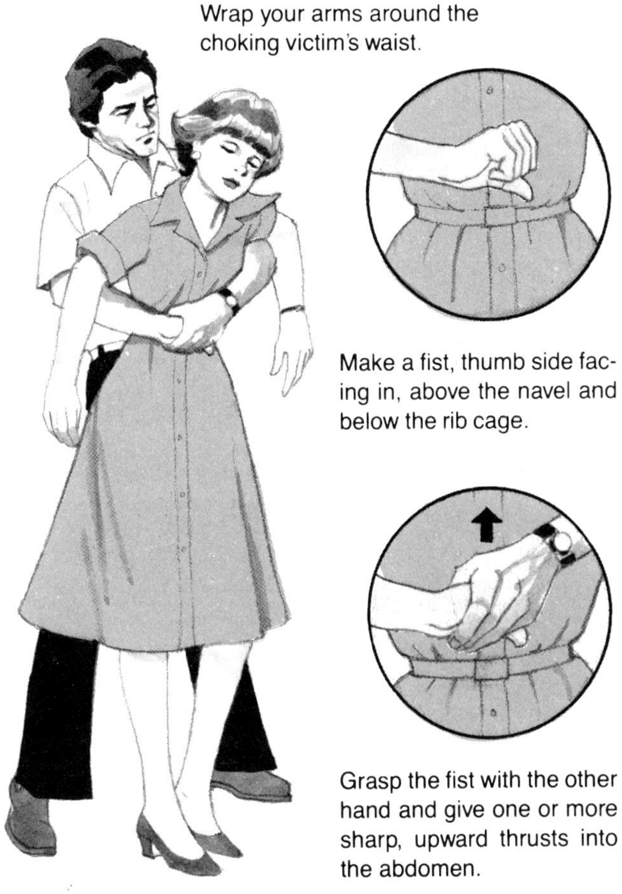
Wrap your arms around the choking victim's waist.
Make a fist, thumb side facing in, above the navel and below the rib cage.
Grasp the fist with the other hand and give one or more sharp, upward thrusts into the abdomen.

Procedure as recommended for adults and older children.

Prostaglandin production. A study by Massachusetts researchers found that smoking causes a temporary decrease in the amount of prostaglandin that protects the lining of the stomach and the duodenum. The researchers examined ten nonsmokers and ten smokers. The lining of the stomach and duodenum was looked at with a flexible instrument called an endoscope. (The smokers first smoked four cigarettes over an hour.) The researchers took snips of tissue from the stomachs and duodena of both the smokers and the nonsmokers to measure the amount of a prostaglandin in the tissue. Half of the smokers were subsequently examined a second time, after not smoking for 12 hours. By comparison with these individuals, the other smokers—who did not refrain from smoking—showed significantly lower amounts of prostaglandin. There was no difference between the level of prostaglandin in nonsmokers and the level in those who had refrained from smoking. In other words, the decrease that occurs in prostaglandin production from smoking appears to be temporary.

Digestion. Meanwhile, researchers in Pennsylvania reported on certain smoking-related changes in the digestive system that may contribute to ulcers: the effects of cigarette smoking on motility in the stomach and duodenum (that is, on the muscle contractions of the organs' walls that cause food and liquids to move through the intestinal tract); on the amount of acid in the duodenum; and on secretions from the pancreas, the gland that makes digestive enzymes.

Five smokers with a history of ulcers, and ten nonsmokers without, were studied. Each individual smoked one cigarette every 20 minutes for an hour; there was no smoking the hour before and the hour after. In both groups motility was slowed by 50 percent after smoking. Furthermore, in the individuals with ulcers—who also smoked outside the study—there was more acid in the duodenum that in those who hadn't had ulcers and who didn't normally smoke.

The researchers also performed blood tests to see if the levels of certain hormones that affect pancreatic secretions were altered by smoking. They found that smoking increased the amount of pancreatic polypeptide (a hormone that inhibits pancreatic secretion) in the blood. The researchers speculated that the slowed contractions caused by smoking may allow bile to seep into the stomach from the duodenum, a process thought to contribute to stomach ulcer formation. In addition, the increased level of the pancreatic polypeptide hormone may inhibit the production of pancreatic bicarbonate, a substance that has an important role in neutralizing acid in the duodenum.

Blood flow. A Japanese study of cigarette smokers found that blood flow to the lining of the stomach and duodenum was reduced during smoking. Moreover, the amount of oxygen in the blood in the lining decreased. Many scientists have noted that a strong blood flow to the lining of the intestinal tract is an important factor in preventing the development of ulcers and in healing any ulcers already there.

Irritable Bowel Syndrome

New research indicates that dextromethorphan, an ingredient of over-the-counter cough and cold preparations, can relieve abdominal pain in persons suffering from the puzzling condition called irritable bowel syndrome (IBS). No cause has been identified for this condition, which comprises a group of symptoms that include abdominal pain and a change in bowel habits. People with IBS frequently complain of constipation or diarrhea—in some cases both may occur by turns.

In a study involving four medical centers in the United States, dextromethorphan was administered to one group of IBS patients, and a placebo (an inert substance) to another. About four-fifths of the patients who were given the drug experienced pain relief, but fewer than half of those given the placebo. Four-fifths of the patients receiving dextromethorphan showed significant overall improvement in their condition, including more normal bowel movements in some cases, but only half of those receiving the placebo did. Side effects were minor.

Inflammatory Bowel Disease

New forms of treatment for inflammatory bowel disease (IBD)—a general name for two serious digestive disorders, Crohn's disease and ulcerative colitis—have been found to effectively relieve symptoms with few side effects. The main drug used to relieve IBD symptoms—which include intestinal ulcers, diarrhea, cramping, fever, and weight loss—has been sulfasalazine (Azulfidine). The drug's two components, 5-aminosalicylic acid (5-ASA) and sulfapyridine, are split apart by bacteria in the colon (which, together with the rectum, makes up most of the large intestine). Although sulfasalazine is effective against IBD, its use may be limited by its side effects—such as headache, nausea, and skin rashes—which are due to the sulfapyridine component. The drug's benefits come from the 5-ASA, which acts on the lining of the colon. The new forms under study do without the sulfapyridine component. They include an enema containing 5-ASA; a pill form of 5-ASA that, once swallowed, releases the drug slowly; and a capsule containing disodium azodisalicylate (Dipentum), which is composed of two linked molecules of 5-ASA.

Italian researchers used 5-ASA enemas on 144 patients with mild to moderate ulcerative colitis and reported positive results in 88 percent. While about a third of the patients in the study could not tolerate or were allergic to sulfasalazine, only a few could not tolerate the 5-ASA enemas, complaining of rashes, fever, or diarrhea. The researchers also compared 5-ASA to hydrocortisone enemas, another standard treatment for ulcerative colitis. While only about half of the 42 patients receiving the hydrocortisone improved, nearly all of the 44 patients receiving 5-ASA did. The 5-ASA enema appears to be most effective when the disease is limited to the lower parts of the large intestine.

A Canadian study found that a type of 5-ASA pill with a special hard "enteric" coating is effective for treating ulcerative colitis. When an uncoated 5-ASA pill is taken by mouth, the drug is absorbed in the upper small intestine and excreted in the urine, and so does not reach the colon to produce its beneficial effect on the lining. The coating of the enteric pill form of 5-ASA (Asacol) keeps it from dissolving quickly. The pill does not dissolve until it reaches the last part of the small intestine (ileum) and the colon. The Canadian study tested enteric-coated 5-ASA on 31 patients with ulcerative colitis who had developed side effects while taking sulfasalazine. Only one major side effect caused by sulfasalazine, pericarditis, an inflammation of the covering of the heart, recurred when 5-ASA was taken, and it showed up in only one patient.

The new oral drug disodium azodisalicylate is a means of delivering 5-ASA to the colon with doubled potency. The two molecules of 5-ASA are split apart by bacteria in the colon. To evaluate how readily patients tolerate the drug, Swedish researchers administered it for six to eight months to 160 people with ulcerative colitis, all of whom had experienced side effects when given sulfasalazine. Close to a third of the patients had at least one side effect with the new drug, and about 12 percent with severe diarrhea dropped out of the study. The researchers concluded, however, that overall the side effects were mild compared to those of sulfasalazine and that disodium azodisalicylate was effective. (The new 5-ASA treatments are still being tested and are not yet on the U.S. market, though Asacol is available in Canada.)

Heimlich Maneuver

What is the best way to help a person who is choking on a piece of food or other foreign object? A long-running dispute over this issue ended in July 1985 when the American Red Cross and the American Heart Association endorsed the Heimlich maneuver, or "abdominal thrust." Both organizations had previously recommended that a rescuer give four sharp slaps to the back of a choking victim before trying the Heimlich technique. In September the U.S. surgeon general also endorsed the Heimlich maneuver as best.

To perform the maneuver, the rescuer reaches around the choking person, puts a fist—thumb side against the abdomen—at the bottom of the victim's rib cage, and grasps the fist with the other hand. With the victim bent forward, the rescuer gives one or more quick upward thrusts into the abdomen, pumping air out of the lungs to expel the foreign material.

In early 1986 the American Academy of Pediatrics recommended a modified form of the maneuver as the first move to help choking victims over 1 year old and up to the age of 12 to 15, depending on size: the child is placed on his or her back, and the rescuer kneels alongside and, with the heel of a hand, delivers six to ten sharp thrusts to the bottom of the rib cage. This technique may also be used for unconscious adults or in cases where the victim is so much larger than the rescuer that the standard technique is difficult. (Infants under one year, according to the academy, should be dangled upside down and struck on the back before thrusts to the rib cage are tried.)

Dr. Henry Heimlich, who developed his technique in the early 1970's, had argued that, in general, back blows could force the foreign body deeper into the throat. A study of 1,600 choking cases in fact found that slaps quadrupled the victim's risk of complications, including death.

See also the feature article COLON CANCER: PREVENTION AND TREATMENT *and the Spotlight on Health article* HIGH-TECH SURGERY. DANIEL PELOT, M.D.

Drug Abuse

Dangers of Cocaine During Pregnancy • Cocaine Addiction Therapy • Debate Over Ecstasy • Hazardous Designer Drugs

Cocaine

Effects in pregnancy. Cocaine abuse by pregnant women can have an adverse effect on the unborn child. One study published in 1985 showed that pregnant women who abused cocaine had an increased incidence of spontaneous abortion (miscarriage) during the first three months of pregnancy and of premature detachment of the placenta with the onset of labor (a condition called abruptio placentae). In addition, some infants born to women who abused cocaine appeared to go through a drug withdrawal episode, characterized by jitteriness, poor interaction with their mothers and others, and impaired ability to respond to their environment. They also tended to have abnormal breathing.

Researchers have also noted at least one case of a child born paralyzed on one side. The baby's mother had been a heavy cocaine user during pregnancy, and it appeared that the child had had a stroke while in the womb.

Eliminating the craving. A prescription drug normally used to treat Parkinson's disease and infertility and to stop the secretion of breast milk can also help ease the cocaine addict's craving and relieve withdrawal symptoms. As a result, the drug—bromocriptine, sold as Parlodel—could help wean addicts from cocaine.

One of the serious effects of cocaine on the brain is the rapid depletion of dopamine, a neurotransmitter (or "messenger" chemical). Low levels of dopamine are believed to cause a craving for cocaine, which often makes it difficult for former addicts to stay off the drug. Bromocriptine activates specific areas on nerve cells—called receptors—that are sensitive to dopamine, making it easier for these cells to accept traces of dopamine left unaffected by cocaine. By making lower levels of dopamine more adequate for the brain, bromocriptine could help prevent an abuser's cocaine craving.

When they are not high, cocaine abusers may experience severe depression, which often leads to further cocaine use. To end this cycle, researchers are using medications called tricyclic antidepressants, such as desipramine (sold under the brand names Norpramin and Pertofrane) and imipramine (Tofranil), to treat the depression. The antidepressants also may prevent people from becoming high and thus seem useful in therapy for cocaine use. Careful studies currently under way will provide more exact information in this area.

Dangerous Codeine Combination

Several metropolitan areas have noticed a significant rise in a hazardous way to use codeine—in combination with the drug glutethimide (also sold as Doriden). Glutethimide is a sedative-hypnotic that was developed as a substitute for barbiturates but is prescribed infrequently today because of its potential for abuse. Narcotics abusers sometimes combine it with codeine, either in the form of a cough syrup or Tylenol with codeine. The combination heightens the euphoric effects of each drug; addicts say that the feeling produced is very similar to that of heroin.

It is a highly dangerous abuse pattern. Both glutethimide and codeine depress the respiratory system, and deaths have resulted from accidental overdoses. In addition, the dependency is extremely difficult and expensive to treat; patients must usually be hospitalized for two weeks or longer.

Controversy Over Ecstasy

A drug popularly known as Ecstasy or Adam was banned for one year as an emergency measure by the U.S. Drug Enforcement Administration, effective July 1, 1985. This action temporarily placed the drug on the DEA's Schedule I, a list of "controlled substances"—including heroin and LSD—deemed to have no medical use and high abuse potential.

Ecstasy is actually called MDMA (for 3,4-methylenedioxymethamphetamine). It is chemically related to both mescaline and the amphetamines. The drug is a stimulant, produces euphoria, and also has hallucinogenic properties if taken in large doses. For these reasons MDMA has become very popular, with a reported street value of about $8 to $20 for a 100-milligram tablet.

MDMA was patented in 1914 but grew appreciably in popularity only over the past decade. MDMA users say it makes them feel "warm," "relaxed," and "in touch with people." In recent years some physicians—probably no more than 200—have used MDMA, administering it to relieve cancer patients of pain and prepare them emotionally for death or to accelerate the psychotherapeutic process by reducing patients' defensive feelings and encouraging openness between subject and therapist. Cases of abuse and adverse effects—including a small number of deaths—have been reported, however. The side effects seem related to excessive stimulation of the cardiovascular or nervous systems. Another danger cited by pharmacologists is that the effective dose and the lethal dose are very close—so that the margin for safety is extremely narrow.

Adverse mental effects brought on by MDMA, such as anxiety, depression, paranoia, loss of reasoning ability, and hallucinations, are similar to those seen with LSD. One study of MDA, a street drug that is a close chemical cousin of MDMA, showed permanent brain damage in animals. This last discovery raises questions of similar problems in humans, although a direct comparison between animal experiments and recreational or abusive use by people is not possible.

It is interesting to note that the kind of positive statements being made by some today about MDMA are almost identical to early reports about LSD and MDA, including the alleged ability to reduce psychological defenses and serve as a "catalyst" in therapy. Actual subsequent experience did not support these claims, and neither LSD nor MDA was shown to have legitimate therapeutic uses. Instead, each was shown to have serious negative effects, and each was abused by segments of the population.

The advisability of extending the DEA's ban on MDMA beyond July 1986 was being debated early in 1986, with the DEA considering testimony by mental health experts in favor of the drug. In the meantime, researchers could work with it but only after obtaining permission from the U.S. Food and Drug Administration.

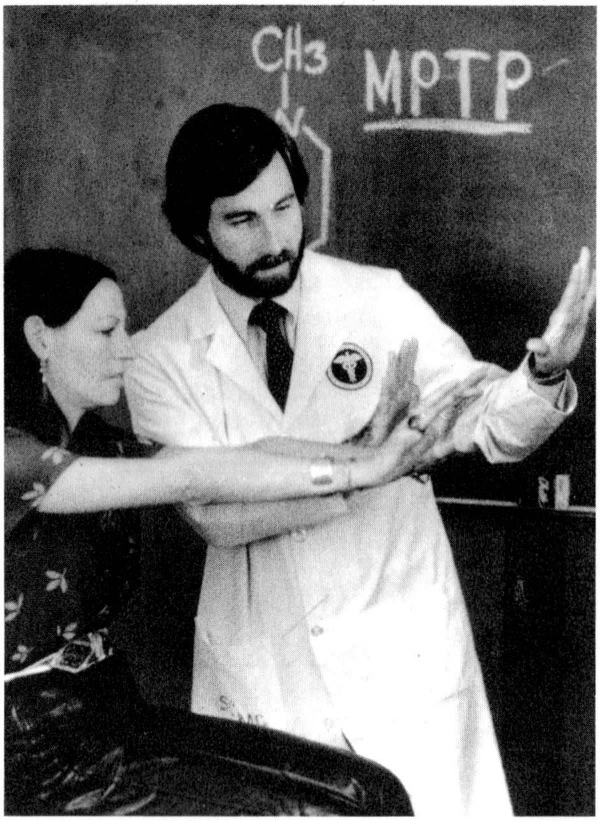

Dr. William Langston of the Santa Clara Valley Medical Center examines a patient who shows symptoms like those of Parkinson's disease; her condition was caused by taking MPTP, a dangerous substance produced accidentally in making the "designer drug" MPPP.

Deadly Designer Drugs

Skilled chemists, most of whom appear to be operating in California, have been creating deadly narcotics that are technically not illegal under current U.S. laws. These so-called designer drugs are produced by making slight alterations in the molecular structure of an abusable drug, resulting in a product whose formula is not included on the DEA's Schedule I of controlled substances. These manufactured drugs are thus legal to produce, sell, and use.

Since 1984 the DEA has invoked emergency measures to temporarily ban certain designer drugs, including several variants of the surgical anesthetic fentanyl (Sublimaze), which in the past were sold to heroin addicts. It was estimated that nearly 100 people died from taking this synthetic heroin in the period between 1979 and mid-1985.

Another designer drug is MPPP, a variant of the painkiller Demerol (meperidine hydrochloride) that also has effects like heroin. In producing MPPP, laboratories may turn out a contaminant called MPTP—which has caused several deaths and stiffness, paralysis, and other symptoms like those of Parkinson's disease.

Improving Drug Abuse Treatment

The use of the painkiller buprenorphine (Buprenex) is being investigated with an eye to narcotic substitution therapy (in which doctors help addicts withdraw from dependence on a substance like heroin by substituting another, safer drug, like methadone). Buprenorphine has some narcotic effects, but it blocks the euphoria caused by most narcotics and produces little physical dependence. Much work must still be done to determine exactly how it can be used. Meanwhile, how best to use methadone is being examined. A large study is in progress that examines differences in the staffing patterns and clinical practices of methadone treatment programs. Methadone maintenance programs vary greatly, and describing and defining these variations may serve as a way to predict which programs will be most effective with certain types of patients.

GEORGE E. WOODY, M.D.,
CHARLES P. O'BRIEN, M.D., PH.D.,
and A. THOMAS MCLELLAN, PH.D.

Drugs

See MEDICATIONS AND DRUGS; DRUG ABUSE.

Ears, Nose, and Throat

Implants to Help the Deaf Hear Speech • Interferon to Fight the Common Cold? • Microsurgery for Blocked Sinuses

Helping the Deaf Hear Speech

An electronic device now being tested, the multichannel cochlear implant, may become the first device available that allows totally deaf people to hear and understand speech. The totally deaf are generally not helped by conventional hearing aids which essentially just amplify sound. A device called a single-channel cochlear implant was approved by the U.S. Food and Drug Administration in November 1984, but this implant allows the deaf person to hear only simple sounds like sirens, telephones, and doorbells; it can also sufficiently discriminate changes of pitch and volume to be an aid to lip reading. The multichannel implant, however, can transmit many complex differences in sound. Studies have indicated that the new implant could help some deaf people understand about 60 percent of speech without lip reading.

Both types of implants operate on the same principle. They take over the function of defective hair cells in the cochlea, the snail-shaped organ of the inner ear—cells that convert sound vibrations to electrical impulses that the cochlear (auditory) nerve then transmits to the brain. The implants use a miniature microphone and sound processor (perhaps worn in a shirt pocket, on eyeglasses, or in the outer ear) to pick up sound and convert it to electrical signals. The signals are then sent to a receiver implanted under the skin near the ear. One or more wire electrodes carry the signals from the receiver to nerve cells in the cochlea for transmission to the brain, bypassing the defective hair cells.

The single-channel implants now in use have only one electrode (channel) going to the cochlea. The potential key advance in the experimental multichannel implants is the use of numerous electrodes, producing the range of pitches necessary to re-create speech. But the recreation is not perfect. One implant user reported that the speech he hears has a "Louis Armstrong quality." Researchers are trying to improve the multichannel implant to better refine speech sounds and to eliminate unwanted background sounds and noises that are picked up and amplified by the device.

Even if perfected and approved for general use, multichannel implants will not be able to help all profoundly deaf people, and efforts are being made to identify the best candidates for receiving the device. First, the patient should not have nerve damage in the inner ear that would prevent the implant's electrical signals from being picked up for transmission to the brain. Other poor candidates for implants are people who were born deaf or lost their hearing very early in childhood, before they developed speech and language skills.

Interferon: New Uses

Nasal spray to prevent colds. An experimental nasal spray containing a type of interferon may help prevent the spread of the common cold. Research teams in the United States and Australia reported in early 1986 that the nasal spray reduced the incidence of colds sig-

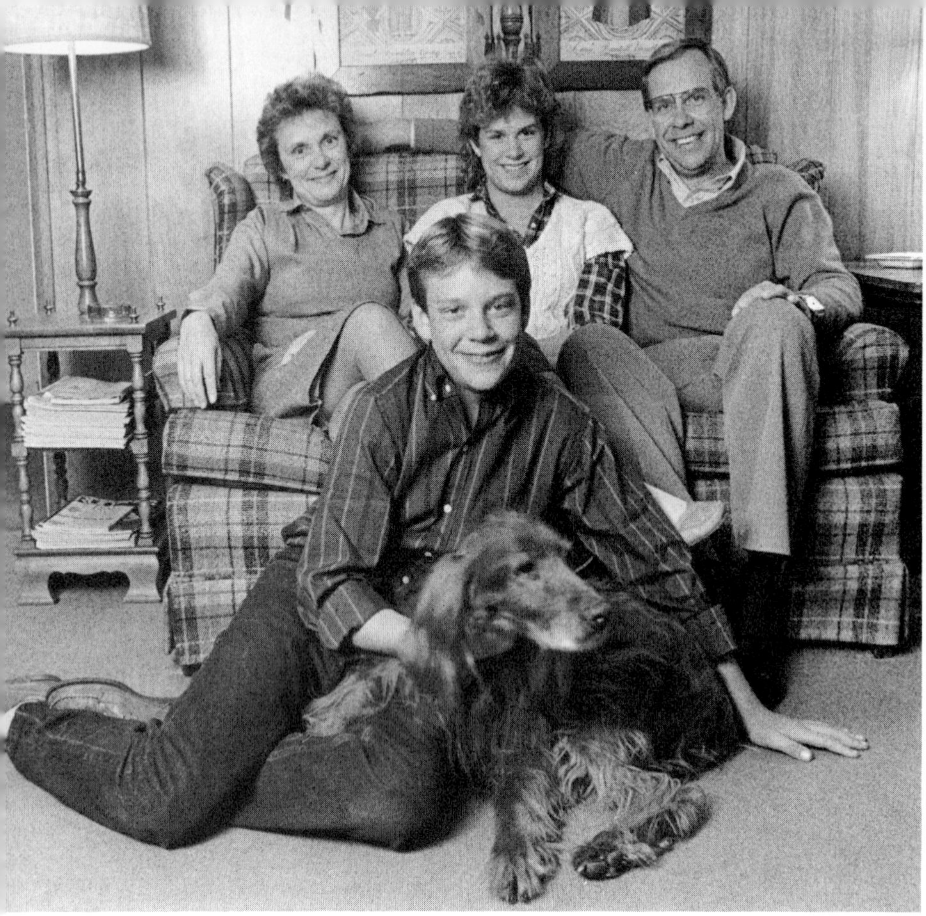

The Lear family of Virginia is one of 106 family groups who participated in studies testing the effectiveness of an interferon nasal spray against the spread of the common cold.

nificantly in healthy family members who used it after one person in the family had already developed a cold. One treatment a day for one week often prevented the spread of cold viruses, without producing the negative side effects (such as minor bleeding or a stuffy nose) found in earlier experiments in which interferon sprays were used for a longer time. The spray was most effective against rhinoviruses, the most common cause of colds. It reduced the overall incidence of respiratory illness by about 40 percent and the incidence of colds caused by rhinoviruses by over 80 percent.

Interferon is actually a group of substances produced naturally in the body in minute quantities to fight invading viruses, among other things. It has become more available for research and for medications such as the nasal spray because it can now be manufactured on a large scale by genetic engineering techniques.

Preventing growths. Interferon may also be effective against a viral disorder that has defied long-lasting treatment, recurrent respiratory tract papillomatosis. In this condition, which is most common in children, wart-like growths called papillomas develop in the trachea (windpipe) and bronchi, the divisions of the trachea leading into the lungs. If the condition is not treated, these growths may eventually cause complete blockage of the airway and death. No consistently reliable method for treating this disease has been available. The standard therapy has been surgical or laser removal of the papillomas, but new growths often soon occur. In studies in which interferon treatment was combined with growth removal, however, some patients were totally cured while others had longer periods of remission than were routinely reported after surgery alone—giving more lasting relief to many patients. The drug is administered subcutaneously (beneath the skin) on a daily basis for one month and then three times a week for six months.

A Clear View of Nasal Problems

A special fiber-optic endoscope, a light-carrying tube that allows a physician to see inside the body, is being used to improve diagnosis and treatment of difficult nasal problems. The scope, small enough to be inserted into the nose and through a sinus opening less than 1/4 inch wide, enables doctors to view areas in the nose and nasal sinuses previously visible only through surgery or extensive X-ray procedures.

The new ability to detect small amounts of drainage within the nasal cavity or the accumulation of pus or small growths within the sinuses has made the diagnosis of many nasal disorders more accurate. Tumors can be detected while they are still in an early stage; previously, they generally were not diagnosed until they became so large that they produced extensive bleeding or deformed the nose or face. The endoscope has also allowed nasal specialists to more easily distinguish between allergic conditions and infections.

With more accurate diagnosis has come improved therapy. Surgical instruments can be inserted beside the endoscope, allowing the removal of diseased tissue or the opening of blocked sinuses with no external surgical incision. The instruments can also be used to cut small pieces of tissue for biopsy, a laboratory examination of the tissue to check for cancer.

See also the Spotlight on Health article High-Tech Surgery.

Head and Neck Tumors

Refinements in the techniques for diagnosing and treating tumors of the head and neck region are benefiting more and more patients. Equipment for computerized tomographic scanning (CT, or CAT, scanning) and for magnetic resonance imaging, two sophisticated diagnostic techniques, has been improved, allowing better depiction of the exact site of a tumor. There has been comparable improvement in radioisotope diagnostic procedures, the use of a radioactive substance to locate a tumor.

In the area of treatment, techniques are being perfected that allow total surgical removal of tumors while preserving normal adjacent tissue, to minimize subsequent disability or disfigurement. For example, small tumors in the voice box (larynx) are no longer always treated by total laryngectomy, or complete removal of the voice box. Other therapeutic advances include a greater understanding of how best to use chemotherapy or radiation in the treatment of head and neck tumors.

Improved lasers are now available for head and neck surgery, and lasers are being increasingly used to destroy tumors. Using lasers with operating microscopes connected to endoscopes, physicians have been able to remove tumors from areas that were previously inaccessible or difficult to reach except by major surgery; these areas include the larynx, the base of the skull, and the middle and inner ear.

Improvements in rehabilitation after surgery include new implants of bone or artificial materials, to recreate the jawbones in patients who have had these removed in cancer operations. Among other prosthetic devices now being employed are artificial eyes, external ears, and portions of the face that have been fashioned by prosthetic consultants adept at matching shape and skin tone to the individual patient. For patients with disability resulting from the removal of nerves, nerve stimulators are being perfected to activate paralyzed muscles needed for swallowing or speaking.

Relief for Facial Pain

Sophisticated bioelectronic devices can help pinpoint the cause of and successfully treat the facial pain and jaw stiffness known as myofacial pain dysfunction (MPD). The disorder, which includes the condition called temporomandibular joint (TMJ) syndrome, is caused by an abnormality in the relationship between the teeth and the joints, muscles, and nerves of the face. It can affect people of all ages. Most commonly, improper alignment of the teeth puts undue pressure on the sensitive tissue lining the temporomandibular, or jaw, joints. In an attempt to correct this misalignment, the muscles that move the jaw are overactive and thus subject to painful strain or spasm.

Researchers have found significant improvement in MPD patients who were diagnosed and treated with electronic devices. For diagnosis, an instrument called a mandibular kinesiograph measures movement of the jawbone by tracking electromagnetic forces from a small magnet temporarily attached to the teeth. In addition, bioelectrical equipment is used to detect hyperactivity or spasm of the muscles that move the jawbone.

After the appropriate diagnosis is made, a therapeutic device called a myomonitor is used to produce electric stimulation of nerves, through the skin, in order to induce relaxation of the muscles. A program of periodic stimulations can induce a state of muscle relaxation for

Hearing problems can be diagnosed in newborns with the new Auditory Response Cradle (ARC), which monitors the infant's reactions to sound stimuli.

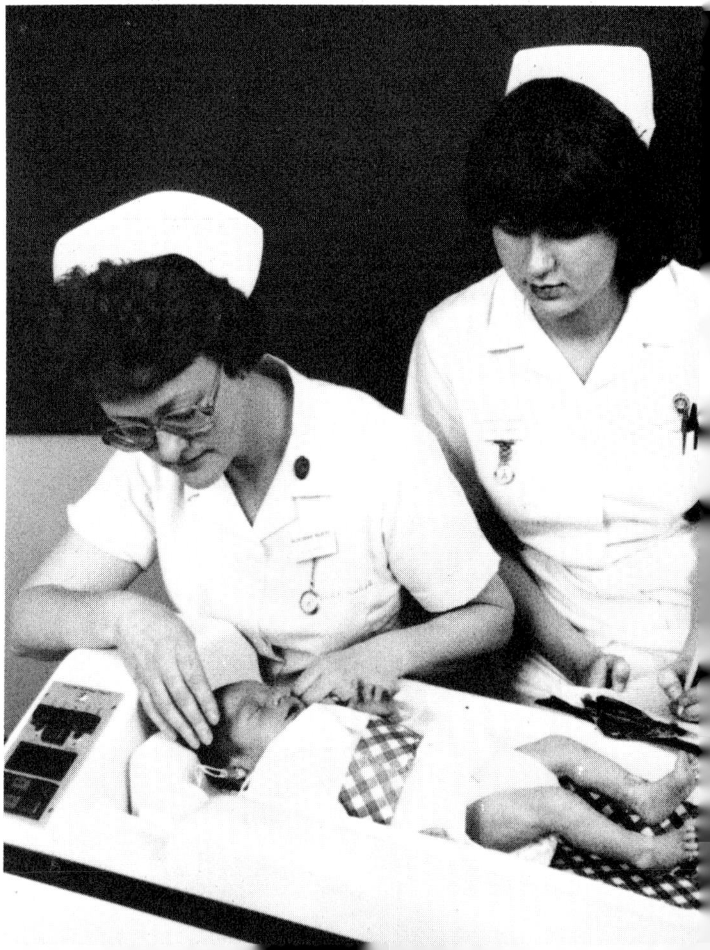

brief periods. Relaxation is used to determine the most "rested position" of the jawbone—a reference point for establishing a new position of dental occlusion (the way the teeth come together when the jaws are closed) involving well-balanced muscle function. This new position is initially established for the patient with a precision acrylic "appliance" worn 24 hours a day on the lower back teeth.

Drug Warnings by Computer

Computers may be able to assist physicians in rendering safer and more up-to-date patient care by making readily available the most recent information about potential drug interactions—that is, undesirable and sometimes dangerous side effects produced when two or more different medications are taken simultaneously. With the great increase in the number of prescription and nonprescription drugs, it has become almost impossible for physicians to know all of the potential drug interactions that may occur. A standard soft computer disk, however, could store readily retrievable information regarding over 300 potential drug interactions of concern to ear, nose, and throat specialists. New information could easily be added to the computer disk as soon as it becomes available.

See also the Spotlight on Health article HAY FEVER.

FRANK E. LUCENTE, M.D.

Environment and Health

Focus on Indoor Pollution • Protecting Water Supplies • Health Risks on the Job • Concern About Chemical Accidents • Light Can Be Hazardous • Illnesses From Animals

Air Pollution—Indoors and Out

Throughout 1985 there was growing concern about air pollution inside the home or workplace—a switch from the long-standing emphasis on outdoor emissions.

Radon contamination. High concentrations of the radioactive gas radon have been found in people's houses in several states. Radon occurs naturally in the radioactive breakdown of uranium, which is found in certain rock formations. The gas can enter a building through cracks in the foundation; colorless and odorless, it can build up to potentially dangerous levels in closed areas. (It disperses in the open air.) Long exposure to radon can lead to lung cancer, and scientists at the U.S. Centers for Disease Control believe that high radon levels may cause up to 30,000 lung cancer deaths in the United States each year.

Following the discovery of higher than expected radon levels in Pennsylvania, New Jersey, and New York, the U.S. Environmental Protection Agency (EPA) in the fall of 1985 announced plans to conduct a national survey on radon and present a five-year plan to lessen the health hazard. Pennsylvania became the first state to help its residents measure radon levels and increase ventilation to disperse it.

Other indoor pollution. Air inside a home or workplace can also be contaminated by many other things, including carbon monoxide, which results from incomplete burning of fuel and causes numerous deaths each year; nitrogen dioxide, produced during burning of natural gas, which may be linked to increased respiratory problems in children in winter; and formaldehyde, which is used in building materials and foam insulation and may cause cancer.

The EPA, in a five-year study of homes and factories in New Jersey, North Carolina, and North Dakota, found that 11 toxic air pollutants occur in high concentrations in the home. Domestically, the chemicals occur as ingredients or by-products of common items such as cleansers, construction materials, and cigarettes. Concentrations of the same chemicals outdoors were relatively insignificant, even around the plants where the chemicals are produced.

Greater effects on children. Children inhaling polluted air get a higher relative dose than adults and therefore suffer a greater health risk from lead and other contaminants found in it, according to recent research. Research involving children and young people who died from accidents and diseases not affecting the lungs showed that the younger the child, the greater the harm from pollution. This is because children inhale more air per unit of body weight, their nasal passages are relatively larger, and their lungs have fewer areas for exchanging oxygen and wastes, so that they get higher concentrations of pollutants.

Water Contamination

Sinking pesticides. Pesticides and other hazardous contaminants can move farther down through the soil and at faster rates than previously believed, meaning that their threat to underground water supplies may also be greater, scientists have found. Soil physicists at the University of California at Riverside, performing

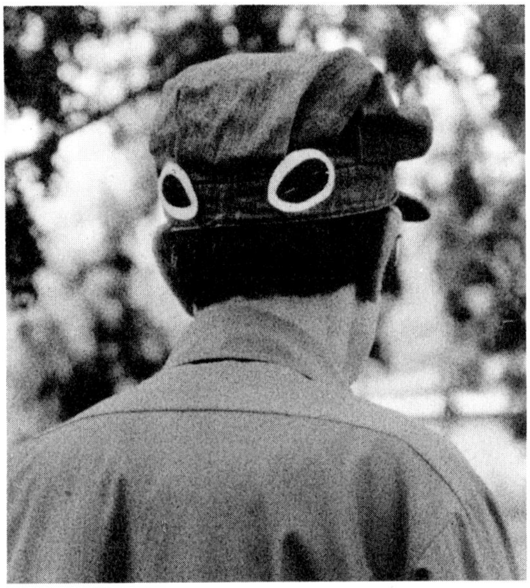

JOGGERS, LOOK UP!

Heart attacks, frostbite, heatstroke, and motor vehicle accidents are just some of the dangers faced by joggers. To this list of conventional plagues must be added a somewhat odd phenomenon: bird attacks. Letters to the *New England Journal of Medicine* in 1985 told of avian assaults in Switzerland, Australia, Minnesota, and Chicago, with the perpetrators a variety of bird species. The injuries were mostly scratches and lacerations on the victim's scalp.

A frequently offered reason for the attacks was that the birds were protecting their homes during nesting season. Other suggestions were that the birds were collecting hair for their nests, had been raised in captivity and were desirous (albeit in bird-brained fashion) of human contact, and, in the case of red-winged blackbirds, were threatened by bright-red running shorts into thinking a territorial challenge was at hand.

Since birds usually attack by diving from behind, one jogger tried protecting himself by putting fake eyes on the back of his cap—insects naturally adorned in this way startle predatory birds. After he made two attack-free walks, and one "eyeless" walk in which an attack occurred, the nesting season and the birds' aggressiveness came to an end, putting the experiment on hold.

one of the first actual field tests ever conducted in this area, found that a significant fraction of pesticides applied to crops reaches a depth ten times greater than predicted by laboratory studies. In a one-acre test application of a typical pesticide that was supposed to go no further than 8 inches below the surface, scientists found 20 percent of the substance as far down as 6 feet. These results may also apply to heavy metals and other wastes. Pesticides designed so that microorganisms will break them down in the surface layers of soil fail to decompose at greater depths because the microorganisms do not exist there.

Nitrate buildup in groundwater. Nitrates—chiefly residues from fertilizers, animal wastes, and septic systems—have been found in high and in some cases dangerous concentrations in tests of nearly 124,000 water wells conducted by the U.S. Geological Survey. The buildups were especially prevalent in the East and Northwest. More than 6 percent of the wells contained nitrate amounts above the permissible level of 10 milligrams per liter for drinking water. While relatively harmless in themselves, nitrates can be converted by the body into nitrosamines, which may cause cancer. Also, in the intestines of newborns, nitrates can be converted into nitrites, which can result in the serious condition methemoglobinemia.

Threats to Great Lakes residents. Residents of the Great Lakes region are exposed to more toxic substances than many other residents of Canada and the United States, a joint U.S.-Canadian study group has found. Surface runoff is one of the major sources of contamination in the Great Lakes. While there has been some success in controlling industrial discharges, levels of certain agents, like the long-banned pesticide DDT, have decreased only slightly, if at all. The toxic substances that get into the water pose special dangers since they accumulate in the food chain.

Groundwater radium and leukemia. Recent research suggests that radioactivity in groundwater can be a health hazard and may cause leukemia. A study by public health experts in Florida found that leukemia was significantly more common in areas where the groundwater had a high level of radioactive radium than in areas with low levels. The radium comes from phosphate ores, abundant in parts of south Florida, that contain uranium and its byproducts, including radium and radon; in some areas the groundwater used as a source of drinking water is contaminated with radium. More work is needed to prove the radiation from radium causes leukemia, but the findings are suggestive.

Occupational Health

An increase in on-the-job injuries and illnesses helped focus attention recently on continuing health threats in the workplace. The U.S. Labor Department reported in late 1985 that 1984 had seen a jump in work-related illness and injury for the first time in years—overall, there was an 11.7 percent rise over 1983 to a total of 5.4 million. Part of the rise was accounted for by increased employment, but the rate of illness and injury was also up, from 7.6 to 8 per 100 workers.

Work-related risk of birth defects. The National Institute for Occupational Safety and Health reported that close to 15 million U.S. workers are currently exposed to substances or conditions that may cause birth defects:

- 9 million—exposed to radiofrequency or microwave radiation, used for heating and drying; associated with embryo deaths and decreased fertility in laboratory animals.
- 2 million—exposed to antifreeze (ethylene glycol) and related substances, used as paint and paint solvents and brake fluids; may be toxic to sperm.
- 1.7 million—exposed to formaldehyde, emitted by plastics and some building materials; suspected of causing cancer.
- 1.4 million—exposed to lead, which can cause brain, liver, and kidney damage.
- 200,000—exposed to anesthetic gases and ethylene oxide, which is used in producing pharmaceuticals and pesticides; both associated with an elevated risk of spontaneous abortions (miscarriages).
- 500,000—exposed to other potentially dangerous substances.

Workers insulate the basement of a Berks County, Pa., house where extremely high levels of radon gas were found; the radioactive gas was produced by natural underground uranium deposits.

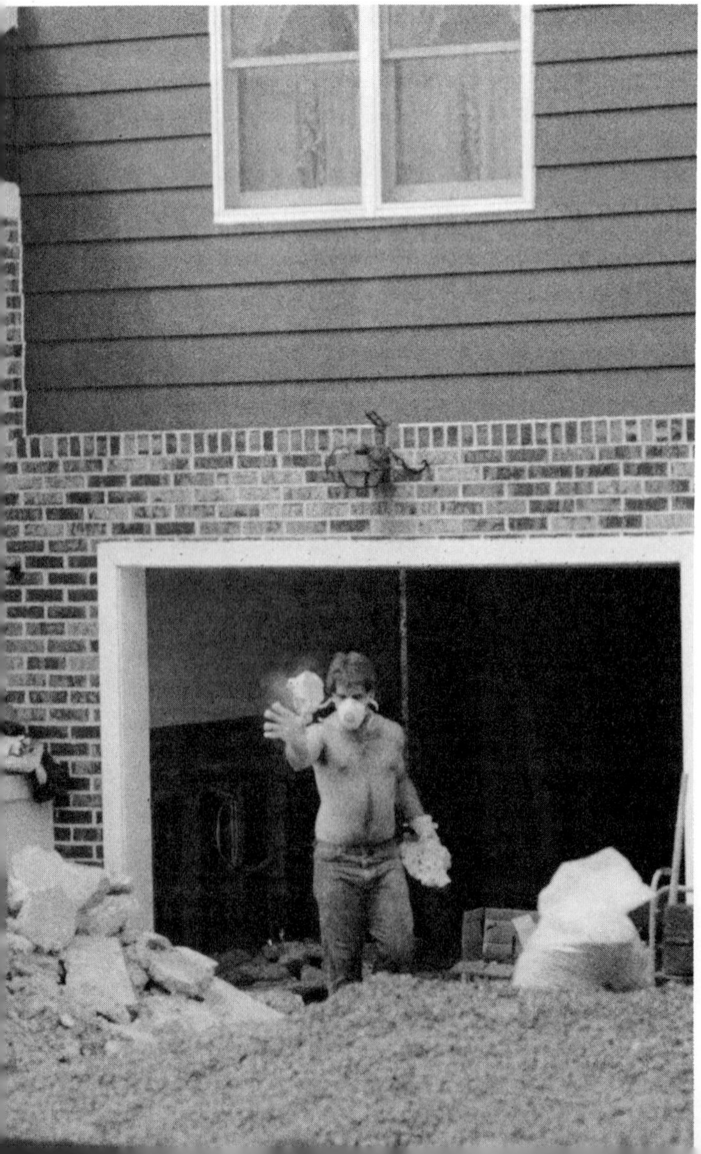

Formaldehyde and benzene regulation. OSHA in December 1985 proposed new rules for worker exposure to benzene and formaldehyde—both of which are believed to cause cancer. The exposure standard for benzene, used in producing plastics, dyes, detergents, and insecticides, would be reduced from 10 parts per million of air to 1 ppm, reducing cancer risks by about 90 percent. Two different proposals were made for formaldehyde, a component of foam insulation, wood products, and plastics; they would lower allowable exposure from the current limit to 3 ppm to either 1.5 ppm or 1 ppm, reducing cancer risks, it was estimated, by roughly 85 or 95 percent, respectively. The ultimate decision on formaldehyde exposure standards may be affected by a four-year U.S. National Cancer Institute study reported in early 1986. The data indicated slight increases in certain cancers in workers exposed to the substance but did not show "a consistently rising risk with level of exposure."

Asbestos Phaseout Proposed

In January 1986 the EPA proposed the banning of asbestos, which causes lung cancer and other lung diseases when inhaled. If the rule is approved after public hearings are held, the prohibition would be immediate for those products—roofing, floor tiles, cement piping, and clothing—for which there are already satisfactory asbestos substitutes. Other products—brake and clutch linings, for example—would be phased out over the next ten years as manufacturers develop substitutes and retool their manufacturing for asbestos-free production.

Chemical Accidents

In the aftermath of the December 1984 industrial disaster at a Union Carbide plant in Bhopāl, India, and the report of continuing health problems among its victims, more attention was paid in the United States and other countries to the dangers of accidental release of dangerous chemicals. Initial optimism on the part of U.S. experts that an accident of the scale of Bhopāl—which involved the release of tons of the highly toxic substance methyl isocyanate (MIC) and killed more than 2,000 people—could not occur in the developed world gave way to increasing concern about potential dangers as several less severe chemical releases occurred in the United States.

Bhopāl's continued suffering. In the first weeks after the Bhopāl disaster, there were several reports that fears of long-term health damage to the 200,000 or more people injured seemed to be unfounded. As research into the effects of the accident continued, however, it became clear that many of the victims did indeed suffer continuing health problems, particularly with the eyes and lungs, and also with the kidneys, liver, nervous system, blood, and female reproductive organs. Assessing the long-term damage was complicated by the extreme poverty in which most of the victims lived; in the case of eye damage, for example, vitamin A deficiency because of poor nutrition is probably a contributing factor. Still, the effects of the gas itself now appear to be both serious and long-term, if not permanent—though final results of many medical studies have not yet been published.

U.S. accidents. After the Bhopāl disaster, Union Carbide temporarily shut down a plant it operated in Institute, W.Va., where MIC was also produced. The company spent five months and $5 million reviewing the safety of the unit that produced MIC, installing new safeguards, and revising manufacturing procedures before reopening the plant in May 1985. But on August 11, a tank near the MIC unit leaked about 500 gallons of a chemical called aldicarb oxime, along with some other substances but not MIC. Six plant employees were injured, and about 135 local residents were treated at a nearby hospital for eye, throat, or lung irritation; their injuries were generally minor. But the leak, at a plant that had received such intensive scrutiny, was worrisome despite Union Carbide's explanation that the incident was caused by the revised and not yet fully tested manufacturing process. Shortly after the Institute leak, a spate of chemical accidents took place across the United States, adding to public concern.

In October 1985 the New York *Times* reported that a draft of a partial survey commissioned by the EPA found that there had been at least 6,928 chemical accidents in the United States over the last five years, killing more than 135 people and injuring nearly 1,500. Close to three fourths of the accidents occurred at plants, the remainder during transportation. One of the consultants involved in preparing the study said the true number of toxic chemical accidents was probably 2½ to 3 times as many as found by the survey.

Rising worries. Bhopāl, and then Institute—an accident that had many features in common with the Indian disaster—led to a new concern about toxic leaks. Most of the laws and regulations governing chemical plants were designed to deal with routine or periodic releases of small quantities of toxic substances, rather than relatively large, unintentional escapes. What is more, regulatory responsibilities are divided confusingly among state governments and several federal agencies. In general, in the wake of the Bhopāl disaster, the larger chemical companies did intensify their safety efforts, but many smaller companies—operating on narrow profit margins, often with older equipment that has fewer safety features than current designs—were unlikely to be able to afford major changes.

Another worry is the safety level in many plants—like nuclear facilities—that handle hazardous chemicals but are not identified or regulated as chemical plants. This concern was exemplified by the leak of a highly poisonous and mildly radioactive hydrogen fluoride gas at a uranium-processing plant in Gore, Okla., in early January 1986. One worker was killed, and scores of people were hospitalized.

One step the EPA took in late 1985 to try to guard against the worst effects of a possible disaster was to issue a list of some 400 extremely toxic chemicals and their health effects if released into the air, in order to help local communities develop emergency plans to cope with a leak. The lack of such plans was cited as a problem in both Bhopāl and Institute. The EPA did not provide information on where the chemicals were produced and stored, however, leaving localities to make that determination for themselves, with the help of EPA guidance. Moreover, the 400 chemicals listed represent a fraction of the thousands of potentially hazardous chemicals produced by modern industry.

Specific regulations. Certain chemicals are coming under tighter government regulation. In 1985 the EPA announced its intention to list ethylene oxide and chloroform as "hazardous air pollutants" under provisions of the Clean Air Act. Chloroform, once used as an anesthetic, is now used principally in producing refrigerants. It can also be produced by the reaction of chlorine with other substances in the process of water purification. The EPA also announced its intention to list butadiene, a compound used in piping, tires, and appliances, as an occupational hazard and a carcinogenic air pollutant. By these actions the EPA has several years to determine the source of emissions of the three substances and to devise regulations for controlling them. (Declaring a substance hazardous outright requires the EPA to initiate regulation within a year.)

Three widely used pesticides, used to fumigate stored crops, were banned because they could cause cancer. The EPA removed carbon tetrachloride, carbon disulfide, and ethylene dichloride from the market as of December 31, 1985. But farmers have been permitted to use stocks on hand until June 30, 1986.

Health Hazards of Light

Two studies published in 1985 indicate the hazards to the eye of exposure to excessive amounts of light.

Sunlight and eye cancer. A study of 500 patients with intraocular malignant melanoma, the most common malignant eye tumor in adults in the United States and Europe, has found a link between the disease and exposure to sunlight and ultraviolet radiation. Risk levels are also related to eye color, but not to complexion or hair color. In the United States the disease is seen almost exclusively in Caucasians.

People with blue eyes were found to have the highest risk, followed closely by those with green, gray, or hazel eyes. The risk for people with brown eyes was only 60 percent of that for those with blue eyes. Persons born in the South were found to have about 2½ times the probable risk of the disease of those born elsewhere, suggesting that greater exposure to sunlight, particularly in childhood, was linked to the disease. Other factors associated with increased risk were freckles, frequent sunlamp use, sunbathing, and lack of eye protection when in the sun.

Nursery lights and infant eye damage. Recent research suggests that the bright lighting in intensive-care nurseries for premature infants may contribute to an increasing number of cases of damage to their retinas that can result in blindness. The condition, called retinopathy of prematurity, is associated with excess oxygen administration and—as the name implies—occurs in premature infants. But light levels in the nurseries where premature babies are treated, which have increased five or ten times since the 1960's, also seem to have an effect. A comparison was made of the frequency of the disease in infants weighing 2.2 pounds or less at birth and exposed either to the standard nursery lighting or to light at about half that level. The researchers found an 86 percent risk of the condition in the babies who were exposed to the higher level of light and only a 54 percent risk for those kept in lower light. The researchers suggested that cycled lighting—dark/dim or dark/light—may be especially protective against scarring of the retina. As to the legitimate need in some circumstances for bright lights—which in hospital nurseries are generally left on 24 hours a day—another researcher has proposed that it could be met instead with spotlights.

Health of Minorities

A U.S. government study notes significant health differences in black and white adults. According to this report, 60,000 deaths annually would have been preventable if minorities had the same low death rates as whites. Six categories accounted for approximately 80 percent of the disparity: 18,000 from heart disease and stroke, 11,000 from homicides and accidents, 8,100 from cancer, 6,100 from infant mortality, 2,150 from cirrhosis, and 1, 850 from diabetes. The incidence of lung cancer was found to be 45 percent greater in black men than in white men, cancer of the esophagus three times greater, and the death rate from prostate cancer twice as high. Hypertension among black men under 45 was ten times higher than among white men. Among women, the death rate from cervical cancer was 2½ times higher in blacks, and coronary deaths twice as frequent.

Animal-Carried Health Hazards

Scientists have recently surveyed a number of diseases transmitted by animals and noted the latest methods for controlling them or minimizing their effects.

Dengue fever. Dengue fever is a tropical disease caused by a virus carried by the yellow fever mosquito. It is characterized by fever, rash, and enlarged lymph glands. Prevalent in the Caribbean and Central America, dengue fever now threatens the United States. Fortunately, another mosquito that is harmless to humans and animals preys on the yellow fever mosquito. This "good" mosquito, combined with chemical control methods, was successful in wiping out 98 percent of the yellow fever mosquitoes in a pilot project, say investigators at the U.S. Department of Agriculture's Research Service. As a result of this achievement, the New Orleans mosquito control agency has begun breeding and releasing the predator mosquitoes as part of its own control program.

Salmonellosis from pet turtles. Pet turtles exported from the United States are an important potential means of spreading salmonellosis, a disease that causes fever and intestinal problems, researchers say. Salmonellosis has been growing more frequent worldwide from various sources, including contaminated food as well as turtles (pet turtles were first associated with salmonellosis in 1962). Though the pet turtle industry has tried to eliminate the problem by breeding animals free of *Salmonella* bacteria, researchers studying turtles say that these efforts have not succeeded. The turtles can also carry other germs, and the scientists conclude that they are not good pets for small children.

Other pet-associated illness. There are an estimated 110 million pet dogs and cats in the United States alone, and over 30 human illnesses can be linked to these pets. These diseases are rarely contracted, but preventive practices can cut the incidence still further. Toxoplasmosis, caused by an intestinal parasite of cats, can cause birth defects if contracted by pregnant women. To avoid the possibility pregnant women should wear gloves when cleaning litter boxes and avoid cats that go outside. Bacterial infections, including brucellosis (or undulant fever) and salmonellosis, can be contracted by contact with the urine, blood, or feces of pets. Diseases transmitted by parasites on pets include the tick-spread Rocky Mountain spotted fever and Lyme disease; tularemia (or rabbit fever), carried by ticks and flies; and plague, contracted from infected fleas. Ringworm and other fungal infections can also be passed from pet to person.

Pet bites, particularly dog bites, can transmit various infective agents, and prompt first aid or emergency care is recommended to minimize the problem. Rabies from and in pets is rare—most rabies is seen in skunks and other wild animals.

In general, the researchers urge the following preventive measures:

- Do not leave small children unsupervised with large dogs.
- Children should be taught not to startle feeding or sleeping pets or to approach strange animals.
- New pets should be wormed, and all pets' food supplies should be controlled.
- Animals should not defecate in play areas or public places, and feces should be promptly removed to prevent transmission of intestinal parasites.
- Pets should not be allowed to forage where plague-carrying fleas are known.
- Tick collars have limited effectiveness but can be used when going into areas where ticks are found in large numbers.

ELLEN THRO

Epidemiology

See PUBLIC HEALTH; WORLD HEALTH NEWS.

Eyes

Lasers Treat Diabetic Eye Disease • Surgery for Nearsightedness Assessed • Injectable Lens Implants for Cataracts

Lasers and Diabetes

Treating macular edema. Early laser treatment can reduce the vision loss caused by a condition often found in people suffering from diabetes, according to a national study whose results were reported in December 1985. The condition, called diabetic macular edema, is marked by swelling in the portion of the eye's retina most responsible for the precise vision needed for reading, driving, and other common activities. (While macular edema does not usually cause a severe decrease in visual sharpness, it can have a dramatic effect on a person's quality of life.)

The swelling of macular edema is caused by leakage of fluid and fatty material from capillaries (small blood vessels) in the eye that have been weakened by diabetes. To treat the condition, laser energy is directed at the leaking capillaries: the heat coagulates the blood and seals the vessels.

The new findings—which came from a large-scale trial sponsored by the National Eye Institute (NEI) of the U.S. Department of Health and Human Services—show that the appropriate use of an argon laser can reduce significantly the risk of visual loss in such patients. In the study, done at 23 medical centers, 754 eyes of patients were treated at the first sign of leakage and swelling, while 1,490 eyes of patients were not treated. If a patient showed swelling in both eyes, only one eye was treated immediately. After three years, only 12 percent of those given early treatment had experienced significant vision loss; among those not treated, 24 percent had comparable vision loss.

Preventing complications of diabetes. The report issued in December is the latest in a series of long-term national studies aimed at protecting persons with diabetes from blindness and vision loss, a major side effect of the disease. The results from this study substantially increased the number of people with diabetes who might benefit from examination by an ophthalmologist. Primary care physicians should ask their patients if they have been experiencing decreased vision in either eye and should refer anyone reporting vision problems to an ophthalmologist for evaluation.

The findings also underscored the importance of early detection and treatment; laser treatment is effective only for patients who are referred to an ophthalmologist in time. Also, the common eye exam in which a patient simply reads letters from a chart may not indicate that a problem exists until it is too late. For early detection an ophthalmologist must look at the retina inside the eye.

An editorial in the *Journal of the American Medical Association* noted that with the release of the late 1985 report, it is now possible to reduce by at least half the amount of moderate to severe visual loss caused by diabetes. For instance, diabetic retinopathy—in which abnormal blood vessels grow and bleeding occurs in the retina—can be treated effectively with lasers. Elimination of the remaining visual risk posed by diabetes will require further evaluation of laser techniques and the exploration of treatments other than the laser. Clinical trials on the effects of aspirin or tight control of blood sugar levels may reveal new techniques for preventing some of the complications of diabetes. Until these or other techniques eliminate diabetic eye diseases, laser treatment remains the principal means of preventing vision loss.

Nearsightedness Surgery

Radial keratotomy, a surgical procedure to correct nearsightedness, or myopia, was again in the news in 1985. Myopia occurs in an eye that is too spherical. In the surgery, a series of four or eight very thin, spokelike incisions are made in the periphery of the cornea; as the incisions heal, the eye becomes more flat. The procedure was developed by a Soviet eye surgeon in the early 1970's and has been performed on almost 150,000 Americans since 1978.

In 1985 the second compilation of results were released from a large-scale study sponsored by the NEI on the long-term results following radial keratotomy. Two years after surgery, 75 percent of the patients had achieved substantial improvement in their visual sharpness when they did not wear glasses, and two thirds of the patients had relatively stable vision. One fourth of the patients showed a continued decrease in the amount of myopia, indicating a continuing effect of the surgical procedure. In some cases, it should be noted,

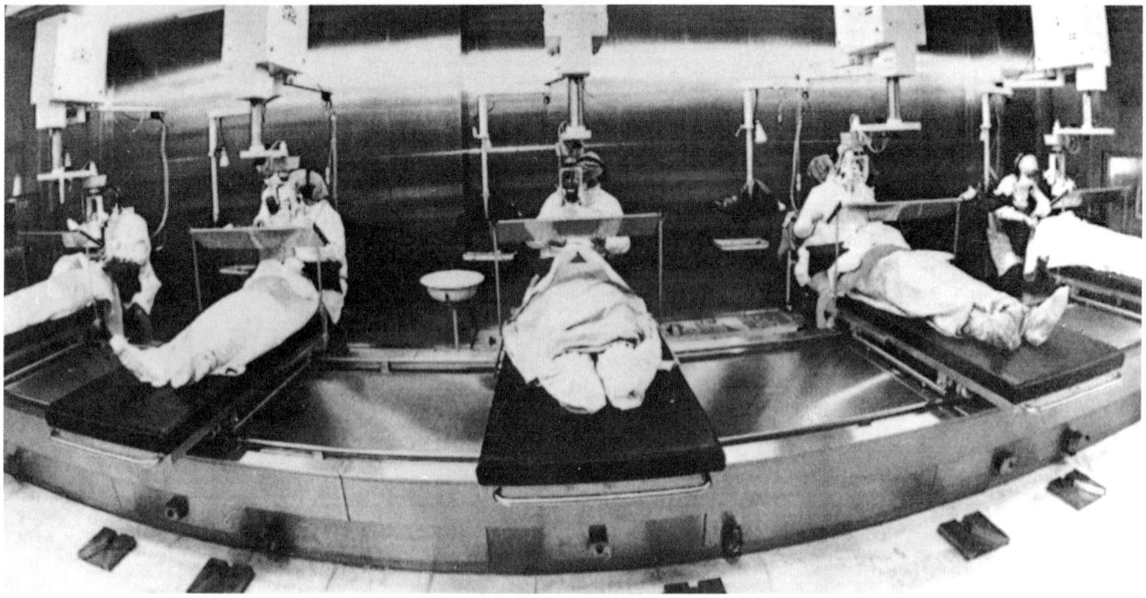

MEDICINE ON THE MOVE

Eye surgery, unlike automobile manufacturing, is not usually associated with the assembly line. But an assembly line is precisely what Dr. Svyatoslav Fyodorov has set up at the Moscow Research Institute of Eye Microsurgery. His "medical factory" performs cataract removal, glaucoma surgery, implantation of lenses, and radial keratotomy, a procedure that was developed by Fyodorov over a decade ago and that corrects nearsightedness with tiny incisions in the cornea.

In the institute's operating theater, patients lying in cots are rolled by conveyor to five work stations where each surgeon performs a specific part of the operation. The radial keratotomy procedure, the factory's most popular, takes about 15 minutes; in all, 60 to 70 operations can be performed a day. (A single surgeon could do only about seven.)

If Fyodorov has his way, some day robots will be used to perform certain routine steps and such operations as appendectomies and coronary bypass surgery will be automated. As for patients who feel uneasy without the comforting presence of "Doc Aibolit" (Russian version of the "old family doctor"), Fyodorov says, "We can probably create a holographic image of him for the operating theater."

vision may grow worse in the years following radial keratotomy because of a return to myopia or the development of farsightedness (hyperopia).

Cataract Breakthrough Possible

The surgical technology used in treating cataracts has evolved rapidly during the last decade. An injectable lens implant may be the next breakthrough. In this technique, a very small hole would be made in the lens affected by the cataract; the cloudy interior portion of the lens would be removed, leaving only the surrounding external capsule in place. Researchers at the University of Southern California are working to develop an experimental substance that could be injected in gel form with a needle through a small opening in the eye into the capsular bag. It would harden into the shape of the natural human lens within an hour or two after injection.

Researchers point out that great progress has been made with injectable lenses, especially in the last few years. Work still needs to be done, but investigators are optimistic that an injectable intraocular lens will be available in the near future. To date, such lenses have been used only experimentally in animals and not in any human surgery. With this approach cataract surgery would become even less invasive than it is now, and the normal focusing power of the eye that is used for reading might be preserved in younger people.

Cataract surgery is one of the most commonly performed surgical procedures in the United States; it is estimated that 750,000 cataract operations are performed annually. A cataract is a clouding in the lens of the eye that reduces the transmission of light rays to the retina, the light-sensitive tissue at the back of the eye.

In the most common technique of cataract surgery, extracapsular cataract extraction, a tiny incision is made in the eye, and the contents of the lens are removed except for the posterior capsule of the lens, which is left in place. Following removal of the lens material, a plastic lens is implanted. With this procedure, improvement in vision occurs about 90 percent of the time.

"Living Lens" Results

Another approach to restoring vision following cataract surgery showed continued promise in 1985. The procedure, called epikeratophakia, involves the cornea—the transparent membrane at the front of the eye that, by its convex surface, acts with the lens to focus light on the retina. In epikeratophakia a piece of cornea from the eye of a deceased person is frozen and then shaped on a small lathe into a "living contact lens," which is sewn onto the patient's cornea.

The preliminary results of an ongoing nationwide study involving about 250 surgeons and more than 1,400 patients indicate that the procedure is safe, predictable, and effective in the treatment of adults and children who have undergone cataract surgery or who have severe myopia.

The study, begun in 1984, is sponsored by American Medical Optics of the American Hospital Supply Corporation. These findings were reported 30 days after suture removal following performance of the epikeratophakia procedure:

- Eighty percent of the adults and children who had suffered from cataracts were within 30 percent of correction without glasses.
- Seventy-five percent of those who had been nearsighted were within the 30 percent range.
- It was necessary to remove the new lens tissue from only 6 percent of the patients. (In most such cases the tissue is replaced with another graft.)

Lasers in Corneal Surgery

The possible use of so-called excimer lasers in corneal surgery has been investigated intensively during the last two years. Excimer lasers are a distinctive class of lasers that produce short pulsed, high-power ultraviolet radiation. The first commercial excimer lasers became available at the beginning of this decade.

These lasers were at first used in scientific research and materials processing. But the discovery that the excimer laser beam could be used to etch precise microscopic patterns in polymer films (a property that may be of use in the manufacture of semiconductors) prompted a number of researchers to explore the possibility of making very precise, clean incisions into human tissue with the excimer laser. Experiments were initially carried out by researchers on the cornea and on the skin and have since been performed in the removal of tumorous plaque (found in blood vessels) and of bone.

Studies have shown that radiation from one particular type of excimer laser can be used to produce very thin incisions in the cornea with a high degree of control. Other laser sources remove tissue by heating it, but it has been hypothesized that the ultraviolet radiation of the excimer laser works by directly breaking the chemical bonds in the materials that make up the tissue. It may be possible to use the excimer laser to make incisions such as those made in radial keratotomy or for cataract surgery. At present, while the excimer laser remains an experimental tool in ophthalmology, some investigation into developing actual therapeutic devices is under way.

See also the Spotlight on Health article WHY YOU NEED EYE EXAMINATIONS. CARMEN A. PULIAFITO, M.D.

Food

See NUTRITION AND DIET.

Genetics and Genetic Engineering

Alternative to Amniocentesis • Birth Defects—Closing In on Bad Genes • Genetic Fingerprints to Fight Crime

New Test for Genetic Defects

Microbiologists at Michigan State University have devised a blood test technique for detecting birth defects that promises to be safer and cheaper than amniocentesis and can be carried out earlier in pregnancy. Amniocentesis, in which a needle inserted into the womb draws a sample of the amniotic fluid around the fetus, carries a slight risk of nicking the fetus or causing a spontaneous abortion. It is ordinarily done around the 16th week of pregnancy. The new technique, dubbed alternative to amniocentesis or ATA, can be used as early as the eighth week and is expected to cost less than half as much. If its initial promise is borne out, the test may soon be available for general use.

ATA involves the study of fetal trophoblast cells, which transport nutrients across the placenta. Some of these cells—about one per 2.5 million red blood cells—are found in the mother's bloodstream during pregnancy. Carrying out the test requires obtaining a concentrated sample of fetal trophoblasts from the mother's blood. The trophoblasts are then broken open to free their chromosomes—individual packets of the basic genetic material DNA (deoxyribonucleic acid). A laser is used to separate the chromosomes into 23 or 24 piles, each for a particular chromosome. (Every cell in the human body, except reproductive cells, normally has 22 pairs of identical chromosomes and a 23rd pair with one X chromosome and one Y chromosome in males and two X's in females.)

This sorting produces some immediate information. If Y chromosomes are present, the fetus is known to be a boy. If the amount of chromosome number 21 exceeds that of the other chromosomes by more than 50 percent, the fetus has Down's syndrome (mongolism), a relatively common birth defect characterized by mental retardation and a distinctive physical appearance. The sorted chromosomes can be subjected to a variety of tests to identify other genetic defects.

The Signposts of Birth Defects

Scientists working to pinpoint the sources of birth defects have recently found new markers—telltale pieces of DNA that signal the presence of defective or abnormal genes—for some diseases and appear to have spotted the faulty genes responsible for a few others.

Cystic fibrosis. A number of researchers have identified genetic markers closely linked to the gene defect responsible for cystic fibrosis. In this disease a thick mucus clogs the airways of the lungs, giving rise to respiratory infections. Most persons with cystic fibrosis die by early adulthood.

The markers are not the faulty gene itself and probably do no harm. However, they lie so close to the defective gene on a particular chromosome—the seventh—that they are passed on to offspring along with that gene. Identification of the markers should speed the search for the faulty gene and may make it possible to detect cystic fibrosis before birth. Some 10 million Americans carry one copy of the defective gene, but only people who inherit it from both parents contract cystic fibrosis.

Down's syndrome. Two new markers associated with an increased risk of having a child with Down's syndrome have been discovered. Although most Down's children are born to women over the age of 35, the new research suggests that heredity plays a major role in causing the syndrome.

Scientists at the Medical College of Virginia found a chromosomal abnormality that they believe can identify 30 percent of the people at risk of having a Down's child. The abnormality is a duplication of a specific region on five chromosomes. In the group studied, 30 percent of the parents of Down's children had the marker, while the incidence of the marker in the general population is less than 2 percent.

A different abnormality was identified among Greek families by geneticists at the Johns Hopkins School of Medicine. They observed that an abnormal form of chromosome 21 was present in 45 percent of Greek families with Down's children but in only 20 percent of Greek families with normal children. The research is being extended to other ethnic groups.

Gene linked to miscarriages. A single gene may be linked to miscarriages, premature births, and possibly to birth defects of the spine, according to researchers at the Case Western Reserve University School of Medicine. In a study of over a thousand white couples in the Cleveland area, the scientists found that parents who carried a specific gene, called C-3, were at least 1,000 times more likely to suffer a miscarriage in the first three months of pregnancy than were parents who did not have the gene. (Blacks were not included in the study, because they very rarely have the gene.)

The C-3 gene is found on the third chromosome in about 10 percent of all whites; it occurs in one or both members of a white couple 17 percent of the time. Nearly half of the Cleveland couples who suffered a miscarriage had the gene. The researchers also suspect a link between the C-3 gene and spina bifida, in which a newborn's spinal cord is not completely enclosed by the bony spine.

Tay-Sachs disease. Scientists at the U.S. National Institutes of Health isolated the DNA sequence responsible for the production of a crucial part of an enzyme called hexosaminidase A. A deficiency in that enzyme results in Tay-Sachs disease, a rare, devastating genetic disorder that causes the buildup of fatty deposits in the brain, leading to early death.

Tay-Sachs disease strikes primarily Jews of Eastern European extraction (Ashkenazi Jews), and one in 30 is thought to be a carrier of the defective gene. The new discovery was expected to help in identifying individuals at risk of developing the disease and in plotting the course of the inherited defect through the population.

Adult Susceptibility to Disease

Work on genetic factors associated with the development of diseases that typically occur later in life has also recorded dividends. Recent advances include markers that may indicate higher than normal chances of having a heart attack and new tests for arthritis and Huntington's disease.

Heart disease. Biochemists at California Biotechnology, Inc., of Mountain View found several genetic markers in the blood that might help pinpoint individuals who are at increased risk of having heart disease. The markers are associated with atherosclerosis, the clogging of arteries that, when it affects those leading to the heart, can cause heart attacks.

The scientists initially studied 196 heart patients in West Germany. One of their findings was that 37.5 percent of the patients had a specific defect in a gene associated with a protein that carries cholesterol—a substance that plays a major role in the development of atherosclerosis—through the blood. In contrast, only 16 percent of the general population had the defective gene. The company is now engaged in a study of several thousand Americans to confirm and elaborate on its findings. The markers might eventually be used to develop a test for identifying people who should take special precautions, including dietary restrictions, to reduce the risk of heart disease.

Rheumatoid arthritis. Physicians at Stanford University produced a simple blood test to identify individuals who have a high genetic risk of developing one form of rheumatoid arthritis. The test may also speed up diagnosis for patients with this form, making early treatment possible. The basis of the test is that people with a high susceptibility to the illness have certain genes in common, even though the genes might not cause the disease.

Huntington's disease. Biochemists at Johns Hopkins University developed a new test that makes it possible to predict whether people from families with a history of Huntington's disease (also known as Huntington's chorea) will get the fatal brain disorder themselves. Huntington's is characterized by uncontrollable body movements and mental deterioration. The researchers did not isolate the gene that causes the disor-

Dramatic progress has been made in cystic fibrosis research and treatment—shown here, a victim of the usually fatal childhood disease, Toronto nurse Susan McKellar, who has lived to have a child of her own. Researchers have identified genetic markers that should help to locate the defective gene responsible for CF.

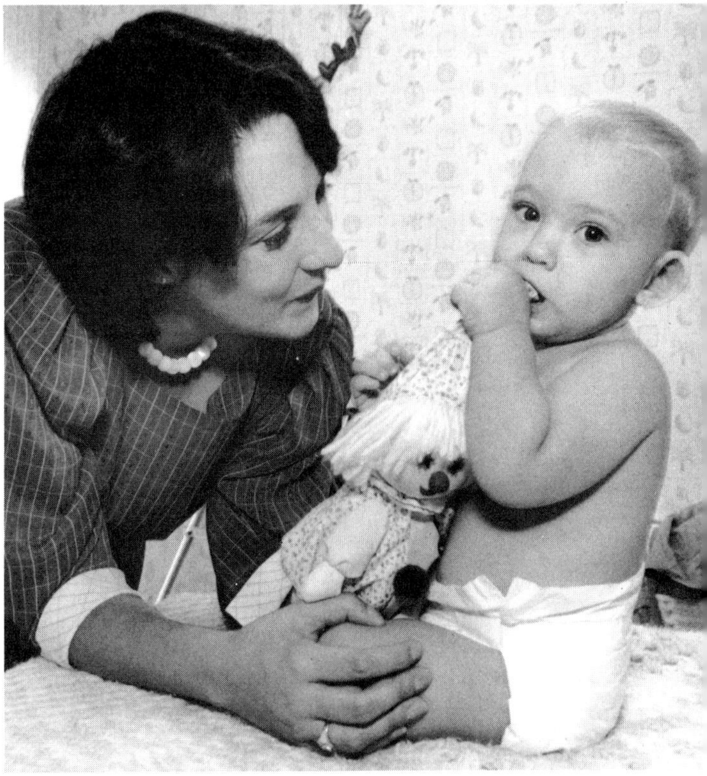

HEREDITY AND CRIME

Are criminals born or made? Debate erupted again with the publication of *Crime and Human Nature* by political scientist James Q. Wilson and behavioral psychologist Richard J. Herrnstein of Harvard. The authors focus on street criminals—persons who hit, mug, steal, rape, and murder.

According to Wilson and Herrnstein, the evidence shows that the social environment is not crucial in explaining such crime. The crucial roles are played by such largely hereditary factors as personality, intelligence, and even anatomy—as well as by parental behavior. Many studies have shown that criminals tend to be muscular young men with lower-than-average IQ's who possess impulsive, "now"-oriented personalities that make it difficult to plan or even think about the future.

Critics of the book argue that much of the evidence cited is ambiguous and inconclusive. Does, for example, the observed difference in IQ's between offenders and nonoffenders really mean that criminals are less intelligent? It may simply be that low-IQ criminals tend to get caught more often.

der, but they did identify a specific piece of DNA that contains the gene.

Children of individuals carrying the Huntington's gene have a 50 percent chance of developing the disease. Because symptoms of the disease do not usually appear until after the child-bearing years are over, many children of Huntington's patients forego having children. The new test could tell them whether they have the gene while they are still young enough to have children.

Obesity Tied to Genes

For years scientists have debated whether heredity or family environment has more to do with the occurrence of obesity. A recent large-scale study—the first of its kind—found that heredity is the principal and perhaps the only factor in determining a person's tendency to be fat or thin.

The study, conducted in Denmark, focused on 540 adults who had been adopted, most within the first few months of life, and who ranged from thin to obese in degree of fatness. Information was also obtained on their biological and adoptive parents. With respect to degree of fatness, the adoptees closely resembled their real parents; no statistical relationship was found between the adoptees and their adoptive parents.

It has long been known that obesity runs in families, but many authorities believed—and some limited earlier studies appeared to show—that if children of fat parents were fat it was simply because they picked up the habits of heavy eating and physical inactivity from their parents. The significance of the new findings, if they are correct, is that efforts directed toward reducing the incidence of obesity can now be concentrated on children identified as having the highest genetic chances of becoming obese. The findings do not mean, one of the researchers warned, that people with too many pounds should give up trying to lose weight on the ground that the attempt is doomed to failure by their genes. The study's results mean, rather, that people with overweight parents need to work harder to control their weight and shed excess pounds.

Growing New Blood Vessels

A team of Harvard University scientists has used genetic engineering techniques to isolate and determine the structure of a protein that induces new blood vessels to grow in living tissue. The protein, which they call angiogenin, is the first material known to promote the growth of an organ. The discovery of angiogenin suggests that substances that promote the growth of other organs may also be found.

Angiogenin has many implications for medical science. The ability to stimulate growth of blood vessels is crucial to the healing of wounds, the development of embryos, and other physiological processes. Angiogenin may eventually be used to promote wound healing or to increase the blood supply in individuals who have heart disease or have suffered a stroke. The identification of angiogenin should also make possible the development of substances that inhibit its action, thereby preventing the growth of blood vessels. Potential applications would include new forms of contraception and new treatments for diseases like cancer, rheumatoid arthritis, diabetic retinopathy, and psoriasis, which involve the formation of new blood vessels.

Genetic Fingerprints

British scientists have used genetic engineering techniques to produce DNA "fingerprints" of human blood, hair, and semen that appear to be unique for every individual (except identical twins). The new technique could allow police to match blood, hair, or semen samples obtained at crime sites to specimens obtained from a suspect. According to some experts, the principal criminological use of the new test may be in rape cases, since sperm are largely made up of DNA and present methods of identifying the origin of semen have severe limitations.

Current methods of matching specimens in crime investigations merely eliminate a suspect when a match is not found; they cannot say conclusively that a specific individual was the source of the specimen. The new technique can make that identification. It could also be used to help establish paternity or maternity in legal disputes, as well as to trace the path of hereditary diseases.

Practical use of the DNA fingerprint test is limited for the time being. The test is very complicated and time-consuming, and interpreting the results—which appear as bands on photographs made through a radioactive process and resemble the bar codes on food packages in supermarkets—demands great care and expertise.

Genetically Engineered Materials

The year 1985 saw testing in humans begin for a number of new products of potential use in treating disease that are made through genetic engineering techniques. One is epidermal growth factor: it promotes the healing of wounds and may prove helpful for burns and peptic ulcers. Another is superoxide dismutase, which acts to reduce damage to tissues deprived of their blood supply when an artery is blocked or blood flow is interrupted during transplants. The new products also include alpha-1-antitrypsin (a protein that may be able to block the development of emphysema) and protein A, which binds tightly to antibodies and might therefore be used to remove excess antibodies from the blood of victims of antoimmune diseases such as arthritis.

Renin, an enzyme that leads to a rise in blood pressure and plays a key role in the body's blood pressure regulation system, was produced synthetically by biotechnologists in 1985. This promises the availability of considerable amounts of renin for research. Scientists now hope to develop a substance capable of inhibiting the enzyme's action in the body. Such an inhibitor could be useful in treating high blood pressure.

In December 1985, genetic engineering scientists reported the production of apolipoprotein E (apo-E), a protein that helps speed the body's removal of cholesterol from the blood. The following month it was announced that protein C had been successfully produced. In the body, this protein helps regulate the formation and the breakdown of blood clots and stimulates the clot-dissolving substance called tissue plasminogen activator (TPA).

See also the feature articles WHAT IS GENETIC COUNSELING? *and* THE NEW VACCINES.

THOMAS H. MAUGH II, PH.D.

Glands and Metabolism

How the Body Controls Cholesterol • Synthetic Growth Hormone to Treat Dwarfism • New Hormones Discovered

Controlling Cholesterol

Improved understanding of how the body regulates cholesterol in the blood is producing better treatment for high cholesterol levels—a major risk factor in heart attack and stroke. In 1985 two researchers who contributed significantly to that improved understanding, Drs. Joseph Goldstein and Michael Brown of the University of Texas Southwestern Medical School, were awarded the Nobel Prize in physiology or medicine.

Cholesterol is a fatlike substance that is essential to some bodily processes. But when cholesterol occurs at high levels in the blood, some of it is deposited on the walls of blood vessels, narrowing them in a process called atherosclerosis. If the narrowing is severe enough and affects an artery nourishing the heart or the brain, a heart attack or stroke may result.

Cholesterol in the blood comes from two sources; some is manufactured in the body, mostly by the liver, and some originates in the diet. It had been known for some time that rising levels of cholesterol in the blood inhibit cholesterol manufacture (or synthesis). Thus, when dietary intake of cholesterol is high, a decrease in synthesis slows the rise in blood cholesterol that might otherwise occur; conversely, a low cholesterol intake leads to increased synthesis, providing the cholesterol needed to maintain cell membranes and other essential body structures. How the body achieved this regulation of cholesterol synthesis was poorly understood, however, prior to the research of Drs. Goldstein and Brown. They discovered on cell surfaces, most notably in the liver, sites called receptors that bind (in essence, capture) low-density lipoprotein (LDL); LDL is the name given to the particles—composed chiefly of protein and cholesterol—that carry most of the cholesterol in the bloodstream. Following this receptor binding, LDL is transported through the cell surfaces into the cells, thereby inhibiting cholesterol synthesis.

When the receptors are absent or defective and cholesterol cannot enter cells, cholesterol in the blood may rise to extremely high levels. There are several genetic

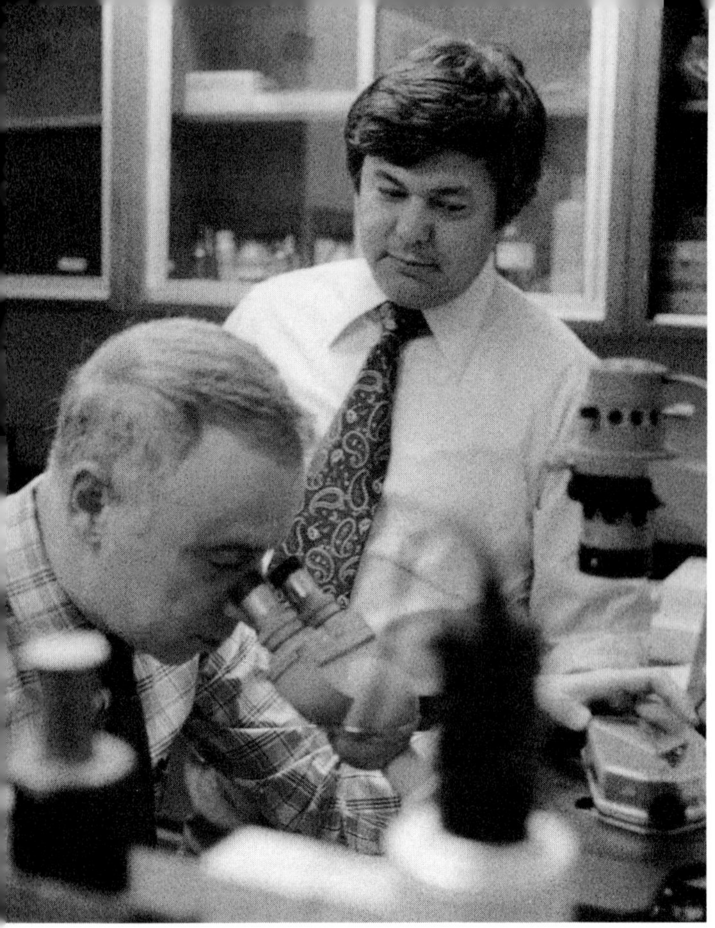

Drs. Joseph Goldstein (left) and Michael Brown of the University of Texas Southwestern Medical School were awarded a Nobel Prize for their discovery of the mechanism by which the body regulates its cholesterol synthesis.

disorders in which LDL receptors are insufficient in number or have a defective structure, resulting in an inherited tendency to high levels of cholesterol in the blood, a condition called familial hypercholesterolemia. People with this condition are at high risk of developing atherosclerosis, and therefore of suffering either a heart attack or a stroke.

In patients with partial receptor defects, combinations of drugs can now be prescribed to lower cholesterol, and these drugs also stimulate production of LDL receptors. Such treatment can bring cholesterol levels to near normal. One particularly effective combination includes a drug that binds dietary cholesterol and similar compounds in the small intestine, so that the cholesterol is eliminated by the body; examples of such a drug are cholestyramine (sold as Questran) and colestipol (Colestid). The second drug in the combination is one that blocks cholesterol synthesis, such as nicotinic acid (niacin, sold under various brand names).

In the rare cases in which LDL receptors are totally absent, a disorder that causes extremely high cholesterol levels and often results in heart attacks in childhood, liver transplants to provide a normal number of LDL receptors have produced striking initial improvement in cholesterol regulation by the body.

The attack on atherosclerosis has also moved forward in other ways—from techniques to widen partially blocked arteries to a better understanding of the role of diet. For example, studies have shown that people who eat large amounts of fish have a lower incidence of atherosclerosis of the arteries nourishing the heart. *See also the feature articles* HEART ATTACKS: REDUCING DEATHS *and* FISH IN THE DIET.

Growth Hormone

The possibility of contamination of U.S. growth hormone supplies, used to treat short stature (dwarfism) in children, led the federal government to halt distribution of the hormone. Only a few months later, however, a synthetic version—a product of genetic engineering techniques—became available.

Growth hormone is secreted by the pituitary gland. If the amount secreted is inadequate, dwarfism results. About three decades ago doctors concluded that the only effective and feasible treatment for this disorder was to administer growth hormone derived from human or other primate sources (growth hormone from most animals was found to be ineffective). The National Hormone and Pituitary Program—an outstanding cooperative venture—was established in the United States to collect human pituitaries removed during autopsies and send them to central laboratories, so that the growth hormone could be extracted and prepared for use in therapy. The program yielded enough growth hormone to treat many cases of hormone deficiency, and the treatment appeared entirely safe.

However, three deaths between November 1984 and April 1985 among about 10,000 people in the United States who had been treated with growth hormone were attributed to a rare virus-induced disease of the brain, Creutzfeldt-Jakob disease—which generally causes about one of every million deaths. These three cases raised the suspicion that some lots of growth hormone were contaminated with the virus. The pituitary is located at the base of the brain, to which it is connected by a stalk of nerve tissue; thus, it could become infected with viruses from the brain. After the third death was reported, the distribution of pituitary-derived human growth hormone in the United States was halted by the federal government in April 1985. Canadian distribution of human growth hormone was also halted.

Some scientists felt the ban was an overreaction; they were confident that the problem occurred with older methods of preparing growth hormone and that current purification procedures do exclude the virus. In an effort to prove this, researchers are testing, in monkeys, new lots of growth hormone as well as samples of older lots. However, the incubation period for Creutzfeldt-Jakob disease is apparently 18 months or longer, meaning that it will be some time before evidence concerning the safety of the current preparations is obtained.

Meanwhile, a synthetic human growth hormone gained government approval for general use in the United States. In 1979 growth hormone was first synthesized through recombinant DNA technology, or genetic engineering, in which bacteria or other microorganisms are genetically altered to produce substances normally made only by higher animals. After testing for safety and effectiveness, a synthetic growth hormone called somatrem (Protropin) was approved by the U.S. Food and Drug Administration in October 1985. It may obviate the need to use growth hormone derived from human pituitaries. Canadian authorities have begun clinical trials of another synthetic version of the hormone.

A second new approach to treating dwarfism is to give patients a synthetic form of the recently discovered growth hormone releasing hormone (GHRH), a substance made in the hypothalamus (a portion of the brain near the pituitary gland) and carried via special blood vessels to the pituitary, where it stimulates secretion of growth hormone. GHRH is a relatively simple compound that can be chemically synthesized. It has been shown that some growth hormone-deficient patients respond to synthetic GHRH, producing sufficient growth hormone to restore normal growth. There is hope that the occasional patient who does not reach normal stature with growth hormone treatment will have a more satisfactory response to GHRH.

WEREWOLVES AND VAMPIRES

They were the stuff of terrifying folktales in the Middle Ages, the subject of ghost stories and horror movies. Now researchers are giving vampires and werewolves a basis in medical fact: they could have been victims of a rare genetic disease called porphyria. Porphyria impedes the body's ability to create heme, needed for hemoglobin. One extreme result is sensitivity to sunlight: such sufferers learn to avoid the daylight hours. Other symptoms may include excessive hair growth, tightened gums (which make the teeth look more prominent and animal-like), and disfigurement. Since lack of heme is the major problem, Canadian biochemist David Dolphin suggests that in the old days porphyrics might have instinctively tried to get blood by biting other humans—as vampires are said to do. The odd habits and features of porphyria victims could have been the starting-point for the horrifying stories of night-stalking blood-drinkers called vampires and half-wolf, half-human creatures called werewolves.

Opponents of the theory, particularly spokespeople for the American Porphyria Foundation, point out that porphyria victims do not develop a thirst for blood, and that in fact drinking blood does not help the disease (although heme injections may). Only one form of porphyria causes disfigurement; this most rare form has been seen in only about 60 people around the world. The roughly 5,000 Americans who suffer from porphyria can be treated (though not cured) and lead normal lives. Although they must still be careful to avoid sunlight, there is little else that would link them to the night-roaming creatures of legend.

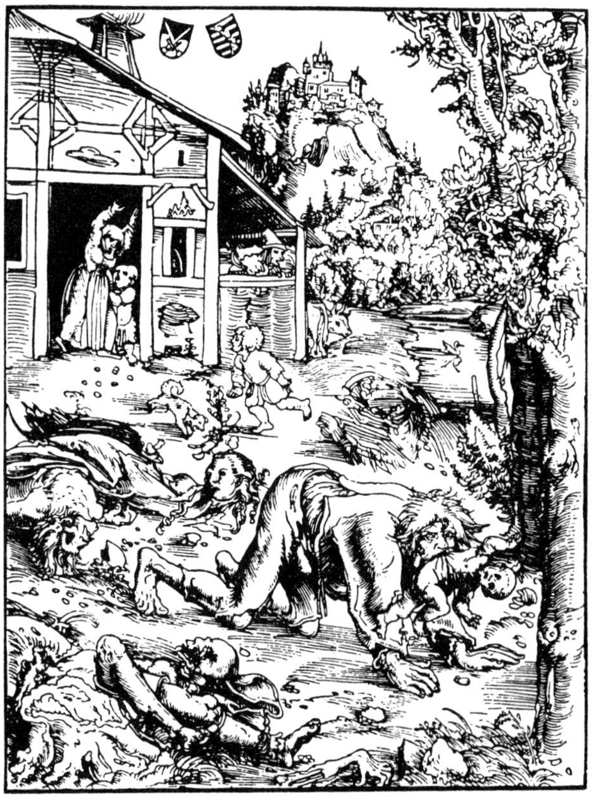

Werewolves terrorize the populace in a woodcut (c. 1512) by Lucas Cranach the Elder.

New Hormones

New hormones continue to be discovered, enhancing physicians' understanding of how the body works and perhaps leading to better treatment of various conditions. GHRH, for example, was isolated only about three years ago. More recently, another hormone produced in the hypothalamus was identified, one that inhibits the secretion of prolactin, the pituitary hormone that controls milk production. This newly discovered hormone may be an important part of the intricate hormonal feedback system that governs reproduction.

There have been preliminary reports of the identification of a hormone (called beta-carboline) that causes anxiety. It appears to be chemically related to the tranquilizers diazepam (often sold as Valium) and chlordiazepoxide (Librium), but it has the opposite effect. Research into the way the substance works may help scientists better understand the relation between brain chemistry and emotional states such as fear and anxiety. Still another newly isolated hormone, called tumor necrosis factor, appears to cause regression of cancer. Clinical tests of the substance's possible effectiveness as an anticancer medication began in Japan in 1985. Its usefulness may be limited, however, since it seems to be identical or nearly identical to a protein that causes severe weight loss in people with cancer or chronic infections. In general much more study will be required to determine more precisely the natural roles of these new hormones and to test their possible therapeutic uses.

WILLIAM L. GREEN, M.D.

Government Policies and Programs

UNITED STATES

Moves to Improve Healthcare • Controlling Medicare Costs • Faster Drug Approvals

Ensuring Quality of Care

Concerns about the quality of doctors who care for U.S. veterans and active military personnel have led to tougher licensing requirements. Quality control in the medicare program, which benefits 30 million elderly and disabled Americans, has been tightened. Attention has also focused on the problem of safeguarding the public from impaired or incompetent doctors.

Veterans' healthcare. Veterans will have access to better healthcare services while the federal government saves money, if legislation signed by President Ronald Reagan in December 1985 lives up to its intent. The measure makes it easier for veterans to obtain outpatient care in Veterans Administration facilities and to receive treatment in non-VA facilities. In addition, it strengthens the VA's quality assurance program and bars the agency from cutting the number of mid-level healthcare workers it employs. A pilot program of paying for chiropractic services takes the VA healthcare program a step toward consistency with medicare, which does pay for chiropractic services.

Physicians without valid and unrestricted state-issued licenses will no longer be able to work for VA hospitals, according to a September announcement. Although such licenses have always been required by law, the VA admitted to not having previously checked the names against lists of those whose licenses had been revoked, suspended, or restricted.

Military medicine. The U.S. military medical system was the subject of several reports of substandard practice in 1985. In a July directive the Pentagon said physicians who move directly from medical school into the military would have to have a state license. State licenses had not previously been required for such doctors. About 22 percent of the military's nearly 13,000 physicians on active duty did not hold state licenses when the directive was issued; they were given three years to comply with the new requirement. Military dentists, nurses, and clinical psychologists are also covered by the licensing directive.

In January 1986 it was disclosed that the Defense Department would for the first time have the quality of military medicine reviewed by civilians. The nonprofit Commission on Professional and Hospital Activities was awarded a contract to monitor the care delivered by doctors in military hospitals around the world.

Medicare disciplinary action. The "peer review organizations" (PRO's) that monitor the care provided by the medicare program have begun taking a more aggressive stance against low-quality and unnecessary care. A federal regulation adopted in May 1985 requires the organizations to impose sanctions on physicians and hospitals giving substandard or unneeded care. PRO's are empowered to suspend physicians or institutions from participation in medicare if complaints against them prove to be well-founded. The review process takes some months, and as of January 1, 1986, disciplinary proceedings had been initiated against nearly 1,000 doctors and 200 institutions.

State actions. State-issued licenses to practice medicine in Pennsylvania can now be immediately suspended when there is "immediate and clear danger to the public health and safety." Under legislation originally passed in May 1985, doctors accused of criminal activity or incompetence can be stopped from practicing (a hearing must be held within 30 days). Two physicians who allegedly were narcotic dependent—one accused of manslaughter in the death of his wife and another accused of attempted homicide for randomly firing a weapon in his neighborhood—were suspended the month after the legislation was passed.

Nursing homes and medicaid were the focus of a California law passed in March. The medicaid program—jointly funded by the states and the federal government but administered by the states—provides healthcare for poor and low-income people. The California measure increased medicaid payments to nursing homes, prohibited discrimination against medicaid patients, strengthened penalties for abusing nursing home patients, and provided for better state inspections of the facilities. The law stated that the increased payments to the homes must be used to increase wages and improve staffing levels.

The Cost of Benefit Programs

Medicare. In the 1985 fiscal year (ended September 30) the U.S. government spent more than $70 billion on medicare. About two-thirds was for hospital care; most of the remainder was for physicians' services.

During the last months of 1985, Congress extended until March 1986 the freeze imposed in 1984 on doctors' charges to medicare patients. The freeze was intended to help hold the line on the burgeoning cost of the medicare program and complemented Congress's 1983 adoption of the so-called diagnosis-related group (DRG) system for reimbursing hospitals; under this system, the diagnosis under which a medicare patient is being treated, rather than the length of hospital stay, determines the payment the hospital receives. Congress was expected to further extend the freeze.

A Massachusetts law, passed in November 1985, mandates that all physicians licensed in that state must agree to accept "assignment" for services that they provide to medicare beneficiaries—that is, they must agree to accept the fee levels set by medicare as payment in full for their services. Both the American Medical Association and the Massachusetts Medical Society immediately announced court challenges to the legislation's constitutionality, arguing that federal law preempted any state regulatory authority over medicare fees. Litigation was expected to continue for some time.

Medicaid. Despite the pressure of rising healthcare costs, a survey in mid-1985 found that no state had implemented new restrictions on eligibility for medicaid. In fact, 19 states expanded medicaid eligibility, and 13 added benefits, during the first six months of the year; some of the state moves were made to comply with federal requirements.

States did make an effort in 1985 to control the program's cost, which was expected to reach $40.9 billion and benefit 22 million people during the year. Michigan and Washington brought to six the number of states that reimburse hospitals for care of medicaid patients according to the DRG formula used for medicare reimbursement. Several states initiated competitive bidding for contracts to care for medicaid patients.

Social security disability review. In December 1985 the Reagan administration announced it would begin a second attempt to determine whether recipients of social security disability payments were still eligible for the benefits, which are paid to those unable to work because of physical or mental disabilities. An earlier review of the disability rolls, begun in 1981 but never completed, had occasioned considerable outrage. Federal judges reinstated over half of 491,000 people whose benefits were cut off. Critics said the way the review had been carried out revealed the administration's lack of compassion in its drive to cut spending. Now, under legislation passed by Congress in 1984, proof is required that a medical condition has improved before benefits can be halted, and benefit checks will continue to arrive during any appeal. Some 50,000 letters informing benefit recipients that their status was under review were mailed in January 1986, with the size of future mailings to be determined by progress in resolving cases.

Federal Funding Developments

Health appropriations. After some last-minute cuts—to ensure acceptance by President Reagan—Congress in December 1985 passed an appropriations measure for labor, health, and education spending for the 1986 fiscal year. Although the measure still had a total that exceeded the administration's request, the president signed it. The Department of Health and Human Services was budgeted at $81.9 billion—about $1.5 billion more than the administration had requested. (Those figures do not include medicare or social security, which are funded separately.)

Budget-cutting legislation. Also in December, however, Congress passed a sweeping budget-cutting measure. While regarding the bill as "constitutionally suspect," President Reagan signed it. Had he refused, the federal government would have faced defaulting on its debts. The legislation, known as the Gramm-Rudman-Hollings bill, was designed to reduce the annual budget deficit in stages to zero over five years. It was quickly challenged in federal court.

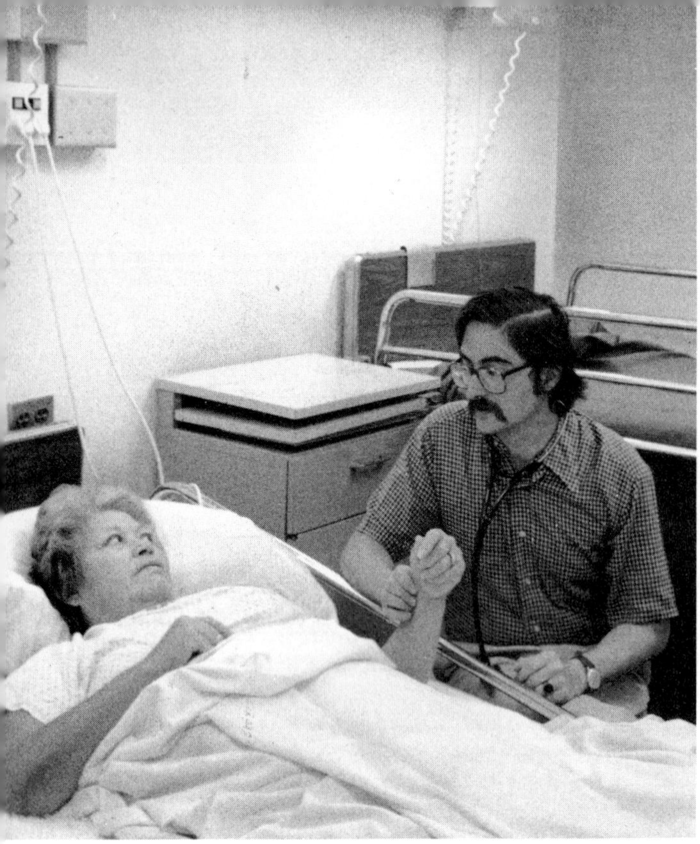

Dr. Laurence Fuortes treats an Indian patient at a Cass Lake, Minn., facility under the auspices of the National Health Service Corps. The program awards scholarships to persons studying to be doctors and other health professionals in return for their commitment to work for a period in areas with insufficient medical personnel.

The historic measure mandated automatic budget cuts in many federal programs if the president and Congress should fail to agree on how to meet the deficit reduction targets, but it limited the amount that certain programs could be cut. These programs included medicaid, medicare, Indian and veterans health, and community health centers. The automatic aspect of the budget cuts was struck down by a federal district court panel in February 1986 as unconstitutional. The ruling was appealed directly to the Supreme Court. However the Court decides the issue, health programs will doubtless feel a budget crunch for years to come. Meanwhile, the first round of budget cuts, affecting the 1986 fiscal year, took effect on March 1.

Aid to medical education. Federal support for training healthcare professionals was renewed in several different forms in 1985. During the fall President Reagan signed bills authorizing aid to medical schools and to nurse-education programs. The bills contained provisions to ensure that students would repay federally subsidized loans they received.

In 1985 the educational and service program known as the National Health Service Corps provided a record number of graduates—1,340. But the number was expected to decline in subsequent years because of funding cutbacks. Established by Congress in 1970 in response to shortages of medical personnel in prisons and in areas like inner cities, rural communities, and Indian reservations, the program offers scholarships to students aspiring to be physicians, dentists, podiatrists, and nurses—in exchange for their commitment to work in such places when they complete their training.

New Department Head

Margaret M. Heckler, U.S. secretary of health and human services for two and a half years, resigned that post in October 1985 to become ambassador to Ireland after a much-publicized request by President Reagan that she do so. The move followed widely reported rumors of increasing friction between Heckler and the White House staff over her management of the Health and Human Services Department and her alleged lack of commitment to administration policy positions. Dr. Otis R. Bowen, a professor of family medicine and former governor of Indiana, was named to succeed her and confirmed by the Senate in December. He is the first physician to head the massive government agency, which has 140,000 employees.

National Institutes of Health

The Republican-dominated Senate joined the Democratic-controlled House of Representatives in late 1985 to override the president's veto of legislation affecting the research activities of the National Institutes of Health. The measure set spending targets for NIH, to serve as a guide for actual appropriations, and reauthorized two of the constituent institutes. (The National Cancer Institute and the National Heart, Lung, and Blood Institute, unlike the other nine institutes in NIH, were established on a temporary basis by the legislation that brought them into existence and had to have their congressional mandate renewed.)

The Reagan administration, backed up by NIH officials and others in the medical community, complained that portions of the bill represented excessive meddling by Congress in managing the agency and in setting research priorities that ought to be the province of medical professionals. For example, the legislation required a greater emphasis on preventing disease and specified the creation of particular job classifications in the NIH to further that goal. It also established a new National Institute for Arthritis and Musculoskeletal and Skin Diseases and a National Center for Nursing Research. Critics charged that setting up these two new administrative structures would serve mainly to increase management costs rather than truly aiding research. There was also some question about just what nursing research might be—research on caring for patients or medical research done by nurses.

Food and Drug Administration

Action plan. In July 1985 the U.S. Food and Drug Administration released an "action plan"—developed after meetings with representatives of health professions, consumer groups, and the drug industry—to chart the FDA's course in coming years.

Among the specific points announced were innovations in the drug review process—such as standardized application formats and greater use of data from testing performed abroad—designed to cut six months from the two years the FDA took, on the average, to approve new drugs. Complementing this was a program to speed up the processing of the 40,000 reports received by the FDA every year on adverse reactions to drugs already on the market: doctors would report such reactions directly to the FDA instead of to manufacturers. Improvements to speed the review process for new medical devices were also announced.

Another goal of the action plan was to ensure the safety of the nation's food supply. In line with this policy, the agency announced in November a reorganization and strengthening of its food-monitoring program and an improved system for reviewing and evaluating possible health hazards of food additives and contaminants.

Congressional criticism of animal drugs. The FDA came under sharp criticism from a congressional subcommittee in a report released in January 1986. The report charged that the agency had failed to adequately monitor the use of potentially toxic drugs and nutrition supplements in livestock. The substances are a boon to farmers, helping to keep animals healthy and promote growth. But residues of such substances, some of which have been linked with cancer, genetic damage, and other conditions, have been found in meat, poultry, and dairy products. FDA rules and monitoring procedures are designed to prevent high levels of these residues, but the congressional report charged that enforcement had been lax and that the FDA had not developed adequate testing techniques for many substances.

Among other charges in the report, many farmers were said to be using substances that were no longer legal or had never been approved by the FDA, sometimes buying unregistered drugs illegally imported from abroad. The FDA was accused of illegally failing to restrict or ban several animal drugs that were reported to cause cancer.

The FDA and the $2 billion animal drug industry acknowledged that the concerns expressed in the report were legitimate. Industry representatives, however, defended their products' safety. An FDA official characterized the report as "very much an overstatement of old, chronic problems that don't affect the public's health." The FDA did say it would increase its efforts to identify and inventory the animal drugs in the marketplace.

Abortion Update

The debate on the right to abortion continued in the courts and at the state government level. In mid-1985 the Reagan administration reiterated its opposition to abortion when it submitted a friend of the court brief in two Supreme Court cases concerning the extent to which states may regulate abortion. The administration asked the Court to overturn its 1973 *Roe* v. *Wade* decision, which determined that women have a constitutional right to an abortion. The Court, however, declined to allow the administration to join in oral arguments on the issue, held in November.

In March the governor of Michigan vetoed legislation that would have banned state funding of abortions for recipients of medicaid. This was the 14th such veto by a governor of that state in 12 years; none of the vetoes have been overridden by the Legislature.

In New Jersey, a federal district court judge ruled in July that the state could not require that abortions after the 16th week of pregnancy be performed only in hospitals. The judge overturned the restriction because the higher cost of a hospital abortion might deprive some women of their right to the procedure.

In another abortion-related court action, the Illinois Appellate Court ruled in April that the state's Public Aid Department did not have to give an antiabortion group records identifying physicians who perform medicaid-funded abortions. In its decision, the court noted the fear of violence by extremist antiabortion groups against abortion providers. The antiabortion group in the case appealed the decision.

Health Insurance

The U.S. Supreme Court ruled in June that states may require employer-provided insurance plans to pay for treatment of mental health problems. The decision was seen as a precedent for upholding similar laws in many states requiring coverage of treatment for alcoholism, drug abuse, and birth defects, as well as of outpatient kidney dialysis and reconstructive surgery for insured mastectomies. The issue was brought to the Court when two insurance companies doing business with Massachusetts employers claimed that federal laws preempted the state's right to require mental health benefits in employer-provided insurance.

See also BIOETHICS *and* HEALTH PERSONNEL AND FACILITIES.

BARBARA SCHERR TRENK

CANADA

Controversy Over Health Act • Heroin Legal as a Painkiller • Breast-Feeding Encouraged

Canada Health Act

The Canadian Medical Association has mounted a court case challenging the 1984 Canada Health Act. The controversial law penalizes provinces that allow doctors or hospitals to charge user fees—additional fees paid by the patient above those reimbursed by medicare, Canada's publicly funded health insurance system. The suit by the 40,000-member association, filed in 1985 in the Supreme Court of Ontario, charges that the Canada Health Act exceeds the constitutional jurisdiction of the federal government and violates the nation's 1982 Charter of Rights and Freedoms. Health care in Canada has been a provincial matter since the country was formed in 1867. According to the CMA suit, the federal government does not have the authority to pass legislation that sets conditions on medicare payments. It also states that the act restricts the freedom of patients to choose their own doctors and infringes on the professional and economic freedom of physicians.

The CMA went to court after surveying 2,800 of its members, a majority of whom wanted to fight the federal legislation. The challenge, likely to be carried to the Supreme Court of Canada, could take several years.

The Canada Health Act allows Ottawa to withhold $1 in medicare grants to the provinces for every $1 that patients pay to doctors or hospitals in user fees. The provinces that permit doctors enrolled in medicare to charge patients more than provincially authorized rates have lost federal funding in amounts ranging from $100,000 a month in Manitoba to $4.8 million a month in Ontario (Canadian dollars throughout). Only Nova Scotia, Prince Edward Island, Newfoundland, the Yukon, and the Northwest Territories have escaped the penalties. Furthermore, user fees for hospital beds, emergency ward treatment, or ambulances have led to penalties for New Brunswick, British Columbia, Newfoundland, Alberta, and Quebec.

In an attempt to persuade provinces to ban extra-billing, the federal government promised to release withheld funds to provinces that act before April 1, 1987. Saskatchewan and Manitoba banned the practice in September 1985, and each reclaimed about $1.5 million of withheld medicare funding. In December 1985 the government of Ontario proposed legislation to force its doctors to stop extra-billing or face fines of up to $10,000. If it passes, Ottawa will transfer more than $84 million in outstanding payments to Ontario.

In New Brunswick, Ontario, and Alberta, the only provinces where extra-billing is still officially sanctioned, doctors can choose to bill the medicare system for the basic cost of treatment and then charge the patient for an additional amount. Where the practice is banned, however, doctors must either bill within medicare rates or opt out of the system entirely and bill all their patients directly for the total fee.

Heroin for Pain Relief

In October 1985 the federal government upheld a long-standing promise and made heroin legal for the treatment of pain. It is available only in hospitals, and its use is at the discretion of the attending physician. Jake Epp, the minister of Health and Welfare, had planned to restrict its use to treatment for cancer pain and only after other pain-relieving drugs had failed. Following intense lobbying by the medical establishment, however, no such restrictions were imposed.

Canada banned heroin in 1954 as a part of a crack-down on the black market for drugs. However, supporters of the medical use of the drug have consistently claimed it to be the most potent agent against pain.

Members of the Ontario Medical Association address reporters after a conference during which Canadian doctors challenged the 1984 law that discourages provinces from allowing doctors to charge additional fees above medicare reimbursements.

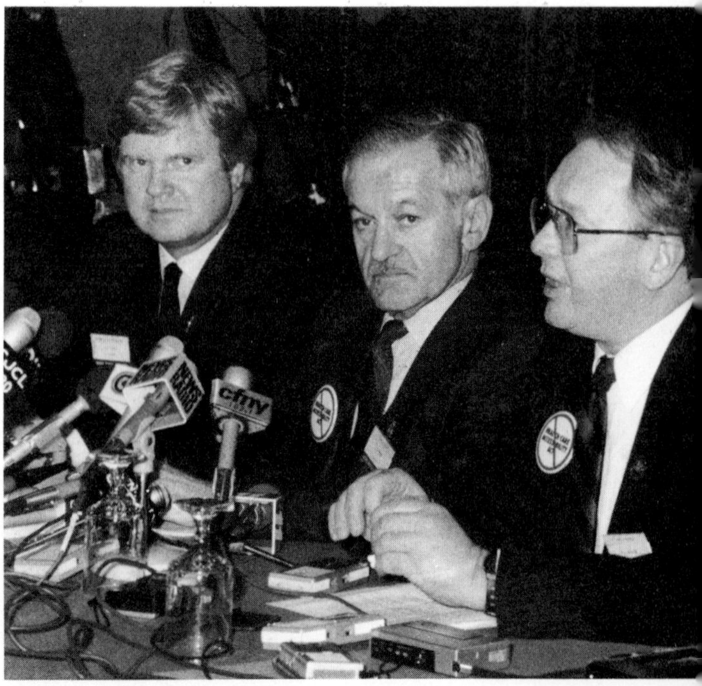

The Government and Smoking

Mixed signals. In a new effort to crack down on smoking, the federal Department of Health and Welfare joined forces with the provincial health ministries and several nongovernment organizations and launched a national antismoking campaign aimed at young people. The program includes $1.5 million in advertising with a rock video style of message.

However, Ottawa appears to be helping both sides in the smoking war. While the Department of Health and Welfare oversees its advertising campaign against smoking, the Department of Agriculture has provided $90 million to help tobacco farmers, most of whom live in Ontario, to cope with a declining market for their crops.

Public puffing. The antismoking lobby won a victory in late 1985 in the grievance between a Health and Welfare Department employee and his employer. The arbitration decision declared that the federal government breached a dangerous substances safety standard by failing to confine workplace smoking to areas with separate ventilation. The ruling, which applies only to workers under federal jurisdiction, would force all smokers working in federal government buildings to be segregated into designated smoking areas. Many experts believe the precedent could eventually apply to all workplaces. The federal government appealed the decision to the Federal Court of Appeal.

Encouraging Breast-Feeding

The federal health department has stepped up a national breast-feeding program. In collaboration with the Canadian Institute of Child Health, the Canadian Pediatric Society, the Canadian Hospital Association, the Canadian Medical Association, the Canadian Nurses Association, and the La Leche League, the government stepped up its encouragement to maternity hospitals to promote breast-feeding. Federal Health Minister Epp said he sees Ottawa's involvement as part of Canada's commitment to the International Code of Marketing of Breast Milk Substitutes, a World Health Organization effort "to protect breast-feeding from undue commercial interference."

Pilots and Medical Care

A new amendment to the Aeronautics Act requires pilots to identify themselves as such to any physician who cares for them. The law also requires physicians to report to designated Department of Transport medical examiners information on any condition of their patients that is likely to constitute a hazard to aviation safety. Failure to comply could result in a maximum fine of $5,000 and up to one year in jail. Pilots could also lose their licenses. This new reporting requirement supplements the periodic medical exams pilots already undergo as a requirement for licensing.

Representatives of the professional associations of both the physicians and the pilots claim the law invades the privacy of pilots and the doctor/patient contract. It forces pilots to practice self-incrimination, they say, and forces physicians to violate medical ethics and a law mandating confidentiality of medical records.

RHONDA BIRENBAUM

Gynecology

See OBSTETRICS AND GYNECOLOGY

Health Personnel and Facilities

Cost Containment Revolution • Decline in Hospital Use • Malpractice Controversy

Healthcare in Flux

A full-scale revolution is sweeping through the U.S. healthcare industry. Triggered mainly by private and government efforts to rein in skyrocketing costs, it is prompting rapid reorganization of healthcare delivery and threatening to render much hospital-based care and the independent physician increasingly obsolete.

Government cutbacks. The most recent developments take place against a background of U.S. government steps to contain healthcare costs that began in 1983. That year Congress adopted a new system for reimbursing hospitals for treatment of the elderly and disabled under medicare; the system set flat rates for care based on 468 (increased to 471 as of early 1986) predetermined "diagnosis-related groups," or DRG's. Patients are classified by diagnosis, and the payment received by the hospital is determined by the DRG to which the patient is assigned, rather than actual services rendered, as in the old system. With the exception of hospitals in New Jersey, Massachusetts, and Maryland, states that have obtained permission from the federal government to use their own similar payment systems, all of the nation's 5,800 community hospitals—that is, nonfederal, short-term general hospitals—are now subject to the new system, called prospective payment. If hospitals can provide care for less than a given DRG reimbursement level, they now pocket the difference; if not, they must swallow the loss. As a result, unlike the cost-based reimbursement system that preceded it, prospective payment has encouraged hospitals to undertake a wave of cost cutting in order to maintain their financial health.

In July 1984, Congress also acted to contain physicians' charges for treating medicare recipients. Medicare's rates for physicians were frozen at 1982 levels for the 1985 federal fiscal year (ended September 30); in addition, doctors had to specify whether they would participate in a program requiring them to accept medicare's allowable rates for all their medicare cases. Medicare actually paid the doctor 80 percent of those rates; doctors were required to bill patients for the rest, and, if they charged more than the rate set by medicare, for the additional amount. For almost all doctors, accepting "assignment"—as sticking to the official medicare rates is called—resulted in lower fees for treating medicare patients. Nonetheless, approximately 30 percent of the nation's doctors signed up for the program, partly in exchange for the promise of fee increases once the freeze was lifted. In late 1985, however, Congress extended the freeze until March 1986. A further extension of the freeze was expected.

A budget-balancing measure known as the Gramm-Rudman-Hollings act, which became law in late 1985, threatened further cutbacks in federal health programs through automatic spending cuts if Congress failed to reduce the federal budget deficit to required levels. The provision for automatic cuts was ruled unconstitutional in February 1986 by a federal court, a decision that was appealed to the Supreme Court. But even if the Supreme Court upholds the decision, cuts in some health programs seem certain to occur in coming years. Meanwhile, budget cuts imposed for the 1986 fiscal year took effect on March 1.

The problem of premature discharges. There were fears in many quarters that the prospective payment system was leading to a decline in the quality of healthcare for the elderly in the United States. The average medicare-covered hospital stay fell from 9.5 days before the system began to 7.5 days in the 1985 fiscal year, and there were a number of reports of patients being discharged prematurely from the hospital because, they were told, their medicare benefits had run out. Federal officials stressed that the average lengths of stay envisioned in the DRG's were not to be taken as a maximum, as had apparently happened in some instances. They pointed out that early discharges had by no means been unknown before prospective payment and maintained that there was no firm evidence such discharges had increased.

In September 1985, however, the Senate Select Committee on Aging said that an investigation by its staff had found considerable evidence that medicare patients were being "inappropriately and prematurely discharged from hospitals." The following month the inspector general of the U.S. Department of Health and Human Services, which operates the medicare program, also reported there was growing reason to believe that the prospective payment system was being abused through premature discharges.

In January 1986 federal officials announced that hospitals would be required to inform medicare patients that they have the right to challenge their discharge if they believe it is premature. A patient would appeal such an impending discharge to the local "peer review organization"—a professional group charged with overseeing the care given medicare patients. The organization would have to make its decision in three days.

Slower healthcare inflation. In addition to cost cutting by government, many private employers and insurance companies have been trying to cut their healthcare costs, by imposing higher deductibles on employee health-insurance coverage, by adopting plans in which employees share more of the tab, by requiring second opinions from physicians for surgical procedures, or by paying for tests and other procedures to be performed outside the hospital in less expensive settings.

The result of all the pressure by industry and government has been some slowing in the rise of healthcare costs. According to the U.S. Department of Labor's Bureau of Labor Statistics, the price index of all medical goods and services rose 6.7 percent during 1985—nearly twice as fast as overall consumer-price inflation, but well below the rates of increase in healthcare costs in the 1970's and early 1980's.

Decline in hospital use. Perhaps more striking, the changes have stimulated a dramatic decline in hospital use, which accounts for about half of all healthcare costs. According to the American Hospital Association's National Hospital Panel Survey, community hospital occupancy in 1984 fell nearly 8 percent, to 66.6 percent; data for 1985 show a further drop, to 63.6 percent, which is the lowest level since the AHA began keeping records in 1963. In addition, community hospital admissions fell 3.7 percent in 1984 and 4.9 percent in 1985.

The roughly 2,900 rural hospitals in the United States were especially hard hit by declines in occupancy. Because rural communities have older-than-average populations, they treat higher percentages of medicare patients. Many older, public, inner-city hospitals, which depend heavily on medicare patients, have also been hurt by declining occupancy.

The falloff in hospital use is now prompting swift consolidation within the industry. Some 3 percent of the nation's community hospital beds were eliminated during 1984 and 1985.

Alternative care organizations. Just as competition for the available healthcare dollars has led to some shrinkage with the hospital industry, it has stimulated the growth of alternative ways of delivering healthcare. Among these are health maintenance organizations (HMO's), which offer comprehensive medical care for a set fee paid in advance; preferred provider organizations, or groups of doctors and hospitals who agree to provide care at predetermined rates; and a small but growing number of "exclusive provider" arrangements, in which providers contract to provide all care to a group of patients. HMO enrollment rose 24.9 percent, to 18.9 million members, between June 1984 and June 1985, while the number of HMO's increased 28.9 percent, to 393. Meanwhile, from a standing start in the early 1980's, preferred provider organizations have grown rapidly as well. The American Medical Care and Review Association estimates that 12 million Americans had access to healthcare from approximately 300 operational preferred provider organizations as of December 1985.

While no two of these alternative care organizations are exactly alike, many are organized around several common operating principles. Foremost for HMO's is the desire to restrict inpatient hospital care. A well-run HMO cuts hospital use in about half by delivering as much care as possible in physicians' offices or in ambulatory-care centers. Many HMO's, preferred provider organizations, and exclusive provider arrangements also rely heavily on screening mechanisms—such as certification that a hospital stay is really necessary—to make certain that patients receive no more than appropriate levels of care.

Whether these alternative approaches will be able to hold down healthcare costs, or insure a high quality of healthcare, is uncertain. Various studies have sug-

Empty Hospital Beds

Percentage of Beds Filled in U.S. Hospitals, 1980-1985

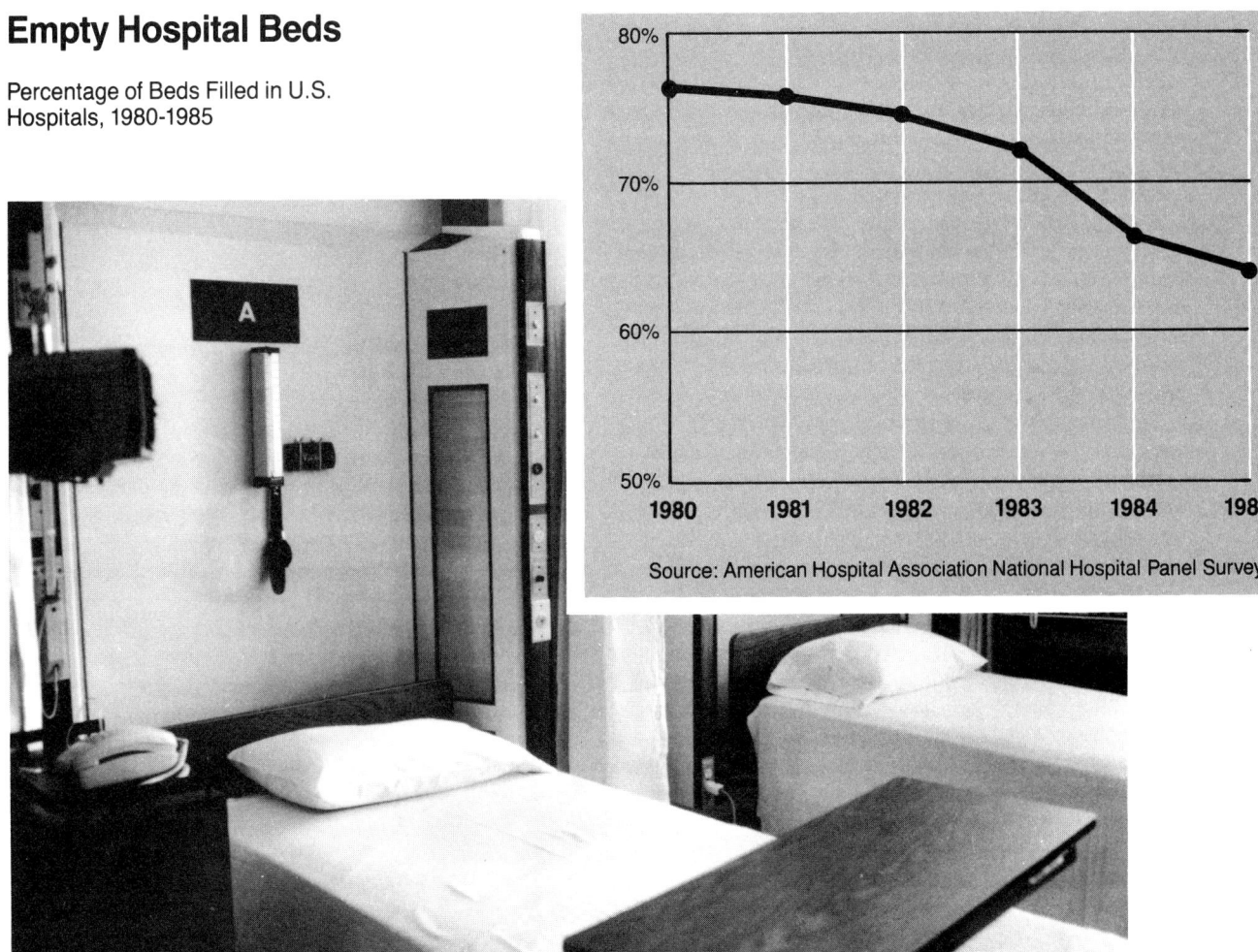

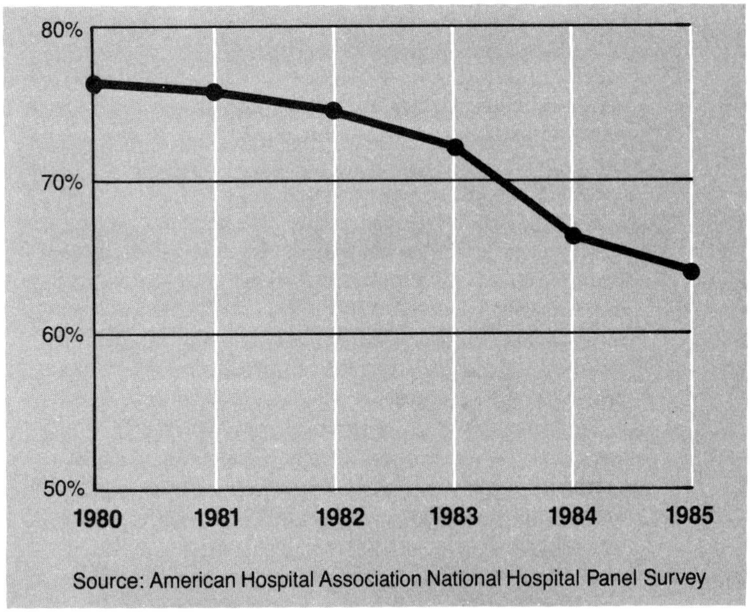

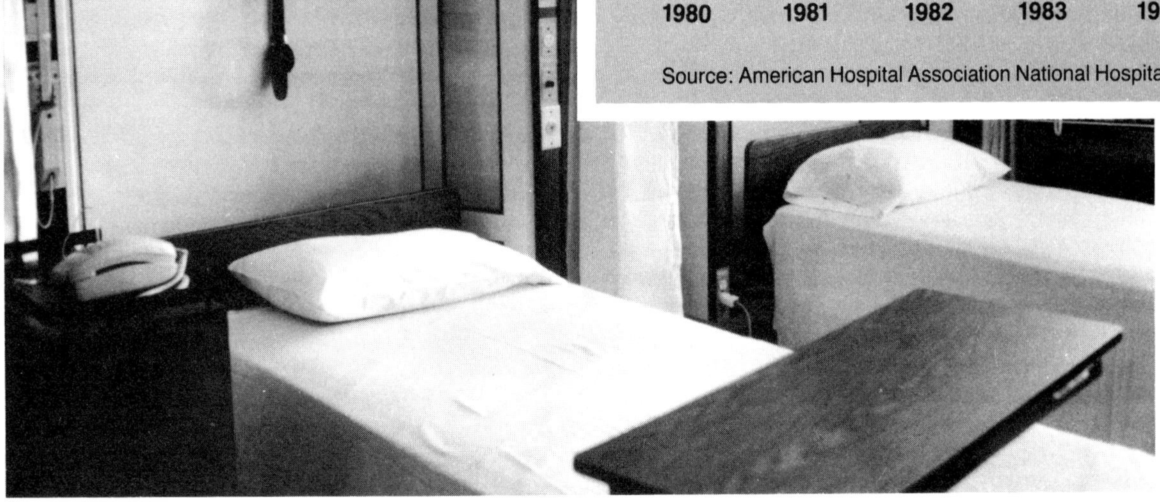

gested that HMO costs are already rising as fast as traditional "fee-for-service" medical care, and employers are now encouraging the creation of objective standards to measure the true quality of healthcare that various systems deliver.

The growth of the alternative organizations is blurring the traditional lines between the providers and the payers of healthcare. Some hospitals or healthcare companies have acquired insurance licenses in order to set up HMO's or offer other forms of health insurance, in part to attract more patients. Groups offering such plans include the largest for-profit hospital chains in the United States and nearly 500 not-for-profit hospitals linked together as the Voluntary Hospitals of America. In addition, some insurance companies have developed their own HMO's or preferred provider organizations. While there is little consensus on the long-range impact on the healthcare industry, some experts have forseen the development by the mid-1990's of perhaps 20 "supermeds"—large, integrated healthcare companies providing healthcare to half or more of all Americans.

Healthcare Jobs

For those who work, or plan to work, in the healthcare industry, the revolution in how medical care is provided has profound implications. But other factors will also influence the employment picture in the coming years. One is the steady increase in the number of older people, who require more healthcare services. At the same time, the population appears to be getting healthier as lifestyles and habits change. In the opinion of a number of medical experts, an emphasis on fitness, quitting smoking, and other ways of promoting health is lowering demand for healthcare services.

Assuming moderate growth in the economy, a U.S. Bureau of Labor Statistics study published in 1985 predicts that healthcare employment outside of hospitals (not including doctors and dentists) will be the fastest area of job growth in the coming decade, climbing 4.3 percent annually. Overall, the bureau foresees that healthcare in 1995 will have 1.9 million more jobs than in 1984—about one out of every nine new jobs created.

The numbers of jobs available will vary widely within the healthcare field. Employment of all hospital personnel, from lab technicians to janitors, dropped in 1984 for the first time since the Bureau of Labor Statistics began following trends in the area in 1958. The bureau projects hospital employment to grow on the average only 0.7 percent a year through 1995.

The growing surpluses of physicians in recent years in many specialties and many areas of the country suggest a continued slowing of the need for new physicians. Even so, the bureau estimates that the number of employed physicians will rise 23 percent by 1995.

Faster-than-average growth is predicted for workers in nursing homes, doctors' offices, and outpatient care facilities. The rosiest outlook is for people with versatile and flexible training and talents, such as registered nurses, physicians' assistants, and medical assistants and technicians.

Hospital Death Rates

In March 1986 the U.S. Department of Health and Human Services released lists of hospitals with unusually high or low death and discharge rates. The move, which was praised by consumer groups, came after requests for the data had been made under the Freedom of Information Act. The lists were based on medicare records for 1984.

Many healthcare professionals condemned the release on the grounds that the data were flawed and misleading. Federal officials said that the lists did not fully take into account such factors as severity of patients' ailments (a hospital might have a high mortality rate because it routinely treats people who are sicker than average) or hospital record-keeping errors. There seemed to be wide agreement, however, that the lists showed that people undergoing surgery are less likely to die in hospitals where the operation is frequently done.

Malpractice Crisis

The frequency of medical malpractice cases filed against doctors has more than tripled over the last decade, as has the average amount awarded to plaintiffs in cases doctors lose. Premiums for malpractice insurance have followed the growth in claims, reaching as high as $100,000 a year for certain high-risk specialists in localities where suits are common. Many doctors say that the growth in malpractice suits has forced them to protect themselves against legal challenges by ordering extra diagnostic tests and treatment procedures—a practice known as defensive medicine that the American Medical Association estimates to cost $15 billion to $40 billion annually.

Early in 1985 the AMA published an "action plan" for stemming the rise in malpractice costs. The plan included public education, efforts to aid the defense in malpractice suits, and programs to reduce risks and raise the quality of medical care, in part by weeding out incompetent physicians and in part through peer review of treatment decisions. More controversially, it also called for legislative action, largely on the state level, to limit attorneys' fees and the size of "noneconomic" awards (those for pain and suffering), to set up pretrial screening panels to make a preliminary decision as to whether a case has merit and so discourage weak cases from going to court, and to itemize verdicts so they could be more closely related to actual injuries and costs incurred.

Legal groups, notably the Association of Trial Lawyers of America, objected that such moves amounted to special-interest legislation and would deprive those injured by medical negligence of their legal right to relief. Nonetheless, legislatures in many states have passed bills implementing some of the AMA's proposals. In October the U.S. Supreme Court upheld a California law limiting damage awards for pain and suffering in malpractice cases, and a month later it upheld another California law limiting attorneys' fees.

See also GOVERNMENT POLICIES AND PROGRAMS.

SUSAN DENTZER

Heart and Circulatory System

Artificial Hearts: Progress and Problems • Aspirin for Heart Attack Prevention • New Device for Irregular Heartbeat

Artificial Hearts

A new role has emerged for artificial hearts, the mechanical devices originally intended as a permanent replacement for a diseased heart. They are now also being used as a temporary "bridge" for people awaiting a human heart transplant—either when a suitable donor heart is not immediately available or when the patient needs time to recover from conditions which make a transplant inadvisable. Of eight artificial heart implants in 1985, five were done on a temporary basis, as were others performed in early 1986.

One reason permanent implantation began to seem less desirable to some physicians was the disturbingly high number of strokes suffered by recipients of the Jarvik-7 artificial heart (the most commonly used model). Although Dr. William C. DeVries, who performed four of the five permanent implantations done by the end of 1985, continued to support use of the artificial heart on a permanent basis, other specialists recommended that such use be deferred until improvements could be made in the devices themselves and in postoperative patient care.

In December 1985 a panel of experts named by the U.S. Food and Drug Administration recommended that DeVries be allowed to perform the remaining three of the seven permanent Jarvik-7 implants he had earlier been authorized by the FDA to do, but also recommended that reporting requirements be tightened and that DeVries be required to obtain case-by-case clearance for the implants. The FDA officially adopted the panel's recommendations in January 1986.

On the other hand, a panel of experts convened by the U.S. National Heart, Lung, and Blood Institute issued a report in May 1985 that strongly endorsed research on permanent artificial hearts, with the ultimate goal of a completely implantable heart—that is, one that would not require compressed-air tubes leading outside the chest to a power source, as the present hearts do. The panel concluded that up to 35,000 Americans a year might be candidates for an artificial heart, for an annual cost of more than $5 billion.

The long-term risks of an implanted artificial heart in humans are still being determined, but at least for presently available models, the risks seem considerable. The Jarvik-7 had an excellent safety record when tested in animals. Among more than 100 calves, sheep, and goats receiving the Jarvik-7, only three animals had strokes, and these strokes were related to infections, not blood clots that originally formed in the heart and then traveled to the brain. However, the incidence of stroke in the human recipients has been extremely high. Moreover, the anticoagulants given to artificial heart recipients to try to prevent strokes may themselves produce serious complications.

Of the first five recipients of permanent artificial hearts, three suffered strokes. William J. Schroeder, who received a Jarvik-7 in November 1984, suffered three strokes within the next year. Murray P. Haydon, who like Schroeder had his implant done by DeVries at the Humana Heart Institute in Louisville, Ky., suffered a stroke in June 1985, less than three months after getting his Jarvik-7. A Swedish patient, Leif Stenberg, was given a Jarvik-7 by Dr. Bjarne Semb at the Karolinska Institute in Stockholm in April 1985. Stenberg died in late November of vascular and respiratory failure, less than three months after suffering a severe stroke.

Dr. Barney Clark, the world's first permanent artificial heart recipient, died in March 1983, after 112 days with a Jarvik-7, of complications from preexisting kidney and lung disease. Jack Burcham, the fifth recipient of a permanent Jarvik-7, died in April 1985, ten days after the implant, when bleeding in his chest caused clots that blocked blood flow to the artificial heart.

The first FDA-authorized temporary use of an artificial heart occurred in August 1985 at the University of Arizona Medical Center in Tucson. Dr. Jack G. Copeland implanted a Jarvik-7 into Michael Drummond, a

25-year-old Arizona man suffering from a severe viral heart infection. Seven days after the operation Drummond suffered a series of mild strokes, necessitating an urgent human heart transplant. He left the hospital with his new heart in November. The Jarvik-7 was later found to have blood clots on its left side, where the main pumping chamber joins with the aorta.

In October 1985, Anthony Mandia, age 44, of Philadelphia became the first person to receive the so-called Penn State heart. It had been approved in March by the FDA for temporary use. Developed at Pennsylvania State University's Hershey Medical Center, the Penn State heart, unlike the Jarvik-7, is made entirely of plastic (the Jarvik-7 contains some metal) and has no inner seams. Theoretically these differences reduce the risk of strokes. Mandia received the implant on an emergency basis when his condition deteriorated while he awaited a human heart donor. He received a human heart ten days after the implant, but he died of an infection in November.

In December 1985 surgeons at Abbott Northwestern Hospital in Minneapolis implanted an artificial heart in a woman for the first time. Mary Lund, age 40, received a smaller version of the Jarvik-7 after a virus attacked her heart muscle. She received a human heart 45 days after the implant.

A second woman received a small-sized Jarvik-7 on a temporary basis in early February 1986. She underwent a human heart transplant after less than a week on the "mini-Jarvik," but when complications developed, she was again given an artificial heart—the first person to receive two such implants. Both were done on an emergency basis by Dr. Copeland in Tucson.

In March 1986, Dr. Emil Buecherl of the Free University of Berlin's Charlottenburg Clinic implanted an artificial heart of his own design in Hans Holzwig, age 39. Holzwig died of kidney failure six days later, soon after receiving a human heart.

Aspirin and Heart Attacks

In October 1985 the FDA officially recognized and approved the regular use of aspirin by patients who have had a heart attack or suffer from the condition known as unstable angina. (The Canadian Ministry of Health had already endorsed regular aspirin use following a heart attack.)

Between 1974 and 1981, six large-scale studies involving over 10,000 heart attack survivors demonstrated an overall 21 percent reduction in second heart attacks for patients who took aspirin daily. In another study, aspirin was shown to reduce by half the number of heart

In October 1985, Anthony Mandia became the first recipient of the Penn State artificial heart, which is made entirely of plastic and has no inner seams. He was later given a human heart, but then died in November.

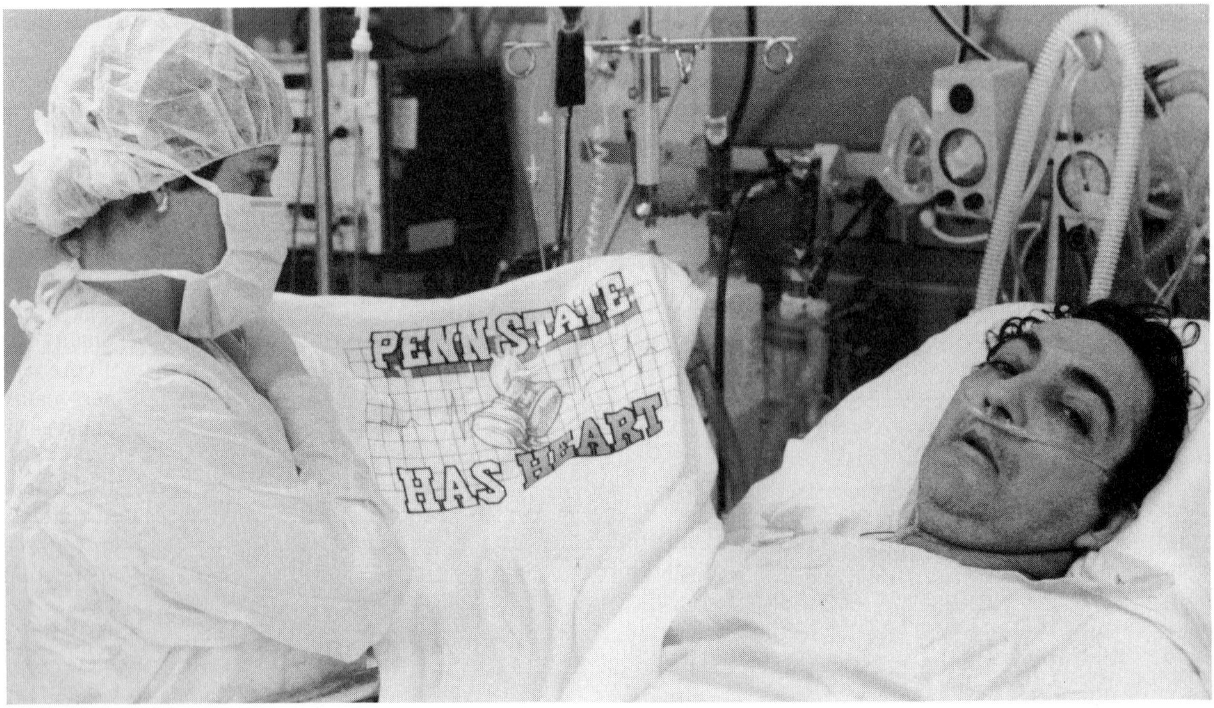

attacks in men with unstable angina, rapidly worsening episodes of chest pain caused by narrowed arteries impeding blood flow to the heart.

Aspirin has also been shown to be beneficial for patients who have undergone coronary artery bypass surgery, in which narrowed sections of arteries supplying blood to the heart are literally bypassed, using veins taken from a leg or arteries from the chest. Up to 20 percent of all bypass grafts develop a clot within them during the first year after surgery. Studies have confirmed that treatment with aspirin—either alone or in combination with another drug, dipyridamole (also sold as Persantine)—can reduce the incidence of clots by half.

The success of aspirin is probably related to its ability to inhibit the action of platelets. Platelets are sticky components in the blood which initiate clotting and control bleeding. Under certain circumstances, platelets can start to form clots in places where there is no bleeding. This can occur in narrowed sections of the arteries nourishing the heart, blocking the flow of blood and causing a heart attack. The dose of aspirin recommended by the FDA is one adult tablet (325 milligrams) daily. Some experimental data suggest that even lower doses, such as one baby aspirin (80 milligrams) a day, may be not only sufficient but possibly better.

Conflicting Estrogen Studies

Two studies on the effects of estrogen taken by women after menopause—both carefully done and both reported in October 1985—reached totally opposite conclusions. Estrogen is the overall name for a group of female hormones, and at menopause the body's natural production of estrogen drops greatly. However, up to 30 percent of postmenopausal women in the United States take estrogen (prescribed by a physician), in part to prevent the bone loss of osteoporosis.

The consequences of estrogen therapy are not fully known. It has been speculated that estrogen may to some degree protect against atherosclerosis, the buildup of fatty deposits on artery walls that can lead to serious narrowing of the arteries supplying blood to the heart (coronary heart disease). This hypothesis is based in part on the observation that women are at considerably greater risk for atherosclerosis after menopause. In addition, estrogen tends to lower the levels of fats in the blood.

One of the studies published in 1985 followed over 1,200 postmenopausal women for 12 years—and found a 50 percent higher risk of cardiovascular disease for those who took estrogen. The greatest risk was among those women who both smoked cigarettes and took estrogen. The other study followed 32,000 women over a four-year period. It demonstrated a 50 percent reduction in coronary heart disease among the women who took estrogen. There was no immediate obvious explanation for these differences, and the true risk or benefit of undergoing estrogen therapy after menopause remains unknown.

Fat in the Diet

In general, the unsaturated fats in vegetable oils tend to lower blood cholesterol, while the saturated fats found, for example, in red meat and dairy products tend to raise it. Scientists had commonly assumed that polyunsaturated fatty acids, such as those that predominate in, say, corn and safflower oil, are more effective in lowering cholesterol than the monounsaturated type characteristic of peanut and olive oil. Recent evidence, however, has cast doubt on this assumption. A study involving 20 patients demonstrated that a high proportion in the diet of one of the monounsaturated fatty acids was as effective as a diet rich in a polyunsaturated fatty acid in reducing total cholesterol in the blood. Moreover, the bloodstream's level of HDL cholesterol, the so-called good cholesterol that is considered to help protect against coronary heart disease, was better preserved by the monounsaturated fatty acid.

Other researchers have linked polyunsaturated fatty acids to cancer in animals. Although doctors generally agree that the current level of saturated fats in the American diet should be reduced, it is not entirely clear how best to replace them.

See also the feature article FISH IN THE DIET.

Personality and Heart Disease

A study reported in 1985 contradicted the theory—which had received support from some earlier studies—that an aggressive, hard-driving personality makes it more likely that someone who has had a heart attack will have a repeat attack. Research in this area has focused mainly on the so-called Type A personality, characterized by a strong sense of operating under time pressure, by easily aroused hostility and aggression, and by a dedication to achievement. Type A personality has been linked to the premature development of coronary heart disease. The more easygoing Type B personality has been found to be somewhat protective against early heart disease.

In the new study, more than 500 patients underwent personality scoring within two weeks of a heart attack, and their progress was then monitored for up to three years. Type A behavior was found to have no effect on long-term complications in or the survival of these patients. A number of doctors questioned the study's methods and results, however, and the controversy over Type A behavior and heart attacks is sure to continue.

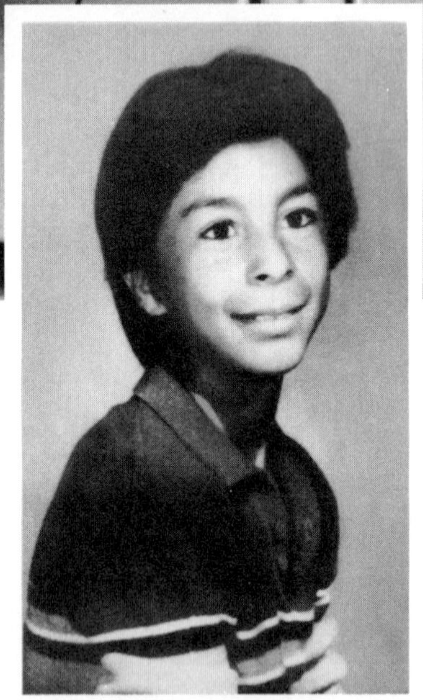

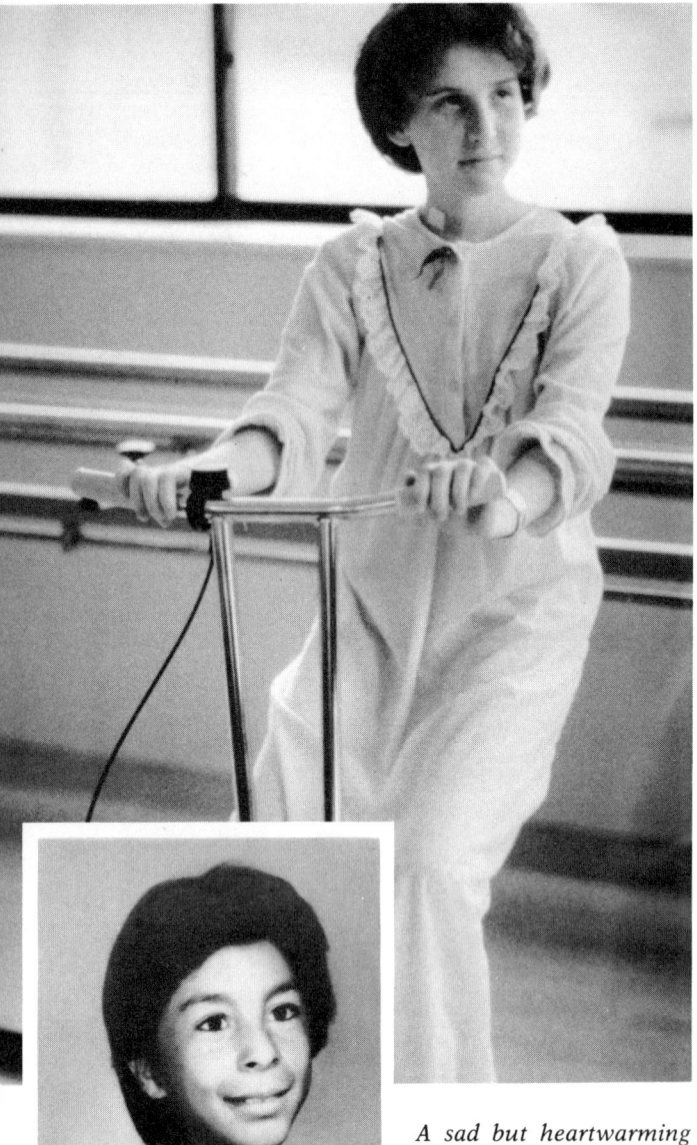

A sad but heartwarming story: Fifteen-year-old Felipe Garza (inset) in a premonition of his own death, instructed that his heart be given to his sick school friend Donna Ashlock. A month later Felipe died; above, Donna recovers with her transplanted heart.

Irregular Heart Rhythm

A device approved by the FDA in October 1985 may dramatically reduce the death rate among patients who have heart rhythm abnormalities that do not respond to drug therapy. Such abnormalities can result in a state called ventricular fibrillation, in which the heartbeat becomes extremely rapid and the heart does not effectively pump blood. Although most patients with heart rhythm abnormalities do respond to drug treatment, the new device, called an implantable defibrillator, has been shown in several studies to reduce tenfold the annual death rate among the substantial minority who are not helped by medication—a reduction from about 40 percent to 4 percent.

The device is surgically implanted in the abdomen, and electrodes are attached to the heart through the diaphragm. A special microcomputer allows the defibrillator to sense and identify a life-threatening irregular heart rhythm and to rapidly deliver an electric discharge that shocks the heart back into a normal rhythm. There are still some problems with the device. For example, an "innocent" heart rhythm could occasionally trigger the defibrillator by mistake. Moreover, at present the battery must be surgically replaced every two years in a minor operation.

See also the feature article HEART ATTACKS: REDUCING DEATHS *and the Spotlight on Health article* HEART MURMURS.

BRUCE D. CHARASH, M.D.,
and JEFFREY FISHER, M.D.

Medical Technology

Robots in the Operating Room • Substitutes for Human Bone • Little Cards With Big Memories

A Robot Assistant

Robots have become commonplace in industry, lending their speed and precision to myriad tasks from welding car parts to assembling circuit boards. Now they have moved into the operating room. In April 1985, for the first time, a robot assisted in surgery when doctors at the Memorial Medical Center of Long Beach in California used a computer-guided robot arm to assist them in a delicate brain tumor biopsy—the collection of tissue for examination. This marriage of sophisticated computer and robotic technology can help surgeons locate and sample brain lesions faster, more accurately, and, some say, more safely than ever before.

By the end of the year, the Long Beach neurosurgeons had used their off-the-shelf industrial robot, which is controlled by specially designed computer programs, to pinpoint and collect brain tissue samples from seven patients. The flexible, six-jointed arm is not much larger than a human arm. Capable of holding either a drill or sampling needle, it can precisely guide these instruments as surgeons penetrate the patient's skull in order to zero in on a suspected tumor or other lesion.

The doctors secure the patient's head within a "stereotaxic frame," a device used by surgeons for decades to help locate positions in the brain. A CT (computerized tomographic) scanner then generates a series of pictures on a display screen that show "slices" of the brain, revealing the site of a suspected lesion. Using scale markers on the stereotaxic frame and data from the CT scanner, a computer calculates the coordinates of the lesion's precise location in the brain. After the surgeons decide which of several paths through the brain the needle should take, all the needed information is fed into the robot's computer memory. The robot is attached to the head frame, then whirs the surgical drill point into the correct position on the skull.

Although the robot arm aims the drill, a doctor applies the pressure needed to pierce the skull. Similarly, once the arm has angled a biopsy needle and determined how deep it must penetrate to reach the lesion, it is the surgeon's hands that gently push it into the brain to collect tissue for analysis. The engineer who developed the system emphasizes that the doctor's sense of touch is indispensable in surgery; the robot does not replace but complements the surgeon's skill.

Because of the arm's remarkable precision—it can pinpoint locations in the brain to within 1/2,000 inch—the surgeon needs only a 1/8-inch-diameter opening in the skull to obtain sample tissue, instead of the 1/2-inch hole required in conventional neurosurgery. A narrower path means fewer disturbed blood vessels and less risk of damage to brain areas that control functions like speech and vision. Consequently, the patient's recovery time is shortened. The robot's precision also means that less time is needed for the surgery.

The system's developers think that the arm could eventually be used to drain abscesses, repair blood vessels and damaged cartilage and ligaments, insert electrodes, biopsy bone, and even deposit cancer-killing radioactive pellets directly into tumors.

Lasers and Clogged Arteries

Researchers in 1985 reported promising results from the first U.S. clinical trials of laser techniques for opening up arteries obstructed by atherosclerosis. Millions of North Americans suffer from this condition, in which hardened fatty deposits called plaques build up on artery walls. Plaques clogging coronary arteries—the vessels that supply oxygen-rich blood to heart muscle—can lead to heart attacks. A potential drawback of using lasers to clear clogged arteries is the danger of puncturing the wall of the vessel. Scientists are trying a variety of strategies to avoid this problem, including chemical pretreatment of the plaques and the use of "cool" lasers called excimers that work at lower than usual temperatures (they emit energy bursts lasting only billionths of a second).

Enhancing blood flow to the heart. In one technique, called laser coronary endarterectomy, a laser destroys plaques in coronary arteries. Using a small carbon dioxide laser, surgeons at the Texas Heart Institute in Houston had by late 1985 succeeded in vaporizing plaques in 16 arteries in eight people. They completely opened 12 of the vessels without damaging the artery walls—a complication that had occurred in some animal experiments. (Similar experiments with humans had earlier been carried out in France.)

As performed by the Texas heart surgeons, the technique is an adjunct to coronary bypass surgery. This is a procedure in which a graft of a blood vessel from elsewhere in the body is used to reroute blood to the heart around a blocked artery. During the operation,

HEALING BY HAND

The ancient healing art known as the laying on of hands, often considered the domain of quacks, charlatans, and religious fanatics, is now being seriously investigated by medical researchers. They do not claim it can work miracles: "People don't throw down their crutches or get cured of cancer," says one leading investigator. But scattered preliminary studies suggest that a method of "therapeutic touch" not involving actual contact may be able to relieve pain, reduce anxiety, and alleviate babies' respiratory problems.

In this method, a trained therapist combines "centering" (a form of mental concentration) with hand motions a few inches above the patient's body. It has been proposed that the results claimed, if valid, are the work of an electromagnetic force—biomagnetism—that exists in the body's tissues and can be transferred from one person to another. Under a three-year grant from the U.S. National Institutes of Health, a University of South Carolina researcher is examining how therapeutic touch affects anxiety in individuals scheduled for heart surgery.

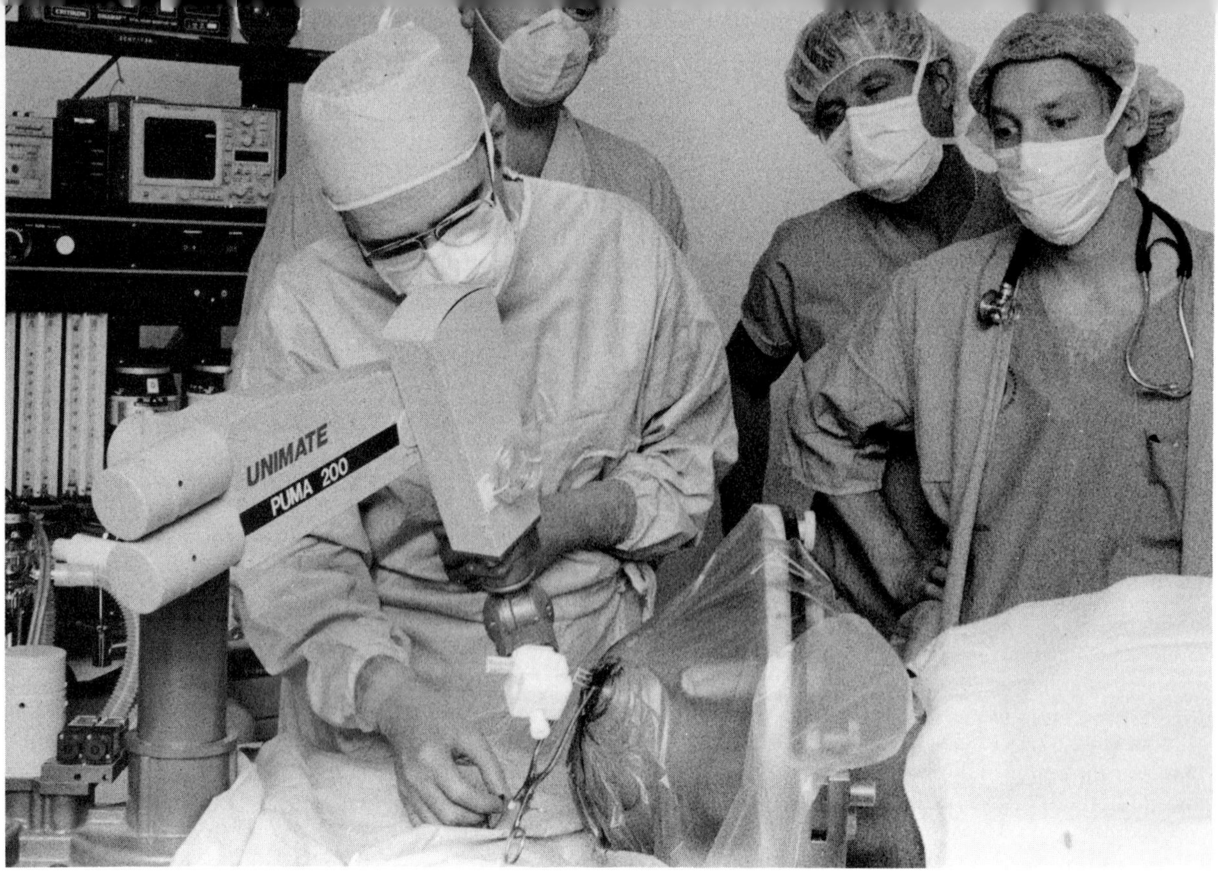

A computer-guided robot arm is used by doctors at California's Memorial Medical Center of Long Beach to pinpoint and collect brain tissue for a biopsy.

the laser technique is used to clear blockages upstream from the planned bypass. The surgeon threads the three-inch long, spaghetti-thin tip of the hand-held, pistol-sized laser through an opening sliced into the clogged artery, running a thin fiber-optic tube, or catheter, alongside the laser barrel so that the laser's progress can be seen. When the laser's tip nears the plaque, the surgeon fires short bursts of infrared laser light, burning clean, wedge-shaped cuts in the mass. Vapor is removed from the site by suction, and tissue debris is flushed out with a solution.

Many bypass patients have blockages in numerous small, branching arteries as well as in the larger vessels being bypassed. Once perfected, laser coronary endarterectomy may allow surgeons to clear obstructed arteries that are too numerous or thin to bypass or that would otherwise need to be sliced open for manual cleaning with a scalpel. (Studies are still needed to determine if the arteries remain open for prolonged periods following laser therapy.) The procedure would not replace the 200,000 coronary bypass operations performed in the United States each year. Rather, the Houston investigators hope the technique will improve the success of bypass operations by further improving blood flow to the heart muscle.

Laser-assisted balloon angioplasty. A different laser device has also been used to clear plaques from patients' arteries. A rounded, metal tip on the optical fiber that delivers the laser's energy cuts the risk of puncturing the artery wall. The tip emits energy in a diffuse pattern, rather than as a narrow beam that might be more likely to cut through the wall. The probe also has a guidance system that permits improved control of its path. Researchers at Boston University are using the probe with an argon laser, but the device works with any type of laser that has a fiber-optic delivery system.

At present, the device is being tested as an adjunct to balloon angioplasty, another procedure for opening blocked arteries, in vessels that are either completely closed or too narrow to permit initial insertion of the tiny balloon. The physician snakes a fiber-optic catheter, down which the laser is to be fired, through a small incision in the thigh and into a large artery to the site of the blockage. When the laser is fired, the probe tip heats up to 750° Fahrenheit and vaporizes the plaques. After the laser has opened a thin channel in the blocked artery, a balloon is inserted into the artery and then inflated to flatten the remains of the plaques, thus creating an opening through which blood can flow.

In testing the system in 40 patients, the Boston University researchers succeeded in partially clearing 39 out of 42 vessels. Without this procedure, patients with completely blocked arteries might have required major bypass surgery or even leg amputation. In future applications, the laser system may be used alone, without balloon angioplasty, depending on the size and other characteristics of the vessel being reopened.

A Bubble for Obesity

To help extremely overweight people lose poundage and stay trim, doctors have tried such radical methods as stapling off a portion of the stomach or wiring the jaws shut. Another approach is to put a plastic balloon into the stomach, and 1985 saw the first approval of such a device, the Gastric Bubble, by the U.S. Food and Drug Administration (FDA). The balloon produces a feeling of fullness that makes it easier for the patient to follow a low-calorie diet. The Bubble is carried to the stomach by a tube inserted down the patient's throat. Once the balloon is inflated, to about the size of a small juice can, the tube is withdrawn. The device is left in place for up to four months, then deflated and removed—or replaced. Intended as a temporary aid for achieving a modification of eating behavior, the Gastric Bubble is said to work only with well-motivated patients.

Artificial Bone

Researchers have long sought a substitute for bone tissue lost through accidents, disease, and surgery. Today, doctors often resort to grafting pieces of a patient's own rib or hip bone to replace bone lost elsewhere in the body. Progress has been made, however, in devising substitutes that greatly simplify the problem of bone replacement.

Glasslike replacement for bone. An easy-to-mold bone substitute called Bioglass received FDA approval early in 1985 for marketing as a replacement for the delicate bones of the middle ear. Developed by a ceramics engineer at the University of Florida in Gainesville, the material is a kind of modified glass in which calcium and phosphorus occur in the same proportions as in natural human bone (other constituents are quartz, silica sand, and sodium oxide). In one study, a Bioglass implant achieved good restoration of hearing in 13 of 16 patients with defective middle ear structures. The material appears to bond well to neighboring tissue within about ten days of implantation, without problems of toxicity or rejection. Testing for other uses of Bioglass is planned—for example, as a resurfacing material for hip replacements and as a jawbone replacement.

A scaffolding for new bone. A ceramic and plaster material developed by a surgeon at the dental school of the University of North Carolina in Chapel Hill, working with biomedical engineers at the university, has emerged as a promising bone substitute that acts as a scaffolding for the regrowth of healthy tissue. By early 1986 the researchers had successfully tested this still-experimental "artificial bone" on some 90 periodontal surgery patients and about ten cancer patients who had suffered bone damage as a result of their disease.

The puttylike material is a mixture of hydroxyapatite (a calcium phosphate that is a key component of bone) baked into hard ceramic particles, and plaster of paris (calcium sulfate). The mixture can be shaped right at the damaged site or molded before surgery. Gradually, the body absorbs the plaster in the implant and replaces it with a "mesh" of blood vessels, connective tissue, and collagen (the nonmineral constituent of bone), which surrounds the ceramic particles to maintain the shape of the implant. The body can not absorb the ceramic, and eventually the collagen entrapping these particles turns into bone, a process called ossification. Although most work to date has been done on jawbone repair, the developers of the material anticipate it will ultimately prove even more useful in work on the skull and facial bones.

LifeCard

Health Management Systems, a part of Blue Cross/Blue Shield of Maryland, in 1985 announced the development of LifeCard, a practically indestructible credit card-sized medical file. The card, which draws on the same optical laser technology that made possible videodisks and compact audio disks, can store—and offer nearly instant access to—the equivalent of 800 typewritten pages of information. Besides holding a person's medical history and details of health insurance coverage, LifeCard can store X-ray and CT images, electro-

The equivalent of hundreds of pages of an individual's medical history (including X rays), as well as insurance coverage, can be stored on this credit card-sized LifeCard developed by Blue Cross/Blue Shield of Maryland.

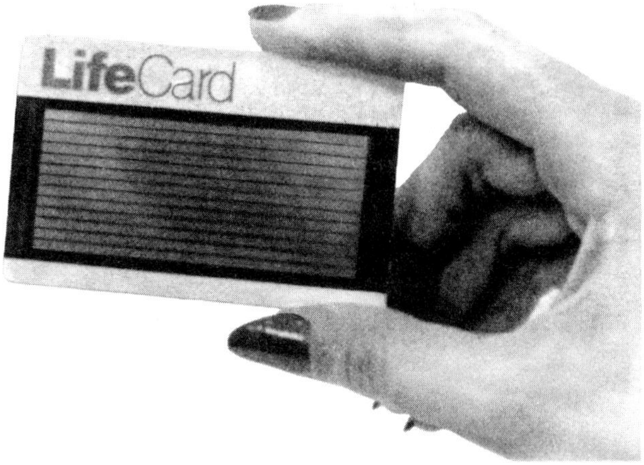

cardiograms, electroencephalograms, and magnetic resonance imaging scans, as well as facsimiles of a patient's photograph and signature. The card is made of Lexan, the same material as bullet-proof glass. The information stored on it can be read and updated with a laser device connected to a desktop computer.

Blue Cross/Blue Shield of Maryland plans to begin distributing LifeCard to its 2 million subscribers in mid-1986 and is marketing the card to insurers in other states as well. The card is expected to save time and improve accuracy in record keeping, diagnosis, and treatment. Most important, in emergency situations it can provide vital medical data that an injured or unconscious person is not able to. GARDINER MORSE

Medications and Drugs

New Antibiotics to Fight Infection • Help for Prostate Cancer • Gold Aids Arthritis Patients • Poisoned Tylenol

New Antibiotics

New antibiotics that strike at an increasingly broad spectrum of infection-causing bacteria were recently approved for use by the U.S. Food and Drug Administration, the Health Protection Branch of Health and Welfare Canada, or both. The antibiotics, which are all administered only by injection, offer better treatment for almost every kind of serious infection.

In 1985, five antibiotics of the beta-lactam class (drugs belonging to the penicillin, cephalosporin, and related families) were approved by the FDA; not all are yet on the market in Canada. Two of the new antibiotics are classified as third-generation cephalosporins: ceftazidime (marketed as Fortaz and Tazidime in the United States and as Fortaz and Magnacef in Canada) and ceftriaxone (sold in the United States as Rocephin). Like four previously developed third-generation cephalosporins, ceftazidime and ceftriaxone are active against certain strains of disease-causing bacteria that are resistant to drugs of the first and second generation of cephalosporins. Both these new antibiotics are useful against a wide range of bacteria responsible for infections of the respiratory and urinary tracts, bones and joints, skin and soft tissues, and the central nervous system.

Ceftazidime is especially effective against *Pseudomonas aeruginosa*, bacteria that often cause fatal infections in hospitalized patients whose resistance has been reduced by other diseases. This new antibiotic is said to be superior to the several other previously available cephalosporins and penicillins with antipseudomonal activity. It has helped patients with cystic fibrosis (a chronic illness that affects the lungs) recover from pneumonia caused by the *Pseudomonas* species or by bacilli (rod-shaped bacteria) that are often resistant to other infection-fighting drugs.

The most important property of the second new cephalosporin, ceftriaxone, is its long duration of action. Often a single daily dose is effective for 24 hours. Once-a-day dosage significantly reduces the cost of treating patients hospitalized for chronic conditions, like the bone infection osteomyelitis, that require long-term treatment. And some patients can even be sent home, where a visiting nurse or a relative can administer the patient's single daily injection.

Both ceftazidime and ceftriaxone can be used in treating meningitis (inflammation of the membranes that cover the brain and spinal cord) in newborn infants, older children, and young adults. The drugs penetrate the inflamed membranes and reach high enough levels in the cerebrospinal fluid to kill the bacteria that most commonly cause meningitis—meningococci, pneumococci, and *Haemophilus influenzae*. Ceftazidime is also effective against meningitis caused by species of *Pseudomonas* bacteria, which does not respond to treatment with ceftriaxone.

The new cephalosporins are also active against the microorganisms that cause gonorrhea. Ceftriaxone seems especially effective; a single, relatively low dose is claimed to be able to cure 100 percent of cases, including those caused by resistant strains of gonococci. This is because ceftriaxone resists breakdown by the so-called beta-lactamase enzymes with which gonococcal bacteria destroy most other beta-lactam antibiotics.

Two of the new antibiotics now on the market in the United States combine penicillins with enzyme-inhibiting compounds that enhance their antibacterial activity. One of these, sold as Timentin, combines the broad-spectrum, penicillin-type antibiotic ticarcillin with potassium clavulanate, a substance that inactivates the beta-lactamase enzymes that make some strains of bacteria resistant to ticarcillin. Thus, this combination product helps cure infections of the lungs, skin and soft tissues, bones and joints, and urinary tract caused by ticarcillin-resistant species of *Staphylococcus aureus*, *Escherichia coli*, and *Haemophilus influenzae*.

The second new combination product, called Primaxin, contains the new antibiotic imipenem together with the enzyme inhibitor cilastatin. Primaxin is being promoted as having the broadest antibacterial spectrum of all available anti-infection medications and as being effective against bacterial infections in almost every part of the body. Many strains resistant to other antibiotics are said to succumb to this new combination.

Amdinocillin (sold as Coactin in the United States) is a penicillin, made in part synthetically, that was approved for use in the United States a year after it was approved in Canada for treating urinary tract infections. (The Canadian brand name is Selexid.) The drug reaches high antibacterial levels in the urine when it is rapidly excreted by the kidneys. These high concentrations kill such urinary tract bacteria as *E. coli, Proteus mirabilis,* and species of *Klebsiella* and *Enterobacter.* Amdinocillin is often given together with other beta-lactam antibiotics for treating the serious infections that occur when these bacteria spread to the bloodstream. The combination is more effective than using single drugs. Also, combining amdinocillin with another beta-lactam is claimed to be safer than combinations that contain so-called aminoglycoside antibiotics, drugs that are effective but can cause kidney damage.

Blood Pressure, Heart Problems

The FDA recently approved new medications for normalizing irregular heart rhythms and for lowering high blood pressure. One drug, acebutolol (Sectral), does both. Acebutolol is a beta blocker, a compound that blocks nerve impulses that stimulate the heart and that also affect the functioning of other body organs and structures. Like other beta blockers, acebutolol has proved useful for treating mild to moderate high blood pressure when taken alone or combined with a diuretic (a drug that rids the body of excess salt and fluid). In addition, it is the only beta blocker besides the older drug propranolol (Inderal) that is also approved for treating patients whose heart rhythm is marked by extra heartbeats that occur at irregular intervals, a condition called ventricular premature beat.

Acebutolol is claimed to be less likely than propranolol either to cause an excessive decrease in the patient's heart rate and pumping power or to set off muscle spasms of the bronchial tubes in asthma patients. Yet, as with other beta blockers, doctors must exercise caution in prescribing the drug for patients with bronchospastic disease, a slow heartbeat, or a history of heart failure. Patients on acebutolol seem somewhat less likely to complain of fatigue, headache, sleep difficulties, and other central nervous system side effects than do patients taking propranolol.

The new drug's prolonged action allows most high blood pressure patients to get along on only a single daily dose. It has such long action because when it is broken down in the body, an active product is formed that the kidneys eliminate from the body only very slowly. Of course, this can be a disadvantage for patients with kidney damage. People with impaired kidney function and many elderly patients should receive a smaller daily dosage.

Another medication, enalapril (Vasotec), was approved by the FDA late in 1985 for treating high blood pressure. It is taken in a single daily dose, alone or combined with other hypertension medications. The drug acts by blocking the action of an enzyme that helps to produce a hormone, called angiotensin II, that raises blood pressure. The pressure-reducing effect is increased when enalapril is taken together with a diuretic. Enalapril causes mainly mild, temporary side effects like headaches, dizziness, or fatigue. However, in clinical tests about 2 out of every 1,000 patients developed swelling of the face, tongue, and throat, which can cause fatal asphyxia (lack of oxygen) and shock. Patients who experience this severe response must stop taking the drug permanently.

SWEET MEDICINE

A popular Southern folk remedy—sprinkling sugar on open wounds—has been lifted into modern medical practice by some doctors from Mississippi as well as Europe and South America. In fact, the practice dates back to the ancient Egyptians, who used honey mixed with butter to promote healing.

Dr. Richard A. Knutson of the Delta Medical Center in Greenville, Miss., has successfully treated more than 3,000 cases ranging from bedsores to gunshot wounds and amputations, using a paste of sugar and povidine-iodine (Betadine). The Betadine helps to prevent infection. It is said that wounds heal faster and scarring is less likely with the sugar treatment than with more conventional packing and dressing methods. Knutson claims the treatment is safe even for those with diabetes because little of the sugar is absorbed by the body.

Such reports, however, have not yet been confirmed by careful studies and are not accepted by all doctors. If sugar does work, it is not known why this might be. One theory is that sugar absorbs the water that infectious bacteria need to grow; another that it draws infection-fighting white blood cells to the wound site.

Enalapril is the second antihypertensive drug of a class called angiotensin-converting enzyme, or ACE, inhibitors. In 1984 the FDA lifted restrictions on the use of the first drug of this type, captopril (Capoten), which was approved several years ago only for treating severe high blood pressure that had not responded to treatment with other drugs. Now, captopril can be used to treat mild and moderate degrees of high blood pressure, as well as selected cases of congestive heart failure.

Flecainide (Tambocor) was approved for use in the United States in the long-term treatment of patients with heart rhythm irregularities that affect the ventricles, the heart's main pumping chambers. The drug suppresses the electrical impulses that arise at an abnormally rapid rate in the heart, keeping these signals from triggering ventricular speedups. This normalizes the patient's heartbeat and can help prevent the uncoordinated heart muscle contractions that are the main cause of cardiac arrest and sudden death.

The dosage of flecainide must be tailored to the needs of each individual, since excessive amounts can—as with all other drugs for ventricular arrhythmias—cause congestive heart failure by reducing the pumping power of the ventricles in patients with already weakened heart muscle. It can actually make some kinds of cardiac irregularities worse, but it is claimed to be less likely to do so than the various other agents of its type. The most common noncardiac side effects of flecainide are dizziness and visual disturbances, complaints reported by about 30 percent of patients. These and other side effects, including headache, nervousness, muscle tremors, abdominal pain, and nausea, caused 6 percent of patients to discontinue it during tests.

Prostate Cancer

The drug leuprolide (Lupron) is now available in both the United States and Canada for treating men with advanced prostate gland cancer. The patient can inject the single daily dose required by himself, in much the same way people with diabetes inject themselves with insulin. Leuprolide works by first stimulating and then suppressing production of pituitary gland hormones that control secretion of the male hormone testosterone by the testes. Because testosterone stimulates the growth of prostate cancer tissue, this drug's inhibitory action on pituitary and testicular hormones helps to reduce the size of tumors that have spread to the patient's bones and elsewhere in his body.

Leuprolide seems safer than diethylstilbestrol (DES), the synthetic female sex hormone that until now has been the principal medication used to treat prostate cancer. Unlike DES, leuprolide produces relief of bone pain and other symptoms without increasing the risk of dangerous blood clots, and it does not cause the painful and disfiguring swelling of male breast tissue sometimes seen during long-term DES treatment. The only significant side effects of the new drug are its tendency to cause discomforting "hot flashes" and a temporary worsening of some patients' condition during the first weeks of treatment. These effects last only until the drug's initial stimulation of hormone secretion ends, a phase followed by its persistent suppression of hormone production. *(See also the Spotlight on Health article* PROSTATE PROBLEMS.)

Potent Pain Reliever

Buprenorphine, a potent pain reliever prepared by chemically modifying an opium plant constituent, came onto the U.S. market as Buprenex. Injected in very small doses, the drug keeps moderate to severe pain under control for up to six hours—almost twice as long as when morphine or meperidine (Demerol) is given. The new drug is also said to be safer in several ways than these standard narcotic pain medications. For example, buprenorphine has a built-in ability to block the effects of overdosage: because of the way the drug functions, its early effects are counteracted by its later effects. Thus, high doses do not ordinarily depress breathing or blood pressure excessively. However, even normal doses can cause severe respiratory depression in patients with conditions like emphysema that are marked by impaired breathing. Caution is needed in such cases, and patients who receive the drug after recovering from general anesthesia or after receiving other drugs that depress respiration need to be carefully monitored to watch for any breathing problems.

Patients who take buprenorphine for chronic pain are said to be less likely to become addicted to it or to suffer withdrawal symptoms when they stop taking it than patients taking conventional pain medications. Another common side effect, constipation, also occurs less often. However, drowsiness develops in two out of three patients, and some complain of dizziness and nausea. Patients who are not hospitalized are warned not to drive, operate dangerous machinery, drink alcohol, or take tranquilizers while receiving buprenorphine.

Hay Fever and Asthma

Terfenadine (Seldane), an antihistamine drug that has been available in Canada for a number of years, received FDA approval in 1985 for use in relieving symptoms of hay fever (seasonal nasal allergy). This drug differs from all previously available antihistamines in one key respect: it rarely makes patients drowsy when taken in doses that control sneezing, runny nose, and other allergy symptoms. This may be because terfenadine does not readily pass from the circulating blood into the brain. Another difference from some other antihistamines is that terfenadine is available only by prescription.

Bitolterol, a drug that widens the bronchial tubes of people with asthma or other conditions causing bronchial spasms, was also approved by the FDA. The drug is marketed as Tornalate and comes in an inhaler that releases measured doses of mist into the patient's mouth. Actually, bitolterol itself is inactive until enzymes in the lungs convert it to an active component called colterol. This substance then produces a prompt improvement in breathing and prevents constriction of the bronchial tubes for five to eight hours or longer.

When used to relieve and prevent bronchial spasms, bitolterol is claimed to cause less stimulation of patients' heart rates than earlier bronchodilators. Nevertheless, patients are warned to avoid inhaling bitolterol too often since too much can lead to adverse cardiovascular effects, particularly in people with coronary artery disease or high blood pressure. Patients complain most commonly of tremors of the skeletal muscles (the muscles attached to bones), but these are said to lessen with continued use of the medication.

Gold Capsule for Arthritis

A pill that contains gold was recently approved in both Canada and the United States for treating rheumatoid arthritis. The medication, called auranofin (Ridaura), is specifically for patients who fail to improve after treatment with full doses of aspirin or nonsteroidal anti-inflammatory drugs like ibuprofen (Motrin). These are the so-called first-step agents in treating rheumatoid arthritis. Even after patients begin to take daily doses of auranofin capsules, they should continue taking one of these first-step drugs and keeping up their prescribed program of exercise and rest.

Gold has long been available in injectable form as a second step in treating progressive, disabling rheumatoid arthritis. However, patients must visit their arthritis specialist weekly for the injections and for laboratory tests of their blood and urine, since injected gold often causes kidney damage and deficiencies of blood platelets and red or white blood cells. But because gold taken orally is relatively safe, patients require blood and urine tests only about once a month. Only rarely do they stop treatment because of side effects, since problems like itchy skin rash, sore mouth, or conjunctivitis are much less likely to occur. However, if patients do have such complaints or develop bleeding gums or skin bruises, they should see their doctor promptly. In addition, oral gold is more likely to cause certain adverse effects than is the injectable form; these include diarrhea, abdominal cramps, and other gastrointestinal complaints.

Patients taking auranofin are advised not to become discouraged if they do not see rapid improvement and not to stop taking the drug or raise its dosage on their own. It may take three or four months or more before the joint pain, tenderness, and swelling of rheumatoid arthritis start to lessen.

Chemotherapy Side Effects

Dronabinol (Marinol), a synthetic form of the main active ingredient in marijuana, was approved for U.S. use in preventing the nausea and vomiting that often occur during cancer chemotherapy. Dronabinol is as effective as most of the antivomiting drugs routinely used for this purpose, and perhaps even more so. However, because it can cause disturbing mental effects, it is best reserved for patients who fail to respond to treatment with previously available medications.

About one in four patients taking dronabinol experiences a typical marijuana-type "high," while some suffer disturbing psychiatric reactions. Patients should be told that such mental changes are possible so that they do not become alarmed if they begin to feel anxious, depressed, or disoriented or experience hallucinations.

While dronabinol is usually used in hospitals, it is occasionally prescribed for outpatients to take at home for a few days. These patients should be watched closely by a responsible friend or relative. Also, because dronabinol is a central nervous system depressant, it commonly causes drowsiness and can impair motor coordination. Outpatients should not drive when taking dronabinol, nor should they drink alcohol or take sedatives or sleeping pills together with it.

Dissolving Gallstones

Monooctanoin (Moctanin), a drug that can dissolve cholesterol-containing gallstones (the most common kind of gallstones), received FDA approval for use in some patients with stones left behind in the bile ducts following surgical removal of the gallbladder. About a third of the time, all the remaining stones dissolve when monooctanoin, a liquid compound, is allowed to flow continuously into the bile duct under low pressure through a tube inserted into the common bile duct. Another third of the time, the stones become small enough to pass into the upper intestinal tract and be eliminated in the feces. When successful, this treatment spares the patient from further surgery or other risky procedures.

Monooctanoin is a so-called orphan drug—one for which the FDA seeks sponsoring companies willing to undertake development and testing, since the medication is needed by so few patients that it is not likely to prove commercially profitable. About 2,000 Americans annually may benefit from monooctanoin.

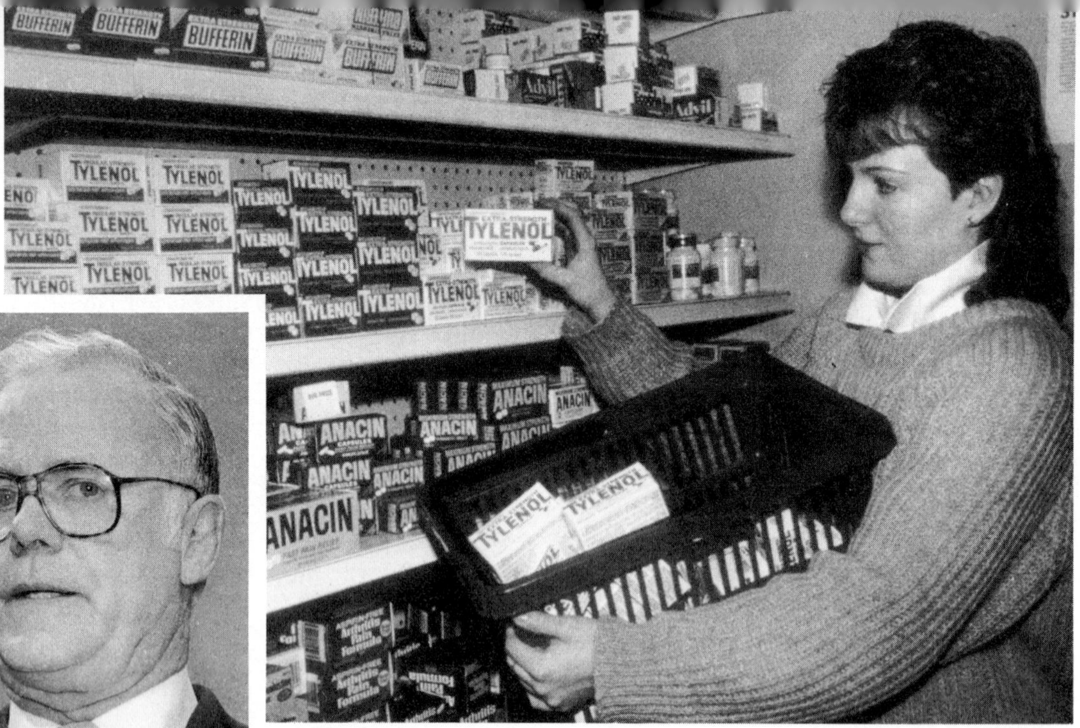

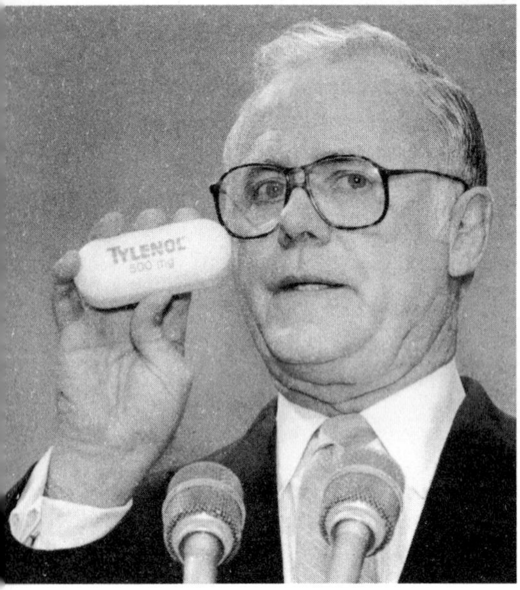

After a New York woman who had taken Extra-Strength Tylenol capsules died of cyanide poisoning, a national alert was issued and the capsules removed from drugstores. Manufacturer Johnson & Johnson discontinued all of its over-the-counter capsules, producing Tylenol only as tablets and "caplets" (left, Chairman James Burke with an oversized model).

Chelation Pills Banned

In July 1985 the FDA notified manufacturers and distributors of oral chelation products that they must stop selling these unapproved drugs. At the same time the agency warned consumers against taking these products to prevent or treat cardiovascular and other diseases. A chelation agent is one that combines in the body with a heavy metal like lead or with calcium to speed removal of an excess of the essential element. The chelation products that have been widely sold by mail, in retail stores, and door-to-door are mixtures of vitamins, minerals, and amino acids. Their promoters claim that the tablets or capsules help to prevent buildup of plaque on the walls of arteries, thus improving blood flow and preventing or relieving coronary heart disease and other disorders caused by clogged arteries. The FDA refuted such claims, saying these unapproved oral chelation products are of no proven benefit. (These products, it must be emphasized, should be distinguished from approved chelation agents, which are usually injected by a doctor to treat metal poisoning and digitalis overdoses.)

Poisoned Tylenol

Death came out of a Tylenol bottle in early 1986, raising new questions about the safety of over-the-counter medications in capsule form. On February 8 in Yonkers, N.Y., a 23-year-old woman died of cyanide poisoning after taking two capsules from a freshly opened bottle of Extra-Strength Tylenol that had been purchased at a supermarket in nearby Bronxville. A few days later investigators found five cyanide-tainted capsules in a similar bottle from a Bronxville dime store.

It was the second time in less than four years that Extra-Strength Tylenol's manufacturer, Johnson & Johnson, had faced a poisoning crisis. (Tylenol is the company's brand name for the painkiller acetaminophen.) In 1982, seven Chicago-area residents died after taking Extra-Strength Tylenol capsules laced with cyanide. That case was still unsolved when the 1986 poisoning occurred. Investigators believed that in all the poisonings Tylenol bottles were, for unknown motives, removed from a store and then—after some capsules were filled with cyanide—replaced on store shelves. The 1982 incidents led to a rash of copycat poisonings of other food and drug products, and the FDA mandated tamper-resistant packaging for over-the-counter drugs. Johnson & Johnson exceeded the FDA packaging requirements. The company introduced a "triple safety seal," consisting of glued end flaps on the cardboard carton, a plastic shrink wrap over the cap, and an inner seal of foil over the mouth of the bottle. The possibility remained, however, that a determined and skillful individual could successfully breach and replace the seals. The FBI announced in late February 1986 that its scientists had in fact found signs of tampering with the safety seals of the two Bronxville bottles that contained cyanide.

Shortly after the second tainted bottle of Tylenol was found, Johnson & Johnson announced that it was discontinuing the manufacture and sale of the capsule form of all its over-the-counter drugs. Tylenol would be produced only as tablets and "caplets"—tablets that are capsule-shaped and coated to be more easily swallowed. Tablets, including caplets, are much more resistant to poisoning than most capsules, which can simply be pulled apart, emptied, and filled with poison. Dipping a tablet in a poison solution would probably cause discoloration or decomposition.

Other drugmakers were reluctant to give up the capsule form. But about six weeks after the Yonkers woman died, questions about the future of capsules were again being asked as a new tampering incident occurred. The drug manufacturer SmithKline Beckman received warnings that packages of its capsule products had been poisoned. Small amounts of warfarin, an anticoagulant substance used in rat poison, were indeed found in several capsules of the cold medicine Contac, the allergy remedy Teldrin, and the appetite suppressant Dietac. SmithKline immediately recalled the products from the market.

See also the feature article THE NEW VACCINES *and the Spotlight on Health article* NEW WAYS TO TAKE MEDICINE. MORTON J. RODMAN, PH.D.

Mental Health

Treating Depression in New Ways • Reaction to the Space Shuttle Disaster • Is Cancer Affected by Emotions?

New Ideas on Depression

Treatment with sleep and light. There is growing evidence that certain physical methods can help alleviate some kinds of depression. With one method, people suffering from depression are forced to alter their sleep cycle by what is called phase advance, in which patients go to sleep earlier at night than their customary time. Since people with serious depression often wake up too early in the morning, getting them to bed earlier advances their sleep cycle and gives them more sleep. This leads to improvement in the depression. When these patients go back to their unstructured sleep patterns, however, they again become depressed.

Another experimental treatment for depression has been "phototherapy" for people who tend to get depressed when the amount of daylight is greatly reduced in the winter. This disorder has been given the appropriate acronym SAD, for seasonal affective disorder. The treatment involves, in essence, extending the period of daylight by exposing the patient to bright lights before dawn and/or after dusk. One study showed a significant improvement in depression for patients exposed to bright light but not to dim light. Discontinuation of the bright-light treatment resulted in a recurrence of the depression two to four days later.

The effects of diet. While many so-called health food preparations have been oversold as remedies for psychological disturbances, investigators are finding some evidence that eating foods rich in substances used by the body to build neurotransmitters, the chemicals that communicate between nerve cells, may help the body correct certain deficits related to these disorders. Some of these substances are precursors of norepinephrine and serotonin, neurotransmitters whose levels in the body are reduced in some kinds of depression. Including large amounts of the precursors of these substances in the diet has helped some patients with depressive disorders.

The food and depression connection may be a factor in the serious eating disorder bulimia, the "binge-purge" syndrome whose victims periodically gorge themselves and then induce vomiting of what they have just eaten. Attempts to link what is known about the clinical course of bulimia with knowledge of brain function have been enhanced by the observation that bulimics often respond well to treatment with antidepressants, which work by elevating levels of neurotransmitters in the brain. This response to antidepressants suggests that bulimia may be an atypical form of depression. Several recent studies have, in fact, indicated that bulimic behavior, especially the compulsive eating of large amounts of carbohydrate-rich food, may be a kind of self-medication, since this carbohydrate loading has been found to elevate neurotransmitter levels in some patients. Binge eating is hardly recommended as a treatment for depression, but such studies show great promise in providing a more coherent picture of the relationship between brain and behavior.

Suicide. An interesting study of the Old Order Amish people of southeastern Pennsylvania that was published in 1985 demonstrated a remarkably strong genetic link for suicide. This inbred religious community has very few of the usual risk factors for suicide. The community has little alcohol or drug abuse and no unemployment. Family structures are intact, with two or three generations living in a home, and the Amish have strong community ties. The study, which covered the period from 1880 to 1980, found that serious depressive disorders and suicide ran in certain families. Of 26 suicides, 7 occurred in one group of relatives and 5 in another. Most of the remaining suicides occurred in two other family groups. Thus, the study provides evidence of a strong genetic component to serious depression and related suicidal behavior.

The Space Shuttle Disaster

The explosion that destroyed the space shuttle *Challenger* on January 28, 1986, killing all seven astronauts on board, elicited an outpouring of emotion throughout the United States and the world. Disbelief yielded to shock and grief as people witnessed television film of the explosion and experienced the loss of the five men and two women, one a schoolteacher and the first "ordinary American" sent into space. Several factors seemed to account for the intensity of the response. For many people the space program had come to represent humanity's loftiest goals, the dream of using technology to transcend our human limitations. In addition, we often handle anxiety about death through a preoccupation with reaching goals, as though by our doing the right thing death will be indefinitely held at bay. The loss of the shuttle was a painful reminder that all human endeavors, no matter how noble and well-planned, have their limitations, and that no one is invulnerable. Also, unlike other national tragedies, there was no identifiable enemy for Americans to blame, no images of arrogant terrorists to deflect attention from the sense of helplessness that accompanies every loss.

In the United States there was widespread concern that children would be especially affected by the loss, since many schools had made the planned flight the focus of an intensive educational experience, with lessons to be taught from space by "teachernaut" Christa McAuliffe. While some mental-health professionals warned that children might suffer increased anxiety, sleeplessness, and, especially among young children, fears about the loss of teachers and parents, there was no evidence of long-term effects. The news media and schools emphasized the importance of collective grieving and sharing the loss openly; this process was led by President Ronald Reagan, who delayed his State of the Union address for a week and spoke movingly of the tragedy in several public statements. The task in grieving is to acknowledge, bear, and put into perspective the loss, and the collective public mourning helped to make the loss real in psychological terms while "normalizing" the strong emotional response to it.

Emotions and Cancer

The results of a major study published in 1985 have intensified an ongoing debate about whether psychological factors, such as the way one handles emotional and social stress, have any effect on the development or the

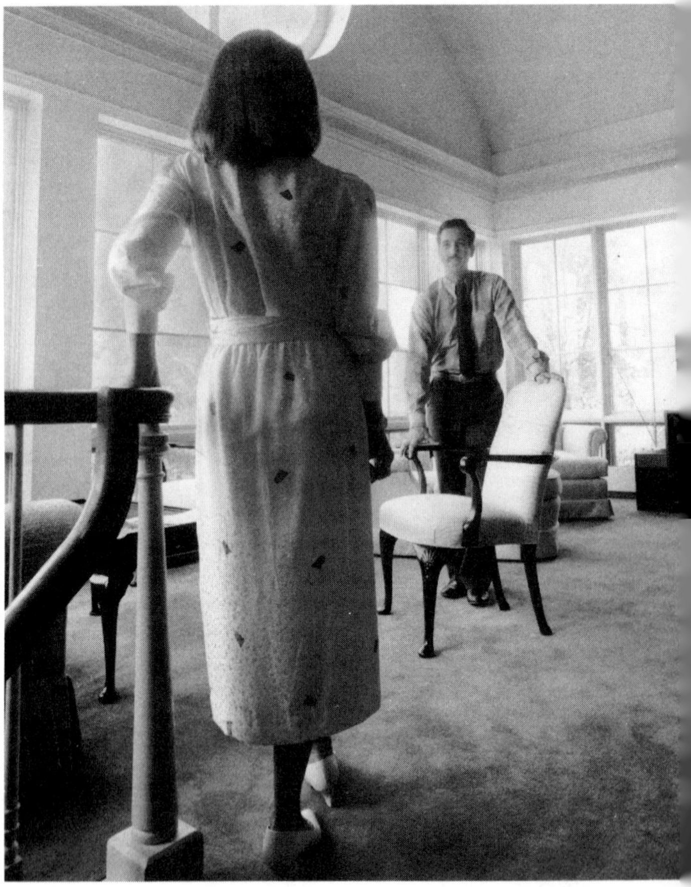

progression of illnesses such as cancer. A number of cancer studies in the past decade have suggested that suppression of one's natural emotions, especially anger, may result in a worse outcome. In one study, for example, women who came for breast biopsies and were found to have cancer tended to be less expressive of anger than women whose breast lumps turned out to be noncancerous. Another study showed that uncooperative patients—those who were rated by their doctors as less compliant and more troublesome—turned out to live longer than those who received better "grades." In the latter study, however, the uncooperative patients had received only half as much chemotherapy as the more compliant ones and therefore were probably somewhat healthier to begin with.

These speculations that suppression of feeling may somehow be related to vulnerability to cancer have sparked enormous interest, including an editorial in the prestigious British medical journal *The Lancet* that endorsed a new field known as psychoimmunology. The theory behind this field is that under various kinds of stress the body's immune function, its ability to fight invading bacterial and viral organisms, is impaired somehow. Research has demonstrated quite convinc-

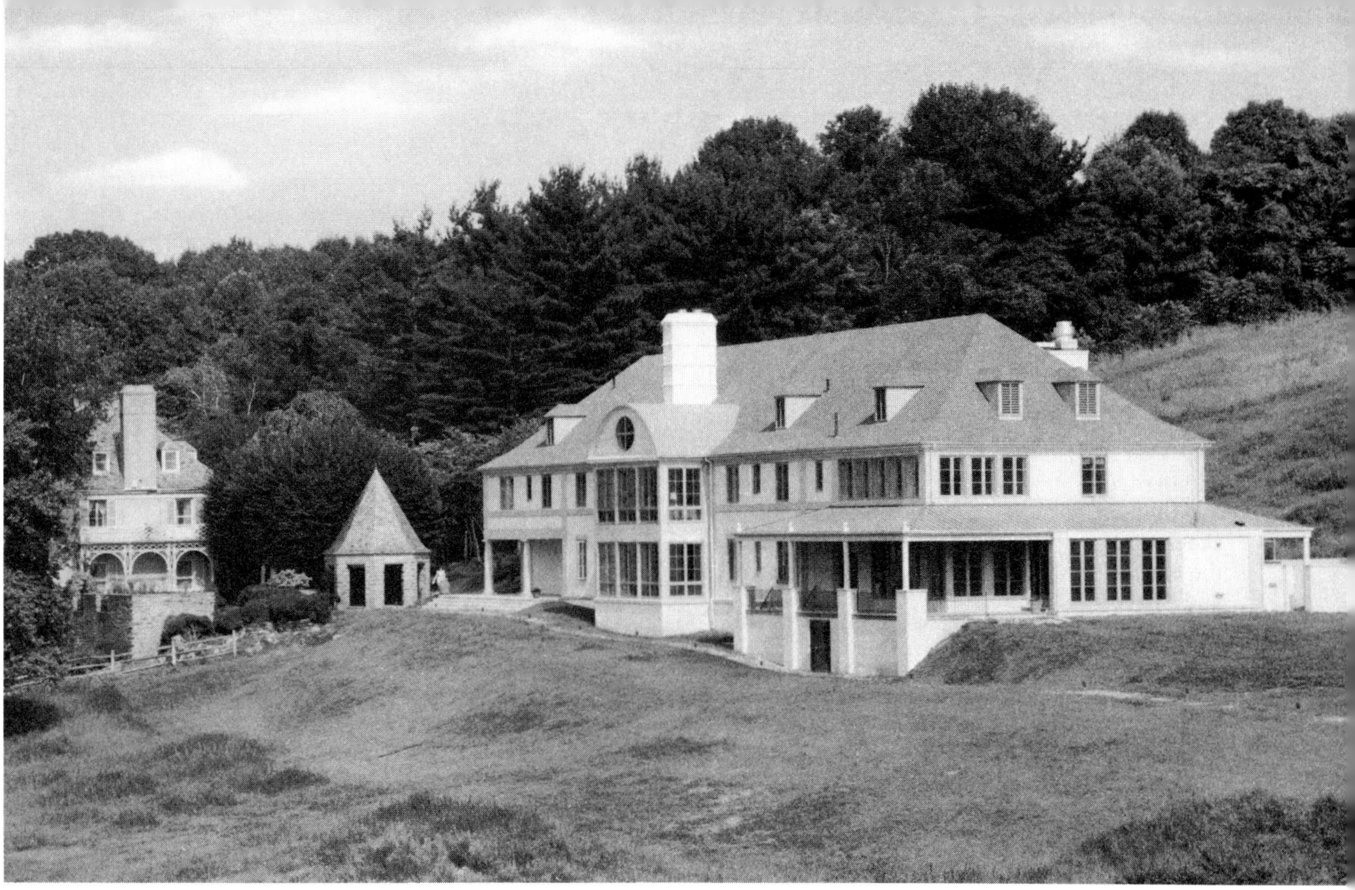

New Treatment Center for Eating Disorders

In June 1985 the first freestanding residential facility devoted exclusively to the treatment of anorexia nervosa and bulimia was opened—the Renfrew Center in Philadelphia. Left, Dr. Leonard Levitz conducts a counseling session with a bulimic patient.

ingly that laboratory animals can be conditioned, using stimuli such as smell or taste, to change the way their immune systems function. In humans, it has long been observed that certain kinds of stress, such as the death of a spouse, increase the risk of becoming ill and dying. Research has also shown that job stress may be related to lowered immune function and that immunity rises during sleep, perhaps partly explaining the restorative effect of sleep in helping people fight disease.

In theory these changes in immune function could influence vulnerability to infectious disease, autoimmune diseases such as arthritis, and possibly the development or progression of cancer. One theory of cancer, known as the immune surveillance theory, holds that the body is producing cancerous cells all the time but that the immune system identifies and kills them. Some breakdown in this immune surveillance would allow cancer cells to develop into tumors, which eventually may become lethal. There are problems with this theory, in that animals and humans with compromised immune responses are not necessarily more vulnerable to cancer, but the idea is intriguing and has caught the attention of the public.

However, a study published in the *New England Journal of Medicine* in June 1985 concluded that psychosocial variables, such as a feeling of helplessness, could account for none of the differences in disease progression or longevity among the 359 cancer patients studied. Only biological variables—the stage, or severity, and type of disease—accounted for the progress of the illness. Thus, the scientific literature has so far provided no definitive proof that psychological variables affect the development or progress of cancer. It must be borne in mind that more mundane variables such as delay in seeking treatment and health-related habits like smoking and diet are more obvious and important ways in which personality and social support can influence a person's health or the course of an illness.

Nonetheless, some have been quick to use what evidence there is to justify a series of psychotherapeutic measures intended to treat cancer itself rather than its symptoms. Both group and individual psychotherapies using techniques ranging from hypnosis to drug therapy have been helpful in controlling the anxiety, depression, and pain often associated with cancer. But no studies have convincingly shown that such treatment prolongs life, even though it makes patients more comfortable. This is especially important to keep in mind since cancer patients, because of the seriousness of their illness, will cling to any hope that something they do will help control its course. While this attitude sounds positive, it can have the corrosive effect of making patients feel guilty if the disease progresses despite their efforts. As the editorial that accompanied the *New England Journal of Medicine* study pointed out, this can turn into a process of blaming the victim, in which a patient with one problem, cancer, is now saddled with a second problem, being made to feel responsible for getting the disease in the first place or having it spread.

Studying the Brain

High-tech approaches to analyzing activity in the brain continue to reveal information about the physical basis of various mental functions and disorders. One such method, called brain electrical activity mapping or BEAM, gives a computerized picture of electrical activity throughout the surface of the brain. This approach builds on the traditional electroencephalogram (EEG), which measures electrical activity in the brain at specific points on its surface, and the cortical evoked potential, which is the electrical activity evoked in the brain by a stimulus such as a flash of light or a sound. In one study among normal volunteers capable of experiencing the profound changes in perception called hallucinations while under hypnosis, it was found that there were changes in their brain electrical activity during the hallucinations. The hypnotized subjects were instructed to visualize a cardboard box blocking their view of a television screen. They reported seeing a vivid image of the box obscuring their view of the stimulus lights flashing on the screen, and during this experience their brains showed decreased electrical activity in response to the lights. Thus, the hallucinated experience of decreased view of the lights was accompanied by a reduction in brain electrical response to them. Furthermore, this suppression of response was significantly greater in the right than in the left hemisphere of the brain, suggesting that the focus on an internally generated image, that of the hallucinated box, is a function more of the right than of the left hemisphere.

Another type of brain image, made by the computerized X-ray technique called positron emission tomography (the PET scan), has recently shown that patients with serious psychiatric illnesses such as schizophrenia and manic-depressive (bipolar) disorder have a shift in the balance of brain activity from front to back, that is, less activity in the front of the brain and relatively more in the back. Since the frontal cortex is involved in purposefulness, the planning and integration of functions occurring elsewhere in the brain, it makes sense that there would be relatively less frontal function in these illnesses in which purposeful activity is in fact impaired. The back of the brain is more involved in the interpretation of sensory perception, especially vision. The relative increase in activity at the back of the brain may indicate some kind of hypervigilance in patients with serious psychiatric disorders. Furthermore, in schizo-

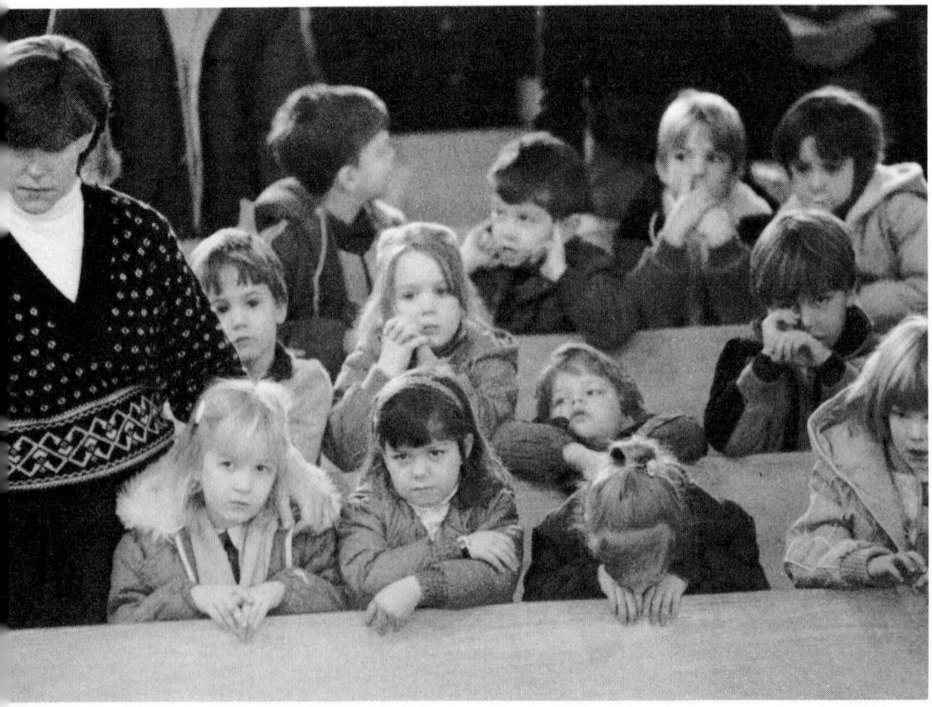

Open discussions and communal grieving (shown here, a Concord, N.H., prayer service) helped children handle the grief and terror caused by the explosion of the space shuttle Challenger *and the loss of "teachernaut" Christa McAuliffe.*

phrenics these abnormalities in brain activity have been found to diminish when the patients are treated with medication, although some deficit in activity in the front part of the brain seems to persist.

Automated Aids for the Elderly

Ingenious information-processing equipment is being applied to help elderly people with memory loss or mental disorders. Computerized telephone systems, for example, automatically signal for help if an older person living alone does not perform normal daily functions such as opening the refrigerator. Small computer notebooks are being used to aid people with memory problems, and even pill boxes with memories have been developed. These automated devices provide the same kind of assistance for those with mental problems that mechanical supports such as wheelchairs and robots provide for those with physical handicaps.

Psychiatry and the Law

In April 1985 the American Medical Association and the American Psychiatric Association issued their first joint statement on the so-called insanity defense, which underscored many points of agreement between the two groups despite some continued differences. Both associations, the statement said, start with the belief that the criminal justice system must ensure a balance between the public's need to be protected from potentially violent offenders and the mentally ill defendant's right to humane treatment. The two groups agree that mental impairment should be a rare defense. Furthermore, the statement said, individuals with serious mental illnesses who have committed acts of violence should be given proper medical and psychiatric treatment—treatment that the AMA and APA believe is now often inadequate. The statement also asserted that physicians, particularly psychiatrists, who testify in court need to have an appropriate role that is consistent with the adversary system of justice but is that of a participant, not an advocate, in the adversary proceeding; for example, they have to take care not to stretch their opinions to support their side of the case. Both the AMA and the APA acknowledge that this is a difficult role which requires careful and thoughtful involvement from both the legal and the medical sides. (The dangers of using medical opinions in the legal system were once lightheartedly referred to by Supreme Court Justice Felix Frankfurter as the "cross-sterilization of disciplines.")

In previous years the APA had recommended tightening guidelines so that the insanity defense could be used only when defendants had severe mental illness that impaired their ability to understand either what they had done or that what they had done was wrong. (Earlier versions of the insanity defense had more general standards for deciding that actions were the product of mental illness.) The AMA, on the other hand, had recommended that the insanity defense be abolished altogether, although it acknowledged that mental illness may affect criminal intent. A decision on intent is important in distinguishing, for example, between first-degree and second-degree murder and manslaughter, as well as in determining the right actions to be taken once guilt has been established.

Mental Health Care Costs

Two recent reports make it clear that the lack of a public policy in the United States to actively support mental health research and treatment will have serious social as well as economic costs. One of the reports, a major review of the relationship between psychiatric and other kinds of medical care, concluded that individuals who had received outpatient psychiatric treatment subsequently made less use of other medical services than they had before the treatment. This pattern was especially strong among patients over 55 years of age. Thus, appropriate psychiatric treatment may not only help patients cope with psychological problems, the effects of physical illness, and social isolation; it may also reduce the overall cost of healthcare by decreasing the amount of time spent in the hospital.

Evidence of the cost benefits of psychiatric treatment is especially important at a time when a major reorganization in the delivery of medical services is occurring in the United States. Many prepaid health plans and standard medical insurance plans are reluctant to provide anything more than minimal psychiatric services, fearing costly overuse. However, such a stance not only fails to address the psychiatric needs of patients but may ultimately cost more.

In a related development, a comprehensive report released by the Institute of Medicine raised concerns about the federal government's reluctance to support mental health research and treatment. According to the report, mental disorders and substance abuse affect 30-45 million people in the United States each year, requiring direct expenditures of $20 billion and a total economic cost of $185 billion. Research has already improved both drug and psychosocial treatments for some mental illnesses and addictions, the report noted, and since many of these conditions are severe and chronic, even small advances in treatment have great social benefit. In addition, the report said, research on both brain function and health-related behavior (such as coping with stress, exercise, smoking, and eating or drinking habits) has become increasingly important as it is recognized that many serious illnesses can be prevented or better treated by sustained changes in behavior. However, federal funding for research on mental health disorders has declined in real terms over the past two decades, and the report recommended a funding increase.

DAVID SPIEGEL, M.D.

Nutrition and Diet

New Nutrient Guidelines Postponed • Should Children Eat Less Fat and Cholesterol? • Importance of Good Nutrition Before Pregnancy • The Calcium Craze

Nutrient Guidelines Controversy

Proposed changes in the Recommended Daily Dietary Allowances (RDA's) for some vitamins and minerals provoked sharp debate among scientists in 1985. In September the New York *Times* reported that a draft report by the Committee on Dietary Allowances of the U.S. National Academy of Sciences recommended reducing the RDA's for vitamins A, C, and B_6, magnesium, iron, and zinc and raising the calcium RDA's for women. In October the academy's president announced that revised RDA's would not be issued "at this time" because "an impasse" had developed between the committee and the nutrition scientists who reviewed the report. He said that many reviewers believed that the committee's recommendations for some nutrients were not fully justified by the evidence it presented. The academy had never experienced such a deadlock over its guidelines on dietary allowances, issued every four or five years since 1943.

The RDA for any particular nutrient is the average daily amount that should be consumed over a period of time to maintain good health in the majority (95 percent or more) of healthy Americans. Separate RDA's are determined for age groups from infancy through old age and for males and females in the groups after early childhood. Special RDA's are set for pregnant and breast-feeding (lactating) women.

The RDA's are of much more than academic importance. Many food programs are based on them. The federal school lunch program requires that each meal contain one-third of the RDA for several nutrients. Food stamp allotments are designed to permit the purchase of a combination of foods that supplies 100 percent of the RDA's. The federal Women, Infants, and Children Program takes the RDA's into account in determining the food supplements it provides to pregnant and nursing women and young children in low-income families. Labels on food packages give the quantities of certain nutrients in the product as percentages of the U.S. Recommended Daily Allowances (U.S. RDA's), which are derived by the Food and Drug Administration from the RDA's set by the National Academy of Sciences.

How did the impasse over revising the RDA's come about? How could well-qualified scientists presented with the same information come to such divergent conclusions? The answer lies partly in the definition of the RDA's as the amounts of nutrients needed to maintain good health. The concept of good health is imprecise. To some people it means the absence of any overt signs of disease—in this case, disease stemming from a nutrient deficiency. To others it means that the body's reserves of particular nutrients are maintained at a maximum level. To still others, it means that particular nutrients are being consumed in amounts sufficient to offer maximum protection against diseases like cancer and the common cold that are not caused by a deficiency of these nutrients. Clearly, recommendations as to how much of a nutrient is needed will vary according to which definition of good health is used.

On the whole, medical science is moving toward a broader definition of good health. Most doctors would agree that a person who does not have enough of a nutrient stored up in the body to cover periods when the need for that nutrient may increase is not in the best possible health. Nor could a person who is not consuming enough of a nutrient to offer maximum protection against, say, cancer or heart attacks be considered in the best health. Women, for example, should consume enough iron not only to prevent anemia but also to protect them if their need for iron should increase because of abnormal bleeding or pregnancy. The same is true for calcium. Individuals should take in enough of this mineral not only to guard against such problems connected with calcium deficiency as rickets and osteomalacia but also to prevent, to the extent possible, the development of osteoporosis—the brittle bones of old age.

Still, there are many matters over which experts will disagree. A number of scientists have advised Americans to consume more foods containing vitamins A and C to ensure maximum protection against certain cancers. But how much more must be consumed to offer maximum protection? The answer is not known. In this and some other cases, scientists charged with establishing RDA's must try to derive a precise number from inadequate data. They must use their judgment, and the judgment of reasonable people can differ.

From a practical standpoint the academy's decision to delay revising the RDA's was a good one. Since changes in the RDA's would affect many federal and state food programs, they should not be made unless the need for them is clearly and objectively documented. The scientific differences may be resolved in the next year or so. The establishment of new RDA's may then follow. In the meantime, the existing RDA's, issued in 1980, will remain in use.

Fat, Cholesterol, and Children

How much fat and cholesterol young children should consume is another issue that has recently provoked controversy. In 1984 a panel of experts convened by the U.S. National Institutes of Health recommended that Americans over the age of two change their diets so that no more than 30 percent of total calories comes from fat (the existing average then was about 40 percent), with no more than 10 percent of total calories from saturated fat. In addition, the committee urged that the intake of cholesterol be kept to 300 milligrams a day or less. But a number of scientific groups, including the American Academy of Pediatrics, did not accept the inclusion of young children in the recommendations. The basic question was whether the benefits of cutting dietary fat and cholesterol outweighed the risks.

The panel's recommendations reflected evidence suggesting that reducing fat and cholesterol intake might help ward off or delay the deterioration and clogging of arteries known as atherosclerosis. When this condition affects coronary arteries—those leading to the heart—it can lead to heart attacks.

It is clear that atherosclerosis can begin relatively early in life. Signs of its development have often been seen in autopsies on young soldiers killed in wars as well as on young adults killed in accidents. It would seem logical, therefore, to introduce preventive measures, such as dietary changes, at as early an age as possible.

Those who argue against applying the fat and cholesterol recommendations to children point out that the effects of such changes have not been systematically studied in this age group. Very young children (ages two to five) might actually benefit if they took in more than 30 percent of their calories as fat and consumed more than 300 milligrams of cholesterol a day. In addition, some scientists fear that endorsing the recommendations might encourage parents to reduce the fat and cholesterol intake of infants.

For young children, no studies have shown that lowering the levels of cholesterol in the blood would affect the incidence of coronary artery disease. At the same time, scientists agree that very young infants have a relatively higher fat requirement than adults. They need energy in a concentrated form, and they need specific fatty acids. They probably also have a greater requirement for cholesterol. These extra needs are in part due to the rapid growth of the brain in early life; the sheaths surrounding the nerves and the areas around some of the nerve connections are made up largely of fat and contain large amounts of cholesterol. Breast milk has half of its calories in the form of fat and is high in cholesterol. Although nobody is recommending dietary modifications for very young infants, the age at which such modifications should be made is not clear, and some scientists think that two years is too young.

In my judgment, not all young children need be placed on a modified-fat, low-cholesterol diet. Changes in diet are called for, however, when children are at risk of developing heart disease because of family history or because of high cholesterol levels in the blood. Parents and health professionals must determine which children are at risk.

LOOKING BACKWARD

Could it be that the best cure for what ails us is to return to the diet of our Stone Age ancestors?

An anthropologist and a physician at Emory University in Atlanta, investigating the eating habits of the Paleolithic people who lived before the dawn of agriculture, have pointed out that this diet was mostly game, fruits, tubers, and nuts. Although the Stone Age people ate considerable meat, it was from wild game and lean. They ate no dairy products but obtained substantial calcium from other sources. In general, the diet was high in fiber content and rich in vitamins, minerals, and protein.

The researchers were able to figure out the Stone Age diet by studying the eating practices of the few remaining hunting/gathering societies, which are mostly free from the so-called diseases of civilization—high blood pressure, diabetes, heart disease, and certain types of cancer.

Although we hope we have progressed a great distance, culturally, from the first humans of 40,000 years ago, we're constitutionally the same and may very well be genetically programmed for their diet. At any rate, the Stone Age menu bears some startling resemblances to the current nutritional recommendations of such health experts as the American Cancer Society and American Heart Association.

Nutrition Prior to Pregnancy

During the past decade extensive research has shown how important good nutrition is to pregnant women. More recently it has become clear that the health of both the pregnant woman and her fetus depend to a large degree also on the woman's eating habits and general state of health before the child is conceived.

Good nutrition is important before conception for two reasons. First, if a woman waits until she knows she is pregnant before adopting good eating habits, she will have missed the first few weeks of fetal development. During this early period, when a great deal of fetal growth occurs, good nutrition can provide major benefits. Second, certain nutrients will be drained from the mother's body during pregnancy, and so adequate stores of these nutrients should be built up beforehand.

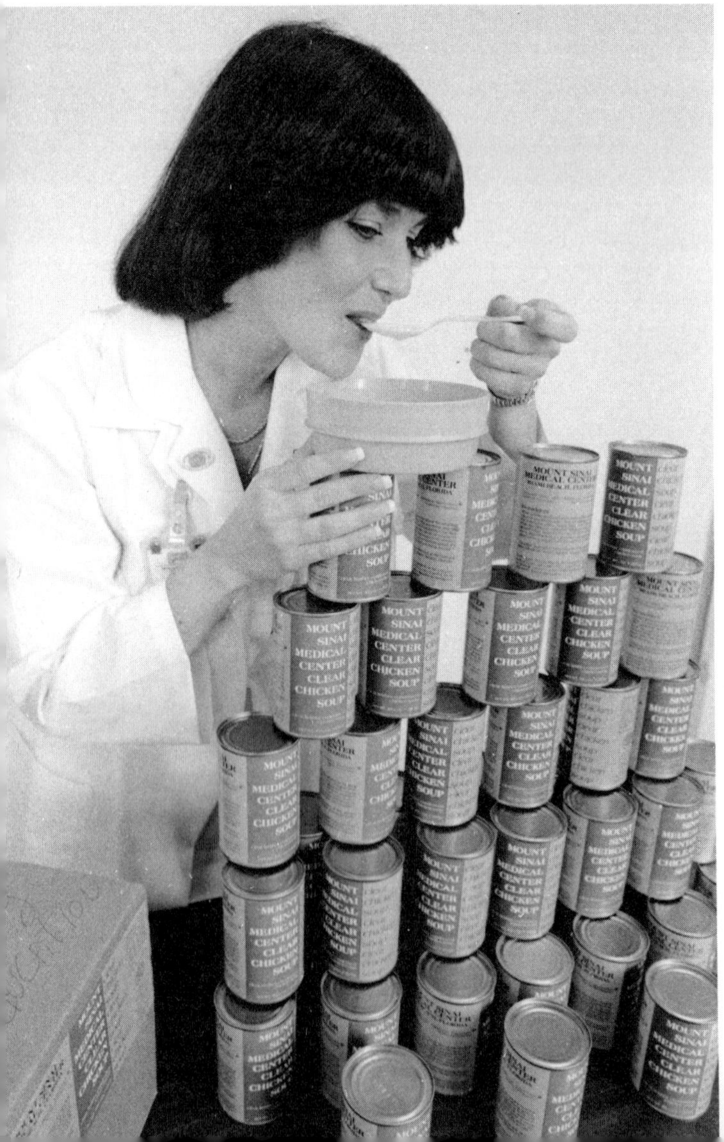

Mom's chicken soup, the favorite all-time remedy for colds and flu, became available in new packaging at the gift shop of Mount Sinai Medical Center in Miami Beach, Fla., after a study showed that hot chicken soup really is effective in relieving congestion. What is possibly missing: Mom's tender loving care?

Today, more and more women are planning their pregnancies. The mother-to-be can take certain simple steps to help insure a smooth course for both herself and her infant. Before becoming pregnant, she should try to bring her weight to within 10 percent of her ideal body weight. The woman who is near her ideal weight before pregnancy should gain about 25 to 30 pounds while pregnant. For an underweight woman, it is easier—and may be healthier—to catch up to the ideal body weight before becoming pregnant. If a woman is overweight, she must still gain at least 15 pounds during pregnancy. The time to lose weight, therefore, is before pregnancy. Weight loss during pregnancy should never be attempted.

A woman needs more of all vitamins and minerals when she is pregnant. During the earliest stages of pregnancy the vitamin called folic acid is especially important for the developing fetus. Consequently, the woman planning a baby should make sure her intake of this vitamin before conception is adequate. Some oral contraceptives interfere with the absorption and processing of folic acid by the body; women who have been taking these contraceptives may be at increased risk for folic acid deficiency. For this reason, a woman planning to become pregnant should begin taking a prenatal vitamin preparation. The preparation should also contain iron. Many American women do not consume enough of this nutrient. Moreover, the body's reserves of it can easily be depleted during pregnancy.

An intolerance of lactose (milk sugar) is a common problem, and many pregnant women find it difficult to consume large enough amounts of dairy products to meet their increased requirement for calcium. Such women are now routinely prescribed calcium supplements while they are pregnant and nursing. Again, it is better for them to start taking the supplements before they become pregnant so that they can build their reserves of calcium and cover the early period of pregnancy.

The Calcium Phenomenon

Calcium emerged as a hot ticket in supermarkets, health food stores, and drug stores in 1985. The dairy and drug industries rushed to meet an explosion in demand. Sales of calcium supplements (now available in a potpourri of forms—powders, tablets, liquids, gels, gums, mints) were up sevenfold from 1980.

Nutrition experts have always recognized the mineral's importance to good health. The new craze for calcium probably owes its origins to a well-publicized conference on osteoporosis that was convened by the National Institutes of Health in 1984. The conference

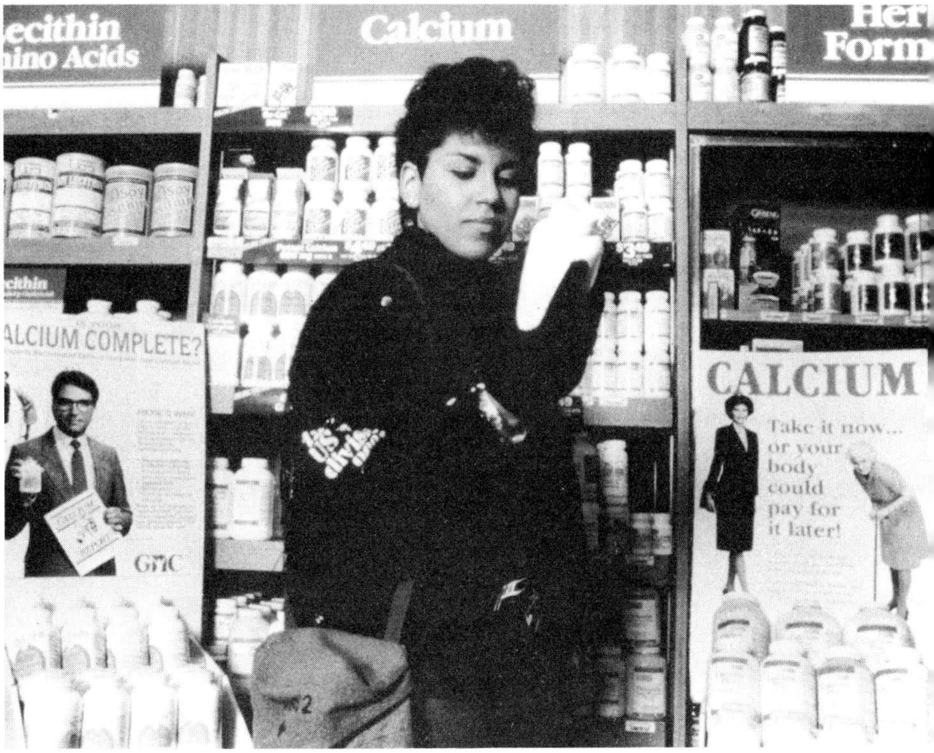

The sales of calcium supplements boomed as the public became aware of the role of calcium in helping to prevent the bone disease osteoporosis.

called calcium and the female hormone estrogen the "mainstays of prevention and management" of the disease. The public's interest was further stimulated by high-power marketing campaigns conducted by the dairy industry and calcium supplement makers. Also fueling the calcium boom were tentative research findings suggesting that adding more calcium to the diet might protect against high blood pressure and colon cancer in some people.

The craze for calcium has a dark side. Some supplement products contain lead and other toxic metals. There is also the danger that users of supplements may consume excessive amounts. Too much calcium may upset the body's absorption of iron, zinc, and manganese, may be constipating, and may cause kidney stones.

Many individuals, it is true, are not now getting enough calcium, but very often a change in diet is all that is needed. The present RDA is 800 milligrams for most people. (It is 1,200 milligrams for adolescents aged 11 to 18 and for pregnant and lactating women.) Many authorities believe all women need more than 800 milligrams, especially after menopause. Dairy products are the most obvious dietary sources of calcium. A single glass of milk provides over 290 milligrams; a single cup of plain, low fat yogurt, 415. Other foods high in calcium include tofu, raw oysters, sardines with bones, broccoli, and collard greens.

Regulating Appetite

Scientists are devoting more and more attention to the processes by which appetite is controlled. Such research has the potential to substantially increase doctors' understanding of, and ability to control, such problems as obesity, anorexia (the "self-starving illness"), and bulimia (uncontrolled binge eating). A number of recent studies on appetite regulation have focused on the potential roles played by certain chemical substances produced in the body.

Because the hypothalamus has long been known to be the area of the brain that controls appetite, some researchers have sought to determine the role, if any, played by endorphins. These chemicals, which resemble morphine in their effects, are produced by the hypothalamus and are involved in the processes by which pain is perceived and blocked. Studies with animals have found a link between increased levels of endorphins and increased feeding behavior. In addition, it appears that certain external factors can directly affect the release of endorphins and indirectly influence appetite. In animal experiments, for example, increasing the carbohydrate content of the diet stimulated the release of endorphins. Thus, feeling hungry or sated after eating may largely depend on what is eaten, which influences the release by the brain of special chemicals involved in appetite regulation.

The gastrointestinal tract also produces substances involved in the control of appetite. Cholecystokinin, a hormone secreted by the wall of the small intestine, acts to depress appetite. Animal experiments have shown that cholecystokinin is able in some way to signal the brain to alter feeding behavior. The signal seems to be transmitted through the vagus nerves, which run to the brain.

Irradiation of Pork Approved

The use of low-level radiation on food as an alternative to chemical preservatives has taken a major step toward general acceptance in the United States. The sale of irradiated pork to consumers was approved in January 1986 by the U.S. Department of Agriculture. The Food and Drug Administration (FDA) had given its preliminary approval in 1985, and late in the year it also gave preliminary approval to the irradiation of fresh fruits and vegetables. The go-ahead on pork was the first U.S. authorization for irradiation of food sold directly to the consumer. In 1983 approval was granted for the irradiation of spices.

In the irradiation process, the food products are transported on a conveyor belt to a chamber where they are exposed to gamma rays, usually from cobalt-60, an isotope produced in nuclear reactors. The food products do not become radioactive. In pork, the process kills an organism that causes trichinosis.

Although food irradiation is in use in over two dozen countries, it remains controversial. Proponents argue that it uses far less energy than freezing or canning and claim it is safer than chemical additives. Opponents say the technique destroys certain nutrients in foods and has not been adequately tested for safety.

Medical Schools Faulted

American medical schools provide too little instruction about food and nutrition, according to a mid-1985 report from the Committee on Nutrition in Medical Education of the National Academy of Sciences. The report, based on a survey of over a third of the medical schools in the United States, followed an explosion of new information in recent years linking good nutrition to the maintenance of health and the prevention of disease—information that physicians must be able to use to benefit their patients. Doctors' general lack of training in nutrition, coupled with a lack of interest in the subject on the part of many physicians, has led the public to seek alternative sources of nutrition information. Of all health fields, nutrition is the one most saturated with self-styled experts. Much of their advice is not based on any scientific data, and some of it is dangerous.

The committee recommended that medical schools provide a minimum of 25 to 30 hours of basic nutrition information. (A fifth of the schools studied were offering less than 10, and the average was 21.) The panel also called for more nutrition research and more and better-organized nutrition departments. The recommendations are being widely discussed by medical educators, and some are already being implemented.

See also the feature articles THE FACTS ABOUT SWEETENERS *and* FISH IN THE DIET *and the Spotlight on Health articles* PREVENTING OSTEOPOROSIS, HOW TO READ FOOD LABELS, *and* THE IMPORTANCE OF IRON.

MYRON WINICK, M.D.

Obstetrics and Gynecology

Ultrasound Guidance Helps In Vitro Fertilization • What Should Be Done With "Surplus" Frozen Embryos? • First U.S. Septuplets

Harvesting Egg Cells

New technique. An ultrasound-guided, nonsurgical method of collecting egg cells has been developed for use in "test-tube" fertilization (actually called in vitro fertilization). The new technique has several advantages over laparoscopy, the traditional surgical method used to harvest egg cells. While laparoscopy is still the favored means in North America, several U.S. centers are adopting the new method, developed in Europe and called transvaginal oocyte (egg cell) retrieval.

As with all techniques for harvesting eggs, in transvaginal oocyte retrieval the woman first takes a hormone that stimulates her ovaries to produce a number of eggs instead of only one. Several days later, an ultrasound monitor is passed over the woman's abdomen to pinpoint the precise location of the maturing oocytes within the ovaries. After administering a local anesthetic, the doctor inserts a needle through the vaginal wall (again using ultrasound to guide the needle's path) to the spot where fluid containing the oocytes can be sucked up into the needle and withdrawn from the body. In contrast, laparoscopy is more invasive and expensive and requires general anesthesia. A viewing instrument—the laparoscope—is inserted through an incision in the abdominal wall to enable the doctor to see the ovaries. A needle is inserted through a second incision to suck up the egg cells.

The egg cells collected in either way are incubated for several hours to allow them to mature, and then they are fertilized with the husband's sperm. Several of the fertilized eggs are inserted with a needle into the woman's uterus where, it is hoped, at least one will lead to a healthy pregnancy and delivery.

Raising ethical problems. Improved harvesting techniques have made it practical for in vitro fertilization specialists to remove up to 25 egg cells from a woman at one time. After fertilization in the laboratory, those not immediately implanted in the woman's uterus can be frozen using the method of cryopreservation, first developed in Australia. They can then be stored for possible future use—for example, if the first attempt at achieving pregnancy fails. Experience with cryopreservation has shown that most of these fertilized eggs can survive the freezing and thawing processes and still develop into normal fetuses.

A still unresolved question is the fate of any "surplus" frozen embryos. Although they are simple organisms, consisting of perhaps four to eight cells, each is nevertheless endowed with a specific genetic makeup and is capable of developing into an individual if placed in the uterus of a willing recipient. While society debates such questions, innovative methods like transvaginal oocyte retrieval are helping to sustain the remarkable pace of progress that in vitro fertilization specialists have achieved.

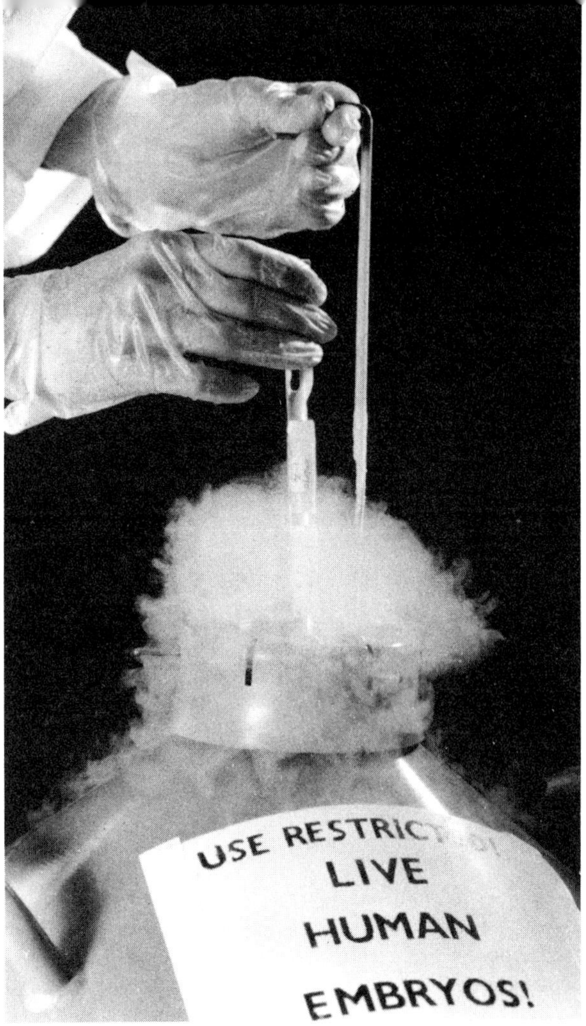

In the freezing technique called cryopreservation, a vial containing a human embryo is submerged in a tank of liquid nitrogen. The frozen embryos can be safely stored until they are thawed and implanted in a woman's uterus.

First U.S. Septuplets

On May 21, 1985, in the largest multiple birth ever recorded in the United States, Patti Frustaci of Orange, Calif., gave birth to seven diminutive infants; the last to be delivered, a girl, was stillborn. The babies were delivered by cesarean 12 weeks prematurely; the surviving two girls and four boys weighed from 1 pound, 1 ounce, to 1 pound, 13 ounces. Mrs. Frustaci and her husband, Sam, had been treated at an infertility clinic, and she had been given Pergonal, the same fertility drug that had enabled her to have her first child (a single pregnancy). About 20 percent of pregnancies achieved with Pergonal are multiple births, usually twins.

The six newborns all suffered from medical problems associated with their premature birth, the most serious of which was hyaline membrane disease, a condition of immature lungs. By mid-June, three of the six had died. The surviving three finally were able to leave the hospital, but they continued to need constant monitoring and ongoing medical attention. In October 1985 the Frustacis filed a $3.2 million suit against their fertility specialist and the clinic they had attended, accusing the defendants of having incorrectly administered Pergonal and of having failed to properly monitor Mrs. Frustaci's progress on the drug.

Risks of Multiple Births

Obstetricians appear to be rediscovering a fact that has long gone unheeded—that while twin and other multiple births are relatively uncommon, they account for a disproportionately large number of perinatal (fetal and newborn) deaths and medical problems. Multiple-birth babies are vulnerable in a number of ways. They are more likely to be born underweight, a major risk factor in perinatal deaths, and more likely to be born prematurely. Also common are breech or other abnormal birth presentations, in which a part of the body other than the baby's head emerges first, and other delivery problems. The mother is more likely to suffer from complications of pregnancy, like anemia and high blood pressure, that sometimes affect the babies.

With the growing awareness that multiple-birth mothers have special needs both before and during birth, various measures that their physicians can take are receiving particular emphasis. A series of ultrasound scans should be performed in the later stages of pregnancy to determine whether the fetuses are growing normally. So-called nonstress tests of each fetus are advisable in late pregnancy. Here, the mother, with the help of an instrument called a fetal monitor, counts how often the baby moves during a certain time period; the number of movements is an indicator of whether the baby is developing normally. The obstetrician should also decide in advance, at least tentatively, whether the babies will be delivered by cesarean or by normal vaginal delivery, usually based on considerations that include the position of the babies in the uterus and the size differences between the twins.

Patti Frustaci, shown with her husband visiting one of their newborn children, gave birth to seven babies in the largest multiple birth ever recorded in the United States. One of the infants was stillborn; three others died soon after birth.

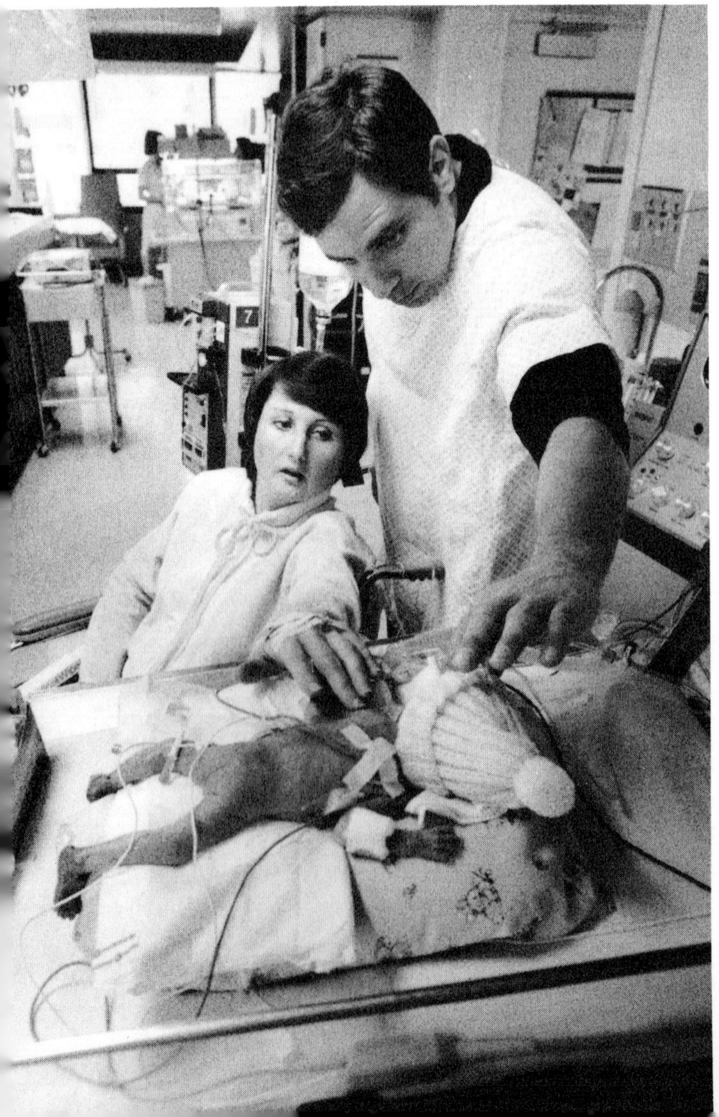

Treating Preeclampsia

A combination of drugs shows promise in treating preeclampsia, a condition of late pregnancy that affects 5 to 10 percent of pregnant women (particularly those pregnant for the first time). Preeclampsia is characterized by a rise in blood pressure, blurred vision, and "puffiness," a signal that too much body fluid is being retained. It may be related to the retarded growth of some fetuses, since chronic high blood pressure in the mother decreases the supply to the fetus of oxygen and nutrients carried in the mother's bloodstream. Preeclampsia may develop into full eclampsia, a potentially life-threatening disorder to mother and baby.

Although some experts continue to emphasize traditional findings indicating a relationship between malnutrition and the development of preeclampsia and eclampsia, the cause of these conditions remains essentially unknown, and investigators have expanded their efforts to identify hereditary, immunologic, and circulatory factors that might play a role. At the same time, a possible way to effectively manage the high blood pressure that occurs in preeclampsia was suggested by an Australian study published in 1985. These workers reported that they treated women with the blood pressure drugs clonidine (sold as Catapres and Combipres) and methyldopa (Aldoclor, Aldomet, and Aldoril) and with hydralazine, a drug with various brand names, which widens blood vessels. If started before the 32nd week of pregnancy, the medications appeared to ensure relatively normal growth and development of the fetus and to result in fewer fetal and newborn deaths. These findings, if confirmed by other investigators, suggest that treatment with antihypertension drugs, while inadvisable and potentially dangerous for the fetus after the 32nd week, may be useful in treating women who have not yet reached that point in their pregnancy.

New Delivery Method

The year 1985 witnessed modest progress in the United States (though not in Canada) toward greater use of the vacuum extractor, an instrument for assisting difficult vaginal deliveries. The vacuum extractor has already largely replaced forceps in virtually all other parts of the world. The vacuum extractor consists of a small suction cap that is attached to the baby's head. A vacuum is created by means of a pump connected to the cap, permitting gentle suction to be applied in order to draw the rest of the body out of the birth canal.

In the extractors used outside the United States, the cap is generally made of metal, but plastic, "soft-cup" extractors are the ones gaining in popularity among U.S. obstetricians. Several recent studies of deliveries with this type of extractor reported less damage to the

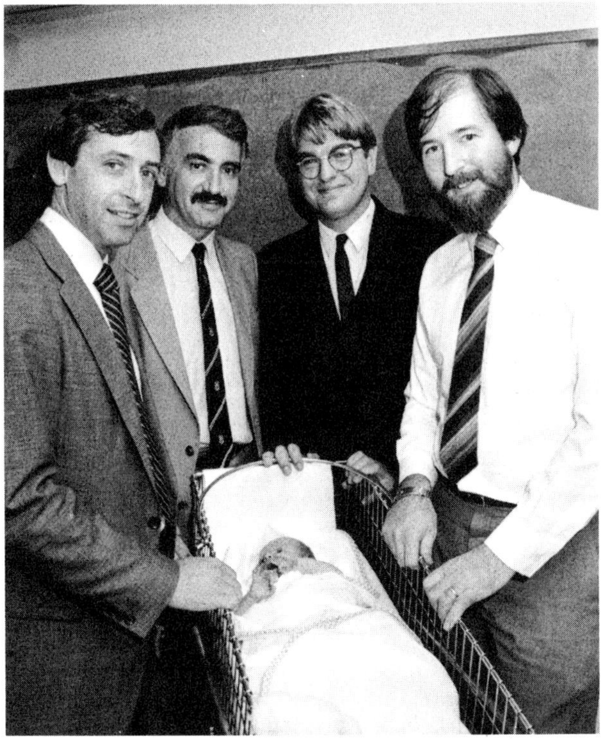

The Melbourne medical team responsible for baby Joseph.

ANOTHER IN VITRO FIRST

Joseph, born on March 28, 1985, in Australia, was not among the first "test-tube" babies, but he was unusual nonetheless. This was apparently the first time that in vitro fertilization was used successfully to overcome an infertility problem in a man rather than a woman.

Because of a vasectomy that could not be reversed, Joseph's father was unable to ejaculate sperm. A normal male ejaculation has over 100 million active sperm, enough to make it reasonably likely that some will manage to traverse the arduous course into the fallopian tubes to reach an egg cell waiting to be fertilized.

Doctors at Melbourne's Monash University decided to try the in vitro technique (in which fertilization takes place in laboratory glassware) because it requires relatively small numbers of sperm. They extracted a moderate quantity from the father-to-be and combined it with eggs taken from his wife. One egg was successfully fertilized and then inserted into her womb. The happy result, weighing 7 pounds at birth, was Joseph.

mother's vaginal tissues and less maternal blood loss than with forceps delivery, as well as fewer cases in which the baby's scalp was affected.

Understanding Difficult Labor

Growing attention is focusing on understanding and preventing shoulder dystocia, a serious problem that leads to the impairment and even death of babies during childbirth. Dystocia is a general medical term meaning difficult labor. During a normal delivery, the baby's shoulders, arms, and trunk follow the head rapidly out of the birth canal. But in shoulder dystocia, the birth process appears to be delayed—arrested—after the head has emerged but before the shoulders have followed.

Recent reports emphasize several factors that may cause arrest of the shoulders during birth. These include fetal macrosomia (the medical term for a very large fetus); administering oxytocin, a drug that stimulates the uterus to contract, to the mother during an earlier stage of labor (this exhausts the uterus to the point where it cannot continue to contract); labor (in which oxytocin has not been used) that seems to come to a stop; and treatment of the last with difficult forceps extraction procedures. A consensus of opinion has developed among obstetrical experts that a cesarean should be performed in most cases if a fetus weighs 10 pounds or even approaches that weight. In addition, physicians should understand that in the normal process of delivery, expulsion of the head and of the rest of the body normally require two separate uterine contractions. Many tragic cases of shoulder dystocia could probably be prevented if, after the baby's head has emerged, obstetricians waited for the next uterine contraction to occur before trying to extract the baby's body. The force of this contraction can be increased by giving oxytocin for the first time at this point.

Tubal Pregnancy

Would many of the tubal pregnancies that have not reached the stage of rupture simply resolve themselves naturally, without surgery? This surprising concept was recently presented about a dangerous problem that has been widely reported as occurring with increasing frequency in virtually all populations of the world.

A tubal pregnancy is one type of ectopic pregnancy,

the medical term describing a fertilized egg that becomes implanted outside the uterus, usually in a fallopian tube. Symptoms include persistent and worsening abdominal pain and vaginal bleeding; internal bleeding may also occur and lead to shock. The developing egg can cause the tube to rupture, which may cause severe internal bleeding, threatening the life of the mother. For this reason, a diagnosis of ectopic pregnancy has traditionally been followed by surgery to remove the fetus—since it cannot survive—and either repair or remove the tube. Since the symptoms that signal ectopic pregnancy can also be caused by other conditions, and since the outcome of these pregnancies is potentially grave, accurate and early diagnosis is both difficult and important.

Against this background, information presented in 1985 indicating that without surgery, most ectopic pregnancies would subside by themselves, is of great interest. It has long been known the "occult" (hidden) ectopic pregnancies do occur—in other words, that occasionally an ectopic pregnancy begins and ends without the patient (or her doctor) ever being aware of it. It is also a well-established fact that most human conceptions end in "occult abortion"; the fertilized egg simply fails to survive. If it turns out that, rather than being the exception, most ectopic pregnancies do indeed end on their own, then many prevailing concepts concerning human reproduction in general and ectopic pregnancy in particular are bound to change.

This new observation also suggests that the increasing incidence of ectopic pregnancies reported over the past several decades is not a true increase; rather, it results primarily from physicians' improved ability to diagnose ectopic pregnancy. This could mean that the majority of cases in which gynecologists performed "life-saving" surgery in recent years might have abated by themselves. Such a view is likely to raise considerable controversy and perhaps lead to a useful reconsideration of the entire subject of ectopic pregnancy.

Childbirth Risks in Older Women

With a growing number of women waiting until their 30's to have children, encouraging news was reported in January 1986: pregnancy-related deaths in women 35 and older are declining. For every 100,000 live births among this age group in the United States in 1974-1978, there were 47.5 maternal deaths; by 1982, the rate had dropped by about 50 percent to 24.2. In comparison, the maternal death rate for all age groups over the same time period declined by 34 percent.

The researchers attributed at least part of the decline to the fact that an increasing proportion of mothers 35 and older have relatively high incomes and educational levels. Medical advances in treating complications of pregnancy and childbirth also account for some of the decline, in this and all age groups. Despite the declining death rate, women 35 and older are still approximately three times more likely to die from pregnancy-related cases than younger women. Furthermore, the data must be interpreted with the awareness that U.S. maternal death rates are known to be underreported.

See also the Spotlight on Health articles CESAREANS: WHEN ARE THEY NEEDED? *and* IUD'S.

LESLIE IFFY, M.D.

Pediatrics

A Vaccine for Meningitis • Breathing Help for Premature Babies • New Ways to Diagnose Ear and Throat Infections • Baboon Heart Transplant Assailed

New Meningitis Vaccine

A vaccine against the leading cause of bacterial meningitis was approved for general use in the United States in 1985 and in Canada in early 1986. This disease, which occurs when bacteria invade the lining of the brain and spinal cord, can have effects ranging from seizures and hearing loss to mental retardation and death. The vaccine prevents infection with a bacterium known as *Haemophilus influenzae* type b (or *H. influenzae*), which in addition to meningitis can cause a variety of other serious infections. This organism most often attacks children under five years of age and can be spread from one child to another. The vaccine is particularly important because treatment of *H. influenzae* disease with antibiotics is not always successful, and by the time symptoms of the disease appear, the infection may have already done permanent damage.

Scientists have known for many years that the body defends itself against *H. influenzae* by producing protective substances called antibodies that attach to the outer coating, or capsule, of the bacterium, eventually destroying it. The new vaccine, which contains purified pieces of the coating from killed *H. influenzae* bacteria, prevents disease by stimulating the body to form such antibodies. Studies in Finland, using an identical vaccine to immunize thousands of children, have shown that the product is extremely safe. The major drawback of the *H. influenzae* vaccine (officially called Haemophilus b polysaccharide vaccine) is that it does not prevent disease in children less than 18 months old, since they usually cannot produce antibodies against *H. influenzae* bacteria. On the other hand, the vaccine is highly effective in children two years of age or older, and possibly effective in those 18 to 23 months old. On the basis of this information, two major advisory groups—the American Academy of Pediatrics and the U.S. Centers for Disease Control—have recommended that all children be immunized routinely with Haemophilus b polysaccharide vaccine at two years of age or shortly thereafter.

Although the vaccine undoubtedly will prevent thousands of cases of *H. influenzae* illness, a more effective vaccine is needed for children under two years of age. Researchers currently are testing several promising vaccines that may protect children in this age group.

Premature Infants

A study reported from Toronto in 1985 found that early treatment of premature infants with surfactant may help prevent or alleviate a disease caused by the absence of this substance in their lungs. The disorder, one of the most common and serious illnesses afflicting premature newborns, is called hyaline membrane disease or respiratory distress syndrome.

Surfactant ordinarily coats the surface of the lungs and keeps the smallest air passages open. Without this essential ingredient, which a premature infant's lungs are too undeveloped to produce, portions of the lungs tend to collapse, preventing the newborn from receiving an adequate amount of oxygen. Standard treatment of hyaline membrane disease involves supplying additional oxygen and, often, mechanical ventilation (a machine that "breathes" for the infant). Although these measures may be life-saving, they can produce a number of side effects, such as eye disease or long-term damage to the lungs.

The idea of preventing hyaline membrane disease by treating immature lungs with surfactant has appealed to scientists for a long time, but only recently has this strategy been carried out in premature newborns. In the Toronto study, one group of 39 premature newborns had surfactant from an animal source sprayed directly into their lungs immediately after birth; for comparison, a second group of 33 premature infants were not given surfactant. Each group otherwise received similar treatment. The researchers found that newborns treated with surfactant were able to breathe better; that is, they required less additional oxygen and less time on the ventilator. They also had less evidence of lung damage than babies not receiving surfactant. Although treatment with surfactant was beneficial overall, many of the treated infants still developed hyaline membrane disease. Nevertheless, the use of surfactant represents a major step in treating premature infants.

Detecting Ear Infections

An innovative device called the acoustic otoscope uses sound waves to detect a common affliction of childhood: middle ear infection, or otitis media. Most children have at least one case of otitis media during the first three years of life, and some children experience many episodes. In otitis media, fluid builds up in the middle ear, the cavity behind the eardrum, and becomes infected. Usually a doctor detects the presence of fluid by direct examination of the eardrum, using a device called a pneumatic otoscope. Unfortunately, in many children the small size of their ears or the presence of wax or debris in front of the eardrum prevents the examiner from making an accurate diagnosis.

These small obstructions don't seriously affect the precision of the acoustic otoscope, which works by bouncing sound waves off the eardrum and recording the reflected sound when it returns to the instrument. When the middle ear cavity contains fluid, the eardrum becomes stiff, causing it to reflect more sound than in its normally flexible condition. The acoustic otoscope offers several advantages over the pneumatic device: it's less dependent on the examiner's skill and judgment, faster, more comfortable for the patient, and bet-

The common childhood ailment otitis media (middle ear infection) can now be identified painlessly and accurately by the acoustic otoscope, which uses sound waves to detect fluid in the middle ear.

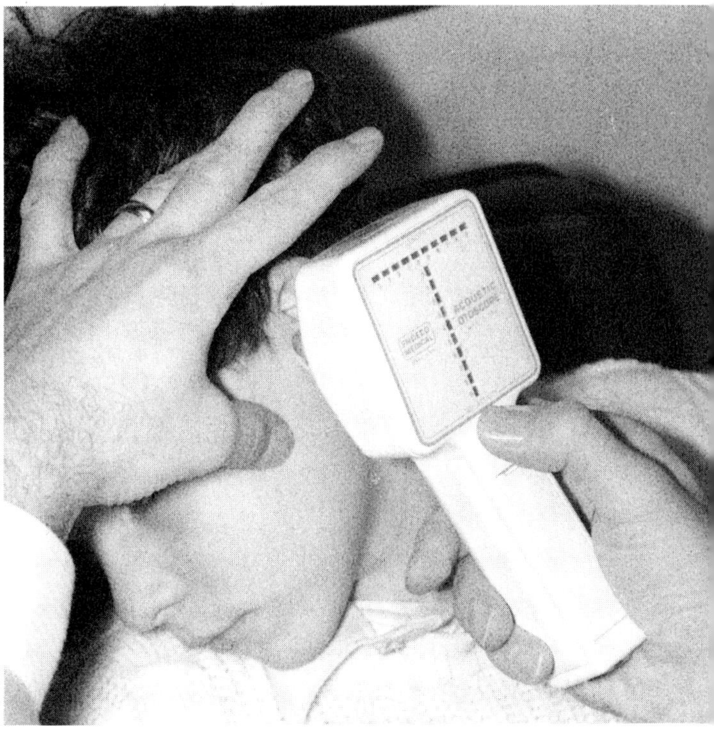

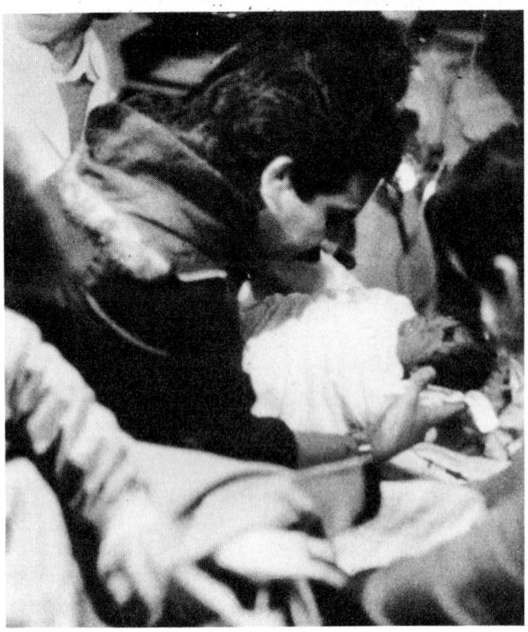

SURVIVAL OF THE FRAILEST

The earthquakes that struck Mexico in September 1985 claimed thousands of lives and left large areas of Mexico City devastated. But amid the rubble there was a sign of hope—the remarkable rescue of at least 45 infants, mostly newborns, trapped in the wreckage of Juárez and General hospitals for up to nine days. Many suffered from dehydration, kidney problems, infections, or fractures, and two died not long after they were found. But the others were expected to make full recoveries, although the possibility remained of some lingering psychological effects.

How did the infants survive the disaster? Speculations were that the babies' small size helped them avoid being hit by falling debris; that they lived off the excess fat and fluids with which babies are born; that some were kept warm for a time by the bodies of dying adults. With their undeveloped minds, the infants may have been immune to the terror and shock experienced by adults; also, fresh from the womb, newborns would be better able to endure a dark and cramped environment. But, as one Mexican physician commented: "The truth is that although we are doctors, we think it is a miracle."

ter able to evaluate the eardrum in the presence of wax. Although it is extremely accurate, occasional false readings occur; therefore it is likely to supplement, rather than replace, the traditional ear examination.

Rapid Diagnosis of Strep Throat

Several quick tests became available in 1984 and 1985 to diagnose throat infections caused by the *Streptococcus* bacterium—infections that are commonly called strep throat. With a quick diagnosis of strep throat, antibiotic treatment can be started right away.

Most throat infections in children are caused by either streptococcal bacteria or viruses. The distinction between the two types of infection is important because antibiotics are effective against bacteria, but not viruses. For many years, the diagnosis of strep throat has been based on the throat culture, in which a specimen from a patient's infected throat is put on a special plate where the *Streptococcus* will grow if it is present. This procedure is accurate but quite slow, often taking 24 to 48 hours to verify the diagnosis. Since many physicians like to confirm the diagnosis of streptococcal infection before prescribing antibiotics, treatment may be delayed for several days. With the new tests, results are usually available within an hour.

Although the individual quick tests vary, all work by recognizing parts of the bacteria called antigens. The specimen is obtained by swabbing the throat with a cotton-tipped applicator, and the antigens are identified directly from the throat swab after the addition of special chemicals. Most of the rapid tests compare favorably to the throat culture, although some tests may miss up to 20 percent of infections.

Ending Epilepsy Treatment

Seizure medications can be safely stopped in most children with epilepsy who have not had any seizures for at least two years, according to a 1985 study from the Johns Hopkins University School of Medicine.

Epilepsy, a brain disorder that affects up to 1 to 2 percent of the population, usually begins in childhood. Epileptic seizures occur when the brain's normal electrical waves become disorganized. In most patients, epilepsy can be controlled successfully with drugs, but unfortunately many of these have undesirable side effects. Although many children appear to outgrow the need for medication as they get older, doctors have tended to continue such treatment for many years to prevent the return of seizures.

In the new study, medications were discontinued in 88 children who had not had any seizures for at least two years, and the children were monitored closely for up to five years. At the end of the study, 66 children (three-fourths of the group) were still free of seizures. By looking at a recording of the brain's electrical activity, called an electroencephalogram (EEG), the type of seizures they had had, and the age when seizures began, the researchers found they could predict which children were likely to remain free of seizures.

See also the Spotlight on Health article TREATING EPILEPSY.

Baby Fae Controversy

The transplanting of a baboon heart into the newborn infant Baby Fae in 1984 was strongly criticized in an editorial published in the *Journal of the American Medical Association* in December 1985. Baby Fae, who had been born with a fatal heart defect, died 20 days after Dr. Leonard Bailey implanted the baboon heart in October 1984. The editorial, written by two other doctors, said that Bailey's belief that an infant's immature immune system wasn't capable of a strong rejection response to foreign tissue was "wishful thinking." Bailey himself had admitted that he had made a grave error when he used a heart from a baboon with a different blood type from Baby Fae. Because of this incompatibility her immune system produced antibodies against the baboon's red blood cells, causing them to clump together and clog the heart and other organs. The editorial concluded that the operation was doomed to failure in any case because baboons are too genetically dissimilar to humans, and that such interspecies transplants are not feasible given the current state of medical knowledge.

In an article in the same issue of the *Journal* and a news conference after its publication, Bailey defended himself strongly, saying his critics' comments were "patronizing" and based on "1960's thinking." He noted that human infant donors are extremely scarce and said that in future cases like Baby Fae's he will look for a human donor but, if none is available, will transplant an animal heart permanently or as a bridge until a human donor is found. The critics from the medical journal agree that an animal heart transplant could be a way to keep an infant alive until a human donor can be found.

Ribavirin Approved

In late 1985 the U.S. Food and Drug Administration granted approval for a drug called ribavirin (brand name, Virazole) to be used in treating a common respiratory infection in infants and young children. The infection, caused by a virus called respiratory syncytial virus, can be fatal, and until ribavirin there was no specific treatment for it, although children did usually recover. Ribavirin acts to prevent the virus from reproducing itself, and in several studies patients who received the drug, in the form of an aerosol mist, recovered significantly more quickly than those who did not. Ribavirin is also being tested against several other viruses.

See also the Spotlight on Health article PROTECTING CHILDREN FROM POISONING.

RAYMOND B. KARASIC, M.D.

Psychiatry and Psychology

See MENTAL HEALTH.

Public Health

Health Warnings Mandated for Smokeless Tobacco • A General Ban on Tobacco Advertising? • Lung Cancer Rate Declines • Measles Outbreaks at Colleges • Mass Food Poisoning From Milk and Cheese

Tobacco and Health

While the public view of public health in the United States in 1985 and early 1986 was dominated by concern about AIDS (acquired immune deficiency syndrome), the long-standing controversy over the use of tobacco, which causes many more deaths and health problems than AIDS or any other communicable disease, heated up considerably. As Congress moved toward legislation that would require health warning labels on smokeless tobacco products and ban radio and television commercials for them, the American Medical Association called for a complete ban on all forms of tobacco advertising. On the other side of the debate, a major tobacco company mounted an advertising campaign to raise doubts about the health risks of smoking and won a product liability lawsuit brought by the family of a deceased smoker. Meanwhile, a historic decline was reported in the incidence of lung cancer among white men, as well as a dramatically higher risk from cigarette smoking among workers who are also exposed to asbestos.

Smokeless tobacco legislation. In early 1986, Congress completed action on legislation mandating health warning labels on containers of chewing tobacco and snuff (finely ground tobacco) and banning radio and television advertisements for these products. The bill required the following three labels to be printed on tobacco tins and pouches on a rotating basis: "This product may cause mouth cancer"; "This product may cause gum disease and tooth loss"; and "This product is not a safe alternative to cigarettes." Most of the tobacco industry reluctantly supported the bill rather than face a diversity of state labeling requirements. The measure was signed into law in late February.

The congressional action came a few weeks after a panel of doctors, dentists, and other experts convened by the National Institutes of Health issued a strong warning against the use of smokeless tobacco. Both the legislation and the convening of the panel reflected growing concern about increased use of smokeless tobacco by young people, especially teenage boys. According to the panel, at least 10 million Americans use chewing tobacco and snuff, and 3 million of these are under the age of 21.

AMA pushes for tobacco advertising ban. The policy-making body of the American Medical Association voted on December 10, 1985, to press for federal laws that would prohibit all promotion and advertising of tobacco products. The association also called for a ban on the sale of cigarettes in vending machines and on the sale of tobacco products to persons under 21.

Although cigarette advertisements have been banned from radio and television since 1971, AMA leaders acknowledged that they faced a difficult task in seeking to have the ban extended to all tobacco products and, more important, to newspapers, magazines, billboards, and other media. After the December 10 vote, the American Civil Liberties Union joined the tobacco, advertising, and publishing industries in denouncing the proposal as an unconstitutional abridgement of the right to free speech. Supporters of a ban contend that advertising, as a form of "commercial speech," is not protected by the First Amendment to the same degree as political, philosophical, or religious speech, and that a total ban on tobacco advertising is justified by the scale of medical and economic damage tobacco causes.

Apart from the constitutional issue, critics of the AMA's proposal have questioned whether such a ban would succeed in its object of reducing tobacco use. Opponents of a ban cite the precedents of Poland and Italy, where such legislation has not been followed by any reduction in the number of smokers. In addition, cigarette advertisers claim that their targeted market is not, as their critics charge, impressionable young people. The ads, they say, are intended to ensure a smoker's allegiance to a brand or to attract smokers away from a different brand, not to promote smoking per se.

R. J. Reynolds and its foes. The second largest U.S. tobacco company, R. J. Reynolds, launched an ad-

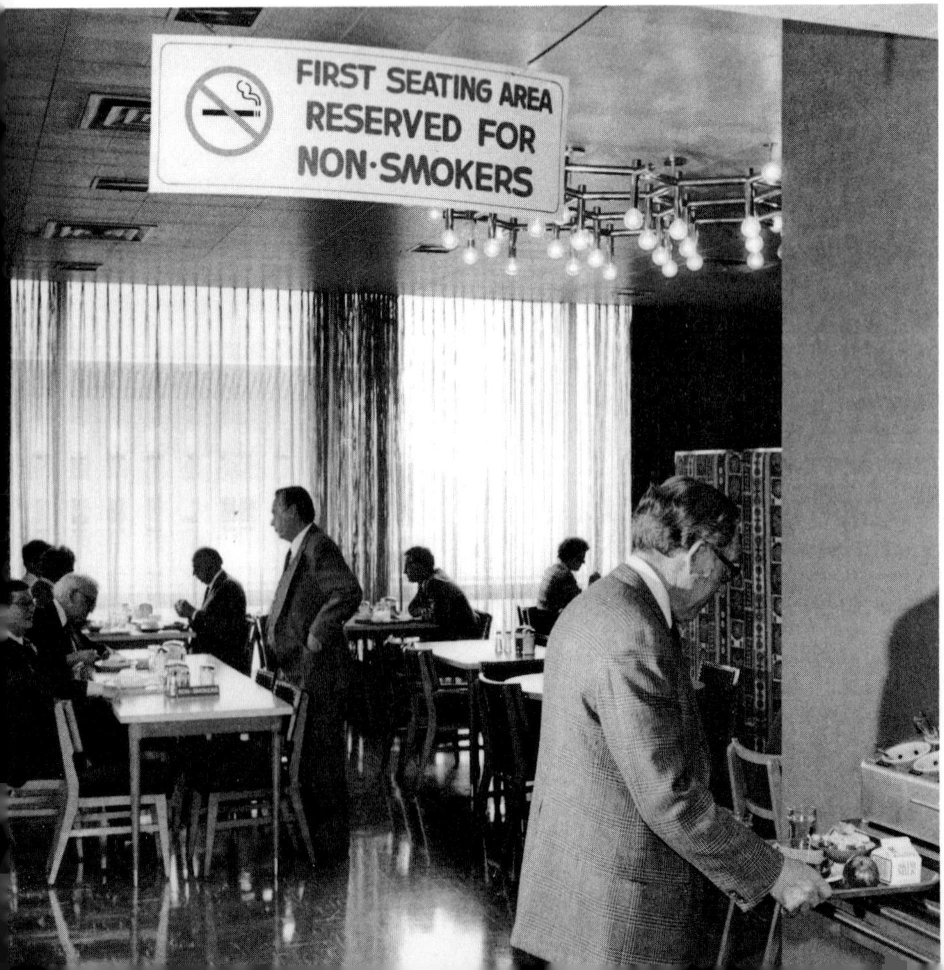

As the nonsmokers' rights movement gains momentum, more restrictions are being placed on smoking; shown here, the nonsmoking section of the employee cafeteria of the Commercial Credit Corporation in Baltimore.

vertising campaign in 1985 that cited a federal study as evidence that "the controversy over smoking and health remains an open one." But the ad came under heavy attack from public health experts, and a coalition of groups including the American Cancer Society, the American Heart Association, and the American Lung Association petitioned the Federal Trade Commission to halt its publication and to force Reynolds to pay for corrective ads.

The ad, which appeared in 25 newspapers and magazines, dealt with a federally funded ten-year study of 13,000 men who were at high risk for heart disease because of high blood pressure, high cholesterol levels in the blood, and smoking. The study was intended to test whether special treatment aimed at reducing these risk factors would lower the men's rate of heart attacks. In fact, the half of the group who received special treatment did reduce these risk factors more than those who got only "usual care," but they did not suffer any fewer deaths from heart disease. The Reynolds ad cited this finding in stating that a link between heart disease and smoking, high blood pressure, and high cholesterol is "an opinion. A judgment. But *not* scientific fact." The company's critics, however, pointed out that smoking was only one of three factors involved and that a third of the men in the study were nonsmokers. Even more significant, they said, was the finding that in both groups those who quit smoking had a nearly 50 percent lower coronary death rate.

On December 23, 1985, a jury in Santa Barbara, Calif., cleared Reynolds of liability in the death of John Galbraith, a chain smoker who had died of lung cancer in 1982. The suit brought by Galbraith's family contended that his lung cancer had been caused by compulsive smoking of Reynolds' Winston, Salem, and Camel cigarettes and that Reynolds had been negligent in failing to warn him that smoking was addictive. Although the tobacco industry has won all of the nearly 150 product liability suits it has faced since the late 1950's, a new wave of suits has been filed in recent years by plaintiffs hoping to benefit from new evidence about the dangers of smoking and a more favorable climate of public opinion. Damage awards are also being sought by former asbestos manufacturers who argue that tobacco companies should share responsibility for the extraordinary occurrence of respiratory disease and cancer in smokers who were also exposed to asbestos.

Surgeon general's report. Support for the asbestos industry's contention came in 1985 from the U.S. surgeon general's annual report on the health consequences of smoking, which was released in December. The report, which focused on cancer and chronic lung disease in the workplace, said that smoking had been found to multiply the risk of lung cancer created by occupational exposure to asbestos. Working with asbestos increases the risk of developing lung cancer fivefold, while smoking increases the risk tenfold. Thus, smokers who work with asbestos are approximately 50 times more likely to develop lung cancer than people who neither smoke nor work with asbestos. The report also said that smoking contributed, though not to the same degree, to lung diseases associated with exposure to silica dust, coal dust, cotton dust, and other substances in the workplace.

In other findings, the report said that blue-collar workers are at higher risk than white-collar workers for developing cancer and chronic lung disease because they smoke more, begin smoking at an earlier age, are less likely in succeed in quitting smoking, and are exposed to more hazardous substances in their jobs. The report also noted that "the work environment may be a major factor capable of predisposing an individual toward or away from becoming a smoker" and urged that employers be required to provide "a work environment that does not promote smoking or interfere with cessation."

The report as a whole, and especially its conclusion that cigarettes pose a greater danger to the health of

WRESTLING WITH TROUBLE

One reason professional wrestling has become so extraordinarily popular is the ability of grapplers like Hulk Hogan and Rowdy Roddy Piper to endure seemingly vicious body slams, eye gouges, and various bone-crunching blows. The wrestlers generally emerge from the ring none the worse for wear, but some doctors are beginning to fear that fans trying to imitate the antics of their favorite hero or villain on living room rugs and front lawns are risking serious injury. In one case, reported in the *New England Journal of Medicine,* a 58-year-old man suffered a ruptured gallbladder, requiring surgery, after being body-slammed to the ground by his son.

Several things save the pros from severe injury. The first, of course, is that wrestling is largely a sham—the action choreographed, the violence faked. But beyond that, the wrestlers tend to be in excellent physical condition, know how to take falls, and perform in a ring with a floor so flexible that—like a trampoline—it can cushion a hard fall. The bottom line is that pro wrestling is best left to the pros.

most American workers than do workplace hazards, was criticized by both the Tobacco Institute (the trade organization of the U.S. tobacco industry) and the AFL-CIO. Both groups charged that the report was an attempt to shift the blame for lung disease from employers to workers, and the Tobacco Institute suggested the attempt was politically motivated.

Another federal agency, the congressional Office of Technology Assessment, estimated in September that $12 billion to $35 billion would be spent in 1985 to treat smoking-related illnesses in the United States. The agency also estimated that such illnesses could cost the U.S. economy an additional $27 billion to $61 billion in lost productivity.

Lung cancer. The incidence of lung cancer among white men in the United States dropped by 4 percent from 1982 to 1983, according to a December 1985 report by the National Cancer Institute. This dramatic decrease, the first significant drop in at least 50 years, was attributed mainly to lower cigarette consumption over the past two decades. The rate of lung cancer among black men remained about 60 percent higher than for white men, but it too showed signs of leveling off. There was no such promising news for women, at least in the short term; although women are also smoking somewhat less, a decrease in either the incidence of or deaths from lung cancer was not expected by the Institute until perhaps the year 2000. Lung cancer, which has one of the highest mortality rates of any type of cancer, surpassed breast cancer in 1985 as the leading cause of cancer deaths among American women.

See also the Spotlight on Health article WHY TEENAGERS SMOKE.

Food Poisoning Epidemics

The largest outbreaks of two bacterial diseases that had ever been documented in the United States occurred during the first half of 1985. Both were transmitted by dairy products: in one case the product was milk; in the other, cheese.

Salmonellosis in the Midwest. In the largest documented food poisoning epidemic in U.S. history, more than 16,000 people in several Midwestern states became ill as a result of drinking milk contaminated with the bacterium *Salmonella typhimurium.* Two deaths were said to be directly caused by the bacterium. At least four persons who were already ill died partly because of additional complications caused by *Salmonella* poisoning. After the first cases were diagnosed in late March, the contaminated milk was quickly traced to a large dairy in Melrose Park, Ill., a suburb of Chicago, which supplied milk to a large grocery chain in Illinois and surrounding states. In early May, a joint federal-state investigative team reported that the *Salmonella* may have ended up in packaged milk because of a valve that allowed *Salmonella*-contaminated raw milk to mix with previously pasteurized milk (during pasteurization milk is heated so as to kill microorganisms.) The outbreak led to new Illinois regulations for dairy processing, including a requirement that pasteurization of milk be the final step before packaging and distribution to stores.

Salmonellosis causes acute diarrhea and often other symptoms, including nausea, fever, headaches, and stomach cramps. It is rarely fatal. The number of cases in the 1985 Midwestern outbreak was more than half the number normally reported annually for the entire country. Especially disturbing to public health officials was the discovery that the strain of the *Salmonella* bacterium that caused the outbreak was resistant to several common antibiotics used to treat the disease. Some experts suggested that the widespread use of antibiotics in livestock feed may have contributed to the development of such resistant strains and thus endangered human health.

Listeriosis from cheeses. An outbreak of listeriosis, a disease caused by infection with the bacterium *Listeria monocytogenes,* led to at least 29 deaths (some press accounts reported the number of dead at close to 100), most of them in southern California, between April and July of 1985. Most of the victims were Hispanic women and their unborn and newborn children, and the outbreak was traced to Mexican-style fresh cheeses produced by Jalisco Mexican Products of Artesia, Calif., a suburb of Los Angeles. Investigators found that the company's factory may have processed more milk than it had the capacity to pasteurize, and the Los Angeles County district attorney said there was a "strong suspicion" that the contaminated cheese had been made at least partly from unpasteurized milk. However, *Listeria* is not always destroyed even by proper pasteurization.

Most people infected with *Listeria* do not suffer any symptoms, but in a small number of cases the infection causes abdominal pain, fever, and severe vomiting. The bacterium can also cause meningitis, an infection of structures surrounding the brain or spinal cord. It is especially dangerous to persons with weak immune systems, including infants and the elderly, and to pregnant women and their unborn children, since it often infects the placenta, the maternal structure that nourishes the fetus.

Measles on Campuses

A series of measles outbreaks on U.S. college campuses in early 1985 reminded public health officials of the need to focus special emphasis on the college-age population in measles-eradication efforts. The major outbreaks occurred from January through March at Ohio State University, with 12 confirmed cases; Boston University, with 82 confirmed cases plus several cases at nearby colleges; and Principia College in Illinois, with 128 confirmed or probable cases out of a student body of 712. At Principia, a Christian Science school where many students had refused immunization on religious grounds, three students died of respiratory complications from measles infections.

Because the national childhood immunization program begun in 1963 took a number of years to implement, many Americans who are now of college age missed being immunized during their early school years but did not catch measles, either. Thus, they have no immunity to the disease, which is highly infectious.

Measles outbreaks at colleges are controlled by providing mass immunization clinics and requiring proof of measles immunity in order to return to classes and campus activities. Prevention of future outbreaks will require proof of measles immunity from all students who wish to enroll in colleges and universities. (A small number of students will need to be exempted for medical or religious reasons.)

Over 2,700 cases of measles were reported in the United States in 1985, according to preliminary data. Before 1963, the annual average exceeded 500,000.

Toxic Exposure Case

In a widely publicized legal case, three Illinois company officials were convicted in June 1985 of murdering an employee who had died in 1983 from inhaling cyanide that he used in his job to recover silver from used film. The three officials—the president of the now-defunct company, the plant manager, and a foreman—were sentenced to 25 years in prison. The murder convictions were thought to be the first ever brought against American corporate officials as a result of a job-related death. (A fourth official was acquitted.)

The employee, Stefan Golab, was an illegal immigrant from Poland who had worked at the plant of Film Recovery Systems in Elk Grove Village, a suburb of Chicago. The judge in the nonjury trial found that the officials had known that working conditions at the plant were extremely dangerous but had failed to provide appropriate warnings for the employees, many of whom could not speak or read English. According to legal experts, the case was the first time that murder charges against corporate executives in connection with a job-related death had even gone to trial; usually officials in such circumstances are charged with the lesser crime of manslaughter. The convictions were appealed.

See also the feature article AIDS: TWO EPIDEMICS.

STEVEN D. HELGERSON, M.D., M.P.H.,
and JAMES F. JEKEL, M.D., M.P.H.

Respiratory System

Treating Lung Cancer With Lasers • Lung Diseases in AIDS Patients • What Causes Asthma? • Breathing Disorders in Sleep Contribute to High Blood Pressure

Laser Therapy for Lung Cancer

Doctors have added laser beams to their arsenal of weapons against lung cancer, the leading cancer killer in the United States and Canada. Lasers can be used to clear airways in the lung that have become obstructed by cancerous tissue. The treatment does not cure lung cancer, but it can ease many of its symptoms. Doctors generally use a type of laser called a YAG laser to deliver a beam through a fiber-optic tube. The light can vaporize tissue blocking the airways. To get to the target, doctors use another fiber-optic tube, a bronchoscope, to see into the lung.

Doctors in Michigan reported the results of treating 55 patients with a YAG laser in 1985. A majority of the patients were helped by the treatment: their obstructed airways were opened, relieving them of breathlessness and pneumonia. But there were some complications, both minor and serious. The greatest danger appears to be an accident in which the laser burns through a major blood vessel, causing severe bleeding. In fact, two of the patients in the Michigan study died when this happened. Researchers in Louisiana reported similar complications in their treatment of patients with lasers, but by injecting a substance that makes blood vessels in the lung more visible to X rays, they were able to reduce the likelihood of bleeding. The laser technique is difficult and requires experienced and skillful doctors.

AIDS-Related Lung Disease

A recent report on respiratory problems in AIDS patients suggests that lung disease plays a crucial role in the outcome of the disease. In AIDS, a virus attacks a certain type of white blood cell that is an essential part of the immune system, leaving the body vulnerable to a host of infections that a healthy person can fight off. Many of these infections affect the lungs.

Of 130 AIDS patients studied by New York doctors, almost half had respiratory abnormalities, either when they were admitted to the hospital or at some point during the four years of the study. Infections were most often responsible for lung disease; they were caused by agents such as *Pneumocystis carinii*, an organism that causes pneumonia only in people whose immune systems are weakened; by cytomegalovirus—a virus closely related to herpesviruses—which sometimes causes severe infections in newborns but is rarely serious in healthy adults; and by a bacterium that sometimes causes a condition resembling tuberculosis. In the later stages of disease, many AIDS patients had more than one infectious organism active at a time. There were also lung problems not caused by infectious agents, notably eight cases of lung cancer caused by the spread of Kaposi's sarcoma, an otherwise rare form of skin cancer that often afflicts AIDS patients.

A report by doctors at Yale University on the results of bronchoscopy (examination of the lungs with a bronchoscope) in AIDS patients suggests a reason why lung disorders may be such a common consequence of the disease. Analysis of fluid from the lining of the lung revealed more abnormalities in the immune system there than in the blood. This means that the lungs may be especially vulnerable and thus may be affected at an early stage of the disease.

Lung disease is often the immediate cause of death in AIDS. During the New York study, 41 percent of the patients who also had a lung disease died. Of course, whether a patient died or not depended on the stage AIDS had reached and the type of lung disease; this was a particularly important factor in the case of infections. Death occurred in all of the patients whose respiratory system deteriorated to the extent that they had to have support from a respirator.

See also the feature article AIDS: TWO EPIDEMICS.

Nutrition and Lung Disease

Doctors have recently begun to understand better how poor nutrition affects the respiratory system, and they have started to place greater emphasis on proper nourishment for patients with chronic lung disease. It has long been known that starvation affects the respiratory system with particular severity. For example, careful records kept by Jewish physicians of the effects of extreme food shortages in the Warsaw Ghetto during World War II show a decrease in breathing frequency and in the volume of each individual breath as starvation progressed. The rate at which the body used oxygen fell, presumably so it would use less food as fuel. Bronchitis, pneumonia, and tuberculosis were common in the ghetto.

Just how starvation causes these respiratory changes is becoming more clear today. The reason for the slowness and diminished volume of breathing is probably that starvation affects the respiratory muscles, especially the diaphragm, the most important muscle for breathing. Malnutrition causes the diaphragm to decrease in size, weight, and strength. It also seems to diminish the drive to breathe and the response to stimuli such as exertion, which would normally increase the rate of respiration.

Malnutrition also affects the immune system, making it less capable of fighting off infections like bronchitis, pneumonia, and tuberculosis. In fact, there is a time-tested medical adage that "death from starvation is death from pneumonia."

The effects of malnutrition on the respiratory system add up to a compelling reason to guard against malnutrition in patients with lung disease and to provide nutritional therapy for poorly nourished patients. Weight loss and malnourishment are particularly common in people with emphysema and other diseases in the group called chronic obstructive pulmonary disease. These people are prone to stomach disorders such as ulcers that impair their ability to eat. In severe cases, breathlessness may be bad enough to interfere with eating. In most cases, however, it is not insufficient intake of food as such that is at the root of the problem. Rather, lung disease patients with poor respiratory muscle strength and lung function have to work hard for each breath, thereby increasing their need for food energy to the point where their intake of calories is not sufficient. Psychological factors like depression may also play a role in nutritional problems for these patients.

All this suggests that an effort should be made to improve nutrition in lung disease patients who show signs of malnourishment, even if there is as yet no proof that improving their nutrient intake will improve their condition. They should be encouraged to take in adequate calories and to vary their diet among the major food groups, with particular attention given to getting enough protein.

New Information on Asthma

Causes of adult asthma. Serious lower respiratory tract infections in children may lead to asthma in later life. This finding was announced by researchers from Harvard University, who reported the first results from a ten-year study of risk factors for the development of obstructive lung disease, especially asthma, in adults. Children from East Boston enrolled in the study were periodically examined for the number and effects of any respiratory infections they had. Doctors have long wondered about the effect of childhood colds—that is, upper respiratory tract infections—on the development of asthma later in life, but the Harvard researchers found a greater correlation between infections in the lower respiratory tract, such as croup, and the later development of asthma. Their report is convincing evidence that severe lower respiratory tract infections in children can have serious consequences in later life.

Colds and asthma. Doctors studying the effects of colds on cases of asthma that are already present have found that the most common type of cold virus—called a rhinovirus—does not often bring on attacks of adult asthma. In the study, volunteers who had asthma were directly infected with rhinoviruses. Although over 90 percent of them came down with colds, most did not have asthma attacks as a result. The researchers suggested that other viruses, such as those for influenza, may be more commonly involved in bringing on asthma and should be evaluated in a similar study.

Asthma and pregnancy. Recent studies of pregnant women with asthma indicate that proper control and treatment of the condition during pregnancy can minimize complications that were common in the past, such as premature birth, low birth weight, and sometimes even fetal or maternal death. This is important news, since asthma is the most common form of obstructive lung disease during pregnancy.

Treatment of a pregnant woman's asthma must be carefully balanced between taking the best possible care of the mother's breathing problem and minimizing the risks posed to the fetus. In protecting the fetus, doctors must remember that dangers are posed by both a poor oxygen supply because of the mother's impaired breathing and the side effects of drugs used to treat it. Fortunately, it appears that most asthma drugs can be safely used during pregnancy, particularly in the later stages. (All drugs should be avoided in early pregnancy unless they are absolutely essential.)

Thus, doctors can now answer more optimistically than in the past one question asked by pregnant women with asthma: "What effect will my asthma have on the outcome of my pregnancy?" Recent data collected from several studies also help to answer another common question: "What effect will my pregnancy have on my asthma?" Unfortunately, the answer seems to be that there is really no way of telling. About half of the women in these studies had no substantial change in their asthma during pregnancy, about a quarter noted improvement, and about a quarter reported a worsening. Also, the state of a woman's asthma during one pregnancy does not seem to have much value in predicting what will happen during a later pregnancy.

Sleep-Related Breathing Disorders

Sleep apnea and high blood pressure. A study reported in 1985 suggests that many people may have high blood pressure at least partly because of sleep apnea, a disorder that most commonly affects middle-aged, often overweight, men, who cease breathing many times during a night's sleep—commonly for about 10 seconds but sometimes for as long as a minute. It has been known that this cessation of breathing lowers oxygen levels in the blood and leads to raised blood pressure. Doctors in Houston decided to find out how many people with known hypertension might have unrecognized sleep apnea. They studied 46 middle-aged and older men and found that 14 of them did indeed have the sleep apnea syndrome. Seven of them were treated for it and had an improvement in blood pressure as well as in the sleep apnea. The researchers do not recommend overnight sleep studies, which are expensive and time-consuming, for all patients with mild hypertension, but they suggest that doctors should be aware of the connection and look for other symptoms of disordered breathing during sleep.

Other causes of breathing disorders in sleep. Articles published in 1985 explored two more reasons for sleep-related breathing disorders. Obstruction of the nose, whether by hay fever, a deviated nasal septum, or even gauze used as packing after a severe nosebleed, is known to cause such disorders, and doctors in Pennsylvania have looked into why this occurs. On the theory that there are receptors in the nose that influence respiration, they applied a local anesthetic spray inside the noses of volunteers taking part in an overnight sleep study. They found a four-fold increase in breathing problems during sleep after the anesthesia, suggesting that these nasal receptors may be important in maintaining a normal breathing rhythm during sleep and that anything that interferes with them can lead to breathing disorders.

Canadian researchers studied the effect of a group of diseases called interstitial lung diseases, characterized by the abnormal collection of cells or scar tissue within the lungs. (They include sarcoidosis, scleroderma, and fibrosing alveolitis.) In 11 patients with these diseases, the quality of sleep was found to be worse, with more fragmented and disturbed sleep, than in healthy people. Apneas were more frequent and blood oxygen levels lower, especially in those with oxygen levels that were already low from the disease itself.

SUSAN K. PINGLETON, M.D.

Sexually Transmitted Diseases

See VENEREAL DISEASES.

Teeth and Gums

Dental Problems of the Elderly • Fluoride for Young and Old • Helping Denture Wearers • Diabetes and Gum Disease

Dental Needs of the Aged

As the "graying of America" becomes increasingly apparent, the dental profession is paying more and more attention to the teeth and gum problems of the growing elderly population. The special problems of the aging include dry mouth, the decay of exposed root surfaces, and—for those without teeth—the need to maintain adequate bony support in order to wear full dentures comfortably.

Treating salivary gland problems. New treatments, including a drug commonly used for eye disease and a type of electrical stimulation, are being developed for dry mouth, or xerostomia, which affects many older people. These developments promise substantial relief, because chronic dry mouth is much more than an annoyance: the lack of saliva produces serious difficulties in eating, swallowing, tasting food, and speaking. In addition, mouth sores, cracking of the lips, yeast infections, erosion and abrasion of the teeth, and rampant dental decay are very common, and those without natural teeth find it difficult to wear full dentures.

Serious dry mouth problems can result from the chronic use of medications that interfere with the functioning of nerves or with hormones that control the secretion of saliva. The medications most likely to produce serious oral dryness include drugs to fight high blood pressure and antidepressants, both prescribed for millions of Americans, as well an antihistamines, decongestants, some ulcer medications, and tranquilizers. It has been estimated that more than 50 percent of U.S. residents over age 65 use medications that cause dryness.

There are diseases that affect the functioning of the salivary glands. The major such disease is Sjögren's syndrome, which results in both dry eyes and dry mouth. The syndrome may appear as part of a generalized connective tissue disorder, most commonly rheumatoid arthritis. In addition, a particularly aggravated form of dry mouth occurs in people who have had radiation therapy for cancer of the head or neck. Any of the salivary glands in the area being radiated may shut down, and in most instances they do so irreversibly.

Some older people also experience dry mouth as a result of age-related changes in the salivary glands—usually those in the floor of the mouth and inside the lip. However, these alterations usually do not generate complaints. Chronic anxiety or other emotional problems and breathing through the mouth instead of through the nose can also contribute to dry mouth.

Treatment of dry mouth mainly addresses the symptoms. Sugar-free candy and chewing gum are used to stimulate the functioning of the salivary glands, and glycerine, mineral oil, and commercially available "artificial saliva" are given to provide some lubrication to protect the soft tissues. Various forms of fluoride are used to protect the natural teeth.

Recent research promises additional help to dry mouth sufferers who have some functional capacity left. A study has been conducted on the use of pilocarpine, a chemical commonly found in eye drops used in the treatment of glaucoma. An oral form of pilocarpine was tested for its effectiveness and safety by researchers at the National Institute of Dental Research. The drug is slowly absorbed into the body, and it stimulates the surfaces of the salivary gland cells to produce saliva. Patients are relieved of the discomfort of dryness for about three hours; they experience no changes in heart rate or blood pressure from the drug as used (these may occur with large doses).

Elsewhere, other researchers are studying the potential benefits of electronically stimulating salivation. A battery-powered device that provides stimulating pulses by means of a hand-held probe is inserted for about three minutes into the mouth, where it stimulates sensors on the tongue and soft tissues. The short-term effects appear to be promising.

Fighting off decay. Decay is usually thought of as a problem of the young, but an increasing number of older people are retaining their teeth—and consequently experiencing tooth decay. Using fluoride and avoiding sugary foods can help prevent the problem.

With increasing age there is a likelihood of gum recession and, as a consequence, more root surfaces may be exposed to the agents of dental decay. Studies indicate that the combination of extended longevity and a greater number of retained teeth leads to an increase in tooth decay. The root surfaces are particularly vulnerable in people with low salivary flow: with the loss of the protective properties of saliva, there is a greater buildup of bacterial plaque and food particles around the teeth, especially at the gum line. To make matters worse, when many people begin to experience dry mouth and want to stimulate the flow of saliva, they often use sour candies, which contain acid, or sweet candies, mints, or gum. Unless they use candies with sweeteners that do not promote tooth decay (such as sorbitol, mannitol, xylitol, or aspartame), they are unwittingly providing the plaque with an ideal environment for the generation of decay-producing acids.

Fluorides are often considered to be of value only to children, but fluoride, which guards against decay, can benefit young and old alike. Fluoridated water supplies have been shown to be effective, and self-applied fluorides, whether in mouthwashes, toothpastes, or prescription-only gels, are valuable in preventing and even reversing early decay. New fluoride preparations aimed at optimizing prevention of cavities are under development (and work is proceeding on a "slow-release device" bonded to a back tooth or a removable bridge), but all of the standard forms of fluoride currently available are beneficial.

Wearing dentures well. Several new techniques have been developed to help people who wear dentures do so more successfully. Although the percentage of people without teeth is declining, there are still many millions in Canada and the United States who rely on full dentures for chewing food. A well-functioning full denture depends on the maintenance of the alveolar ridges, the bony supports in the upper and lower jaws. The pressure exerted by dentures, combined with the loss of stimulation formerly provided by natural teeth, results over time in a narrowing of the ridge and loss of vertical height. Chewing becomes more difficult.

To help preserve the alveolar bone, oral surgeons at Louisiana State University School of Dentistry in New Orleans, have placed hydroxylapatite root implants in fresh sockets left after tooth extraction. The implants are composed of an inert biomaterial that is chemically similar to bone and tooth mineral. It is a nonporous, highly dense, pure polycrystalline ceramic. The surgeons followed the results of implants in 49 patients for up to 31 months after tooth extraction and found that at the implant sites there was twice as much alveolar bone as in sites without the implants.

Hydroxylapatite is also being used for rebuilding alveolar ridges that are either atrophied or shrunk to the point where retaining a denture is difficult; the American Association of Oral and Maxillofacial Surgeons reports that there are several thousand cases where hydroxylapatite has been used successfully to build up the affected ridges. This work often can be done in the dentist's office, and it appears to be a reasonable procedure for many elderly patients. New dentures can be made as soon as four to six weeks following the surgery.

Diabetes and Gum Disease

A group of periodontists from the dental school at the State University of New York at Buffalo have teamed up with diabetes specialists in Phoenix, Ariz., to study gum disease in Pima Indians. This native American tribe has the highest rate of diabetes in the world: 40 percent of the Pimas suffer from diabetes, as compared with 2.5 percent of the U.S. population (diagnosed cases). It has long been known that people with diabetes are highly susceptible to gum, or periodontal, disease and that treatment of these patients is more difficult that in otherwise healthy people.

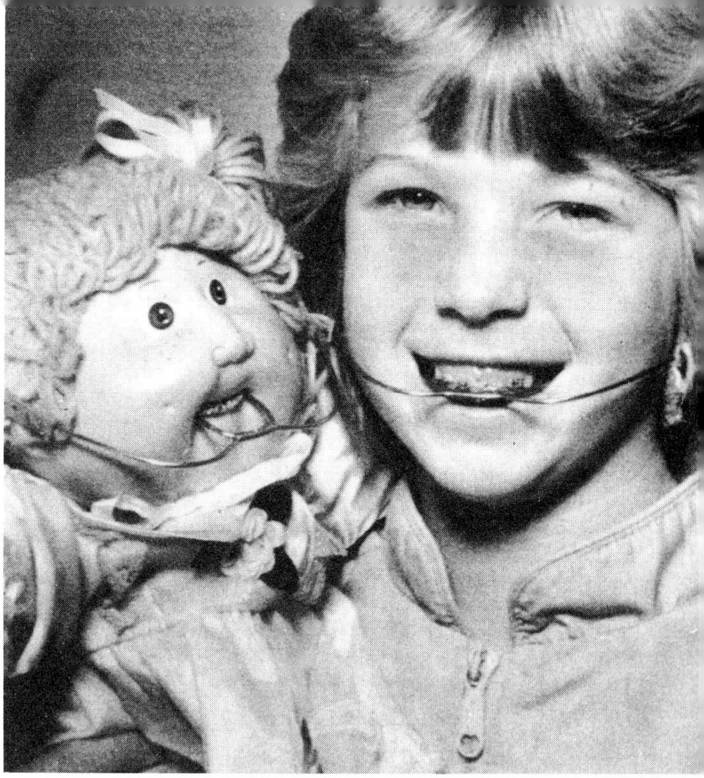

How do you convince a child with a serious overbite to wear braces? Why, says dentist Joe Mitchell of Salinas, Calif., let her set an example for her Cabbage Patch doll fitted with an identical set.

The new research showed that Pima Indians with diabetes were much more likely to have gum disease than members of the tribe who did not have diabetes. In addition, gum disease was much more severe in the diabetic population: one third of the group with diabetes had lost all of their teeth (a common consequence of severe periodontal disease), while only 2 percent of the Indians who did not have diabetes were missing all of their teeth. The researchers found that the periodontal disease started at a much earlier age in the diabetes sufferers and that it was associated with a particular mouth bacterium (*Bacteroides gingivalis*) that has been implicated as a major cause of periodontal disease. It is still not known why this bacterium is able to flourish in the mouths of people who have diabetes.

Few Dental Complaints

A recent nationwide survey provided indirect evidence that most adults are not confronted with acute dental problems. The 1985 survey of over 1,400 adults—the first national study of pain experienced by Americans—found that while 73 percent said they had suffered from

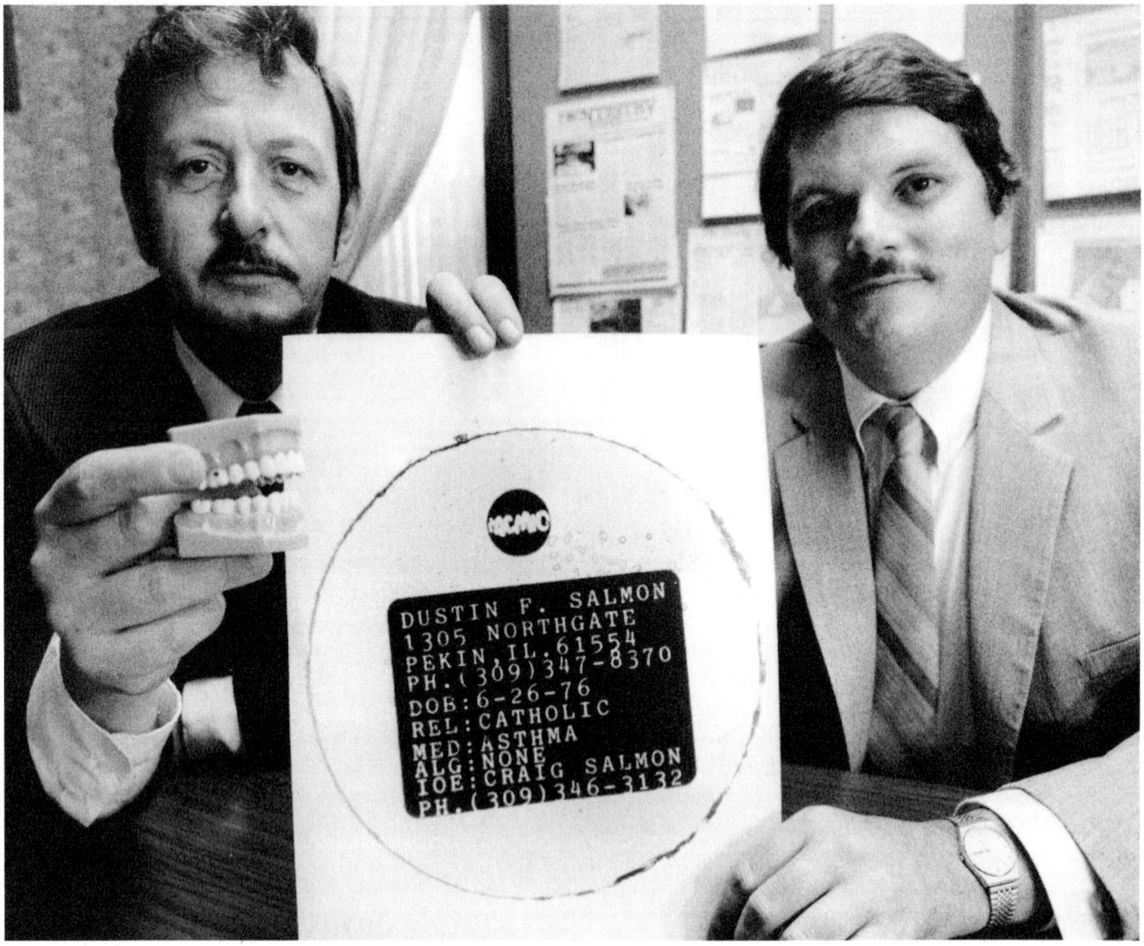
DUSTIN F. SALMON
1305 NORTHGATE
PEKIN, IL. 61554
PH.(309)347-8370
DOB:6-26-76
REL:CATHOLIC
MED:ASTHMA
ALG:NONE
IOE:CRAIG SALMON
PH.(309)346-3132

Detective Jim Conover (left) and Dr. Jeffrey Maxwell demonstrate their ID disk, the small black dot on a back tooth about the size of the letter "o."

DENTAL ID DOTS

One specialized and much publicized use of dental records is to help police and forensic experts identify bodies and comatose accident victims. But dental charts and X rays yield only a probable ID at best, and the improved dental health of Americans in recent years has made it more difficult to distinguish one mouth from another.

Now there is a new tooth-based ID system: a microdisk—a dot of metal or plastic a fraction of an inch in diameter—bonded to a back molar. If microdisks gain broad acceptance, they could be a major help in identifying missing children.

Installed in 15 minutes—without either drilling or anesthesia—the tiny disk cannot be dislodged or damaged by brushing, does not harm the teeth, and lasts about three to six years. The information carried on the disk can be anything from an ID or telephone number to basic personal or medical data. The microdisks that are now available can accommodate as many as 1,000 characters. The characters can be read with a magnifying glass or a microscope after the disk is removed from the mouth. Use of the miniature disks has gained the endorsement of the American Dental Association.

headaches during the past year, and more than 50 percent reported occasional back pain, muscle pain, and joint pain, only 27 percent reported experiencing dental pain. IRWIN D. MANDEL, D.D.S.

Venereal Diseases

Chlamydia—The Most Common Venereal Disease • Gonorrhea That Resists Antibiotics • Do Genital Warts Cause Cancer?

Chlamydia on the Rise

The importance of venereal, or sexually transmitted, disease caused by a type of bacteria called chlamydia has recently been getting increasing recognition. Since chlamydia can have serious consequences, diagnosing and treating it promptly is crucial. It is now believed that there are an estimated 3 million new cases of chlamydia each year in the United States alone—considerably more than the 1.8 million cases per year of gonorrhea, the most common of those sexually transmitted diseases that by law must be reported to U.S. health authorities. (Chlamydia does not fall into this category, known as reportable diseases.)

New diagnostic tests. Growing recognition of the importance of chlamydial infections has stimulated the development of new diagnostic methods. Two new tests recently became available for detecting *Chlamydia trachomatis*, the technical name of the microorganism involved. One test uses genetically engineered antibodies (substances that react specifically with a given antigen, in this case, certain chlamydia proteins), and the other uses so-called enzyme immunoassay techniques, which also detect such chlamydia proteins. The new tests make diagnosis of chlamydia infections both cheaper and more readily available. They have the additional advantage of being able to provide test results in hours rather than the two to four days previously required for diagnosis.

Diagnosing chlamydia was difficult in the past because, unlike other bacteria that can be grown in the laboratory using relatively simple techniques, chlamydia is a parasite that grows within cells, meaning it can only be grown in living cell culture. Because of the cost and difficulty of cell culture—that is, of growing living cells—until recently tests for chlamydia were available only through large laboratories and research programs. This made diagnosis either unavailable or too expensive for most doctors and patients.

The availability and accuracy of the new, less expensive tests now make efforts to control chlamydia possible. In August 1985 the U.S. Centers for Disease Control (CDC) published new guidelines for preventing and controlling chlamydia infections. The guidelines call for screening "high risk" individuals for chlamydia in order to identify infected people who do not show symptoms and who thus might unknowingly spread the infection to their sexual partners. (Those at risk include patients at sexually transmitted disease clinics; chlamydia and other venereal diseases, especially gonorrhea, often occur together. In fact, the guidelines call for treating people diagnosed with gonorrhea for chlamydia automatically.) The availability of the new tests provides an accurate, less expensive means of diagnosing chlamydial infection and is an encouraging step toward controlling this organism. What is more, the two tests currently available are probably only the first generation of non-culture diagnostic tests for chlamydia and will almost certainly be followed by other tests that are still cheaper, more accurate, and easier to perform.

Symptoms and complications. The new CDC guidelines also recommend treating patients who are thought to have chlamydia infections on the basis of their symptoms, even before the chlamydia organism is identified. Chlamydia can cause a wide variety of sexually transmitted disease syndromes similar to those found in gonorrhea. However, gonorrhea usually causes considerable inflammation and results in prominent signs and symptoms, such as a genital discharge or painful urination. In contrast, the inflammation caused by a chlamydia infection—usually in the urinary tract or, in women, the cervix (the mouth of the uterus)—is relatively mild. Infected individuals frequently fail to become aware of any signs and symptoms, and because of this complications may be more likely to occur. These include epididymitis (infection of the testicle and surrounding structures) in men and, more serious, pelvic inflammatory disease (PID, infection of the uterus and fallopian tubes) in women.

As with other sexually transmitted diseases, the consequences of chlamydial infections for women are more far-reaching than for men. Approximately a third of PID cases in U.S. women are due to chlamydial infection, and a first episode of PID leads to infertility in about one of ten women who get it. Furthermore, women who have had PID are seven times as likely as other women to have an ectopic pregnancy (a pregnancy outside the uterus, usually in a fallopian tube). In addition, as with gonorrhea, chlamydia can be passed on to infants of infected mothers during childbirth. Screening of pregnant women for gonorrhea is a routine part of prenatal care, and therefore gonorrhea in newborns is relatively rare. That pregnant women are not routinely screened for chlamydia is probably one reason why chlamydia is the most common cause of eye infections in newborns and a major cause of pneumonia in infants under the age of six months.

Gonorrhea

The development of new antibiotic-resistant strains of the bacterium that causes gonorrhea (*Neisseria gonorrhoeae*) was reported in 1985. Thus far, the new strains have caused sporadic outbreaks of infection, and at least one sustained one. These bacteria are resistant to standard antibiotics such as penicillin and tetracycline—the drugs usually used to treat gonorrhea—on the basis of their genetic makeup.

The strains of antibiotic-resistant gonorrhea doctors have been familiar with in the past produce an enzyme that inactivates penicillin. These bacteria were first recognized nearly ten years ago and can be detected in the laboratory using simple tests. By contrast, the new strains are resistant to antibiotics as a result of the additive effects of several genetic mutations, which have resulted in increased resistance produced by several factors. Because the resistance is on the basis of multiple, separate steps, no easy, single-step method is available for detection of these new strains. Since detection of the new strains is more difficult than for the earlier ones, the intensive methods that have been used to detect and control outbreaks of antibiotic-resistant gonorrhea may not be as effective as in the past. The new strains are not yet a major problem for treatment of gonorrhea in the United States, but they have now been detected throughout the country and could make the current recommended treatments for gonorrhea ineffective at halting spread of the disease.

The continuing development of antibiotic-resistant gonorrhea has stimulated research into new antibiotics for gonorrhea therapy. In the CDC's recently revised treatment recommendations for sexually transmitted diseases, a new antibiotic, ceftriaxone (sold as Rocephin), was recommended as first-choice therapy for gonorrhea. This change is of particular interest, not only because ceftriaxone is among the most effective antibiotics yet tested against gonorrhea, but also because this is the first time in recent years that an antibiotic other than a penicillin or tetracycline has been recommended as a first choice for treating gonorrhea. Other new antibiotics active against strains of gonorrhea resistant to penicillin and tetracycline are the subject of ongoing research. One family of drugs is made up of experimental antibiotics called quinolones, which are highly effective against both chlamydia and gonorrhea. These drugs have the added advantage of being effective when taken orally, as opposed to some of the penicillins and other antibiotics, like ceftriaxone, that must be given by injection.

Genital Warts and Cancer

Recent research suggests that genital warts, which are caused by a sexually transmitted virus, may be related to cancers of the cervix, penis, and anus. Most warts, including genital warts, are actually infections caused by a virus called the human papilloma virus. There are many different types of human papilloma virus, which tend to cause infections at different locations. The types of human papilloma virus that most commonly cause genital warts are known as types 6, 11, 16, and 18. In most cases, genital wart infections tend to heal spontaneously. However, new information suggests that this sexually transmitted disease may be related to cervical dysplasia (abnormal cervical cells that are not cancerous but may progress to cancer) and possibly to the origin of cancer of the cervix, penis, and anus.

At present, the best studies of genital warts and their relation to dysplasia and cervical cancer have been carried out in women with genital wart virus infections of the cervix, where the infection often occurs without signs or symptoms and is detected only in the form of microscopic abnormalities on Pap smears. Using Pap smears as a means of detecting the presence of wart virus infections, several groups of researchers have shown that between 1 and 2 percent of women have wart virus infections of the cervix that are not visible to the naked eye. Researchers have also demonstrated that in many cases of cervical dysplasia or cancer, genetic material (DNA) from the human papilloma virus can be found in the abnormal cells. This suggests that the human papilloma virus may help cause genital tract malignancies. Although the majority of genital warts are caused by human papilloma virus type 6, the genetic material most often detected in patients with cervical cancer is from types 16 and 18.

Important questions still remain, such as what percentage of women with genital warts caused by human papilloma virus 16 or 18 go on to develop dysplasia or cancer, what form of therapy is best for these infections, and how to prevent transmission of the papilloma virus from one person to another. Active research continues, and doctors may soon have new means for detection and cure of precancerous infections, rather than being limited to using the watchful waiting approach currently employed for detection and treatment of genital tract cancers.

See also the feature article AIDS: TWO EPIDEMICS.

EDWARD W. HOOK III, M.D.

World Health News

Meeting the Nuclear Threat • Coping With Disasters • AIDS Cases Around the World • Advances and a Setback in the War on Malaria • Vitamin A Deficiency May Be Fatal

Nuclear War

Physicians work to save lives, putting to good use the findings of scientific research. But sometimes political and social action is required as well. The Nobel Peace Prize committee tacitly acknowledged this in October 1985 when it awarded the prize to the International Physicians for the Prevention of Nuclear War.

The organization, which has 100,000 members in 40 countries, was founded in 1980 by two prominent heart specialists—Dr. Bernard Lown of the United States and Dr. Yevgeny Chazov of the Soviet Union. The group has strongly argued that as the ultimate practice of preventive medicine, the political process must be used to abolish nuclear weapons, because the world as we know it would be destroyed by a large-scale nuclear war, and medicine would have no power against such a disaster. In late 1984, less than a year before the choice for the peace prize was announced, there had come a shocking reminder that humankind can indeed destroy itself in large numbers, if not totally: the leak of a toxic gas at a chemical plant in Bhopāl, India, killed thousands of people. The awarding of the prize to the doctors group was a recognition of the concern felt around the world regarding the threat nuclear weapons pose to everyone. It may also have reflected a desire to send a message to the leaders of the United States and the Soviet Union, who were to meet in a summit conference in November 1985.

Natural Disasters

A series of recent disasters brought home the fact that the therapeutic ability of medical science is severely limited in the face of the powers that can be unleashed by nature. What is needed to hold to a minimum the deaths and adverse effects on health from such calamities is early warning and preventive social action.

In Africa, drought, coupled with a decline in land productivity because of overgrazing and overcultivation, helped bring on a famine that affected much of the continent. The airlifting of food from around the world was able to save only some from death. Nor could health agencies provide more than limited help after the sudden destruction wrought by the September 1985 earthquakes in Mexico, where thousands of people were crushed to death or buried alive; by the mud slides in October near Ponce, Puerto Rico, which buried a village; or by the eruption in November of the volcano Nevado del Ruiz in Colombia, where 25,000 people were drowned by floods or buried in mud slides resulting from the sudden melting of snow and ice by the volcanic heat and from coincidental rains.

Now health authorities are faced with the physical and psychological aftereffects of these disasters. Many children who survived in Africa may be permanently

A grief-stricken father buries his son, one of 25,000 people killed when the Colombian volcano Nevado del Ruiz erupted in late 1985. Such catastrophic natural disasters leave survivors in severe emotional shock, with extreme psychological as well as physical problems.

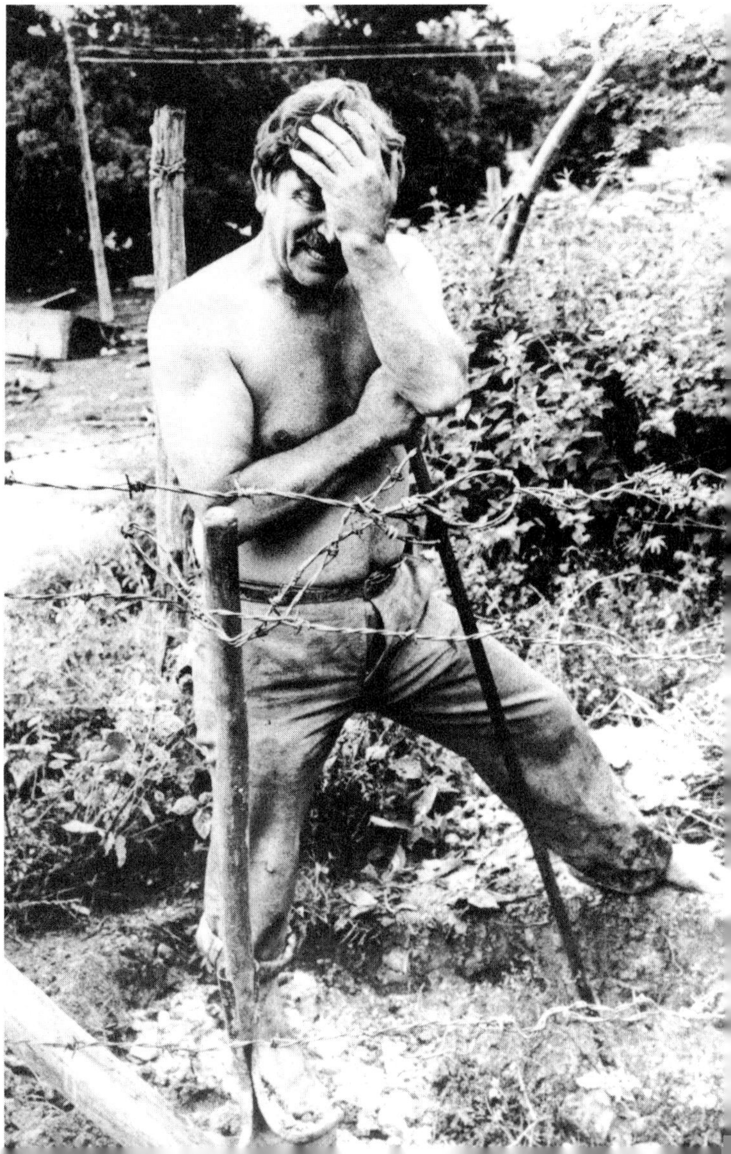

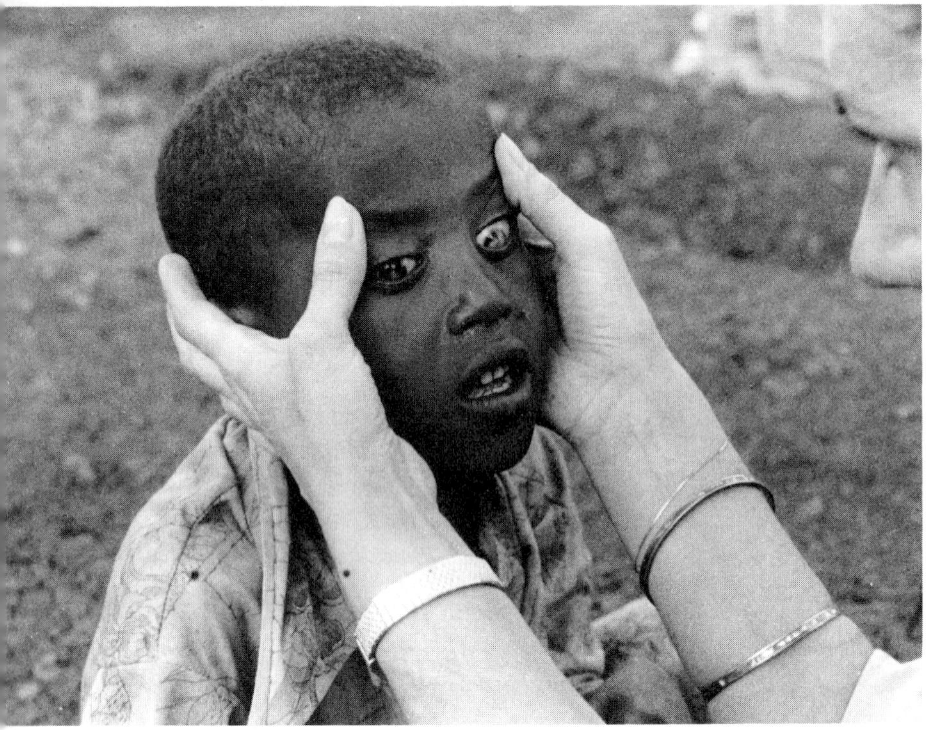

This Ethiopian child is suffering from scarring of the corneas, a result of vitamin A deficiency that can lead to blindness and even death.

impaired physically or mentally. In Mexico, thousands of people became rootless refugees, and many are suffering from severe emotional shock. Psychiatric problems show up both in those who survive a disaster—they may feel guilt, asking "Why did I survive?"—and in rescue workers, who often experience depression and a sense of powerlessness from seeing so much death. Those who have lost loved ones sometimes attempt suicide. The effects of these disasters will last for a long time.

AIDS

First recognized in the United States, the deadly disease known as AIDS (acquired immune deficiency syndrome) has developed into a worldwide concern. By March 1986 the United States had reported more than 18,000 cases, with over 9,500 deaths. Brazil ranked second in number of reported cases, with more than 570. Other countries with sizable numbers of cases reported were, as of late 1985, France and Haiti with almost 400, Canada and West Germany with more than 300, and Great Britain with more than 200. (By March 1986, Canada had over 500 cases.) As of September 30, 1985, there were over 1,570 reported cases in 21 European countries—and nearly 800 deaths.

But such figures do not tell the whole story. Some nations' statistics may be faulty. Some have insisted they have no cases at all, while local doctors have made private assertions to the contrary. The disease is known to be prevalent in the ten or so countries in Central Africa, from Gabon through Zaire to Tanzania, but overall figures are unavailable. In December 1985, Kenya reported ten cases (including eight deaths) to the World Health Organization; this was the first official report by a nation in black Africa.

See also the feature article AIDS: TWO EPIDEMICS.

Malaria

Scientists have reported some advances in the fight against malaria, which in recent years has again become a serious problem in tropical and subtropical areas after a period of fairly good control in most countries.

Tests in humans of two experimental vaccines for preventing the disease were expected to begin in 1986. The vaccines, both developed in the United States, are aimed at the first (sporozoite) phase of the life cycle of the parasite *Plasmodium falciparum*, which causes the most dangerous form of malaria. The vaccines are based on a characteristic protein from the sporozoite that is capable of stimulating the body to produce antibodies against the parasite. In one vaccine the protein is produced through genetic engineering techniques. The other vaccine involves the use of a different approach: chemical synthesis.

In May 1985 researchers reported that severe infections caused by the parasite can be effectively treated on an emergency basis by intravenous administration of quinidine, a heart medication—commonly carried in hospitals—that is related to the malaria drug quinine. The latter drug is not usually carried in hospitals that seldom see malaria and thus is often not available in emergencies.

Meanwhile, the search for new treatments for malaria continued. A report published in May 1985 drew attention to Chinese research on a drug derived from a wormwood plant that, it was suggested, might be the basis for "a totally new class of antimalarials." The drug, called *qinghaosu* or artemisinin, was said to have been successfully used in China on several thousand malaria patients. Swedish researchers reported in January 1986 preliminary evidence suggesting that artificially produced copies of a human antibody to a protein in *Plasmodium falciparum* might some day be the basis for an effective treatment. The scientists used genetic engineering techniques to produce large amounts of human monoclonal antibodies.

Some estimates put the number of new cases of malaria each year as high as 400 million, with perhaps 2 million to 4 million deaths annually; the death toll is particularly high among children. One reason for the current resurgence of malaria is that the mosquitoes that carry the disease-causing parasites have become increasingly resistant to insecticides. Another factor is the parasites' growing resistance to drugs used in treatment. Moreover, spraying with the potent insecticide DDT had been curtailed because it causes serious environmental damage. In response to the growing menace of malaria, the worldwide use of DDT is rising again, but more and more mosquitoes are becoming resistant even to DDT.

See also the feature articles STAYING HEALTHY WHEN TRAVELING *and* THE NEW VACCINES.

Cocaine

The problem of cocaine has taken on more serious dimensions in recent years. More people seem to be smoking ("free-basing") the drug—which provides a faster high, and is more addictive, than snorting it—and the international scope of its use has become clearer. In the United States the estimated number of regular cocaine users is at least 5 million.

The cocaine-producing countries in South America have come to have a drug abuse problem of their own as the use of "coca paste" (cocaine sulfate) has spread rapidly. About 3 percent to 5 percent of the people in some South American nations are believed to be addicted to it. An alternative product in one process for the preparation of "street cocaine," coca paste contains residues of the gasoline used in its manufacture. Ordinarily smoked, it is both toxic to the lungs and highly addictive.

Cocaine abuse is now a serious problem as well in the nations, mostly in the Caribbean, through which the drug makes its way north from South America. This was shown at a 1985 international drug symposium for the Americas held in the Bahamas and sponsored by the Bahamian Ministry of Health and the United States. It was reported that an "epidemic" of cocaine abuse had begun in the Bahamas in 1983, with significant numbers of people seeking treatment for complications of drug abuse. Apparently the cocaine supply markedly increased, and drug sellers started pushing cheaper, free-base cocaine instead of the much less addictive cocaine powder used for snorting.

Meanwhile, concern increased over the growing availability of "crack" in the United States. A purified form of free-base cocaine, crack can be readily smoked. Street cocaine powder, by contrast, needs to be processed by the user before free-basing. A drug dealer arrested in New York in November 1985 was reported to have been producing 2.2 pounds of crack each day for a daily net profit of $500,000.

See also DRUG ABUSE.

Vitamin A Deficiency

Spurred by growing evidence that a diet lacking in vitamin A can be far more dangerous than previously believed, international health authorities in 1985 stepped up efforts to combat the problem. Vitamin A deficiency, to which children aged six months to six years are particularly vulnerable, has long been known to be a major cause of blindness in developing countries. It now appears to be a significant cause of death as well.

Vitamin A deficiency has been reported in most African and many Asian countries, as well as in some areas of Latin America. The number of children who develop health problems because of it has been estimated at several million annually. According to the World Health Organization, over half a million children lose their eyesight each year because they do not get enough vitamin A.

A new indication of how substantial the death toll from vitamin A deficiency may be was revealed in mid-1985 by a Johns Hopkins University professor who headed a large-scale study in Indonesia. Several thousand small children were given large doses of vitamin A at six-month intervals. After a year, it was found that the death rate in the group was as much as 35 percent lower than among untreated children.

In October the World Health Organization established a $50 million ten-year program to fight vitamin A deficiency.

JAMES F. JEKEL, M.D., M.P.H.
and STEVEN D. HELGERSON, M.D., M.P.H.

Contributors

Begley, Sharon. Science Editor, *Newsweek.* HIGH-TECH SURGERY.

Birenbaum, Rhonda. Writer specializing in medicine and science; Regional Correspondent, *Canadian Research* and *The Journal of the Addiction Research Foundation.* GOVERNMENT POLICIES AND PROGRAMS (CANADA).

Carleton, Susan. Editor, *MDA News,* the magazine of the Muscular Dystrophy Association; former Senior Editor, *Rx Being Well.* NEW WAYS TO TAKE MEDICINE.

Charash, Bruce D., M.D. Dan and Elaine Sargent Cardiology Fellow, New York Hospital-Cornell Medical Center, New York City. HEART AND CIRCULATORY SYSTEM (coauthor).

Cooper, Sally. Founder and Executive Director, National Assault Prevention Center; National Training Director, Child Assault Prevention Project. SEX ABUSE: WHAT TO TELL YOUR CHILD.

Dentzer, Susan. General Business Editor, *Newsweek,* specializing in healthcare economics. HEALTH PERSONNEL AND FACILITIES.

Evans, Richard I., Ph.D. Professor of Psychology, University of Houston; Principal Investigator, U.S. Department of Health and Human Services Bio-behavioral Collaboration in Adolescent Health Promotion project. WHY TEENAGERS SMOKE.

Fisher, Jeffrey, M.D. Assistant Professor of Medicine, Division of Cardiology, New York Hospital-Cornell Medical Center, New York City. HEART AND CIRCULATORY SYSTEM (coauthor).

Gaum, Leonard David, M.D. Assistant Professor of Urology, former Director of Urodynamics, Washington University, St. Louis. PROSTATE PROBLEMS.

Green, William L., M.D. Associate Chief of Staff for Research and Development, Veterans Administration Medical Center; Professor of Medicine, State University of New York, Downstate Medical Center, Brooklyn, N.Y. GLANDS AND METABOLISM.

Griem, Katherine L., M.D. Chief Resident, Radiation Therapy, Joint Center for Radiation Therapy, Harvard Medical School. NEW SURGERY FOR BREAST CANCER (coauthor).

Harris, Jay R., M.D. Acting Head, Department of Radiation Therapy, Acting Director, Joint Center for Radiation Therapy, Harvard Medical School. NEW SURGERY FOR BREAST CANCER (coauthor).

Helgerson, Steven D., M.D., M.P.H. Clinical Assistant Professor of Epidemiology and Public Health, Yale University School of Medicine; Medical Epidemiologist, Centers for Disease Control. PUBLIC HEALTH; WORLD HEALTH NEWS (coauthor).

Hook, Edward W., III, M.D. Assistant Professor of Medicine, Division of Infectious Diseases, The Johns Hopkins University School of Medicine; Director of Clinical Services, Baltimore City Health Department. VENEREAL DISEASES.

Hume, Eric L., M.D. Assistant Professor of Orthopaedic Surgery, Jefferson Medical College of Thomas Jefferson University, Philadelphia. BONES, MUSCLES, AND JOINTS.

Iffy, Leslie, M.D. Professor of Obstetrics and Gynecology, Director, Division of Maternal and Fetal Medicine, University of Medicine and Dentistry, Newark, N.J. OBSTETRICS AND GYNECOLOGY.

Jekel, James F., M.D., M.P.H. Professor of Epidemiology and Public Health, Yale University School of Medicine. PUBLIC HEALTH; WORLD HEALTH NEWS (coauthor).

Kales, Anthony, M.D. Professor and Chairman, Department of Psychiatry, Director, Sleep Research and Treatment Center, Pennsylvania State University College of Medicine; Founder, UCLA Sleep Research and Treatment Center. SLEEPWALKING.

Karasic, Raymond B., M.D. Assistant Professor of Pediatrics, University of Pittsburgh. PEDIATRICS.

Kindlon, Daniel J., Ph.D. Research Fellow in Psychology, The Children's Hospital/Judge Baker Guidance Center, Harvard Medical School. WHAT IS HYPERACTIVITY? (coauthor).

Kloner, Robert A., M.D., Ph.D. Professor of Internal Medicine, Wayne State University Medical School, Detroit; investigator, American Heart Association. HEART MURMURS.

Kluger, Matthew J., Ph.D. Professor of Physiology, University of Michigan Medical School. IS FEVER GOOD?

Lindsay, Robert, Ph.D. Director, Regional Bone Center, Helen Hayes Hospital, West Haverstraw, N.Y.; Professor of Clinical Medicine, College of Physicians and Surgeons, Columbia University. PREVENTING OSTEOPOROSIS (coauthor).

Lucente, Frank E., M.D. Professor and Chairman, Department of Oto-laryngology, New York Eye and Ear Infirmary, New York Medical College, New York City. EARS, NOSE, AND THROAT.

Mandel, Irwin D., D.D.S. Professor of Dentistry, Director, Center for Clinical Research in Dentistry, School of Dental and Oral Surgery, Columbia University. TEETH AND GUMS.

Maugh, Thomas H., II, Ph.D. Science Writer, Los Angeles *Times.* GENETICS AND GENETIC ENGINEERING.

McLellan, A. Thomas, Ph.D. Director of Clinical Research, Psychiatric Service, Philadelphia Veterans Administration Medical Center; Associate Professor, Department of Psychiatry, University of Pennsylvania. DRUG ABUSE (coauthor).

Morse, Gardiner. Staff Writer, *Massachusetts Medicine;* former Staff Writer, *Science News.* MEDICAL TECHNOLOGY.

Moses, Hamilton, III, M.D. Assistant Professor and Deputy Director, Department of Neurology, The Johns Hopkins Medical Institutions. BRAIN AND NERVOUS SYSTEM.

Murray, Thomas H., Ph.D. Professor of Ethics and Public Policy, Institute for the Medical Humanities, University of Texas Medical Branch at Galveston. BIOETHICS.

Muss, Hyman B., M.D. Professor of Medicine, Hematology/Oncology Section, Bowman Gray School of Medicine, Wake Forest University, Winston-Salem, N.C. CANCER.

O'Brien, Charles P., M.D., Ph.D. Chief, Psychiatric Service, Philadelphia Veterans Administration Medical Center; Professor, Department of Psychiatry, University of Pennsylvania. DRUG ABUSE (coauthor).

Pellock, John M., M.D. Associate Professor of Neurology and Pediatrics, Director, Child Seizure Clinic, Medical College of Virginia. TREATING EPILEPSY.

Pelot, Daniel, M.D. Associate Clinical Professor, Division of Gastroenterology, Department of Medicine, University of California at Irvine. DIGESTIVE SYSTEM.

Pingleton, Susan K., M.D. Professor of Medicine, Director, Clinical Investigations, Pulmonary Division, University of Kansas Medical Center, Kansas City. RESPIRATORY SYSTEM.

Puliafito, Carmen A., M.D. Assistant Professor of Ophthalmology, Harvard Medical School; Director of Laser Research, Massachusetts Eye and Ear Infirmary. EYES; WHY YOU NEED EYE EXAMINATIONS.

Rodman, Morton J., Ph.D. Professor of Pharmacology, Rutgers University, New Brunswick, N.J. MEDICATIONS AND DRUGS.

Rosen, Mortimer G., M.D. Willard C. Rappleye Professor of Obstetrics and Gynecology, Chairman, Department of Obstetrics and Gynecology, College of Physicians and Surgeons, Columbia University; Director, Obstetrical and Gynecological Service, Presbyterian Hospital, New York City. CESAREANS: WHEN ARE THEY NEEDED?

Schwartz, Howard J., M.D. Clinical Associate Professor of Medicine, Case Western Reserve University School of Medicine, Cleveland; Fellow, American Academy of Allergy and Immunology. HAY FEVER (coauthor).

Shangold, Mona M., M.D. Assistant Professor of Obstetrics and Gynecology, Director, Sports Gynecology Center, Georgetown University School of Medicine, Washington, D.C. PREGNANCY AND EXERCISE.

Sher, Theodore H., M.D. Assistant Clinical Professor of Pediatrics, Case Western Reserve University School of Medicine, Cleveland; Director, Division of Pediatric Allergy, Rainbow Babies and Childrens Hospital, Cleveland. HAY FEVER (coauthor).

Spiegel, David, M.D. Associate Professor of Psychiatry and Behavioral Sciences (Clinical), Director, Adult Psychiatric Outpatient Clinic, Stanford University School of Medicine. MENTAL HEALTH.

Sternheim, William L., M.D. Assistant Professor of Medicine, University of Miami School of Medicine. BLOOD AND LYMPHATIC SYSTEM.

Thro, Ellen. Science writer; member, National Association of Science Writers and American Medical Writers Association. ENVIRONMENT AND HEALTH.

Tohmé, Jack, M.D. Associate Clinical Director, Regional Bone Center, Helen Hayes Hospital, West Haverstraw, N.Y.; Assistant Clinical Professor of Medicine, College of Physicians and Surgeons, Columbia University. PREVENTING OSTEOPOROSIS (coauthor).

Trenk, Barbara Scherr. Writer specializing in health issues. GOVERNMENT POLICIES AND PROGRAMS (UNITED STATES).

Winick, Myron, M.D. R.R. Williams Professor of Nutrition, Professor of Pediatrics, Director, Institute of Human Nutrition, Director, Center for Nutrition, Genetics and Human Development, College of Physicians and Surgeons, Columbia University. NUTRITION AND DIET.

Woody, George E., M.D. Chief, Substance Abuse Treatment Unit, Philadelphia Veterans Administration Medical Center; Clinical Professor, Department of Psychiatry, University of Pennsylvania. DRUG ABUSE (coauthor).

Worner, T.M., M.D. Chief, Medical Section, Alcohol Dependency Treatment Program, Veterans Administration Medical Center, Bronx, N.Y.; Assistant Professor of Medicine, Mount Sinai School of Medicine, City University of New York. ALCOHOLISM.

Yogman, Michael W., M.D. Director, Infant Health and Development Program, The Children's Hospital; Assistant Professor of Pediatrics, Harvard Medical School. WHAT IS HYPERACTIVITY? (coauthor).

Index

Page number in *italics* indicates the reference is to an illustration.

A

B

C

F

G

H

N

O

P

Photo/Art Credits

4: clockwise from right, August Upitis/Shostal; Holly Bower/The Stock Market; Harry Redl/Black Star; **5:** Emil Chendea; **7:** Guy Gillette/Photo Researchers; **8:** Richard Kolar/Animals Animals; 9: Copyright © 1982, Grandma Moses Properties Co., New York. Anna Mary Robertson (Grandma) Moses, born in 1860, began to paint in old age, and by the time she died in 1961 at the age of 101, she had become world famous for her home-spun paintings of the American landscape. In works such as *Sugaring Off,* she provided a record of traditional rural farming practices; **10:** R. Rowan/Photo Researchers; **11:** David Thompson/O.S.F. Earth Scenes; **12:** Paolo Koch/Photo Researchers; **13:** art by Corinne Abbazia Hekker Graphics; **14:** art by Corinne Abbazia Hekker Graphics; **15:** G. D. Searle & Co.; **16:** Cliff Haac/Research Triangle Institute; **18:** Joel Baldwin; **20:** E. T. Archive Ltd.; **22:** Richard Wood/Taurus Photos; **23:** courtesy Gurney's Inn; **25:** top, Wide World; bottom, Peter Arnold; **26:** John Launois/Black Star; **27:** Bruce Silverstein/Peter Arnold; **28:** Christoph Henning/Wheeler Pictures; **30–31:** John Launois/Black Star; **33:** Don Renner; **34:** Olivier Rebbot/Woodfin Camp; **35:** top, Curt Kaufman/Leo de Wys; bottom, Michael Beasley/Click/Chicago; **36:** Focus on Sports; **39:** Harry Gruyaert/Magnum; **42:** Mel DiGiacomo; **43:** Dana Fineman/Sygma; **44:** Sygma; **45:** © 1985 S. M. Owen/Black Star; **46:** Jim Pozarek/Gamma-Liaison; **47:** chart by Martin Eichtersheimer; **48:** top left, chart by Martin Eichtersheimer based on data from U.S. Centers for Disease Control; top right, Lynn Johnson/Black Star; bottom, Alan Reininger/Contact Press; **49:** L. Gubb/Gamma-Liaison; **51:** Lester Sloan/Newsweek; **52:** Brian Reynolds/Sygma; **54:** Don Renner; **57:** Horst Schafer/Photo Trends; **59:** art by Corinne Abbazia Hekker Graphics; **60:** George Tames/New York Times; **61:** Mimi Forsyth/Monkmeyer; **62:** S. Karin Epstein/Camera 5; **64:** Sygma; **66:** American Cancer Society; **67:** art by Judy Skorpil; **68:** art by Judy Skorpil; **70–71:** March of Dimes Birth Defects Foundation; **72:** March of Dimes Birth Defects Foundation; **75:** March of Dimes Birth Defects Foundation; **76:** March of Dimes Birth Defects Foundation; **77:** art by Judy Skorpil; **78:** March of Dimes Birth Defects Foundation; **82:** Van Bucher/Photo Researchers; **84:** left, Lyn Schneider/The Stock Market; right, Shostal; **85:** Jim Pickerell/Click/Chicago; **86:** Emil Chendea; **87:** Shostal; **89:** Doug Wilson; **90:** Porterfield-Chickering/Photo Researchers; **92–93:** Sven-Olof Lindblad/Photo Researchers; **94:** Berlitz; **95:** top, Van Bucher/Photo Researchers; bottom, Charles P. Lemieux/The Stock Market; **96:** Richard Steedman/The Stock Market; **97:** Dave Davidson/The Stock Market; **98:** Wolfgang Kaehler; **100:** Jane Latta; **102:** International Association for Medical Assistance to Travellers; **104–105: Art Seitz/Gamma-Liaison; 107:** art by Judy Skorpil; **108:** Len Kaltman/The Stock Market; **109:** Leo de Wys; **110:** Miguel/Image Bank; **112:** both photos, Skin Cancer Foundation; **113:** Sybil Shelton/Monkmeyer; **125:** Andrew Popper/Phototake; **127:** American Heart Association; **128:** art by Emil Chendea; **129:** Ann Chwatsky/Phototake; **131:** Phototake; **132:** Nick Kleinberg/New York Times; **133:** art by Ruth Adam; **136–137:** Christa Armstrong/Photo Researchers; **138:** chart by Corinne Abbazia Hekker Graphics; **139:** Bettmann Archive; **142:** Eddie Adams/Liaison; **143:** chart by Corinne Abbazia Hekker Graphics; **145:** Morimoto/Gamma-Liaison; **148:** Gail Troussoff/Woodfin Camp; **151:** top left and right, Bettmann Archive; bottom, Wide World; **153:** Oakes/Southwest Foundation; **154:** Hank Morgan/Rainbow; **156:** Collection, The Museum of Modern Art, New York; **159:** art by Corinne Abbazia Hekker Graphics; **160:** Teri Leigh Stratford/Photo Researchers; **161:** Sabine Weiss/Photo Researchers; **163:** art by Emil Chendea; **164:** courtesy of Elizabeth Loftus; **166–167:** Stan Willard/New York University Medical Center; **168:** Suzanne Opton; **169:** printed with permission of the Muscular Dystrophy Association; **170:** Al Giese; **171:** left, Burke Rehabilitation Center; right, Stan Willard/New York University Medical Center; **172:** top, New York University Medical Center; bottom, Jacques M. Chenet/Newsweek; **176:** art by Emil Chendea; photo, Bernard Vidal; **179:** clockwise from top, Jerry Stebbins/© Discover Magazine 1/84, Time Inc.; Fred Ward/Black Star; John Madere/© Discover Magazine 1/84, Time Inc.; **180:** Jim McHugh/PEOPLE Weekly © 1985 Time Inc.; **182:** Bettmann Archive; **184:** Frank Siteman/Taurus Photos; **186:** art by Emil Chendea; **189:** art by Emil Chendea; **191–193:** art by Denise Brunkus; **195:** art by Judy Skorpil; **197:** Boston Symphony Orchestra; **198:** Mimi Forsyth/Monkmeyer; **200:** William Hubbell/Woodfin Camp; **201:** art by Judy Skorpil; **202:** American Cancer Society; **204:** photo, American Association of Poison Control Centers; **205:** © 1985 Eagle/Horowitz Productions, Ltd., Inc.; **207:** art by Emil Chendea; **209:** photo, © Phototake; **210–211:** art by Judy Skorpil; **212–213:** art by Denise Brunkus; **215:** Hirshhorn Museum and Sculpture Garden, Smithsonian Institution; **218:** reprinted with special permission of King Features Syndicate, Inc.; **219–220:** art by Corinne Abbazia Hekker Graphics; **221–222:** art by Emil Chendea; **223:** Rob Nelson/Picture Group; **226:** art by Sally Springer; **228:** Mimi Forsyth/Monkmeyer; **229:** Brian Lanker/© Discover Magazine 3/85, Time Inc.; **231:** Jim Olive; **234:** art by Marvin Friedman; **237:** art by Corinne Abbazia Hekker Graphics; **241:** Mark Gluckman/New York Times; **243:** William E. Sauro/New York Times; inset, UPI/Bettmann Newsphotos; **246:** Press Association Photos; **251:** Wide World; **253:** Stephen Ferry/Gamma-Liaison; **255:** Washington University Photographic Services; **260:** James D. Wilson/Newsweek; **262:** Pamela Price/Picture Group; **263:** reprinted from Popular Science © 1985, Times Mirror Magazines, Inc.; **265:** Thomas Eisner; **266:** Dan Miller/New York Times; **273:** Mirko Petricevic; **276:** University of Texas Health Science Center at Dallas; **277:** The Granger Collection; **280:** National Health Service Corps, U.S. Public Health Service; **282:** Toronto Star; **285:** Eric Kroll/Taurus Photos; **288:** Johy Vastyan/Pennsylvania State University; **290:** Dave Powers/TIME Magazine; inset, Wide World; **292:** courtesy of Memorial Medical Center of Long Beach; **293:** George Tames/New York Times; **298:** left, Yvonne Hemsey/Gamma-Liaison; right, Clarence Davis/New York Daily News; **300–301:** both photos, William E. Sauro/New York Times; **302:** Wide World; **306:** UPI/Bettmann Newsphotos; **307:** Jacques M. Chenet/Newsweek; **309:** Jim Olive; **310:** Barry Staver/PEOPLE Weekly © 1985 Time Inc.; **311:** Patrick McArdell/Australian Information Service; **313:** Margi Ide; **314:** Owen Franken/Picture Group; **316:** Marty Katz/New York Times; **323:** UPI/Bettmann Newsphotos; **324:** Steve Kagan/PEOPLE Weekly © 1985 Time Inc.; **327:** Wide World; **328:** courtesy Helen Keller International